Canine and Feline Nephrology and Urology

Canine and Feline Nephrology and Urology

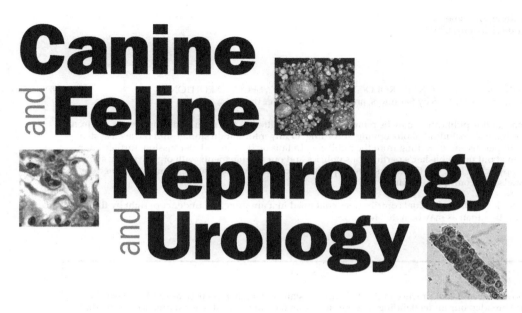

Second Edition

DENNIS J. CHEW, DVM, DACVIM
Professor of Veterinary Clinical Sciences
College of Veterinary Medicine
The Ohio State University
Columbus, Ohio

STEPHEN P. DIBARTOLA, DVM, DACVIM
Professor of Medicine
Associate Dean for Administration and Curriculum
Department of Veterinary Clinical Sciences and Veterinary Administration
College of Veterinary Medicine
The Ohio State University
Columbus, Ohio

PATRICIA A. SCHENCK, DVM, PHD
Endocrine Section
Diagnostic Center for Population and Animal Health
Michigan State University
Lansing, Michigan

ELSEVIER
SAUNDERS

3251 Riverport Lane
St. Louis, Missouri 63043

CANINE AND FELINE NEPHROLOGY AND UROLOGY, SECOND EDITION   ISBN: 978-0-7216-8178-8

Notice

Knowledge and best practice in this field are constantly changing. As new research and experience broaden our understanding, changes in research methods, professional practices, or medical treatment may become necessary.

Practitioners and researchers must always rely on their own experience and knowledge in evaluating and using any information, methods, compounds, or experiments described herein. In using such information or methods they should be mindful of their own safety and the safety of others, including parties for whom they have a professional responsibility.

With respect to any drug or pharmaceutical products identified, readers are advised to check the most current information provided (i) on procedures featured or (ii) by the manufacturer of each product to be administered, to verify the recommended dose or formula, the method and duration of administration, and contraindications. It is the responsibility of practitioners, relying on their own experience and knowledge of their patients, to make diagnoses, to determine dosages and the best treatment for each individual patient, and to take all appropriate safety precautions. To the fullest extent of the law, neither the Publisher nor the authors, contributors, or editors, assume any liability for any injury and/or damage to persons or property as a matter of products liability, negligence or otherwise, or from any use or operation of any methods, products, instructions, or ideas contained in the material herein.

Vice President and Publisher: Linda Duncan
Acquisitions Editor: Heidi Pohlman
Senior Developmental Editor: Shelly Stringer
Publishing Services Manager: Catherine Jackson
Senior Project Manager: Mary Pohlman
Senior Book Designer: Amy Buxton

Printed in the United States of America

Last digit is the print number: 9 8 7 6 5 4 3 2 1

▪▪▪ Preface

anine and Feline Nephrology and Urology is intended to be used by veterinary students, recent
graduates, and seasoned veterinarians who want to review disorders of the urinary system.
Although this manual may have value for specialists and residents training in internal medicine, it was not written specifically for that audience. We have worked together and developed our
approach to dogs and cats with diseases of the urinary tract over the past 30 years at The Ohio State
University Veterinary Teaching Hospital. This book reflects our experience and opinions. Dr. Patricia
Schenck of Michigan State University has brought her organizational skills and generalist's viewpoint
to the final development of the book.

We have taken care to ensure that treatment approaches are reasonable and that drug dosages are
correct. Ultimately, each practicing veterinarian must decide if these approaches to diagnosis and treatment are consistent with his or her own philosophy of practice before implementing specific management plans. Drug dosages should always be double-checked and verified. We would like to hear your
opinions about the approaches we have recommended in this manual. Every book contains errors, so
please make us aware of any you discover.

The second edition includes five new sections that appear at the end of each chapter. We have
enjoyed putting them together and hope that you find them interesting and helpful. These sections are
entitled, *What Do We Do?*, *Thoughts for the Future*, *Common Misconceptions*, *Summary Tips*, and *Frequently
Asked Questions*. *Thoughts for the Future* sections briefly discuss what lies ahead in the areas of urinary
tract research and therapeutics. The other sections, are composed of personal experiences from within
our practices and our interactions with students and fellow veterinarians to present real-life scenarios
to you and to answer the questions we most commonly encounter. The material in this manual is not
extensively referenced, but a suggested reading list is provided for each chapter.

Dennis J. Chew
Stephen P. DiBartola

v

··· Acknowledgments

The wisdom of the original giants of veterinary nephrology and urology is reflected in this manual. We specifically acknowledge the pioneering work of Drs. Ken Bovee, Del Finco, Gerry Ling, Don Low, and Carl Osborne. Likewise, we have been influenced by many contemporary colleagues such as Larry Adams, Tim Allen, Susi Arnold, Jeanne Barsanti, Joe Bartges, Scott Brown, Tony Buffington, Larry Cowgill, Jonathan Elliott, Greg Grauer, Jeff Klausner, John Kruger, Cathy Langston, George Lees, Meryl Littman, Jody Lulich, Dave Polzin, Linda Ross, Mike Schaer, Dave Senior, and Shelly Vaden. We also have learned much from several generations of veterinary students, interns, and internal medicine residents who have trained in OSU's Veterinary Teaching Hospital. Helio deMorais, Bernie Hansen, and Jodi Westropp are previous residents we are happy to have seen adopt our enthusiasm for veterinary nephrology and urology. We hope the subjects discussed in this manual will prompt another generation of veterinary internists to explore and teach nephrology and urology. Replacements for our generation are sorely needed.

Special thanks to Ray Kersey who had the original vision for this manual many years ago. After Ray's retirement, Tony Winkel inherited the project at Elsevier and pushed us to keep the project going. Heidi Pohlman, Shelly Stringer, and Mary Pohlman have been the most recent project managers, and we appreciate their efforts to see the project through to completion. Dr. Amanda Owen deserves credit for organizational writing of the chapters on feline interstitial cystitis and urinary neoplasia. Finally, we appreciate the excellent artwork of Mr. Tim Vojt who has been our colleague all of these years.

Dennis J. Chew, DVM
Stephen P. DiBartola, DVM
Columbus, Ohio

I am particularly grateful to Drs. Arthur Lage and Richard Scott who have had a great influence on my early training in nephrology and urology. Dr. Richard Scott's unique thinking and decision making influence me to this day. "Scotty" always emphasized the importance of examining fresh urinary sediment and passed this practice on to a generation of veterinarians at the Animal Medical Center in the 1970s. He was decades ahead of the veterinary profession in his approach to what we now consider standard practice. He is more recognized today for his development of guidelines for supplementation of parenteral fluids with potassium (called "Scott's Sliding Scale"). Two colleagues at our university who consistently think "outside of the box" deserve special mention. Dr. Larry Nagode's passion for understanding the relationships between parathyroid hormone, calcitriol, and renal patholophysiology has had a major impact on me and has positively affected delivery of advanced patient care. Dr. Tony Buffington deserves tremendous credit for shifting the paradigm of idiopathic/interstitial cystitis of cats from that of a nutritional disease to one of complex neurological, endocrine, and environmental effects. The late Dr. Charles Capen inspired me to advance my understanding of disorders of calcium homeostasis, an area of great interest in nephrology. Dr. Mary McLoughlin deserves recognition as a gifted soft tissue surgeon who has worked extensively to develop surgical procedures for the urinary tract, especially management of ectopic ureters. We shared great excitement for development of diagnositic uroendoscopy and during our work on ectopic ureters.

I am especially thankful that Dr. Stephen P. DiBartola and I were able to develop our thinking in veterinary nephrology and urology together during the past 30 years at The Ohio State University College of Veterinary Medicine. We have had quite a ride together teaching and practicing veterinary urology–vive les néphronauts! We have had a lot of fun (and very few disagreements) in the process–seeing cases, researching projects, writing papers and books, and sharing in the teaching of more than 3500 veterinary students. We both love the pathophysiology of fluid, electrolyte, and acid-base derangements and have been able to be sounding boards for each other on difficult and interesting cases. I feel blessed to have been his colleague, but our relationship extends beyond that of colleagues. Most who meet us think we are very different, but we are surprisingly similar in our approach to life and work. I am thankful for Steve's support and friendship during both the good and difficult times. Dr. Patricia Schenck also has been a great colleague and special friend along my journey.

Dennis J. Chew, DVM
Columbus, Ohio

I echo all of Dennis' comments about the past 30 years of working together. Dennis was the first person I met when I arrived as an internal medicine resident at the College of Veterinary Medicine at the Ohio State University in 1977 and it was his genuine love of nephrology as well as fluid, electrolyte, and acid-base balance that captured my interest and sparked my enthusiasm. Everyone who meets Dennis likes him instantly and instinctively, and I was no exception. However, unlike many others, I was fortunate enough to make a career out of my association with Dennis. In addition, I want to thank my wife Dr. Maxey Wellman for standing by me for more than 30 years despite my quirks and imperfections, and my children, Matthew, Michael, Alex, and Stephanie, for all they have taught me about the most important job in the world–being a parent.

Stephen P. DiBartola, DVM
Columbus, Ohio

I came to The Ohio State University in 1992 with a background in lipid and nutrition research. There I met Dr. Dennis Chew, and I became rapidly drawn into the world of calcium and renal disease. Several positions and many years later, I'm still involved in calcium research with both Drs. Chew and DiBartola. I would like to thank all the four-legged critters in my life that helped me choose the veterinary profession. I am also thankful to all the veterinary students and veterinarians that I interact with and continue to learn from every day. Music is an integral part of my being, and I'm thankful for the musicians that surround me and fill that part of my soul. Special thanks to Dennis Chew who has been my friend for so many years—what a long, strange trip it's been, and I hope there are many more years in the journey! Finally, I am grateful to my parents for their love and support.

Patricia A. Schenck, DVM, PhD
Lansing, MI

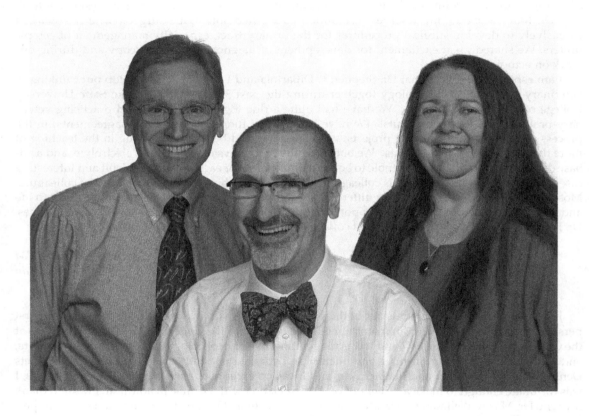

This book is dedicated to
the memories of Neil Presnell
and Paul Dunkle.

■■■ Contents

Chapter 1: Urinalysis, *1*

Chapter 2: Clinical Evaluation of the Urinary Tract, *32*

Chapter 3: Acute Renal Failure, *63*

Chapter 4: Specific Syndromes Causing Acute Intrinsic Renal Failure, *93*

Chapter 5: Chronic Renal Failure, *145*

Chapter 6: Familial Renal Diseases of Dogs and Cats, *197*

Chapter 7: Diseases of the Glomerulus, *218*

Chapter 8: Cystitis and Urethritis: Urinary Tract Infection, *240*

Chapter 9: Urolithiasis, *272*

Chapter 10: Nonobstructive Idiopathic or Interstitial Cystitis in Cats, *306*

Chapter 11: Obstructive Uropathy and Nephropathy, *341*

Chapter 12: Urinary Tract Trauma and Uroperitoneum, *391*

Chapter 13: Disorders of Micturition and Urinary Incontinence, *409*

Chapter 14: Tumors of the Urinary System, *434*

Chapter 15: Approach to Polyuria and Polydipsia, *465*

Chapter 16: Miscellaneous Syndromes, *487*

Canine and Feline Nephrology and Urology

1 Urinalysis

INTRODUCTION

A. Routine urinalysis is simple and inexpensive.
B. Urinalysis not only is helpful in evaluation of patients with urinary tract disease but also in those with systemic disease affecting many other body systems.
C. Results of serial urinalyses can reflect progression or resolution of disease.
D. Abnormalities on urinalysis often occur before changes occur in serum biochemistry (i.e., urinalysis can be very sensitive).
E. Urine should be submitted for analysis at the same time blood is submitted for biochemical analysis.
F. Complete urinalysis consists of three parts: Physical properties, chemical properties, and urine sediment findings.

COLLECTION OF URINE

A. Urine collection technique influences interpretation of the results. Urine specimens should be placed in containers that are clean and free of chemical contaminants (e.g. detergents, disinfectants, bleach). Ideally, collect 10 to 12 mL of urine for analysis. At a minimum, 3 mL should be submitted.

Midstream Voided Sample
1. The goal of this approach is to allow the initial stream of urine to flush contaminants from the urethra and genital tract.

Technique

DOGS
(1) Male dogs may be more difficult to collect due to short duration of voiding (i.e. "marking").

CATS
(1) Use non-resorbable cat litter.
(2) Cellophane wrap over a tilted litter pan containing a gradient of cat litter.

Advantages
a. No risk of complications for the patient.
b. Client can collect the sample.
c. Suitable for initial screening.
d. Method of choice to evaluate hematuria (other collection methods may result in addition of red blood cells [RBCs] to the urine from trauma).

Disadvantages
a. Subject to contamination by the urethra and genital tract despite precautions.
b. Subject to contamination from the environment.

Manual Expression of Urine by Digital Palpation of the Bladder
Technique
   a. Gradually increase pressure in the bladder, compressing the bladder wall by abdominal palpation until urine is expelled.
   b. Many times the animal will void urine after bladder palpation failed to produce a urine sample. Thus, the clinician should be prepared to collect a voided sample.
Advantages
   a. Ease of use in anesthetized patients.
Disadvantages
   a. Not recommended except in anesthetized animals.
   b. Red blood cells (RBCs) and protein may enter the urine sample as a result of the force required to expel urine.
   c. Collection of urine by manual expression carries a risk of bladder rupture.
   d. Infected bladder urine can reflux into the ureters during manual expression thus increasing the risk of upper urinary tract infection (UTI).

Catheterization
Technique
   a. Maintain sterile technique while using a catheter, gloves, and proper patient cleansing and disinfection. A gentle approach is necessary to minimize trauma to the urinary tract. The catheter should never be advanced by force, and a ruptured urethra or bladder can be a consequence of poor technique.
   (1) Male dogs (Figure 1-1): Catheter types include polypropylene, polyvinyl, and balloon-tipped ureteral catheters for use in humans. Softer catheters are chosen for indwelling urinary catheterization. A catheter size of 3.5 to 10 French (1 French unit = 0.33 mm) is recommended, depending on the size of animal. The appropriate length of catheter to insert is chosen by estimating the length from the external urethral orifice to the bladder neck by over-laying the catheter on the animal's body. The patient is positioned in lateral recumbency, excessive hair near the tip of the prepuce clipped, and the penis extruded by an assistant. The penis and external urethral orifice are gently cleansed and rinsed with a mild disinfectant (e.g., benzalkonium chloride) and sterile saline. The packaging containing the sterile catheter can be cut to facilitate manipulation of the catheter without contamination. Liberally coat the end of the catheter with sterile lubricating jelly and insert the catheter into the external urethral orifice. The catheter should be directed parallel to the abdominal wall to facilitate its passage. Resistance may be encountered in the perineal region and also at the level of the ischial arch. If necessary, external perineal palpation or rectal palpation can be used to redirect the catheter tip. To avoid trauma to the bladder, the catheter is passed only as far as needed to obtain urine drainage. In cases of obstruction the catheter may be advanced farther to allow better drainage of urine.
   (2) Female dogs (Figure 1-2): Direct visualization of the urethral orifice using a speculum is preferred over a blind technique so as to avoid contamination of the urinary tract with genital bacterial flora. A variety of types and sizes of specula are available; those with self-contained light sources are preferable. Anuscopes designed for humans are easily adapted for use in most female dogs. Otoscopic and vaginal specula of various sizes also can be used. Catheters described above for use in male dogs can be used in females, as can Foley catheters and metal bitch catheters. Stylets are necessary for polyvinyl catheters and for small-caliber polypropylene

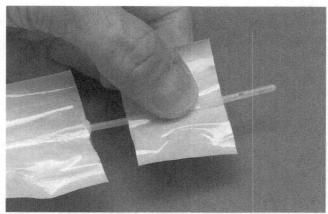

FIGURE 1-1 ■ Sterile handling of a urinary catheter for a male dog. The sterile catheter package has been cut with scissors to facilitate passage of the catheter while at the same time maintaining sterile technique. This technique allows the catheter to be manipulated without the use of sterile gloves.

catheters. The patient usually is placed in sternal recumbency, but different body positions may facilitate catheter passage in some circumstances. The external genitalia should be clipped of hair, cleansed, and disinfected. Pass the speculum or anuscope dorsally and then cranially, minimizing vaginal contamination. It is easier to pass the speculum beyond the urethral orifice and then retract it slowly until the orifice comes into view. Liberally coat the end of the catheter with sterile lubricating jelly and insert it into the external urethral orifice. The urinary catheter is advanced under direct visualization until urine is obtained.

(3) Male cats: Catheter types include medical grade Silastic, Jackson-style (Cook Veterinary Catheters), polyvinyl, and polypropylene catheters. Tom cat catheters are rigid polypropylene catheters available in 3.5 F as open-end or side-holes varieties. The open-end catheter is shorter than the side-hole catheter and consequently is not always reliable for draining the bladder. Polyvinyl catheters are available in 3.5 F or 5 F sizes. The cat is placed in lateral or dorsal recumbency with its hind limbs pulled caudally. The penis should be extended caudally to eliminate the natural curvature of the urethra. A perception of distal urethral obstruction may be created if the penis is not sufficiently extended. Coat the end of the catheter with sterile lubricating jelly and advance it into the urethra until urine is obtained.

(4) Female cats: A small otoscope can be used to visualize the urethral orifice. The vestibule of most female cats can accommodate a small anuscope speculum. Small female cats can be catheterized blindly. Rigid polypropylene or polyvinyl catheters generally are used. Rarely, small Foley catheters are used. Generally, a 6 to 8 F catheter can be accommodated. Female cats almost always require sedation to allow urinary catheterization. The cat is placed in ventral recumbency with its hind limbs over the edge of the table, and the tail extended dorsally. Some operators prefer dorsal recumbency. The catheter should be gently inserted and directed slightly dorsally along the ventral floor of the vestibule to enter the external urethral orifice. A small otoscope speculum can be used to visualize the external urethral orifice and facilitate catheterization passage.

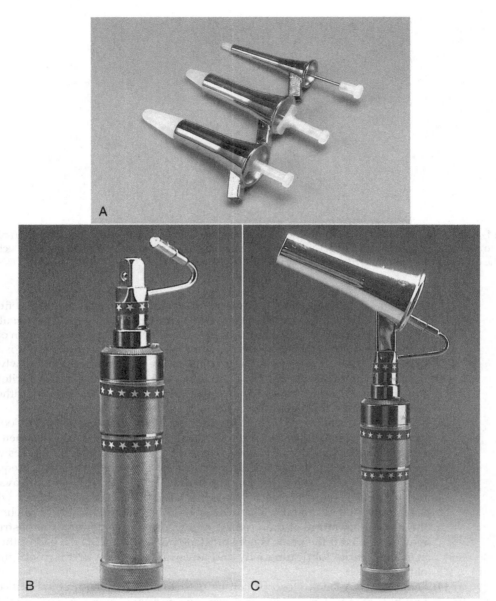

FIGURE 1-2 ■ Anuscopes (Welch-Allyn) to facilitate urinary catheterization in female dogs. **A,** One of three sizes of anuscope will accommodate most female dogs to facilitate passage of a urinary catheter (shown with obturators in place). **B,** The self-contained light source of the anuscope provides an advantage over a vaginal speculum without its own light source. **C,** Assembled anuscope with light source in place.

Advantages

a. Simple to perform in most male dogs.

Disadvantages

a. The normal bacterial flora of the distal urethra can be introduced into the bladder during passage of the catheter.
b. Approximately 20% risk of introducing UTI in female dogs.
c. May result in increased numbers of RBC and epithelial cells in the sediment due to trauma.
d. Rupture of the urethra or bladder may occur if excessive force is used to pass the catheter or if the tissues are friable.
e. Never chosen for routine collection of urine from male cats due to the risk of urethral trauma and subsequent obstruction.
f. Sedation or light anesthesia may be necessary to provide adequate restraint and analgesia.

Cystocentesis

Technique (Figure 1-3)

STANDARD (BLADDER PALPABLE AND CAN BE STABILIZED)

(1) Restrain animal in lateral or dorsal recumbency (cat, small dog) or allow animal to remain standing (large dog).
(2) Sedate aggressive animals as necessary.
(3) Clipping or wetting the hair with water to expose skin at puncture site is preferred by some operators but is not necessary. Do not disinfect the skin before cystocentesis because this carries a risk of contamination of urine by disinfectant and possible false negative culture results.
(4) Stabilize the bladder's position by palpation. Compressing the bladder from the opposite side of the abdomen often facilitates its identification on palpation.
(5) Perform bladder puncture using a 22-gauge needle connected to a 6- or 12-mL syringe. Aim the needle toward the pelvic inlet to minimize bladder trauma because the bladder will decrease in size as urine is aspirated. Gentle negative pressure on the syringe during puncture allows urine to be aspirated immediately after penetration of the bladder lumen.

BLIND (BLADDER NOT PALPABLE)

(1) Restrain animal in dorsal recumbency.
(2) Visualize a point on the ventral midline between the fourth and fifth teats and make needle puncture at this location.
(3) Choose a more caudal insertion site (i.e., closer to the pubis) if the bladder is very small.
(4) Choose a more cranial insertion site (i.e., closer to the fourth teat) if the bladder is very large.
(5) Push the viscera caudally with the fingers of one hand as necessary to allow a slight bulging of the bladder to be seen.
(6) Deflect the penis and prepuce in male dogs to one side before midline puncture.
(7) Blind technique is successful in approximately 50% of attempts in dogs but is not recommended in cats because the position of the bladder in cats is considerably more variable than in dogs.
(8) Ultrasound guidance can be helpful when difficulty is experienced using the blind technique.

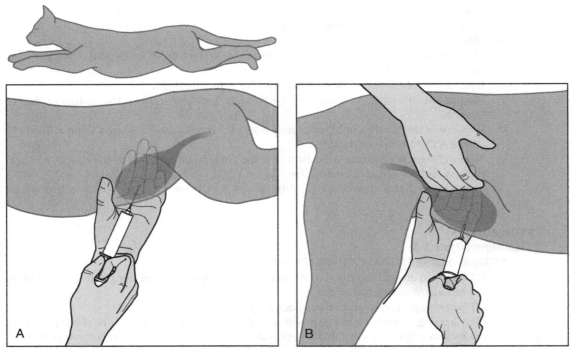

FIGURE 1-3 ■ Cystocentesis techniques in the cat and dog. **A,** Cystocentesis in the cat using lateral recumbency. The cat is restrained in lateral recumbency while the operator stabilizes the bladder followed by puncture with a 22-gauge needle and gentle aspiration of urine. Note that the needle is aimed toward the pelvic inlet to minimize the risk of trauma during the procedure. **B,** Cystocentesis in a large standing dog. The operator stabilizes the bladder just cranial to the hind limb with the left hand while an assistant elevates the skin of flank dorsally and caudally. With the right hand, the operator punctures the lateral wall of the bladder. (Drawn by Tim Vojt.)

Advantages
    a. Contamination from the distal urethra, vagina, vestibule, prepuce, or perineum is avoided.
    b. Simple to perform when the bladder is palpable.
    c. Negligible risk of introducing infection.
    d. Useful in animals at high risk for infection (e.g., diabetes mellitus, hyperadrenocorticism).
    e. Well tolerated by both dogs and cats.

Disadvantages
    a. Should not be attempted if cystotomy has been performed in the past week, if the animal has an atonic bladder, or if transitional cell carcinoma is likely present.
    b. Potential risk of urine leakage if the bladder remains distended after the procedure. Leakage also may occur if the bladder wall is devitalized.
    c. Puncture of other abdominal viscera may occur.
    d. RBCs may be introduced into the sediment due to iatrogenic trauma, which may be confused with pathologic hematuria.

Complications
    a. Complications are rare.
    b. Transient macroscopic or microscopic hematuria.

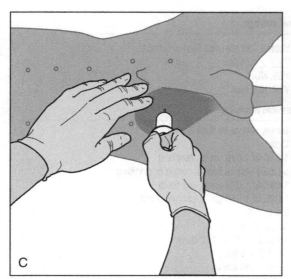
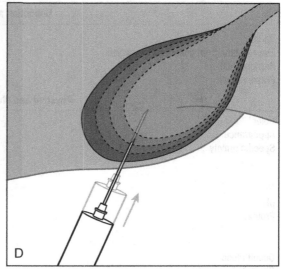

FIGURE 1-3, cont'd ■ **C,** Cystocentesis in a male dog in dorsal recumbency. The penis is deflected from the midline by the operator with the nondominant hand while also pushing the abdominal viscera caudally. This caudal shift of the viscera often causes the bulging bladder to become more obvious as the site to choose for needle puncture. When the bladder is not palpable with either the male or female dog in dorsal recumbency, the needle is advanced on the midline at the intersection of an imaginary "X" drawn from the fourth and fifth teats on each side of the abdomen. **D,** Angle and depth of cystocentesis needle. The needle should penetrate into the bladder lumen sufficiently deep so that the needle stays in the lumen as the bladder contracts in size as urine volume is withdrawn. Theoretically, the needle should enter the bladder at an angle so that a longer transmural tract is created that will seal the needle tract more readily. (Drawn by Tim Vojt.)

    c. Seeding of tumor cells from transitional cell carcinoma potentially can occur, but the frequency and importance of this problem is not known.
    d. Some cats salivate excessively or vomit after cystocentesis (i.e., vagovagal response).
    e. Rarely a cat will collapse after cystocentesis, possibly due to catecholamine release, and this effect may be more severe in cats with underlying cardiovascular disease.
    f. <25,000µ platelet count increases the risk for bleeding; <10,000µ platelet count is an absolute contraindication.
    g. Avoid if the patient is known to have emphysematous cystitis, as this may increase the chances for urine leakage.

PERFORMANCE OF THE URINALYSIS

  A. Examine fresh urine whenever possible to identify elements that are lost over time (e.g., cellular elements) and to avoid artifacts that develop in urine that is refrigerated or held at room temperature (e.g., crystal precipitation).
  B. Collect urine specimens from dogs in the morning to obtain maximally concentrated urine. Timing of collection is not as important in cats.
  C. Refrigerated urine should be warmed to room temperature before performing urinalysis because the color reactions of the chemical reagent pads on the dipstrips are temperature sensitive.
  D. Always note how the sample was obtained on the laboratory report because technique of collection may influence interpretation (Figure 1-4).

Collection and storage	
Source	Voided Catheterized Cystocentesis
Elapsed time from collection to analysis	_____ minutes _____ hours
Refrigeration	YES, NO
Preservatives	YES, NO, Type: _____
Physical and chemical analysis	
Color	Straw, yellow, or light amber
Appearance	Clear
Specific gravity	1.015 to 1.050 (dogs, random)
	>1.030 first AM before eating or drinking
	1.035 to 1.070 (cats, dry food)
	1.025 to 1.050 (cats, canned food)
pH	5.5 to 6.5
Protein	Negative, trace,
	+1 (SG 1.040 to 1.050), or
	+2 (SG > 1.060)
Occult blood	Negative to trace
Glucose	Negative
Ketones	Negative
Bilirubin	Negative to 1+ (dogs, especially males with high SG)
	Negative (cats)
Microscopic sediment evaluation	
Casts (per lpf)—Normal values	
Hyaline	0-2
Granular	0-1
Cellular, RBC	None
Cellular, WBC	None
Cellular, renal epithelial	None
Other (e.g., Hb, Mb)	None
RBCs (per hpf)	
Voided	0-8
Catheterized	0-5
Nontraumatic cystocentesis	0-3
Routine cystocentesis	<10
Traumatic cystocentesis	>50
WBCs (per hpf)	
Voided	<10
Catheterized	<7
Cystocentesis	<3
Clumps?	No

FIGURE 1-4 ■ Urinalysis Form and Expected Results from Normal Dogs and Cats.

Epithelial cells (per hpf)	
Squamous	0 to few
Transitional	0 to few
Clumps	None
Caudate (with tails)	None
Strap or stirrup cells	None
Bacteria (per hpf)	
Voided	Rare
Catheterized	Rare
Cystocentesis	None
Type (if present)	Rods
	Cocci
	Both
Crystals (per hpf)—struvite, oxalate, urate, cystine	
Type (if present)	Struvite
	Oxalate
	Urate
	Cystine—never normal
	Amorphous (unidentified)
	Drug
Number, fresh urine	0 to few
Number, stored urine	Few to many
Size (small, medium, large)	
Free or aggregated	

Hb, hemoglobin; *hpf*, high-power field; *lpf*, low-power field; *Mb*, myoglobin; *RBC*, red blood cell; *SG*, specific gravity; *WBC*, white blood cell.

FIGURE 1-4, cont'd

INTERPRETATION OF THE URINALYSIS

Physical Properties
Color
 a. The normal yellow color of urine is due to urochrome and urobilin.

 b. Very concentrated urine may be deep amber in color whereas very dilute urine may be almost colorless.

ABNORMAL URINE COLORS

 (1) Unusual colors may be due to drugs or their metabolites.

  (a) Deep amber.

   (i) Highly concentrated urine.

   (ii) Increased amounts of bile pigments.

  (b) Red or reddish-brown color.

   (i) Usually due to intact RBC, hemoglobin (from lysed RBCs in urine or systemic hemolysis) or myoglobin.

   (ii) Dry food dye (rare).

   (iii) Porphyrins (rare).

  (c) Dark brown to black color.

   (i) Usually represents conversion of hemoglobin to methemoglobin in acid urine.

(d) Yellow-brown to yellow-green color.
  (i) Usually due to bilirubin.
(e) Green color.
  (i) UTI with *Pseudomonas*.
  (ii) Oxidation of bilirubin to biliverdin.
  (iii) Methylene blue administration results in greenish-blue urine.

Appearance

a. Normal urine usually is clear but occasionally it can be cloudy.
b. Cloudy urine often contains increased cellular elements (white blood cells [WBCs], RBCs, epithelial cells), crystals, mucus, or showers of casts. Bacteria or fungal organisms, sperm, and prostatic secretions sometimes account for cloudy urine.
c. Flocculent urine may contain aggregates of WBCs, epithelial cells, very small calculi, or aggregates of crystals (so-called *sand*).

Odor

a. The normal odor of urine is due to volatile fatty acids.
b. The most common abnormal odor is ammoniacal due to the release of ammonia by urease-producing bacteria.
c. Putrefaction of proteins in urine can also cause malodorous urine.

Specific Gravity

a. Urine specific gravity (USG) is the weight of the urine compared to that of an equal volume of water. It reflects both the total number of solutes and their weight (heavier molecules contribute more to USG than smaller ones).

> ! Urine specific gravity provides the most meaningful information about renal function on the urinalysis.

  (1) 1000 mg/dL glucose increases the USG approximately 0.004.
  (2) 1000 mg/dL protein increases the USG approximately 0.003.
b. USG estimated by dipstrip pads is not accurate over a wide range of USG and should not be used.
c. USG is estimated by refractometry (refraction of light in solution is affected by the number and size of the particles in the solution).
  (1) The refractometer should be temperature compensated for accurate and consistent estimates of USG.
  (2) Dog and cat urine have different refractometric properties, and scales specifically developed for use in dogs or cats should be used for most accurate results.
  (3) Optical and digital refractometers designed for veterinary use have scales that allow determination of USG values up to 1.060.
  (4) Commonly available refractometers designed for use in humans only measure USG up to 1.035.
  (5) USG should not simply be reported as >1.035 in dogs and cats. When the initial USG reading exceeds the refractometer's scale, mix equal volumes of urine and distilled water and determine the USG. Multiply the numbers to the right of the decimal point by a factor of 2 to determine the actual USG.
d. Use the USG as a guide to interpret the relative concentration of abnormal elements or chemical constituents in the sample.
  (1) 4+ (1000 mg/dL) proteinuria in a urine sample of 1.010 USG represents more severe proteinuria than 4+ (1000 mg/dL) proteinuria in urine of 1.045 USG.

(2) 4 WBCs/high-power field (hpf) in urinary sediment from a urine sample of 1.060 USG may be less clinically relevant than 4 WBCs/hpf in urine sediment from a urine sample of 1.015 USG.

e. USG should be determined before treatment with fluids, diuretics, corticosteroids, or other medications.

f. Repeated production of submaximally concentrated urine in dogs and cats usually indicates abnormal renal function (see Chapter 2).

g. The first urine of the morning is most likely to have the highest solute concentration. USG will vary based on diet moisture content, amount of water consumed, excess dietary solutes requiring renal excretion, renal function, and hydration status (see Chapter 15, Approach to Polyuria and Polydipsia).

   (1) First urine of the morning should have USG >1.035 in cats consuming dry foods and >1.025 in cats consuming canned foods.

   (2) Average USG throughout the day should be >1.020 in dogs.

      (a) In dogs, often USG is >1.030 to 1.040 in samples of the first urine of the morning before consumption of food or water.

      (b) The USG of some dogs may vary widely throughout the day presumably as a result of eating, drinking, and activity.

h. Dehydrated dogs and cats should elaborate maximally concentrated urine (>1.040 USG) if the hypothalamic-pituitary-adrenal-renal axis is normal.

Chemical Properties
Dipstrip Evaluation

a. Chemical properties usually are measured semiquantitatively by dipstrip tests (Box 1-1).

b. Reactions for analytes (except pH) should be interpreted with consideration of the USG (i.e., smaller quantitative reactions in dilute urine are potentially of more significance than similar reactions in highly concentrated urine).

c. Dipstrip reactions ideally are performed on the urine supernatant after centrifugation.

d. Heavily pigmented urine (e.g., presence of blood or bilirubin) can make it difficult to accurately read the color reaction of the reagent pads on the dipstrip.

■ BOX 1-1
■ **SOURCES OF POSSIBLE ERROR WHEN USING DIPSTRIP REAGENT PADS**

- Refrigerated sample not returned to room temperature
- Contamination of urine with disinfectant
- Outdated dipstrip reagent pads
- Improper storage of dipstrip reagent pads (e.g., exposed to air)
- Loss of chemicals from dipstrip reagent pads after prolonged immersion in urine
- Leakage of reagent chemicals from adjacent reagent pads if dipstrips are held vertically (i.e., they are designed to be read while holding the strip horizontally)
- Dipstrip reagent pads contaminated by materials from the technician's fingers
- Reading dipstrip reagent pads at incorrect time intervals (i.e., the reagent pads are time sensitive)
- Poor ambient lighting
- Poor visual acuity of laboratory technician to detect color changes
- Difficulty in reading reagent pad color reaction due to highly pigmented urine
- Failure to use positive and negative controls to verify accuracy of new dipstrip reagent pads

pH

    a. Substantial variation occurs between pH values determined by dipstrip as compared to pH meter in dogs and cats and measurement by pH meter is superior.

    b. Normal urine pH of carnivores (dogs and cats) is 5.0 to 7.5.

    c. Urine pH varies with diet and acid-base balance but urine pH is not a reliable indicator of systemic acid-base imbalance.

    d. Causes of acidic urine pH.

        (1) Meat diet.

        (2) Administration of acidifying agents.

        (3) Metabolic acidosis.

        (4) Respiratory acidosis.

        (5) Paradoxical aciduria in metabolic alkalosis with potassium and chloride depletion.

        (6) Protein catabolic states.

    e. Causes of alkaline urine pH.

        (1) Plant-based diet.

        (2) Urine exposed to air for prolonged time at room temperature.

        (3) Postprandial alkaline tide.

        (4) UTI by a urease-positive organism (acidic urine pH however does not rule out UTI).

        (5) Contamination of the urine sample with bacteria during or after collection.

        (6) Administration of alkalinizing agents.

        (7) Metabolic alkalosis.

        (8) Respiratory alkalosis (including stress-induced respiratory alkalosis in cats).

        (9) Distal renal tubular acidosis.

Urine Protein Concentration: Proteinuria May Be Categorized as Prerenal, Renal (Glomerular or Postglomerular), or Postrenal

    a. Dipstrip test results are reported as negative, trace (10 mg/dL), 1+ (30 mg/dL), 2+ (100 mg/dL), 3+ (300 mg/dL), or 4+ (1000 mg/dL).

    b. Randomly collected urine samples with relatively high USG from normal dogs contain small amounts of protein (trace to 1+ or 10 to 30 mg/dL).

        (1) Urine with USG >1.060 may result in +2 (100 mg/dL) reading for protein that does not signify pathologic proteinuria.

        (2) Highly concentrated urine magnifies the concentration of small amounts of protein normally found in the urine.

        (3) In cats, highly concentrated urine may directly activate the dipstrip reagent pad in the absence of pathologic proteinuria.

    c. Commonly used dipstrip methods are much more sensitive to albumin than globulin.

    d. False positives may occur in very alkaline urine (≥ 8.0 pH) or urine contaminated with the antiseptic agent benzalkonium chloride (Zephiran).

    e. False negatives may occur in very acidic or dilute urine.

    f. Results must be interpreted in view of urine specific gravity.

> **!** Proteinuria may indicate a pathologic process anywhere in the urinary tract. It also indicates renal disease when lower urinary tract sources of protein are excluded.

    g. The origin of the proteinuria must be localized (i.e., kidney, ureter, bladder, urethra, genital tract) by careful consideration of the history, physical examination findings, method of urine collection, and urine sediment evaluation.

h. Pathologic renal proteinuria may result from:
   (1) Increased glomerular filtration of protein.
   (2) Failure of tubular reabsorption of protein.
   (3) Tubular secretion of protein.
   (4) Protein leakage from damaged tubular cells.
   (5) Renal parenchymal inflammation.
   (6) Any combination of the above.
i. In diseases of the glomerulus, increased glomerular filtration of protein due to loss of glomerular barrier function is the major cause of proteinuria and albumin is the primary protein lost early in the course of the disease.
j. Persistent, moderate to heavy proteinuria in the absence of urine sediment abnormalities is highly suggestive of glomerular disease (e.g., glomerulonephritis, amyloidosis).
k. If the sediment is active and proteinuria is mild to moderate, consider inflammatory renal disease or disease of the lower urinary tract or genital tract.
l. The finding of proteinuria should be integrated with urinary sediment findings (i.e., RBCs, WBCs, bacteria, epithelial cells, and casts in the sediment may provide clues to the origin of the proteinuria).
m. Causes of prerenal proteinuria include:
   (1) Bence-Jones proteins (i.e., immunoglobulin light chains) in multiple myeloma.
   (2) Hemoglobinuria when hemolysis is present.
   (3) Myoglobinuria when rhabdomyolysis is present.

Glucose

a. Glucose in the glomerular filtrate is almost completely reabsorbed in the proximal tubules and is not normally present in the urine of dogs and cats.
b. If blood glucose concentration exceeds the renal threshold (approximately 180 mg/dL in the dog and 300 mg/dL in cats), glucose will appear in the urine (i.e., glucosuria, glycosuria).
c. Most dipstick tests utilize a colorimetric test based on an enzymatic reaction specific for glucose (i.e., glucose oxidase).
   (1) Peroxide and hypochlorite may give false-positive reactions.
   (2) False-positive reactions on dipstick testing may also be seen in animals receiving cephalexin. If copper-reduction-based testing is used (such as Clinitest), then false-positive reactions may be noted in animals receiving amoxicillin, clavulanate enrofloxacin, or nitrofurantoin.
   (3) Refrigerated urine or urine containing formaldehyde or vitamin C may give false-negative reactions.
d. Causes of glucosuria (glycosuria).
   (1) Diabetes mellitus (most common).
   (2) Stress or excitement (especially cats).
   (3) Chronically sick cats in the absence of hyperglycemia (i.e., altered tubular transport of glucose).

> **!** Glucosuria is an important abnormal finding on urinalysis necessitating prompt diagnosis or exclusion of diabetes mellitus.

   (4) Administration of glucose-containing fluids.
   (5) Renal tubular disease.
      (a) Primary renal glucosuria.
      (b) Fanconi syndrome (e.g., Basenji dogs).

(c) Tubular injury due to acute renal failure.
(d) Tubular injury due to familial nephropathy (uncommon).
(e) Tubular injury due to chronic renal failure (uncommon).
(6) Severe urethral obstruction in some cats — actually is pseudoglucosuria due to some nonglucose oxidizing substance.

Ketones

a. Ketones (i.e., beta-hydroxybutyrate, acetoacetate, acetone) are the products of excessive and incomplete oxidation of fatty acids. They are not normally present in the urine of dogs and cats.
b. Inadequate consumption of carbohydrates or impaired endogenous utilization of carbohydrates for energy can increase oxidation of fatty acids.
c. The nitroprusside reagent pad on the dipstrip reacts with acetone and acetoacetate to produce a lavender color. Nitroprusside is much more reactive with acetoacetate and does not react with beta-hydroxybutyrate.
d. Causes of ketonuria.
(1) Diabetic ketoacidosis in association with glucosuria (most common).
(2) Starvation or prolonged fasting in an immature animal (fasting dogs and cats do not become ketotic as readily as do humans).
(3) Glycogen storage disease (rare).
(4) Low-carbohydrate, high-fat diet.
(5) Persistent hypoglycemia (decreased insulin secretion increases ketone formation).

Occult Blood

a. The dipstrip reagent pad test is based on the ability of hemoglobin or myoglobin to release oxygen moieties from peroxide and this reaction is linked to a chromogen.
b. Dipstick tests are sensitive but do not differentiate among intact erythrocytes, hemoglobin released from RBCs in urine, hemoglobin liberated as a consequence of systemic hemolysis, and myoglobin. A positive test should be interpreted in light of the urine sediment findings (i.e., presence or absence of RBC in the urine sediment) and the color of the serum (i.e., presence or absence of hemolysis). Serum is pink if hemolysis is present but clear if the pigmenturia is a result of rhabdomyolysis. Reagent pads from some manufacturers can distinguish intact RBCs (i.e., speckled color reaction) from free hemoglobin in urine (i.e., diffuse color reaction).
c. If necessary, ammonium sulfate precipitation or urine protein electrophoresis can be used to differentiate hemoglobinuria from myoglobinuria.

❗ The occult blood reaction becomes positive before hematuria is observed macroscopically.

d. Causes of hemoglobinuria arising as a consequence of systemic hemolysis include:
(1) Transfusion reaction.
(2) Autoimmune hemolytic anemia.
(3) Disseminated intravascular coagulation.
(4) Postcaval syndrome of dirofilariasis.
(5) Splenic torsion.
(6) Heat stroke.
(7) Severe hypophosphatemia.
(8) Zinc toxicity.
(9) RBC enzyme deficiencies (e.g. phosphofructokinase, pyruvate kinase).
e. Myoglobinuria is less common but may occur as a result of severe rhabdomyolysis.
(1) Persistent muscular contractions due to status epilepticus.

(2) Crushing injury (e.g. vehicular injury).
(3) Post-exertional (e.g. racing greyhounds).
(4) Heat stroke.
(5) Severe hypokalemia (especially in cats).

f. Dilute or alkaline urine may cause RBC lysis and an occult blood-positive reaction. The urine sediment should contain RBC "ghosts" in this situation.
g. Vitamin C and formalin may produce false-negative reactions.
h. Contamination of the sample with flea feces uncommonly may cause a positive occult blood reaction.

Bilirubin

a. Bilirubin is derived from the breakdown of heme by the reticuloendothelial system. It is transported in blood bound to albumin to the liver where it is conjugated with glucuronide and excreted in the bile.
b. Only direct-reacting (conjugated) bilirubin appears in the urine.
c. The renal threshold for bilirubin is low in dogs, and bilirubin may be detected in the urine in dogs with liver disease before hyperbilirubinemia occurs.
d. Small amounts of bilirubin (trace to +1) may be found in concentrated urine samples from normal dogs (especially males). +2 to +3 reactions are likely to be abnormal in concentrated urine samples and trace to +1 reactions may be abnormal in dogs with dilute urine.
e. Bilirubin is not normally found in the urine of cats, and its presence in feline urine samples should be considered a sign of underlying disease.
f. The kidney of the dog (especially males) can degrade hemoglobin and conjugate bilirubin to some extent.
g. Bilirubin is unstable in urine allowed to stand exposed to air at room temperature. Bilirubin concentration should be determined using fresh, uncentrifuged urine because calcium-containing crystals may adsorb bilirubin and bilirubin can undergo oxidation over time to biliverdin or be hydrolyzed to unconjugated bilirubin, which will not be detected by the reagent pad.
h. Causes of bilirubinuria.
   (1) Hemolysis.
      (a) Autoimmune hemolytic anemia.
      (b) Secondary to liver dysfunction after anemia and hemosiderosis.
      (c) Metabolism of hemoglobin to bilirubin by the kidney in dogs after glomerular filtration.
   (2) Liver disease.
   (3) Extrahepatic biliary obstruction.
   (4) Fever.
   (5) Starvation.

Leukocyte Esterase Reaction (Not Useful in Veterinary Medicine)

a. Indoxyl released by esterases from intact or lysed leukocytes reacts with a diazonium salt and is detected as a blue color reaction after oxidation by atmospheric oxygen.
b. Specific for pyuria in canine urine samples but has low sensitivity (many false-negative results).
c. Very frequent occurrence of false-positive results (low specificity) for WBCs in feline urine.

Specific Gravity Reagent Pad Reaction (Not Useful in Veterinary Medicine)

a. Does not correlate with USG results obtained using a refractometer.
b. Should not be used in veterinary patients.

Urinary Sediment

> ❗ Normal urine contains very few formed elements and little should be seen during microscopic examination.

1. Do not omit the sediment examination as much meaningful information may be overlooked. Evaluation of the urinary sediment is comparable to performing a differential blood count as part of a complete hemogram. Many conditions may go undiagnosed if a complete urinary sediment examination is not performed.
2. A complete urinary sediment examination requires proper identification of cells (RBCs, WBCs, epithelial cells), casts, organisms (bacterial, fungal), crystals, mucus, and artifacts or contaminants.
3. Perform the sediment examination on fresh urine sample because casts and cellular elements degenerate rapidly at room temperature.
4. Centrifuge 5 to 10 mL of urine at 1000 to 1500 rpm for 5 minutes. Too much force will disrupt delicate elements (e.g., cellular casts). Stain with Sedi-Stain or examine unstained depending on preference. Examine under reduced light (i.e., condenser down, reduced diaphragm aperture).
5. Whenever possible, use the same volume when comparing results from the same patient.
6. Keep the method of urine collection in mind because it can influence interpretation.
7. Keep the urine specific gravity in mind.
   a. The USG will influence the relative numbers of formed elements.
   b. High USG will cause crenation of cells in urine.
   c. Low USG will cause ballooning and lysis of cells in urine.
8. Numbers of casts are recorded per low-power field (lpf, 10×) and numbers of RBCs, WBCs, and epithelial cells are recorded per hpf (40×).
9. The presence or absence of bacteria, crystals, amorphous material, lipid droplets and sperm is noted. Positive findings should be further characterized as few, moderate, or many. Results from an average of 10 microscopic fields are reported.
10. Urine sediment examination is facilitated (especially if personnel are inexperienced) if fresh urine and supra-vital staining (Sedi-Stain) are used in evaluation. These procedures will ensure preservation of fragile cellular elements and enhance ability to identify abnormal components in the sediment.
11. It is not always possible to accurately identify all elements in a urinary sediment sample due to the altered morphology of cellular elements that may arise as a consequence of the relatively wide pH and osmolality range of normal urine.
12. Normal values for urinary sediment evaluation cannot be easily provided because of methodological differences among laboratories (e.g., volume of sample processed, time and force of centrifugation, size of drop used in making coverslip preparation, presence or absence of staining).

Red Blood Cells (RBCs) (Figure 1-5)

   a. Occasional RBCs are considered normal in the urine sediment.
      (1) Voided sample: 0 to 8 per hpf.
      (2) Catheterized sample: 0 to 5 per hpf.
      (3) Cystocentesis sample: 0 to 3 per hpf (up to 50 RBCs/hpf may be normal if urine was collected by cystocentesis and the procedure was traumatic).
   b. Excessive numbers of RBCs in urine is called hematuria. Hematuria may be microscopic or macroscopic (i.e., visible to the naked eye). Detection of excessive numbers of RBCs in urine does localize the site of entry into the urinary tract unless RBCs are observed in RBC casts (i.e., renal origin).

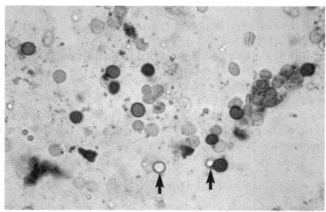

FIGURE 1-5 ■ Red blood cells (RBCs). Note difference in uptake of stain by RBCs. Large numbers of RBCs can enter the urine as a result of trauma, inflammation from infection or urolithiasis, and neoplasia, but can also be an artifact of cystocentesis. *Arrows* point to refractile lipid droplets that are easily confused with RBCs. (Sedi-Stain, ×400).

      (1) Presence of so-called *dysmorphic* RBCs indicates renal origin in humans but this finding has not yet been studied in veterinary patients.

      (2) Precipitates of hemoglobin in the urine sediment can be confused with RBC, but hemoglobin precipitates have a distinctive orange-brown color and vary widely in diameter.

      (3) Lipid droplets are often confused with RBCs, especially in cats.

  c. Hematuria may arise from the kidney, ureter, bladder, urethra, prostate gland, uterus, vestibule, vagina, vulva, penis, prepuce, or perineum. The history, physical examination findings, and method of urine collection all must be considered in localizing hematuria.

  d. Urinary causes of hematuria.

      (1) Trauma (including renal biopsy).

      (2) Urolithiasis.

      (3) Neoplasia.

      (4) UTI.

      (5) Inflammatory disease of the urogenital tract.

      (6) Idiopathic lower urinary tract disease of cats (i.e. feline idiopathic cystitis).

      (7) Chemically-induced lesions (e.g. cyclophosphamide-induced cystitis).

      (8) Systemic diseases associated with hemorrhage.

        (a) Warfarin intoxication.

        (b) Disseminated intravascular coagulation.

        (c) Thrombocytopenia.

      (9) Renal infarction (rare).

     (10) Nephritis or nephrosis.

     (11) Parasites (e.g., *Dioctophyma renale, Capillaria*).

     (12) Renal pelvic hematoma.

  e. Nonurinary causes for hematuria: Genital tract contamination.

      (1) Prostatic disease.

      (2) Penile or preputial contamination.

      (3) Vaginal, vestibular, or vulvar contamination.

        (4) Estrus.

        (5) Uterine disease (e.g., pyometra, endometritis).

White Blood Cells (WBCs) (Figure 1-6)

  a. Occasional WBCs are considered normal in the urine sediment.

      (1) Voided sample: 0 to 8 per hpf.

      (2) Catheterized sample: 0 to 5 per hpf.

      (3) Cystocentesis sample: 0 to 3 per hpf.

  b. WBCs are 2- to 2.5-times the size of RBCs in urine (depending on USG) (Figure 1-7). It can be difficult or impossible to accurately identify WBCs in the urine sediment if cellular degeneration has occurred.

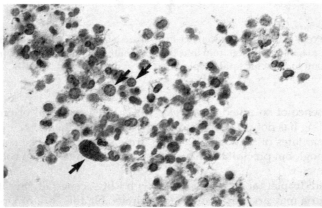

FIGURE 1-6 ■ White blood cells (WBCs). Urinary tract infection (UTI) or inflammation from urolithiasis or neoplasia may cause pyuria. Clumping of WBCs in the urine may indicate infection. *Arrows* point to epithelial cells. (Sedi-Stain, ×400).

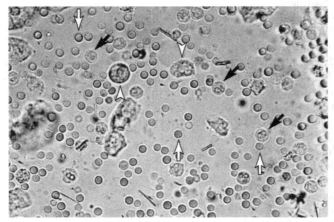

FIGURE 1-7 ■ Urine sediment containing RBCs, WBCs, and epithelial cells. Note that WBCs (*black arrows*) are approximately twice the size of RBCs (*white arrows*), and epithelial cells (*white arrowheads*) are usually twice the size of WBCs. (Sedi-Stain, ×400).

c. Increased numbers of WBCs in the urine sediment is called pyuria and indicates inflammation somewhere in the urinary tract or contamination from the genital tract. It also is important to note clumping of WBCs because this finding may indicate the presence of UTI.

d. Examine the urine sediment carefully for organisms that may account for the pyuria. Bacteria may be visible as free-floating organisms between clumps of WBCs or may be present as phagocytized organisms in WBCs.

e. Fungal organisms or yeast are rarely the cause of pyuria.

f. Swollen WBCs containing intracellular material undergoing Brownian motion have been called *glitter cells*. Their presence has been associated with pyelonephritis, but they also may be observed in patients with USG <1.015 for other reasons.

g. Causes of pyuria.

    (1) Urinary tract inflammation including but not limited solely to UTI. Urinary tract infection, however, is the most common cause of pyuria. WBCs can enter urine from the kidney, ureter, bladder, or urethra.

    (2) Genital tract contamination or inflammation. WBCs can arise from the vulva, vestibule, vagina, uterus, prostate gland, testes, epididymis, vas deferens, penis, prepuce, or perineum.

h. The presence of WBCs in the urine sediment does not localize the site of inflammation or infection unless they occur in WBC casts indicating renal origin.

i. Trauma does not necessarily contribute WBCs to the urine sediment but RBCs are commonly found in the urine sediment as a consequence of trauma.

Epithelial Cells

SQUAMOUS EPITHELIAL CELLS

    (1) Squamous epithelial cells are large, polygonal cells with small round nuclei. They tend to fold on themselves and sometimes are confused with casts. Their large size allows them to be easily distinguished from casts.

    (2) Common in voided or catheterized samples due to urethral or vaginal contamination.

    (3) Small numbers can be a normal finding and increased numbers may be found in the urine sediment of females during estrus.

    (4) Sometimes observed in urine sediment of samples obtained by cystocentesis, presumably as a result of aspiration of epithelial cells from skin.

    (5) Usually of no diagnostic significance.

TRANSITIONAL EPITHELIAL CELLS (Figure 1-8)

    (1) Transitional epithelial cells are variable-sized urothelial cells that enter urine anywhere from the renal pelvis to the urethra.

    (2) Small numbers normally are found in the urine sediment as a result of normally occurring senescence of the urothelium.

    (3) The size of transitional cells increases from the renal pelvis to urethra. Normally, they are slightly larger to twice the size of WBCs. Small transitional cells usually originate from the kidney, but small transitional cells also can originate from the ureter, bladder, and urethra. Large transitional cells do not arise from the kidney.

    (4) Increased numbers of transitional cells may be present in the urine sediment with infection, mechanical trauma (e.g., urolithiasis), chemical irritation (e.g., cyclophosphamide), idiopathic inflammation (e.g., feline idiopathic cystitis), or neoplasia of the urinary tract.

    (5) Rafts are clumps of epithelial cells (either alone or in association with increased numbers of RBCs) observed most commonly in patients with neoplasia. Rafts of epithelial cells also can be observed as a reaction to inflammation, usually in the presence of WBCs and RBCs.

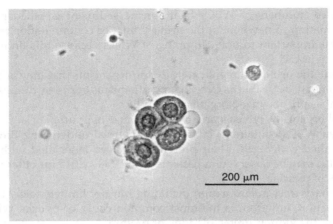

200 μm

FIGURE 1-8 ■ Transitional epithelial cell cells. Transitional epithelial cells can enter the urine as a result of inflammation in the renal pelvis, ureter, bladder, or proximal urethra. They are rarely encountered in cats with idiopathic cystitis. Clumps of transitional epithelial cells can be observed after severe urinary tract inflammation, and can occur in animals with neoplasia. (Sedi-Stain, ×400). (Courtesy Dr. Michael Horton, Fairborn Animal Hospital, Fairborn, Ohio.)

(a) Large nuclei, multiple nucleoli, coarse nuclear chromatin, mitotic figures, and cytoplasmic basophilia are features of neoplasia that can be observed in wet-mount cytological preparations of urine sediment.

(b) Neoplastic epithelial cells are best identified using conventional stains used for hematology (e.g., Wright-Giemsa). Dry mount cytology can be performed on urine sediment with or without supra-vital staining.

RENAL EPITHELIAL CELLS

(1) Renal cells are small epithelial cells that originate from the renal pelvis or tubules.

(2) There is no definitive way to be certain that small epithelial cells observed in the urine sediment have originated from the kidneys. They can only be identified as having a renal origin when observed in cellular casts.

(3) Caudate cells are small transitional cells with tapered ends (so-called *tails*) thought to originate from the renal pelvis.

(4) The presence of renal epithelial cells in urine is abnormal. They are observed most often in patients with ischemic, nephrotoxic, or degenerative renal disease, usually in patients with acute renal failure.

Casts

a. Casts are cylindrical molds of the renal tubules composed of aggregated protein matrix with or without embedded cells. A spectrum from nearly all matrix to nearly all cells or granules may occur depending on the disease state associated with cast formation. Casts are classified on the basis of the predominating component (Figure 1-9).

b. Casts form by precipitation of protein and any intact cells, intracellular organelles, brush border, or cellular debris that may be present in the tubular lumen. They form in the distal tubules as a consequence of maximal acidity, highest solute concentration, and lowest flow rate in this segment of the nephron.

c. Casts are large cylindrical structures with well-defined, parallel borders. The length of the cast is expected to be several times its width. The ends of casts often are rounded. Do not confuse a linear strand of mucus with a cast. Strands of mucus do not have parallel sides.

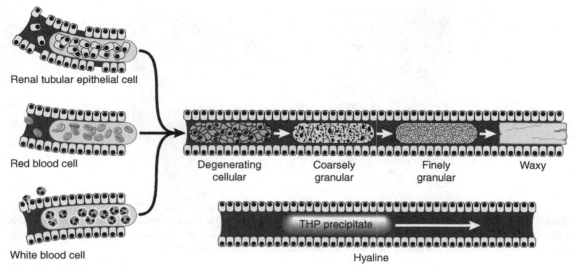

Renal tubular epithelial cell

Red blood cell

White blood cell

Degenerating cellular

Coarsely granular

Finely granular

Waxy

THP precipitate

Hyaline

FIGURE 1-9 ■ Addis theory of cast formation. According to this theory, granular casts result from the breakdown of cells and waxy casts from additional degeneration of granular casts. Hyaline casts are pure precipitates of Tamm Horsfall mucoprotein (THP). (Drawn by Tim Vojt.)

> (1) Very wide casts form either in the collecting duct or in dilated portions of the distal tubule, whereas very thin casts may form in areas of tubular compression associated with interstitial inflammation or edema.
>
> (2) Convoluted casts reflect the course of distal convoluted tubules.

d. The presence of abnormal numbers of casts in the urine sediment is called cylindruria.

e. Cylindruria reflects activity in the kidney and thus is of localizing value.

f. Tamm-Horsfall mucoprotein is secreted by the distal tubular cells and is the most important matrix protein in casts. Increased amounts of this protein in the distal tubules facilitate cast formation. Increased amounts of filtered plasma protein (e.g., albumin, hemoglobin, myoglobin) in the tubular fluid favor precipitation of Tamm-Horsfall mucoprotein.

g. Zero to 2 hyaline casts per lpf and 0 to 1 granular casts per lpf are considered normal, but no cellular casts should be observed in normal urine sediment.

TYPES OF CASTS

Hyaline casts (Figure 1-10)

> (a) Hyaline casts are pure protein precipitates of Tamm-Horsfall mucoprotein.
>
> (b) Are of low optical density and often are not identified in urine sediment as a consequence.
>
> (c) Dissolve rapidly in dilute or alkaline urine.
>
> (d) Are transparent and sometimes confused with waxy casts, which are translucent.
>
> (e) May contain a small number of lipid droplets or granules.
>
> (f) Usually are of minimal pathologic significance and may be formed transiently in many situations (e.g., fever, exercise, passive renal congestion).
>
> (g) Commonly seen in glomerular diseases associated with marked proteinuria (e.g., amyloidosis, glomerulonephritis).
>
> (h) Sometimes seen in renal tubular diseases that decrease reabsorption of proteins or add inflammatory proteins to urine.

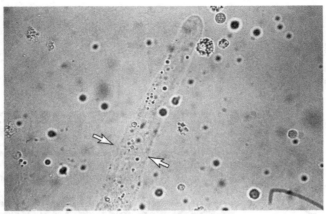

FIGURE 1-10 ■ Hyaline cast. Notice the transparent nature of this hyaline cast. *Arrows* point to the parallel walls of this cast. Hyaline casts are precipitates of the matrix protein that forms them. They are easily missed if the urine sediment sample is examined under excessive transillumination. (Sedi-Stain, ×400).

    (i) Dehydration with loss of negative charge from glomeruli (negative charge of the glomerulus normally repels serum proteins). Cylindroids are hyaline casts that are longer and thinner than normal and have tapered ends. A cylindroid potentially can form when the tubular lumen has been narrowed due to swelling of tubular cells or compression from interstitial edema or cellular infiltrates.

Cellular casts

    (a) Named according to the predominant cell type present in the casts (e.g., WBCs, RBCs, epithelial cells).

    (b) The cells in cellular casts undergo rapid degeneration and the casts themselves disintegrate quickly. Examination of fresh urine sediment (within 15 minutes of collection) usually is needed to verify the presence of cellular casts. Cellular casts will rarely be reported by remote reference laboratories to which urine samples have been shipped.

    (c) WBC casts (*pus casts*) are suggestive of pyelonephritis (Figure 1-11). Acute to subacute interstitial nephritis, nephrosis, and exudative glomerulonephritis (rare) also may be considered. Degeneration of WBCs in the casts can make it impossible to differentiate WBCs from renal tubular epithelial cells. Confusion may arise if WBCs adhere in a linear fashion to strands of mucus or fibrin during centrifugation of the urine sample.

    (d) RBC casts are the most fragile of the cellular casts and are rarely observed in the urine of dogs and cats. They may be seen in acute glomerulonephritis, after renal trauma (e.g., renal biopsy) or after strenuous exercise. RBC casts must be differentiated from free RBCs arranged in a linear fashion in the urine sediment.

    (e) Hemoglobin casts are variants of RBC casts in which the RBCs have lost their cell membranes but the hemoglobin persists (sometimes called *blood casts*). Blood casts are best seen in unstained urine sediment and have the same clinical relevance as do intact RBC casts.

    (f) Renal epithelial cell casts (Figure 1-12) occur most commonly in patients with acute tubular necrosis or pyelonephritis and they imply severe tubular injury.

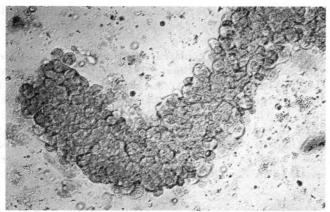

FIGURE 1-11 ■ WBC cast. White blood cell (WBC) casts indicate renal inflammation, often from bacterial pyelonephritis. Care must be taken to be sure the so-called cast is not an artifact arising from the binding of individual WBCs in urine to fibrin or mucus strands. (Sedi-Stain, ×400). (Courtesy of Nancy Facklam, ATH, The Ohio State University, Columbus, Ohio.)

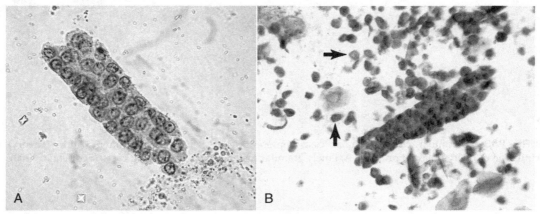

FIGURE 1-12 ■ A, Renal epithelial cell cast from the urine sediment of a dog being treated with gentamicin. The presence of renal epithelial cell casts often indicates severe acute renal tubular injury. B, Another cellular epithelial cell cast comprised of renal tubular epithelial cells. Note free small round epithelial cells (*black arrows*) that are the same size as those within the cast — renal tubular epithelial cells. There is no way to definitively prove the origin of small free epithelial cells in the urine unless they are within a cast. (Sedi-Stain, ×400). (A, Courtesy of Dr. Brian Luria, Florida Veterinary Specialists, Tampa, Fla.)

They often are associated with nephrotoxic or ischemic renal injury but also may be seen with renal infarction, acute interstitial nephritis (e.g., leptospirosis), and pyelonephritis.

(g) Renal fragments are variants of epithelial cell casts that represent portions of the renal tubules that have sloughed into urine without matrix protein precipitation. Their presence indicates severe disruption of tubular basement membranes and more severe renal injury than implied by the presence of epithelial cell casts.

(h) Mixed casts contain more than one identifiable cell type (e.g., WBCs, RBCs, epithelial cells).

(i) Degenerative cell casts refer to casts in which cellular outlines can still be seen, but the cell type cannot be identified because of changes in size and loss of nuclear detail.

(j) Coarsely and finely granular casts (Figure 1-13) represent the degeneration of cells in other casts or precipitation of filtered plasma proteins according to the Addis theory of cast formation. Excessive numbers of granular casts suggest accelerated tubular degeneration, but they also may be seen in patients with glomerular disease when large amounts of filtered plasma protein precipitate in urine.

(k) Fatty casts are coarsely granular casts containing lipid granules and may be seen in patients with glomerular disease or diabetes mellitus.

(l) Waxy casts (Figure 1-14) represent the final stage of degeneration of granular casts and are relatively stable over time in dilute and alkaline urine. Waxy casts

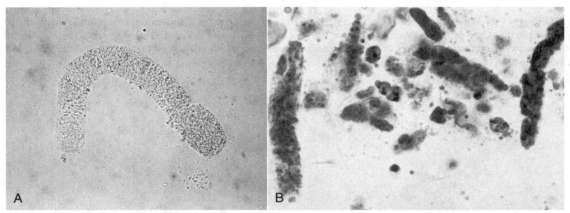

FIGURE 1-13 ■ Granular casts. Granular casts represent renal cellular degeneration (Addis Theory) or precipitation of filtered plasma proteins. **A,** Finely granular cast. **B,** Coarsely granular casts. (Sedi-Stain, ×400).

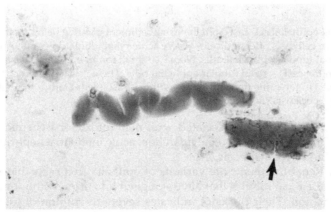

FIGURE 1-14 ■ Waxy casts. Waxy casts are translucent and represent the final transformation of cellular breakdown within the renal tubules. Their presence indicates substantial and prolonged intrarenal stasis. *Black arrow* points to a crack in one of the waxy casts — this is commonly observed because of the brittle nature of the protein that comprises this cast. (Sedi-Stain, ×400).

are easily identified because of their high refractive index and homogenous translucent appearance. They can be convoluted and often contain cracks and blunt ends due to their brittle nature. Staining of waxy casts is variable, but they may appear dark purple when the urine sediment is stained using Sedi-Stain. The presence of waxy casts suggests substantial chronic intrarenal stasis because these casts take considerable time to form. They are associated with chronic renal failure and consequently have been called *renal failure casts*. They are associated with advanced chronic renal disease and their presence is considered an ominous finding.

(m) Broad casts are unusually wide casts that form in the collecting ducts or dilated portions of the distal tubules. Tubular flow normally is rapid in the collecting ducts, making cast formation difficult in this segment. Thus, the presence of broad casts suggests severe intrarenal stasis or tubular obstruction. Abrupt appearance of broad casts may be a favorable prognostic sign when conversion from oliguria to normal urine output or polyuria occurs and previously formed broad casts enter the urine.

Organisms

a. Normal bladder urine is sterile. The distal urethra and genital tract harbor bacteria, and voided or catheterized urine samples may be contaminated with bacteria from the distal urethra, genital tract, skin, or collection container.

b. Contamination of voided or catheterized urine samples by the urethra usually does not result in sufficient numbers of bacteria to be visualized microscopically during urine sediment examination. If however such a specimen is allowed to stand at room temperature these bacterial contaminants may proliferate.

c. To be seen microscopically in the urine sediment there must be:
   (1) >10^4 rods/mL urine.
   (2) >10^5 cocci/mL urine.

d. Large numbers of bacteria in urine collected by catheterization or cystocentesis strongly suggests the presence of UTI (Figure 1-15). Usually pyuria accompanies bacteriuria on urine sediment examination.

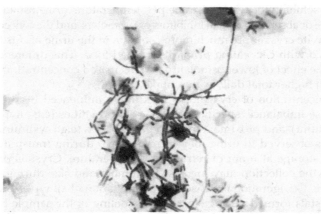

FIGURE 1-15 ■ Bacteria. The bacteria pictured are rod-shaped and filamentous, which facilitates their identification. Many artifacts in urine sediment can resemble bacteria, especially cocci. Suspected cocci should be carefully differentiated from artifacts (e.g., stain precipitates, cellular debris). (Sedi-Stain, ×400).

(1) Rod-shaped bacterial are more easily and accurately identified in the urine sediment than are cocci which sometimes can be confused with particulate debris.
(2) Enteric bacteria sometimes have filamentous morphology in urine which should not be confused with fungal hyphae.
(3) The presence of bacteria without pyuria on urine sediment examination suggests the possibility of bacterial contamination in samples processed without refrigeration or preservatives.
(4) Dogs with hyperadrenocorticism, diabetes mellitus, and those treated with immunosuppressive drugs may have bacterial UTI without pyuria.
(5) Cats with chronic renal failure also may have bacterial UTI without pyuria.
(6) Particulate debris in the urine sediment may be confused with bacteria (especially cocci) and cause false-positive results. Precipitates of stain also may resemble cocci. Finally, stored stain preparations may be contaminated with bacteria. A drop of stain may be examined separately to evaluate this possibility.
(7) Amorphous debris, small crystals, and lipid droplets in urine are subject to Brownian motion and can be confused with bacteria.
(8) Modified Wright-Giemsa staining of dried smears of urinary sediment may facilitate detection of bacteria suspected by evaluation of a wet mount of urinary sediment.
(9) The absence of bacteria on microscopic urine sediment examination does not eliminate the possibility of UTI. Suspected UTI should be confirmed by Gram stain and quantitative urine culture.
(10) Yeast and fungal hyphae in the sediment usually are contaminants. Fungal UTI rarely may occur (e.g., immunocompromised patients treated long-term with antibiotics) and occasionally patients with systemic mycoses have urogenital involvement (e.g., blastomycosis, aspergillosis).

Crystals

a. Crystals are commonly present in urine of normal dogs and cats and often are of little diagnostic significance. Struvite, amorphous phosphate, and oxalate are examples of crystals that may be found in normal urine samples.
b. Persistent crystalluria in fresh urine is a risk factor for recurrent urolithiasis and for urethral plug formation in male cats.
c. Crystal solubility depends on urine pH, temperature, urine osmolality (specific gravity), presence or absence of crystal inhibitors or promoters, and the concentration of crystalloids.
  (1) Struvite crystals are much more common in the urine of cats fed dry foods as compared with cats eating primarily canned food. This difference presumably is due to the effect of lower osmolality and decreased concentration of crystalloids in cats with higher total daily water intake.
d. The concentration of crystalloids in urine is influenced by dietary intake, systemic acid-base imbalance, specific metabolic abnormalities (e.g., hypercalcemia, portosystemic shunt), and proximal renal tubular function (e.g., cystinuria).
e. Crystals observed in urine may form de novo during transport to the laboratory or during storage at room or refrigerator temperature. Crystals present in urine at the time of the collection may increase in number and size during storage at room temperature. Refrigeration increases the precipitation of all types of crystals.
  (1) Crystals formed during storage and cooling of the sample before analysis do not readily go back into solution when the sample is re-warmed.
  (2) Crystals that form after collection of the urine sample are of no clinical relevance for urolith or urethral plug formation.

(3) If the presence or absence of specific crystals in urine is important in the clinical decision-making process, conclusions should be based on immediate evaluation of a fresh urine sample that has not been stored at room or refrigerator temperature.

f. Crystals should be reported according to type (i.e., chemical composition), quantity, size, and whether they are aggregated or individual (i.e., crystal habitat). The time elapsed from sample collection to urine sediment evaluation and whether or not refrigeration was used also are important to note. Large numbers of crystals, crystals that are individually larger, and crystals that have aggregated during evaluation of a fresh sample have more clinical relevance for urolith formation.

g. Crystalluria is not synonymous with urolithiasis.
  (1) Crystals may be present without uroliths.
  (2) Uroliths may be present without crystals.
  (3) When uroliths are present, the type of crystal found in the urine sediment may not match the chemical composition of the uroliths.

> **!** Crystals reported on urinalysis often are artifacts of storage at room or refrigerator temperature. Crystals that form during storage are of no clinical relevance. Crystals may form and increase in number and size during storage.

h. Crystals found in acid urine.
  (1) Uric acid.
  (2) Calcium oxalate (Figure 1-16).
  (3) Cystine (Figure 1-17).

i. Crystals found in alkaline urine.
  (1) Struvite ($MgNH_4PO_4 \cdot 6H_2O$ or so-called *triple phosphate*) (Figure 1-18).
  (2) Calcium phosphate.
  (3) Calcium carbonate.
  (4) Amorphous phosphate ammonium biurate (Figure 1-19).

j. Characteristic crystals also may be found in the urine sediment of animals on specific drugs, especially sulfonamides, enrofloxacin, and amoxicillin.

k. Bilirubin crystals may be found in concentrated samples of normal dog urine.

l. Associations.
  (1) Urates or uric acid: Dalmatians.
  (2) Urates: Liver disease, portosystemic shunt.
  (3) Cystine: Cystinuria.
  (4) Struvite: Normal animals, animals with struvite uroliths.
  (5) Calcium oxalate monohydrate (i.e., whewellite, *hippurate-like* or *picket fence*) or calcium oxalate dihydrate (i.e., weddellite, *Maltese cross* or *square envelope*): Acute renal failure due to ethylene glycol (EG) ingestion.

Miscellaneous Elements and Artifacts

a. Sperm from the urine of normal intact male dogs and cats. Voided samples from recently bred females also may contain sperm.

b. Amorphous debris can arise from small crystals or cellular debris. Large amounts of amorphous debris may be seen in patients with acute intrinsic renal failure, presumably due to necrosis of renal cells.

c. Mucus threads and or fibrin strands may be seen in patients with lower urinary tract or genital inflammation.

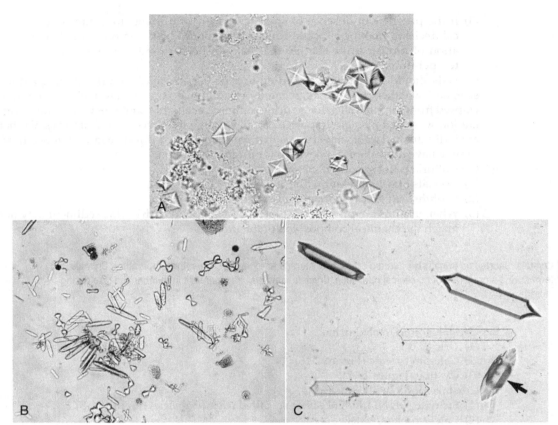

FIGURE 1-16 ■ **A,** Oxalate crystals. The dihydrate form of calcium oxalate is relatively easy to recognize because of its rhomboid shape with internal Maltese cross pattern. There are many different forms of calcium oxalate that are not as easy to identify. Oxalate crystals may be an artifact of storage and refrigeration or may be associated with urolithiasis, hypercalcemia, or EG ingestion. **B,** Calcium oxalate monohydrate crystals can assume a picket fence form. **C,** Calcium oxalate monohydrate. Note the hemp-seed shape to the one crystal in the lower right panel. This crystal also has a budding daughter crystal (*black arrow*). The other picket fence-shaped crystals are another monohydrate form. (Sedi-Stain, ×400). (**A,** Courtesy of Dr. Michael Horton, Fairborn Animal Hospital, Fairborn, Ohio.)

    d. Rarely, ova of the parasites *D. renale* or *Capillaria plica* are seen in the urine sediment. Microfilaria from dogs with dirofilariasis sometimes are observed in the urine sediment if bleeding into the urinary tract has occurred.

    e. Lipid droplets can be seen in patients with cellular degeneration. Lipid droplets often are found in the urine of normal cats. Lipid droplets can be distinguished from RBCs by their refractile nature, which can be identified by altering the depth of focus of the microscopic field. Sudan stain also can be used to confirm that suspected droplets contain lipid.

    f. Foreign material often contaminates urine collected by voiding or catheterization. Plant material, spores, pollen, hair, straw, fecal matter, and talcum powder from surgery gloves may be observed and confused with other urinary elements. Lubricants can contribute refractile droplets to the urine.

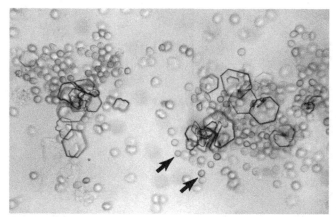

FIGURE 1-17 ■ Cystine crystals. These hexagonal crystals are never normal and are associated with cystinuria or cystine urolithiasis. These crystals may be confused with struvite crystals, but cystine crystals are flat and display little internal architecture. *Arrows* point to RBCs in background. (Sedi-Stain, ×400).

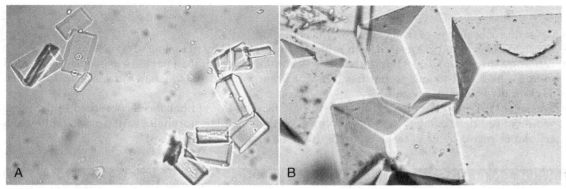

FIGURE 1-18 ■ Struvite crystals. **A,** Struvite crystals have a characteristic *coffin-lid* appearance and are common in urine that has been refrigerated. They also are observed in association with alkaline urine and struvite urolithiasis. **B,** The crystals are much larger and aggregating at the same magnification. (Sedi-Stain, ×400). (Courtesy of Dr. Michael Horton, Fairborn Animal Hospital, Fairborn, Ohio.)

    g. Urinary stain precipitates can be confused with urinary crystals, especially when the stain has been subject to evaporative loss (i.e., low humidity environment). Stain precipitation is most prominent near the edge of the coverslip in wet mount preparations.

    h. Rolled squamous epithelial cells may resemble casts, but they are more intensely stained and much larger than casts.

    i. Clumps of RBCs, WBCs, or epithelial cells can be confused with casts. These clumps usually are more irregular in width and are not linear as expected with casts.

COMMON MISCONCEPTIONS

- Dipstrip tests for identification of WBCs are reliable for detection of WBCs in canine and feline urine samples. (They are not.)
- Dipstrip tests for urine specific gravity are reliable in dogs and cats. (They are not.)

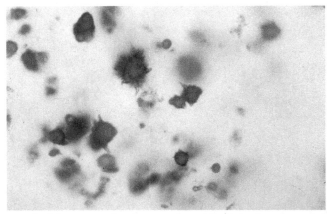

FIGURE 1-19 ■ Urate crystals. These crystals often are found in the urine of normal Dalmatian dogs and in those with urate urolithiasis. They also can be found in the urine sediment of dogs with portosystemic shunts. (Sedi-Stain, ×400).

- Crystalluria is always of major concern. (It is not.)
- Dipstrip pH is highly correlated with urine pH as measured by pH meter. (It is not.)
- Sending a urine sample to a remote reference laboratory is better than having a urinalysis performed in-house by a well-trained technician. (It is not. Transport and storage may introduce artifacts such as clinically irrelevant crystals.)
- The site of origin in the urinary tract of WBCs, RBCs, and or epithelial cells observed in the urine sediment can be accurately determined based on their cellular morphology. (It cannot. Only when cellular elements occur in casts can origin from the kidney be concluded.)

FREQUENTLY ASKED QUESTIONS

Q: Can I re-warm a previously refrigerated urine sample in which crystals have been observed during urine sediment examination?

A: Re-warming the sample will not necessarily allow the crystals to go back into solution.

Q: Why doesn't our laboratory ever report cellular casts from patients suspected to have acute renal failure?

A: Cellular casts are very fragile and frequently degenerate during transport to a reference laboratory. Urine sediment should be examined within 15 to 30 minutes of collection to facilitate identification of cellular casts.

Q: We frequently get reports of bacteria on urinalysis without pyuria and often these patients have negative urine cultures. Do these patients have UTI caused by a fastidious organism?

A: Usually not. Normal urine sediment may contain many artifacts that resemble bacteria. Most often, these reports are false positives. *Corynebacterium urealyticum* is an exception. It is a fastidious, slow-growing organism but usually is associated with very alkaline urine pH, struvite crystalluria, and bladder encrustation with struvite.

Q: Do I really need to use a supra-vital urine stain (Sedi-Stain) to get the most from my urinary sediment examination?

A: In general, using a supra-vital stain makes it easier to identify cells with greater accuracy, especially for novices. Experienced personnel, however, are able to identify elements in urine sediment whether it is stained or not, and some prefer to examine unstained urine sediment under low illumination.

Q: I own a centrifuge with one speed that is designed to centrifuge blood samples. Can I use this centrifuge to process urine samples for sediment examination?

A: Not if you hope to identify delicate sediment elements such as cellular casts, because the force generated for centrifuging blood is very high and will disrupt cellular casts. A centrifuge that generates less centrifugal force is desirable for preparation of urine sediment.

SUGGESTED READINGS

Albasan H, Lulich JP, Osborne CA, et al: Effects of storage time and temperature on pH, specific gravity, and crystal formation in urine samples from dogs and cats, *J Am Vet Med Assoc* 222:176–179, 2003.

Chew DJ, DiBartola SP: *Handbook of canine and feline urinalysis*, St Louis, 1998, Ralston Purina Co.

Chew DJ: Urinalysis. In Bovee KC, editor: *Canine nephrology*, Philadelphia, 1984, Harwal Publishing.

Holan KM, Kruger JM, Gibbons SN, Swenson SL: Clinical evaluation of a leukocyte esterase test-strip for detection of feline pyuria, *Vet Clin Pathol* 26:126–131, 1997.

Heuter KJ, Buffington CA, Chew DJ: Agreement between two methods for measuring urine pH in cats and dogs, *J Am Vet Med Assoc* 213:996–998, 1998.

Osborne CA, Stevens JB, Lulich JP, et al: A clinician's analysis of urinalysis. In Osborne CA, Finco DR, editors: *Canine and feline nephrology and urology*, Media, Pa, 1995, Williams and Wilkins.

Sturgess CP, Hesford A, Owen H, Privett R: An investigation into the effects of storage on the diagnosis of crystalluria in cats, *J Feline Med Surg* 3:81–85, 2001.

Vail DM, Allen TA, Weiser G: Applicability of leukocyte esterase test strip in detection of canine pyuria, *J Am Vet Med Assoc* 89:1451–1453, 1986.

http://www.diaglab.vet.cornell.edu/clinpath/modules/ua-sed/ua-intro.htm

2 Clinical Evaluation of the Urinary Tract

INTRODUCTION AND TERMINOLOGY

A. *Azotemia* is defined as an increased concentration of nonprotein nitrogenous compounds in blood, usually urea and creatinine.
   1. Prerenal azotemia is a consequence of reduced renal perfusion (e.g., severe dehydration, heart failure).
   2. Postrenal azotemia results from interference with excretion of urine from the body (e.g., obstruction, uroabdomen).
   3. Primary renal azotemia is caused by parenchymal renal disease.
   4. Combinations of prerenal with primary renal or postrenal azotemia are common.
   5. The differentiation of prerenal, renal, and postrenal azotemia is summarized in Table 2-1.
B. *Renal failure* refers to the clinical syndrome that occurs when the kidneys are no longer able to maintain their regulatory, excretory, and endocrine functions, resulting in retention of nitrogenous solutes and derangements of fluid, electrolyte, and acid-base balance. Renal failure occurs when 75% of more of the nephron population is nonfunctional.
C. *Uremia* refers to clinical signs and biochemical abnormalities associated with a critical loss of functional nephrons, and includes the extrarenal manifestations of renal failure (e.g., uremic gastroenteritis, hyperparathyroidism).
D. *Renal disease* refers to the presence of morphologic or functional lesions in one or both kidneys, regardless of extent.
E. The following questions should be answered when evaluating patients with suspected urinary tract disease:
   1. Is renal disease present?
      a. Is the disease glomerular, tubular, interstitial, or a combination?
      b. What is the extent of the renal disease?
      c. Is the disease acute or chronic, reversible or irreversible, progressive or nonprogressive?
      d. What is the current status of the patient's renal function?
      e. What nonurinary complicating factors are present and require treatment (e.g., infection, electrolyte and acid-base disturbances, dehydration)?
      f. Can the disease be treated?
      g. What is the prognosis?
   2. Is lower urinary tract disease present?
      a. Does the disease affect the ureters, bladder, or urethra?
      b. Is urinary tract obstruction present (see Chapter 11 for additional information on urinary tract obstruction)
      c. Can the disease be treated?
      d. What is the prognosis?

■ TABLE 2-1
■ ■ **Differentiation of Prerenal, Intrinsic, and Postrenal Azotemia**

Feature	Prerenal	Intrinsic-Renal Acute	Intrinsic-Renal Chronic	Postrenal Obstruction	Postrenal Uroperitoneum
BUN	↑	↑	↑	↑	↑
Serum creatinine	↑	↑	↑	↑	↑
Urine:	>1.030 D	<1.030 D	<1.030 D	Variable	Variable
SG	>1.040 C	<1.040 C	<1.040 C	RBC, WBC, epi	RBC, WBC, epi
Sediment	–	+, – casts	–	+	+
Protein		+, –	+, –		
Renal size	N	↑, or N	↓, or N	↑, or N	N
Hematocrit (anemia)	N	N (early)	↓, or N	N (early)	N
BUN/SCr after IV fluids	Rapid decrease	Little change	Little change	Little change	Little change
PU/PD (long standing)	–	–	+	– (acute)	–
Oliguria	+	+, or –	–, or + (terminal)	Variable	Variable
Hypothermia	–	+ If nephrosis	–	–	–
Renal pain	–	+, –	–	+, –	–, + If renal tear
Ischemic episode	+	+	–	–	+ (trauma)
Nephrotoxin exposure	–	+	–	–	–
Renal ultrasound	N	↑ Echo	↑ Echo/calcinosis	↑ Pelvis/diverticula	N
Contrast urography	N	Absent, or delayed and persistent nephrogram	↓ Excretion	↑ Pelvis/diverticula	Contrast leakage
Serum calcium	N	↓, or N	N, ↓, or ↑ (rarely)	N, or ↓	N, or ↓
Serum phosphorus	N, or ↑	↑	↑	↑	↑
Serum potassium	N	↑, or N	N, or ↓, or ↑ (terminal)	N, or ↑	N, or ↑
Metabolic acidosis	–	Moderate to severe	Mild to moderate	– early, + late	– early, + late
Abdominal fluid	None	+ (if overhydrated)	–	None	+
Blood pressure	↓, or N	N, or ↑	↑, or N	N, or ↑ (chronic)	N, or ↓
Renal biopsy	N	Abnormal	Abnormal	N, early	N

Findings from history, physical examination, serum biochemistry, urinalysis, hematology, radiography, renal histopathology, and special diagnostics may be necessary to distinguish conclusively the type of azotemia. Usually it is relatively easy to decide if azotemia is from postrenal causes after physical examination and routine abdominal radiography. Urinary specific gravity is the most important single test to differentiate prerenal and intrinsic renal azotemia. Urinary sediment, renal size, and hematocrit also are helpful. Results listed in this table are those prior to drug, fluid, or surgical treatments. When two results are listed, the one noted first is most common. Findings will vary in severity according to the stage at which the disease process is investigated. *BUN*, blood urea nitrogen; *epi*, epithelial cells; *N*, normal; *PU/PD*, polyuria and polydipsia; *RBC*, red blood cell; *SCr*, serum creatinine; *SG*, specific gravity; *WBC*, white blood cell; –, negative result; +, positive result; ↑, value increased above normal; ↓, value decreased below normal.

CLINICAL APPROACH

A. The diagnosis of urinary tract disease begins with a careful evaluation of the history and physical examination findings and is further refined by consideration of urinalysis, serum biochemistries, diagnostic imaging, and in some instances histopathology.

History
1. Presenting complaint.
   a. Onset (acute or gradual).
   b. Progression (improving, unchanging, worsening).

  c. Response to previous therapy such as surgery, diet, and drugs (e.g., antibiotics, corticosteroids, non steroidal anti-inflammatory drugs).

Husbandry
  a. Animal's immediate environment (indoor, outdoor, or both).
  b. Animal's use (pet, breeding, show, or working animal).
  c. Geographical origin and travel history.
  d. Exposure to other animals in the household and environment.
  e. Type of diet including type (i.e., dry, canned, semi-moist) and specific brands.
  f. Litter box management for cats (i.e., number and location of litter boxes, litter substrate, cleaning schedule).

Medical History
  a. Information about previous trauma, illness, or surgery (especially of the urinary tract).
  b. Vaccination history (e.g., specific infectious agents, numbers of vaccinations received, time of last vaccination). In dogs, determine the specific leptospiral serovars against which the animal has been vaccinated.

Urination
  a. Frequency and volume.
   (1) Pollakiuria (usually an indicator of lower urinary tract disease).
   (2) Polyuria (usually an indicator of upper urinary tract disease). Normal urine output ranges from 10 to 20 mL/lb/day in dogs and cats.
   (3) Dysuria (usually an indicator of lower urinary tract disease).
   (4) Nocturia (may be an early sign of polyuria, but also can occur as a result of incontinence).
   (5) Oliguria (may be indicative of partial obstruction, dehydration, and some forms of acute renal failure).
   (6) Anuria (often indicates total urinary obstruction or severe acute renal injury)
  b. Initiation of urination. How easily does the animal initiate urination? Difficulty starting the urine stream could be due to partial obstruction, inflammation, or neurologic disease.
  c. Diameter of urine stream, with or without interruption of flow. A narrow stream could indicate partial obstruction, urethral spasm, or neurologic disease.
  d. Hematuria.
   (1) Blood at the beginning of urination may indicate a disease process in the urethra or genital tract.
   (2) Blood at the end of urination may signify a problem in either the bladder or upper urinary tract (kidneys or ureters).
   (3) Dripping of blood unassociated with urination usually indicates a urethral or genital tract source. In intact male dogs, such bleeding often originates from the prostate gland (e.g., benign prostatic hyperplasia).

> ❗ Normal water intake in dogs is up to 40 mL/lb/day, and in cats is up to 20 mL/lb/day.

Water Intake
  a. Dogs: Normal water intake may be as much as 40 mL/lb/day.
  b. Cats: Normal water intake may be as much as 20 mL/lb/day.
  c. A cup is approximately 250 mL, and a quart is approximately 1 liter.
  d. Exposure to nephrotoxins such as ethylene glycol (EG) in antifreeze, Easter lily (cats only), aminoglycosides (e.g., gentamicin), and nonsteroidal anti-inflammatory drugs should be identified. Administration of drugs that could cause polydipsia and polyuria (e.g., glucocorticoids, diuretics) also should be determined.

PHYSICAL EXAMINATION

A. Evaluation of hydration status is important for interpretation of laboratory data, especially urine specific gravity (USG). Dehydration is suggested by decreased skin turgor, dry mucous membranes, and sunken appearance of the eyes in their orbits.

B. Ascites or subcutaneous edema may accompany nephrotic syndrome (i.e., glomerular disease).

C. The oral cavity is examined for ulcers, tongue tip necrosis, and pallor of the mucous membranes that may occur in uremia.

D. Presence of retinal edema, detachment, hemorrhage, or vascular tortuosity noted during fundic examination is compatible with systemic hypertension, which may accompany renal disease. The animal may be blind or have impaired vision.

E. Musculoskeletal evaluation.
  1. Fibrous osteodystrophy may develop in young animals with renal failure, but is rare in older dogs.
  2. Fibrous osteodystrophy is characterized by enlargement and deformity of the maxilla and mandible (so-called *rubber jaw*).
  3. Pathologic fractures are rare.

F. Kidneys.
  1. Both kidneys can be palpated in most cats, and the left kidney in some dogs.
  2. Kidneys should be evaluated for size, shape, consistency, pain, and location.

G. Urinary bladder.
  1. Unless empty, the bladder can be palpated in most dogs and cats.
  2. The bladder should be evaluated for degree of distension, pain, wall thickness, and presence of intramural (e.g., tumors) or intra-luminal (e.g., calculi, clots) masses.
  3. In the absence of obstruction, a distended bladder in a dehydrated animal suggests abnormal renal function or administration of drugs that impair urinary concentrating ability (e.g., glucocorticoids, diuretics).

H. The prostate gland of male dogs and pelvic urethra of males and females are evaluated by rectal examination. The prostate gland should be within the pelvic canal, smooth, bilobed, moveable, and free of pain. Rectal examination is not routine in cats, but should be performed in cats with persistent lower urinary tract signs. The normal pelvic urethra is difficult to identify on rectal palpation.

I. Reproductive organs.
  1. The penis should be exteriorized and examined fully to its base and the testes palpated.
  2. The vulva is examined for any discharge that suggests inflammation elsewhere in the genitourinary tract. Examination of the vestibule and urethral orifice is not part of the routine physical examination.

LABORATORY EVALUATION OF RENAL FUNCTION

Glomerular Function (values for glomerular function tests in the dog and cat are presented in Table 2-2)

1. Glomerular filtration rate (GFR) is directly related to functional renal mass. GFR is the gold standard for the assessment of renal function and detection of renal disease progression. Determination of renal blood flow (RBF) also can be useful in detecting progression of renal disease, but is less commonly evaluated than GFR. Unfortunately, GFR is not routinely measured in the evaluation of renal function. Instead, surrogates for GFR such as blood urea nitrogen (BUN) and serum creatinine concentrations are used because they are more easily determined than is GFR. An ideal substance for estimation of GFR should

■ TABLE 2-2
■ ■ **Normal Values for Clinical Tests of Glomerular Function**

Test (units)	Dog	Cat
Blood urea nitrogen (mg/dL)	8-25	15-35
Serum creatinine (mg/dL)	0.3-1.3	0.8-1.8
Serum cystatin C (mg/dL)	0.5-1.5	NA
Endogenous creatinine clearance (mL/min/kg)	2-5	2-5
Exogenous creatinine clearance (mL/min/kg)	3-5	2-4
Iohexol clearance (mL/min/kg)	1.7-4.1	1.3-4.2
24-hour urine protein excretion (mg/kg/d)	<30	<20
U_{Pr}/U_{Cr}	<0.4	<0.4
Microalbuminuria (mg/dL)	<1	<1

NA, not available.

be produced at a constant rate in the body, have little binding to plasma proteins, be freely filtered, and not undergo tubular reabsorption or secretion.

  a. BUN concentration. Normal BUN concentrations are 8 to 25 mg/dL in the dog and 15 to 35 mg/dL in the cat.
   (1) Renal excretion of urea occurs by glomerular filtration, and BUN concentrations are inversely proportional to GFR. Urea clearance is not a reliable estimate of GFR and, in the face of volume depletion, decreased urea clearance may occur without a decrease in GFR due to increased tubular reabsorption of urea.
   (2) Production and excretion of urea are not constant.
    (a) Production and excretion increase after a high protein meal. A BUN concentration of 30 to 40 mg/dL may occur 4 to 8 hours after feeding a high-protein meal in dogs. Therefore, an 8- to 12-hour fast is recommended before measurement.
    (b) Gastrointestinal bleeding can increase BUN concentration because blood represents an endogenous protein load.
    (c) Clinical conditions characterized by increased catabolism (e.g., starvation, infection, fever) also can increase BUN concentration.
    (d) Some drugs may increase BUN concentration by increasing tissue catabolism (e.g., glucocorticoids, azathioprine) or decreasing protein synthesis (e.g., tetracyclines) but these effects are minimal.
    (e) BUN concentration can be decreased by low-protein diets, anabolic steroids, severe hepatic insufficiency, or portosystemic shunting.
  b. Serum creatinine concentration. Normal serum creatinine concentrations are 0.3 to 1.3 mg/dL in the dog and 0.8 to 1.8 mg/dL in the cat. An individual patient's serum creatinine concentration will increase over time with progression of renal disease, and increasing serum creatinine concentrations should not be ignored even if the results still are within the reference range.
   (1) Methods of measurement.
    (a) Automated colorimetric method (Jaffe reaction): Up to half of the measured creatinine actually may represent noncreatinine chromogens.
    (b) Lloyd's reagent may be used to remove non-creatinine chromogens and provide a more accurate determination of the true serum creatinine concentration.
    (c) Enzymatic methods specific for creatinine also are available to improve the accuracy of the measurement.

(2) Young animals have lower serum creatinine concentrations, whereas males and well-muscled individuals have higher concentrations.
  (a) Serum creatinine concentration in puppies younger than or equal to 16 weeks of age often is 0.4 to 0.5 mg/dL.
  (b) Serum creatinine concentration is slightly lower in very small breed dogs and slightly higher in giant breed dogs.
(3) Cachectic animals that have experienced severe loss of lean muscle mass often have lower serum creatinine concentrations than they otherwise would have if their muscle mass were normal.
(4) Normal reference ranges may differ somewhat among breeds. Greyhound dogs have slightly higher serum creatinine concentrations than do other breeds. In one study, serum creatinine concentrations were 1.8 ± 0.1 mg/dL in greyhounds and 1.5 ± 0.1 mg/dL in other breeds and in another study serum creatinine concentrations ranged from 1.2 to 1.9 mg/dL (mean, 1.6 mg/dL) in greyhounds as compared with 0.6 to 1.7 mg/dL (mean, 1.0 mg/dL) in non-greyhound dogs.

❗ A normal BUN or serum creatinine concentration does not necessarily imply normal renal function.

(5) Serum creatinine concentration (in contrast to BUN concentration) is not affected appreciably by diet.
(6) Creatinine is not metabolized and is excreted by the kidneys almost entirely by glomerular filtration. Serum creatinine concentration varies inversely with GFR.
c. BUN and serum creatinine concentrations often both increase during disease processes. Neither one is more sensitive than the other.
  (1) A normal BUN or serum creatinine concentration does not exclude the possibility of renal disease.
  (2) A normal BUN or serum creatinine concentration implies that at least 25% of renal mass is functional, but how much more renal mass is functional cannot be determined by these tests.
  (3) In some situations, either the BUN or serum creatinine concentration is increased, but not both at the same time. It is not always possible to explain discordant results between BUN and serum creatinine concentrations (Table 2-3).
  (4) Individual patient BUN or serum creatinine concentrations may increase progressively during development of chronic renal disease, but the results still may remain within the normal reference range.

❗ Increases in serum creatinine concentration over time may indicate progressive loss of renal mass even if results still are within normal limits.

  (a) If available, serial test results should be evaluated to identify a trend toward progressively increasing concentrations.
  (b) Considerable variation may occur in serum creatinine concentrations from different laboratories using the same sample but results from the same laboratory typically are very repeatable.
d. The relationship of BUN and serum creatinine concentrations to GFR is a rectangular hyperbola.
  (1) The slope of the curve is small when GFR is mildly or moderately decreased but large when GFR is severely reduced (Figure 2-1). Thus, large changes in GFR early in the course of renal disease cause small increases in BUN or serum creatinine

■ TABLE 2-3
■ ■ **Discordant Results Between Blood Urea Nitrogen (BUN) and Serum Creatinine (SCr) Concentration**

Disproportionate ↑ BUN Relative to SCr	Disproportionate ↑ SCr Relative to BUN
Severe dehydration and volume depletion (common)	Liver disease
Gastrointestinal hemorrhage	Anorexia or low protein diet
Emaciated animal	Massive muscle injury (acute)
Young animal	Well-muscled individual

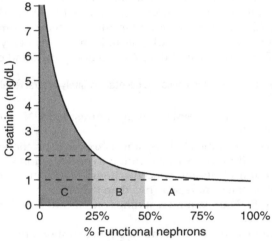

FIGURE 2-1 ■ Steady-state relationship of GFR to BUN and serum creatinine. Note the exponential relationship between loss of functioning renal mass and changes in renal function assessed by BUN or serum creatinine. At least 75% loss of excretory renal function must occur before the BUN or serum creatinine leave the normal range. With more than 75% loss of excretory renal function there are correspondingly larger increases in BUN or serum creatinine while on the rise of the exponential curve. Consequently, small increases or decreases in GFR along this region of the curve can create large numerical change in BUN or creatinine. When two thirds of renal mass has been lost most dogs elaborate urine that is considered isosthenuric (1.007-1.018 USG); many cats with this degree of renal mass loss continue to be able to elaborate urine that is at least moderately concentrated to more than 1.030 specific gravity. The area up to 50% loss of renal mass is referred to as that of decreased renal reserve, from 50% to 75% loss that of renal insufficiency, and 75% loss that of renal failure associated with azotemia. *Area A* represents diminished renal reserve with advancing chronic renal disease (International Renal Interest Society [IRIS] Stage 1). *Area B* represents renal insufficiency (late IRIS Stage 1 and early IRIS Stage 2). *Area C* represents azotemic renal failure (IRIS Stages 3 and 4).

concentration. Small changes in GFR in advanced renal disease cause large changes in BUN or serum creatinine concentration.

(2) An increase in BUN or serum creatinine concentration above normal implies that at least 75% of the nephrons are not functioning.

(a) The magnitude of a single BUN or serum creatinine concentration cannot be used to predict whether azotemia is prerenal, primary renal, or postrenal in origin, and cannot be used to distinguish between acute and chronic, reversible and irreversible, or progressive and non-progressive processes.

        (b) The BUN/creatinine ratio usually is 20:1 to 30:1.
- (i) It may be increased in prerenal and postrenal azotemia as a result of increased tubular reabsorption of urea at lower tubular flow rates or easier absorption of urea than creatinine across peritoneal membranes in animals with uroabdomen.
- (ii) Hyperthyroid cats also may have an increased ratio due to increased GFR and loss of lean muscle mass.
- (iii) It may be increased during cachexia as a result of lower serum creatinine concentration due to loss of lean muscle mass.
- (iv) It may be decreased after fluid therapy as a result of increased tubular flow and decreased tubular reabsorption of urea rather than as a result of a change in GFR.

  e. Normal cystatin C concentration in dogs is approximately 1 mg/dL.
- (1) Cystatin C is a protease inhibitor that is freely filtered by the glomeruli. It does not undergo tubular secretion, and filtered cystatin C is almost completely reabsorbed by the proximal tubular cells.
- (2) Cystatin C is produced at a constant rate in all tissues and its excretion is not dependent on age, sex, or diet.
- (3) Serum cystatin C concentration may serve as a useful marker of GFR.
- (4) Serum cystatin C concentration may be affected by the presence of inflammation or neoplasia.
- (5) Cystatin C determinations are not routinely available from commercial diagnostic laboratories.

Renal Clearance

1. The renal clearance of a substance is that volume of plasma that would have to be filtered by the glomeruli each minute to account for the amount of that substance appearing in the urine each minute. The renal clearance of a substance (x) that is neither reabsorbed nor secreted by the tubules is equal to the GFR. Thus, $GFR = U_x V / P_x$.
2. Creatinine is produced endogenously and excreted by glomerular filtration. Thus, its clearance can be used to estimate GFR.
3. Endogenous creatinine clearance determination:
   - a. Collect all urine for 12 or 24 hours and record volume (failure to collect all urine produced will decrease the calculated clearance value).
   - b. Determine animal's body weight.
   - c. Determine serum and urine creatinine concentrations.
   - d. Normal endogenous creatinine clearance is 2 to 5 mL/min/kg in the dog and cat.
   - e. The main indication for determination of endogenous creatinine clearance is suspicion of renal disease in a patient with polyuria and polydipsia, but normal BUN and serum creatinine concentrations.
4. Exogenous creatinine clearance.
   - a. Administer creatinine (100 mg/kg) SQ or IV to increase serum creatinine concentration approximately 10-fold.
   - b. Approximately 40 minutes later, collect at least 1 timed urine sample using an indwelling urinary catheter (e.g., all urine produced in 20 minutes). The average of three 20-minute collection periods is recommended to minimize collection errors.
   - c. Determine the animal's body weight and serum and urine creatinine concentrations.
   - d. Exogenous creatinine clearance exceeds endogenous creatinine clearance and approximates inulin clearance (the gold standard for determination of GFR) in the dog. In cats, exogenous creatinine clearance may be slightly lower than inulin clearance.

Single Injection Methods for Estimation of Glomerular Filtration Rate

1. Single injection plasma clearance methods using inulin, iohexol, or creatinine have been used to estimate GFR. Inulin clearance is the gold standard, but it is not easily measured and not available at commercial laboratories.

> **▌ Iohexol clearance can be used to estimate GFR clinically.**

2. Plasma clearance of the substance is calculated using the area under the plasma-concentration-versus-time curve.
3. These methods do not require urine collection, but accuracy depends on the number of plasma samples and the timing of their collection.
4. Iohexol is readily available for clinical use, but a laboratory equipped to measure it must be available.
   a. Iohexol is given at dosage of 300 mg/kg IV (using a 300 mg/mL solution), and plasma samples are collected 2, 3, and 4 hours after administration.
   b. Although not specifically reported in dogs and cats, hypersensitivity to iohexol is possible.
   c. Because 1 mL/kg of iohexol is given IV relatively rapidly, caution should be used in overhydrated patients or those with marginal cardiac function.
   d. Several commercial diagnostic laboratories offer iohexol determinations (e.g., Diagnostic Center for Population and Animal Health, Lansing, Mich.).

Effects of Sedatives and Anesthetics on Glomerular Filtration Rate

1. In one study, GFR was similar in dogs sedated with butorphanol and diazepam, acepromazine and butorphanol, and diazepam and ketamine. GFR in sedated dogs was not significantly different from that of awake dogs. Ketamine and acepromazine have minimal effects on GFR in cats.
2. A combination of medetomidine, butorphanol, and atropine has been evaluated in dogs using technetium-labeled diethylenetriaminepentaacetic acid (^{99m}Tc-DTPA) renal scintigraphy as an estimate of GFR and was found to have effects on GFR similar to those observed after saline alone.

Radioisotopes

1. Radioisotopes (e.g., ^{125}I- or ^{131}I-iothalamate, ^{51}Cr-ethylenediaminetetraacetic acid [EDTA], DTPA) have been used to estimate GFR in dogs and cats using both plasma clearance and dynamic renal scintigraphic methods.
2. Plasma clearance of isotopes.
   a. The plasma clearance approach has the same advantages and limitations as described earlier for iohexol or exogenously administered creatinine.
   b. Procedures using radioisotopes require technical expertise and equipment available primarily at referral institutions.
   c. Methods using ^{99m}Tc-DTPA to estimate GFR are clinically useful because the short half-life (6 hours) of ^{99m}Tc allows the animal to be released within 24 to 48 hours after the procedure. Very low dose protocols allow the animal to be released safely on the same day. The percentage of an injected dose of ^{99m}Tc-DTPA extracted by the kidneys over a finite time period correlates well with inulin clearance.
3. Dynamic renal scintigraphy.
   a. This method correlates less well with inulin clearance than does the plasma clearance method in dogs with renal disease. Renal scintigraphy is less accurate than plasma

clearance because a very short sampling period (usually 1 to 3 minutes postinjection) is used, and data obtained over such a short time may not accurately reflect steady state GFR. Characteristics of the gamma camera itself can lead to inaccuracies, and partial obstruction can delay excretion of the tracer from the kidneys and lead to overestimation of GFR.

b. Nuclear imaging using ^{99m}Tc-DTPA has been employed to determine GFR in normal dogs, dogs with renal disease, and in normal cats and those with renal dysfunction.

c. Quantitative renal scintigraphy and determination of plasma disappearance after single-injection using ^{99m}Tc-mercaptoacetyltriglycine have been used to estimate renal plasma flow in dogs. Hepatic uptake of ^{99m}Tc-mercaptoacetyltriglycine in cats may limit the value of this tracer for evaluation of renal plasma flow in this species.

d. The major advantage of this technique is that it is the only method that allows individual analysis of the left and right kidneys.

Serum Phosphorus Concentration

1. Measurement of serum phosphorus concentration can provide information about renal function in addition to that obtained from determination of BUN and serum creatinine concentrations.

2. Increased serum phosphorus concentration is not seen until >85% of the nephrons are nonfunctional.

> **In chronic renal disease, increased serum phosphorus concentration is not seen until > 85% of the nephrons are nonfunctional.**

3. Phosphorus is filtered by the glomeruli and reabsorbed by the tubules. Tubular reabsorption of phosphorus is regulated by parathyroid hormone, and renal secondary hyperparathyroidism maintains serum phosphorus concentration within the normal range by promoting excretion of phosphorus into urine until renal disease is advanced.

4. A serum phosphorus concentration that is disproportionately increased relative to serum creatinine concentration may be observed in acute renal failure. Rust inhibitors in antifreeze products may account for an increase in serum phosphorus concentration in animals shortly after EG ingestion.

5. Thyroxine increases proximal renal tubular reabsorption of phosphate and may contribute to hyperphosphatemia in cats with hyperthyroidism.

6. Serum phosphorus concentrations are 2.5 to 5.0 mg/dL in normal adult dogs and cats. Serum phosphorus concentrations may be as high as 8.5 mg/dL in immature animals as a consequence of bone growth. Most laboratories do not determine separate normal reference ranges for adults and immature animals resulting in a somewhat higher than expected upper limit of normal for serum phosphorus concentration.

Urine Protein

1. The presence of protein in the urine may indicate a disease process anywhere in the urinary tract, or may be a consequence of genital contamination. When the urinary sediment is inactive, the presence of protein in the urine is suggestive of renal disease.

2. Dipstick screening measures mostly albumin and often produces positive results in highly concentrated urine. Trace to +1 proteinuria (i.e., 10 to 30 mg/dl) may be normal in highly concentrated urine. With dipstick screening, a protein concentration of 20 to 30 mg/dL is required for a positive reaction. Dipstick screening for proteinuria may be negative despite the presence of pathologic amounts of protein if the urine is dilute.

> **!** Dipstick screening of urine for protein often produces positive results in highly concentrated urine.

3. If persistent proteinuria is present on dipstick analysis in the absence of hematuria and pyuria, the severity of proteinuria may be assessed by measuring 24-hour urine protein excretion or performing a urine protein-to-urine creatinine ratio (U_{Pr}/U_{Cr}).
4. Urine protein excretion (normal values for 24-hour urine protein excretion and U_{Pr}/U_{Cr} ratio are presented in Table 2-2).
   a. Normal values for 24-hour urine protein excretion in dogs and cats are < 20 to 30 mg/kg/day.
   b. Dogs with primary glomerular disease (e.g., glomerulonephritis, glomerular amyloidosis) often have markedly increased 24-hour urine protein excretion and those with amyloidosis generally have the highest 24-hour urine protein excretion.
   c. 24-hour protein excretion is not often performed due to the requirement for a timed collection of urine.
5. Urine protein/urine creatinine ratio (U_{Pr}/U_{Cr}).
   a. Determination of U_{Pr}/U_{Cr} eliminates the necessity of a 24-hour urine collection and is highly correlated with 24-hour urine protein excretion.
   b. Normal U_{Pr}/U_{Cr} ratios in dogs and cats are < 0.4.
   c. U_{Pr}/U_{Cr} ratios often are normal in animals with high USG and positive dipstick protein reaction. Urine protein and creatinine concentrations are increased to the same extent in highly concentrated urine, and the U_{Pr}/U_{Cr} is unaffected because it is a ratio of the 2 concentrations.
   d. In dogs, U_{Pr}/U_{Cr} results are not affected by differences in sex, method of urine collection, fasted versus fed state, or by time of day of collection.
   e. Pyuria and marked blood contamination of urine samples can result in abnormal U_{Pr}/U_{Cr} ratios in the absence of glomerular disease. Thus, both the urine protein concentration and U_{Pr}/U_{Cr} ratio must be evaluated in conjunction with urinary sediment findings.
      (1) Visibly pink or red urine should not be evaluated by U_{Pr}/U_{Cr} ratio.
      (2) If there are more than 3 white blood cells per high-power field (WBCs/hpf) in concentrated urine, do not evaluate the U_{Pr}/U_{Cr} ratio unless urine culture results are known to be negative, because even a small increase in WBC in the urine sediment can increase the U_{Pr}/U_{Cr} ratio.
   f. Induction of renal failure in experimental studies in cats increased mean U_{Pr}/U_{Cr} ratio from 0.13 to 0.36, and in both groups of cats U_{Pr}/U_{Cr} ratios were higher on 52% as compared with 28% protein diets. Administration of prednisone to normal dogs increased U_{Pr}/U_{Cr} ratios from normal to a mean of 1.2 at 30 days and 0.9 at 42 days.
   g. Dogs with proteinuria on screening urinalysis have increased U_{Pr}/U_{Cr} values. There is overlap between dogs with glomerulonephritis and those with amyloidosis, and renal biopsy remains the only reliable way to differentiate these two diseases.

Microalbuminuria
1. Microalbuminuria may be an early indicator of glomerular damage and loss of normal glomerular barrier function.
2. Microalbuminuria in dogs and cats is defined as a urine albumin concentration of > 1 mg/dL but < 30 mg/dL.

> **!** Microalbuminuria may be an early indicator of glomerular damage.

   a. Methods used in dogs and cats to detect microalbuminuria are based on species-specific enzyme-linked immunosorbent assays (ELISA)[a], and methods used to detect microalbuminuria in humans are not reliable for use in dogs and cats.
   b. Urine is diluted to USG 1.010. Dilution prevents false-positive reactions for protein due to highly concentrated urine.
   c. Urine that is negative for proteinuria on dipstick reaction may be positive for microalbuminuria when evaluated by ELISA.
   d. Results using in-house test kits are reported as negative, mildly positive, moderately positive, or highly positive. Positive results on the in-house test kit should be quantified in mg/dL.
   e. Positive reactions for microalbuminuria should be repeated in 2 weeks to determine if microalbuminuria is persistent.
3. Microalbuminuria has been detected in heartworm-infected dogs and in dogs with familial renal disease (e.g., soft-coated Wheaten terriers with glomerular disease, male dogs with X-linked hereditary nephritis). In these specific disorders, microalbuminuria precedes detection of an increased U_{Pr}/U_{Cr} ratio.
4. The presence of microalbuminuria or increased U_{Pr}/U_{Cr} ratio in the absence of lower urinary tract inflammation provides evidence for glomerular damage but does indicate that progressive renal damage or chronic renal failure will occur.
5. In one study, the prevalence of microalbuminuria in normal healthy dogs was approximately 19%, and prevalence in a hospital population of dogs was 36%. Microalbuminuria was not induced by exercise (i.e., treadmill running) in normal dogs. Microalbuminuria may be associated with increasing age and presence of systemic disease in dogs.
6. It is not known whether seemingly normal dogs with microalbuminuria are at increased risk for development of progressive renal disease. Sequential monitoring of these animals is warranted.
7. Presumably, microalbuminuria precedes the development of overt proteinuria and monitoring is warranted in at-risk individuals (e.g., diabetics, hypertensives).
8. An animal with microalbuminuria should be monitored to determine if the finding is repeatable and whether or not it is progressive. Progressive glomerular injury should be suspected if the magnitude of microalbuminuria increases over time. Other tests of renal function should be considered to determine if increasing microalbuminuria is associated with loss of excretory renal function.

Bladder Tumor Antigen (BTA) Test
1. The first-generation Bard BTA test (V-BTA Test, Bion Diagnostic Sciences, Inc., Redmond, Wash., distributed by Polymedco Inc., Courtland Manor, N.Y.) detects a glycoprotein antigen complex associated with bladder neoplasia in human patients. In a prospective study of 65 dogs with transitional cell carcinoma and other urinary tract disorders, the Bard BTA test had a sensitivity of 90% and specificity of 78%.[b]
2. False positives occur in urine samples with marked proteinuria or glucosuria and in those with pyuria or hematuria.
3. Its most appropriate use is as a routine screening test in geriatric dogs at risk for development of transitional cell carcinoma.
4. Second-generation (BTA Stat) and third-generation (Bard Trak) Bard BTA tests should not be used as these use human monoclonal antibodies that give false-negative results in dogs.

---

a. ERD-Screen Urine Test, Heska Corp., Fort Collins Colo.
b. V-BTA Test, Bion Diagnostic Sciences, Inc, Redmond Wash. (distributed by Polymedco, Inc, Cortlandt Manor, N.Y.).

Tubular Function

1. Normal urinary concentrating ability is dependent upon ability of hypothalamic osmo-receptors to respond to changes in plasma osmolality, release of antidiuretic hormone (ADH) from the neurohypophysis, and response of the distal nephron to ADH. Additionally, medullary hypertonicity must be generated and maintained by the countercurrent multiplier and exchanger systems of the kidney, and an adequate number of functional nephrons must be present to generate the appropriate response to ADH (Figure 2-2).

Urine Specific Gravity (USG) and Osmolality (U_{Osm})

   a. Total urine solute concentration.

      (1) Measured either by USG (estimated by refractometry) or urine U_{Osm}. The latter depends only on the number of osmotically active particles, regardless of their size.

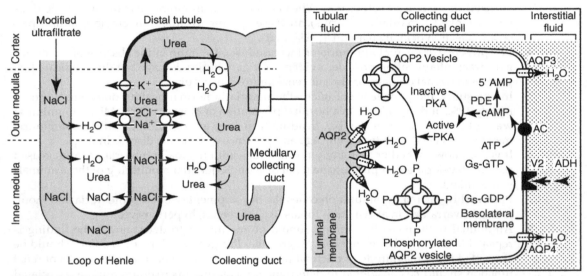

FIGURE 2-2 ■ Factors involved in the elaboration of concentrated or dilute urine. The major factors needed to elaborate maximally concentrated urine are shown in this illustration. A critical minimal number of healthy nephrons is needed to make concentrated urine if the body is capable of making and releasing ADH in adequate quantity. The major stimulus for the release of ADH is an increase in plasma osmolality perfusing the hypothalamus—most animals have evolved to produce concentrated urine for much of the day. The ability to concentrate or dilute the urine centers on the ability of the medullary thick ascending limb of the loop of Henle's ability to actively reabsorb sodium and chloride without water. The ascending limb of the loop of Henle is impermeable to water so that osmolality of tubular fluid progressively decreases during ascent of the loop. At the same time, the osmolality of the interstitium increases. ADH increases the permeability of the cortical collecting duct to water but not urea, so the concentration of urea progressively increases as it descends the collecting duct. ADH increases the medullary collecting duct's permeability to urea, which diffuses into the medullary interstitium, contributing importantly to the hyperosmolality of this region. The presence of a hypertonic interstitium is an overarching requirement to allow water to move out of the descending loop of Henle and out of the collecting duct under the influence of ADH. ADH binds to a specific receptor on the basal side of the collecting duct from the blood, which then activates cyclic adenosine monophosphate (cAMP) and a series of intracellular events that lead to phosphorylation of aquaporins that then migrate to the luminal membrane of the collecting duct, where they are inserted and act as channels to facilitate water transport across these cells. *AC*, adenyl cyclase; *AQP*, aquaporin; *G_s*, stimulatory guanine nucleotide regulatory protein; *GDP*, guanosine diphosphate; *GTP*, guanosine triphosphate; *PDE*, phosphodiesterarse; *PKA*, protein kinase A; *V_2*, vasopressin receptor. (Drawn by Tim Vojt.)

(2) USG is defined as the weight of a solution compared with an equal volume of distilled water and is dependent on both the number and molecular weight of the solute particles. It has the advantage of requiring only simple, inexpensive equipment (refractometer) for measurement.

b. Normally, a roughly linear relationship exists between urine osmolality and specific gravity. If urine contains appreciable amounts of larger molecular weight solutes such as glucose, mannitol, or radiographic contrast agents, these substances will have a proportionally greater effect on USG than on U_{Osm}.

c. Isosthenuria (USG 1.007-1.015, U_{Osm} 300 mOsm/kg) refers to urine of the same total solute concentration as unaltered glomerular filtrate.

! In dogs, urine obtained in the morning has a higher specific gravity than urine obtained in the evening.

d. Hyposthenuria refers to urine of lower total solute concentration than glomerular filtrate (USG <1.007, U_{Osm} <300 mOsm/kg).

e. Hypersthenuria (baruria) refers to urine of higher total solute concentration than glomerular filtrate (USG >1.015, U_{Osm} >300 mOsm/kg).

f. The normal range of total urine solute concentration for dogs and cats is wide (USG 1.001-1.080).

g. Urine samples obtained from dogs in the morning have higher USG values than those obtained in the evening. In dogs, urine concentration decreases with age, but there is no effect of sex on USG.

Water Deprivation Test

a. Indicated in evaluation of animals with polydipsia and polyuria or unknown cause.

b. Most often performed in animals with hyposthenuria (USG <1.007) suspected to have central or nephrogenic diabetes insipidus or psychogenic polydipsia. The water deprivation test also may be useful in evaluation of patients suspected to have partial central diabetes insipidus (USG 1.008-1.017).

c. Water deprivation testing should not be performed on a dehydrated animal that has dilute urine, as these animals have already reached the endpoint of this test and additional water deprivation could be harmful. Failure to concentrate urine likely is due to structural or functional renal dysfunction or administration of drugs that interfere with urinary concentrating ability (e.g., glucocorticoids, diuretics). Water deprivation testing should be performed with extreme caution in animals with severe polyuria, because such patients may rapidly become dehydrated during water deprivation if they have defective urinary concentrating ability and continue to produce large volumes of urine.

d. The water deprivation test also is contraindicated in animals that are azotemic, because the reason for their submaximally concentrated urine already is known. Water deprivation in these instances could result in additional injury to the kidneys.

! Do not perform water deprivation testing if the animal is already dehydrated or azotemic.

e. Water deprivation testing potentially is dangerous in patients with hypercalcemia and should be avoided.

f. Water deprivation testing also is not necessary in patients with underlying disorders (e.g., liver disease, pyometra, *Escherichia coli* pyelonephritis, severe hypokalemia) known to be associated with impaired urinary concentrating ability.

g. Technique.

(1) Placement of an indwelling catheter provides the best opportunity for accurate collection of urine samples and measurement of USG or U_{Osm} and minimizes the opportunity for newly produced concentrated urine to mix with previously produced dilute urine.

(2) Empty the bladder at the beginning of the test, and collect baseline data (i.e., body weight, hematocrit, plasma protein concentration, skin turgor, serum osmolality, U_{Osm}, USG).

(3) Withhold water and monitor these variables every 2 to 4 hours.

    (a) Urine and serum osmolalities are the best tests to follow, but osmolality results often are not immediately available. Thus, USG and body weight assume the greatest importance for decision making during performance of the test.

    (b) An increase in total plasma protein concentration is a relatively reliable indicator of progressive dehydration, but increases in hematocrit and changes in skin turgor are not as reliable.

    (c) Serum creatinine and BUN concentrations should not increase during a properly conducted water deprivation test.

(4) The test is concluded when the patient either demonstrates adequate concentrating ability or becomes dehydrated as evidenced by loss of 5% or more of its original body weight. It is important when weighing the animal to use the same scale each time and to empty the bladder at each evaluation. Maximal stimulation of ADH release will be present after loss of 5% of body weight.

h. Dehydration usually becomes evident within 48 hours in normal dogs and cats, but the time required may vary. Dogs with diabetes insipidus and psychogenic polydipsia usually become dehydrated within 12 hours.

i. By the time dehydration is evident, USG usually exceeds 1.045 in normal dogs and cats.

j. Failure to achieve maximal urinary solute concentration does not localize the level of the malfunction, and a structural or functional defect may be present anywhere along the hypothalamic-pituitary-renal axis.

k. Animals with medullary solute washout may have impaired concentrating ability regardless of the underlying cause of polyuria and polydipsia.

l. ADH challenge.

(1) If there has been a <5% increase in urine osmolality, or <10% change in USG for 3 consecutive determinations, or if the animal has lost 5% or more of its original weight, 0.1 to 0.2 U/lb aqueous vasopressin (Pitressin) (up to a total dose of 5 U) or 5 µg desmopressin (DDAVP) may be given subcutaneously and urinary concentrating ability monitored every 30 minutes for 2 to 6 hours after ADH injection.

(2) Additional increases in U_{Osm} after administration of ADH should not exceed 5% to 10% in normal dogs and cats.

(3) A large increase in U_{Osm} after ADH suggests partial or complete central diabetes insipidus (CDI).

Gradual Water Deprivation

a. Gradual water deprivation can be performed to eliminate diagnostic confusion caused by medullary solute washout.

b. Methods.

(1) Restrict water consumption to 60 mL/lb/day 72 hours before, 45 mL/lb/day 48 hours before, and 30 mL/lb/day 24 hours before the scheduled water deprivation test. In dogs with psychogenic polydipsia, this will promote endogenous release of ADH, increased permeability of the inner medullary collecting ducts to urea, and restoration of the normal gradient of medullary hypertonicity.

■ TABLE 2-4
■ ■ Normal Values for Fractional Electrolyte Clearance (%)

Analyte	Dog	Cat
Sodium	<1	<1
Potassium	<20	<24
Chloride	<1	<1.3
Phosphorus	<39	<73

(2) Reduce water consumption by approximately 10% per day over a 3- to 5-day period (but not <30 mL/lb/day). This approach should only be used in animals that are otherwise healthy on initial clinical evaluation (no evidence of renal disease or dehydration). Dry food should be provided *ad libitum*, and the dog should be weighed daily to monitor for loss of body weight.

(3) A standard complete water deprivation test is carried out after completion of gradual water restriction to restore the medullary gradient.

Fractional Clearance of Electrolytes

a. The fractional clearance of electrolytes is defined as the ratio of the clearance of the electrolyte in question to that of creatinine:

$$FC_x = (U_x V / P_x) / (U_{Cr} V / P_{Cr}) = (U_x P_{Cr}) / (U_{Cr} P_x)$$

This ratio usually is multiplied by 100 and the fractional clearance value expressed as a percentage. Normal values for urinary fractional clearance of electrolytes in dogs and cats are summarized in Table 2-4.

b. The advantage of this measurement is that a timed urine collection is not necessary. In normal animals, the fractional clearances of all electrolytes are much <1.0 (100%), implying net conservation, but values are higher for potassium and phosphorus than for sodium and chloride.

c. The fractional clearance of sodium may be useful in the differentiation of prerenal and primary renal azotemia.

(1) In animals with prerenal azotemia and volume depletion, sodium conservation should be avid and the fractional clearance of sodium very low (<1%).

(2) In animals with azotemia due to primary parenchymal renal disease, the fractional clearance of sodium will be higher than normal (≥1%).

d. Fractional clearance of potassium may be useful in the evaluation of hypokalemic patients to determine if the kidneys are contributing to the hypokalemia.

e. Fractional clearance of phosphorus may be useful during treatment of chronic renal failure (CRF) to see if dietary management and treatment with phosphorus binders have been effective in decreasing the fractional clearance of phosphorus as serum parathyroid hormone (PTH) concentration decreases (see Chapter 5 for additional information about chronic renal failure).

MICROBIOLOGY

A. Clinical signs and urinalysis findings provide supportive evidence, but quantitative microbiology is required to conclusively diagnose urinary tract infection (UTI).

1. The kidneys, ureters, bladder, and proximal urethra of normal dogs and cats are sterile, whereas a resident bacterial flora populates the distal urethra, prepuce, and vagina.

2. UTI occurs when bacteria colonize areas of the urinary tract that normally are sterile.
3. Quantitative bacterial culture of urine allows determination of the number of bacterial colonies (colony-forming units or cfu) that grow from one mL of urine (cfu/mL).
4. Aerobic gram-negative bacteria account for the majority of UTI in dogs and cats, and the remainder are caused by gram-positive organisms. *E. coli* is the most common organism implicated in UTI of dogs and cats. Other organisms isolated include *Proteus* spp, coagulase-positive staphylococci, and streptococci. *Pasteurella multocida* occasionally is isolated from cats with UTI. *Enterobacter* spp, *Klebsiella* spp, and *Pseudomonas aeruginosa* are observed less commonly in dogs and rarely in cats. See Chapter 8 for additional information about UTI.

Method of Urine Collection

1. Voided urine has the greatest potential for bacterial contamination.
   a. Bacterial culture of midstream-voided urine samples from normal dogs and cats often results in growth of $<10^3$ to $\geq 10^5$ cfu/mL. Therefore, culture of voided urine is not recommended in evaluation of patients for UTI.
   b. If, however, no growth is obtained from a voided urine sample, UTI can be excluded as a diagnosis.
2. Catheterization may inoculate the bladder with bacteria from the distal urethra.
   a. Bacterial growth of $\geq 10^5$ cfu/mL may result from culture of urine obtained from catheterization in 20% of normal female dogs. Thus, using 10^5 cfu/mL as indication of UTI in female dogs will result in a substantial number of false-positive results.
   b. Also, the procedure of urethral catheterization itself may result in UTI in 20% of normal female dogs.

> **!** **Urine collected by cystocentesis should be sterile.**

   c. Isolation of bacteria from urine collected by catheterization of male dogs is uncommon, and more than 10^3 cfu/mL is recommended for establishing a diagnosis of UTI in urine samples collected by catheterization from male dogs.
   d. In both male and female cats, growth of more than 10^3 cfu/mL in samples collected by catheterization is considered compatible with UTI.
3. Urine collected by cystocentesis should be sterile in normal animals.
   a. Cystocentesis is recommended for establishing a diagnosis of UTI.
   b. Urine samples obtained by cystocentesis from normal dogs and cats should yield no growth because this procedure bypasses the normal bacterial flora of the urethra and genital tract. Consequently, results obtained by cystocentesis are the standard against which results obtained using voided or catheterized samples are compared.
   c. Small numbers of organisms from the skin or environment occasionally contaminate samples obtained by cystocentesis, and growth of $<10^3$ cfu/mL may be considered suggestive of contamination.
4. Isolation of bacteria from urinary tissues obtained during surgery indicates UTI regardless of number.
5. Urine should be submitted for culture within 30 minutes of collection. If this is not possible, the sample may be refrigerated for up to 6 hours without significant loss of bacterial growth. Some loss of growth can occur after prolonged refrigeration or during transport to a laboratory.
6. Microscopic examination of Gram-stained smears of urine also may be helpful in diagnosis of UTI. In one study, one drop of uncentrifuged urine was allowed to dry, Gram-stained, and examined under oil immersion. The presence of ≥ 2 organisms per field correlated with bacterial counts of $\geq 10^3$ cfu/mL.

DIAGNOSTIC IMAGING

Radiography

1. Radiography provides quantitative information about renal size and shape that frequently cannot be obtained from physical examination. The animal should be properly prepared for abdominal radiography by fasting and enemas to cleanse the colon and maximize the amount of information obtained. Proper positioning is essential to ensure that the kidneys, ureters, bladder, and the entire urethra are visible on the image obtained.
2. To correct for variation in patient size and radiographic magnification, renal size is evaluated in reference to surrounding anatomic landmarks, usually the second lumbar vertebra (L2) on the ventrodorsal view.
3. The left kidney normally is well visualized in the dog, but the right kidney often cannot be seen as clearly, especially its cranial pole. In the dog, the left kidney (near vertebra L2 to L5) is located caudal to the right kidney (near vertebra T13 to L3). In the cat, the kidneys lie near vertebra L3 with the right kidney positioned slightly cranial to the left. Renal size in dogs and cats can be assessed radiographically and compared to the length of vertebra L2. On the ventrodorsal view, the kidney-to-L2 ratio is 2.5 to 3.5 in dogs and 2.4 to 3.0 in cats.
   a. Abnormal renal shape or contour suggests the possibility of renal infarct, cyst, neoplasia, or focal inflammatory change.
   b. Normal renal size does not ensure normal renal tissue.
   c. Marked changes are necessary for renal size to decrease below the lower limit or increase above the upper limit of normal radiographic renal size. Also, the kidneys may become wider in some renal diseases before they exceed the upper limit of normal length.
   d. Small kidney size typically is associated with chronic renal disease.
   e. Enlarged kidneys may indicate acute intrinsic renal failure, neoplasia, polycystic kidney disease, or hydronephrosis.
4. The ureters cannot be seen on plain abdominal radiographs, but radiopaque ureteral calculi may be seen. Radiopaque ureteral calculi are observed commonly in cats. See Chapter 9 for additional information on urolithiasis.
5. The bladder of the dog and cat usually is visible within the abdominal cavity if it is sufficiently full. When more than 50% of the area of a sufficiently full bladder is located within the pelvic canal on the lateral abdominal radiograph, it is referred to as a "pelvic bladder" and this finding may have some clinical relevance in female dogs with urinary incontinence. See Chapter 13 for additional information on urinary incontinence.
6. The urethra often can be seen extending caudally from the bladder neck when gravity pulls a full bladder cranially into the abdomen. This finding is especially prominent in cats.
7. Radiopaque calculi may be identified in the pelvic, perineal, or penile portions of the male urethra. See Chapter 9 for additional information on urolithiasis.
8. The prostate gland may be identified on the lateral abdominal radiograph in intact male dogs.

Excretory Urography

1. Excretory urography is performed by taking sequential abdominal radiographs after intravenous administration of an iodinated organic compound. The contrast medium is filtered and excreted by the kidneys, and the quality of the study is partially dependent upon the patient's GFR.
2. Radiographs should be taken at appropriate intervals (e.g. <1 min, 5 min, 20 min, 40 min) to obtain maximal information about the renal parenchyma and collecting system.
3. Excretory urography is useful in evaluation of abnormalities in renal size, shape, or location; filling defects (e.g., calculi) in the renal pelvis or ureters; certain congenital defects (e.g., unilateral agenesis); renomegaly; acute pyelonephritis; and, rupture of the upper urinary tract.

4. Excretory urography is useful for evaluation of patients suspected to have ectopic ureters. More valuable information is obtained when a pneumocystogram also is performed to provide negative contrast for the ureter as it traverses the bladder. Oblique views facilitate identification of the site of ureter termination.

5. Excretory urography should not be performed in dehydrated patients or in those with known hypersensitivity to contrast media.

6. Decreased GFR may persist for several days after intravenous administration of contrast agents to normal dogs, and acute renal failure (ARF) has been observed rarely in dogs and cats after excretory urography.

7. Ultrasound-guided percutaneous antegrade pyelography can be used to localize ureteral obstruction in dogs and cats and does not depend on GFR for delivery of contrast to the collecting system.

Contrast Urography of the Lower Urinary Tract
Positive Contrast Urethrography
TECHNIQUE

(1) Performed with the bladder full so that the urethra can fill and distend with contrast material.

(2) Typically performed in a retrograde fashion (i.e., from the distal to the proximal portion of the urethra) using iodinated contrast material.

   (a) In males, a balloon-tipped catheter can be placed in the distal urethra (near the os penis) to prevent leakage of contrast material distally.

   (b) In females, the catheter can be placed in the bladder and then withdrawn incrementally into the urethra with injection of contrast material.

(3) Ideally, performed under fluoroscopy to obtain a dynamic study.

(4) Sedation is recommended in males, and sedation with or without anesthesia is necessary in females for good results.

ABNORMALITIES

(1) Intraluminal filling defects (e.g., air bubbles, calculi, blood clots).

(2) Intramural lesions (e.g., neoplasia, inflammation, stricture).

(3) Extramural lesions (e.g., neoplasia, prostatic enlargement).

(4) Ruptured urethra.

(5) Reflux of contrast material into an abnormal prostate gland.

(6) Fistulas (e.g., urethrovaginal, urethrorectal).

Positive Contrast Cystography
TECHNIQUE

(1) Typically performed by passage of a urinary catheter and instillation of iodinated contrast material.

(2) Positive contrast cystography is the procedure of choice when bladder rupture is suspected.

(3) Obtaining oblique views in addition to routine lateral and ventrodorsal views may enhance ability to detect some abnormalities (e.g., ectopic ureters).

ABNORMALITIES

(1) Ruptured bladder.

(2) Intraluminal filling defects (e.g., air bubbles, large calculi, blood clots). Small calculi may be concealed by contrast material.

(3) Intramural lesions (e.g., neoplasia, polypoid cystitis).

(4) Abnormal bladder position (e.g., "pelvic bladder," perineal hernia).

(5) Urachal diverticulum.

(6) Permeation of contrast material into bladder wall with altered permeability (e.g., feline interstitial cystitis).

Double Contrast Cystography

TECHNIQUE

(1) Generally preferred over positive and negative contrast studies due to improved ability to identify and interpret abnormalities, especially mucosal irregularities caused by chronic inflammation or small intramural masses. It allows assessment of bladder wall thickness.

(2) A urinary catheter is passed and a small amount of iodinated contrast material introduced into the bladder followed by gas (e.g., room air) distension of the bladder.

ABNORMALITIES

(1) Mucosal irregularities and intramural lesions (e.g., polypoid cystitis, neoplasia, chronic cystitis).

(2) Intraluminal filling defects (e.g., air bubbles, calculi).

(3) Urachal diverticulum.

Negative Contrast Cystography

TECHNIQUE

(1) Of limited usefulness as a solitary technique.

(2) Provides good assessment of bladder position and wall thickness.

(3) A urinary catheter is passed and the bladder distended with air, CO_2, or nitrous oxide. This technique carries the risk of air embolism. CO_2 and nitrous oxide are preferred because of increased solubility in blood.

ABNORMALITIES

(1) Useful during excretory urography to facilitate identification of ectopic ureters.

(2) Allows assessment of bladder wall thickness (e.g. chronic cystitis).

(3) Not a valuable technique to identify ruptured bladder (positive contrast studies are preferred).

Ultrasonography

Kidneys

ADVANTAGES

(1) Noninvasive imaging technique that does not depend on renal function.

(2) No known adverse effects on the patient.

(3) Allows characterization of internal renal architecture.

ECHOGENICITY

(1) Normally, the kidney is less echogenic than the liver or spleen.

(2) The renal capsule, diverticula, and sinus are the most echogenic structures in the kidney.

(3) The renal medulla normally is less echogenic than the cortex.

(4) There normally is a good corticomedullary distinction.

(5) The hyperechogenicity of renal cortex relative to medulla varies among normal cats and has been attributed to variations in the amount of fat present in proximal tubular cells.

RENAL SIZE

(1) Renal length and volume as determined by ultrasonography are linearly related to body weight in dogs. Guidelines for renal length measurement on ultrasound examination for dogs weighing between 5 and 44 kg are presented in Table 2-5.

(2) In cats, renal length as determined by ultrasonography is normally reported to be between 3.0 and 4.3 cm. However, at The Ohio State University, normal cats typically have a renal length of 3.5 to 4.2 cm.

■ TABLE 2-5
■ ■ **Renal Length on Ultrasound Examination According to Body Weight in Adult Dogs**

Weight (kg)	Number of Dogs	Range of Length (cm)	Mean Length (cm)	Standard Deviation (cm)
5-9	16	3.2-5.2	4.4	0.50
10-14	10	4.8-6.4	5.6	0.60
15-19	20	5.0-6.7	6.0	0.40
20-24	20	5.2-8.0	6.5	0.72
25-29	44	5.3-7.8	6.9	0.58
30-34	32	6.1-8.7	7.2	0.60
35-39	24	6.6-9.3	7.6	0.72
40-44	12	6.3-8.4	7.6	0.54

Adapted from Barr FJ, Holt PE, and Gibbs C: Ultrasonographic measurement of normal renal parameters. *J Small Anim Pract* 1990;31:180-184. Data limited to groups with ≥10 dogs.

    (3) Measurements of renal size determined by excretory urography exceed those obtained by ultrasonography.

UTILITY

    (1) Useful for differentiating solid from fluid-filled lesions (e.g., abscess, cysts) and for determining the distribution of lesions within the kidney (i.e., focal, multifocal, diffuse).

    (2) A pattern of multiple anechoic cavitations is highly suggestive of polycystic kidney disease. Cysts are smooth, sharply demarcated, anechoic lesions that demonstrate through transmission.

    (3) The renal pelvis is dilated with anechoic fluid in hydronephrosis, and the kidney is surrounded by an accumulation of anechoic fluid in cats with perinephric pseudocysts.

    (4) Organized hematomas, abscesses, and necrotic nodules result in a pattern of mixed echogenicity.

    (5) Focal or diffuse lesions of mixed echogenicity that disrupt normal anatomy often are tumors.

    (6) Poorly vascular tumors of homogenous cell type (e.g. lymphosarcoma) may produce hypoechoic lesions that occasionally may be misinterpreted as cysts.

    (7) Diffuse parenchymal renal diseases characterized by cellular infiltration with preservation of normal renal architecture (e.g., chronic tubulointerstitial nephritis) may produce diffuse hyperechogenicity, but occasionally are characterized by a normal ultrasonographic appearance.

    (8) Normal renal ultrasonography does not eliminate the possibility of renal disease or renal failure.

    (9) Fine needle aspiration of focal or diffuse lesions may confirm the diagnosis of lymphosarcoma, renal cyst, renal carcinoma, or renal abscess.

ETHYLENE GLYCOL INTOXICATION

    (1) Within 4 hours of EG ingestion, renal cortical echogenicity can exceed that of liver and approach that of spleen. Medullary echogenicity is increased to a lesser extent.

    (2) Increased cortical and medullary echogenicity with relative hypoechogenicity of the corticomedullary junction and inner medulla results in a "halo" sign that correlates with the onset of anuria. Although unproven, renal hyperechogenicity in EG

intoxication is attributed to deposition of calcium oxalate crystals in the kidneys. The presence of extremely bright echoes from the renal cortex in a kidney that is normal in size is highly suggestive of EG poisoning.

MEDULLARY RIM SIGN

(1) An echogenic line in the outer zone of the medulla and paralleling the corticomedullary junction has been observed in EG intoxication but also in acute tubular necrosis, hypercalcemic nephropathy, granulomatous nephritis due to feline infectious peritonitis, and in chronic tubulointerstitial nephritis.

(2) This lesion also has been observed in normal cats and has been associated with mineralization of tubular basement membranes. Dogs with medullary rim sign as their sole ultrasonographic finding may have no evidence of renal dysfunction. Dogs with medullary rim sign and other ultrasonographic abnormalities (e.g., reduced renal size, increased medullary echogenicity, pyelectasia) often have clinical evidence of renal dysfunction.

INTRARENAL RESISTANCE TO BLOOD FLOW

(1) Intrarenal resistance to blood flow may be assessed and evaluated by calculation of the resistive index.

(a) Values for renal resistive index in normal, nonsedated dogs are approximately 0.6.

(b) Somewhat lower values have been reported in normal, sedated dogs and cats.

(c) Higher-than-normal values for resistive index have been reported in some renal diseases of dogs and cats, but not in experimentally induced aminoglycoside nephrotoxicosis.

COLOR FLOW DOPPLER ULTRASONOGRAPHY

(1) Color flow Doppler ultrasonography can be used to determine the patency of renal arteries, evaluate focal areas of decreased blood flow (e.g., infarcts), and evaluate areas of increased blood flow (e.g., some tumors).

RENAL ULTRASONOGRAPHY

(1) Renal ultrasonography also has been used to monitor the status of renal allografts after transplantation in dogs and cats.

Ureters

a. The normal ureter is not usually identified on ultrasound examination.

b. The ureteral orifice in the trigone region of the bladder normally has a mound-like appearance that can be confused with a mass, especially when the bladder is not fully distended. Intermittent jets of urine being expelled from the ureter into the bladder can be identified using color flow Doppler technique.

c. Dilatation of the ureter proximal to an obstructing calculus may be seen, but it is difficult to image the calculus itself due to the small size of ureteral calculi.

d. Hydroureter can be identified in patients with distal obstruction and in some animals with ectopic ureter.

e. A ureterocele in the bladder rarely may be seen in some patients with ectopic ureters.

Bladder

a. Easily identified when moderately full due to the presence of anechoic urine.

b. Bladder wall thickness may be overestimated when the bladder contains only a small amount of urine.

c. Bladder wall thickness should not exceed 3 mm when the bladder is moderately full. Causes of increased bladder wall thickness include cystitis and neoplasia.

d. Intramural lesions (e.g., neoplasia, polyps) may be identified. Generally, polyps are attached to the bladder wall by a stalk, whereas transitional cell carcinomas have a broader attachment.

e. Intraluminal lesions include cystic calculi (>2-4 mm diameter) and blood clots. Calculi may produce shadowing whereas blood clots do not.

f. A urachal diverticulum is not likely to be identified by ultrasound examination unless it is very large.

g. Echogenic debris may be identified. It may indicate inflammatory material or suspended crystals. In many cases, its clinical relevance is uncertain. Many normal cats have echogenic debris in their bladders that has no clinical explanation.

Urethra

a. The proximal urethra can be visualized by ultrasound examination but the caudal urethra usually cannot be evaluated because of presence of the bony pelvis.

b. Dilatation of the proximal urethra may be identified in patients with distal urethral obstruction.

c. Intramural (e.g., neoplasia, proliferative urethritis) or intraluminal (e.g., calculi, blood clots) lesions may be identified.

Prostate Gland

a. Readily identified on ultrasound examination in intact male dogs and occasionally identified in neutered male dogs. Not identified in intact male cats with the rare exception of prostatic neoplasia in a cat.

b. Size, shape, and echotexture are evaluated. The prostate gland normally is a symmetrical organ with smooth shape and homogenous echogenic pattern.

c. Lesions that may be identified include cyst, abscess, and mineralization.

d. Complex echogenic patterns can be observed in a variety of prostatic diseases (e.g., chronic prostatitis, neoplasia).

CYSTOSCOPY

A. Uroendoscopy is a useful tool for the diagnosis of many lower urinary tract disorders (e.g., ectopic ureter, proliferative urethritis, polypoid cystitis, transitional cell carcinoma). It also is employed in treatment of urethral sphincter mechanism incompetence to allow submucosal injection of collagen in the urethra. See Chapter 13 for additional information on the use of uroendoscopy in patients with urinary incontinence.

Utility

1. Uroendoscopy provides a magnified view of the mucosal surfaces of the vestibule, vagina, urethra, ureteral openings, and bladder.

2. It remains the gold standard for the diagnosis of ectopic ureter, and for accurately determining the termination of ectopic ureters.

3. Uroendoscopy is useful in the definitive evaluation of the lower urinary tract for anatomic abnormalities including stricture, neoplasia, polypoid cystitis, urachal diverticulum, and inflammatory lesions such as proliferative urethritis.

4. Uroendoscopy is very sensitive for the identification of transitional cell carcinoma and can identify the tumor when other techniques such as double contrast cystography and ultrasonography are inconclusive. Biopsy also can be performed to obtain a histologic diagnosis.

5. Uroendoscopy is an important tool in the evaluation of patients with recurrent bacterial UTI in order to exclude the presence of anatomic abnormalities.

6. Uroendoscopy allows visualization of glomerulations (i.e., petechial mucosal bladder hemorrhages) in cats with interstitial cystitis either at low pressure or after a provocative increase in bladder pressure.

Technique

1. Rigid transurethral uroendoscopy is possible in nearly all female dogs and cats weighing more than 3 kg using a rigid cystoscope. It can also be used in males that have had a perineal urethrostomy.
   a. Minimally invasive, requires the least equipment, and readily allows examination of the urinary tract.
   b. General anesthesia is preferred to give adequate muscular relaxation.
   c. Right lateral recumbency is most comfortable for right-handed examiners.
   d. Scrub the perineal region, and wear sterile gloves. Minimize any contamination of the urinary tract.
   e. The scope is advanced by infusing the vaginal vestibule with 0.9% saline. Urine in the bladder is drained and the bladder then distended with sterile 0.9% saline which improves the optical quality of the images.
   f. Antibiotics are administered for 5 days after the procedure to prevent development of UTI.
2. Flexible transurethral uroendoscopy is used in male dogs and cats. It can also be used in larger female dogs.
   a. General anesthesia is preferred.
   b. Flexible scopes are fragile and require careful handling and storage to avoid breakage.
   c. Patient preparation is similar to that for rigid transurethral uroendoscopy. Complete examination of the bladder is difficult due to the small size of the cystoscope.
   d. Antibiotics are administered for 5 days after the procedure to prevent development of UTI.

RENAL BIOPSY

Utility

1. Renal biopsy allows the clinician to establish a histologic diagnosis and should be considered when the information obtained is likely to alter patient management or prognosis. Examples of such situations include differentiation of protein-losing glomerular diseases, differentiation of ARF from CRF, determination of the status of tubular basement membranes in ARF, and establishing the response of the patient to therapy or the progression of previously documented renal disease.
2. A renal biopsy should not be performed until thorough clinical evaluation of the patient has been completed.

Techniques

1. Techniques include blind percutaneous, laparoscopic, open, and ultrasound-guided approaches.
   a. The blind percutaneous technique works well in cats because their kidneys can be readily palpated and immobilized.
   b. Laparoscopy allows direct visualization of the kidney and detection of hemorrhage but requires special equipment and expertise.
   c. If a larger sample is required, or the operator is inexperienced, wedge biopsy via laparotomy is recommended. Advantages of this procedure include the ability to visually inspect the kidneys and other abdominal organs, to choose the specific biopsy site, to take an adequately sized sample, and to observe the kidney for hemorrhage.
   d. Ultrasound-guided needle biopsies can be obtained under sedation. At our hospital, renal biopsy in dogs and cats usually is performed under ultrasound guidance using the Bard7 biopsy instrument with the animal sedated using a combination of medetomidine, butorphanol, and atropine. Alternatively, an intravenous infusion of propofol (with endotracheal

       intubation) or gas anesthesia may be used. If tissue architecture is not considered essential for diagnosis (e.g., renal lymphosarcoma, feline infectious peritonitis), aspiration of the kidney using a 23- or 25-gauge needle may provide sufficient material for cytology.

  e. Before biopsy, an IV catheter should be placed, and clotting ability should be evaluated (buccal mucosal bleeding time and estimation of platelet numbers). Hematocrit and plasma proteins should be determined before biopsy but after adequate rehydration with parenteral fluids. Hematocrit and plasma proteins should be monitored after biopsy to detect hemorrhage.

  f. Biopsy instruments.

    (1) Franklin-modified Vim Silverman needle and the Tru-Cut biopsy needle[c] are most commonly used.

    (2) Avoid penetration of the kidney with the outer cannula prior to penetration of the cutting needle to prevent retrieval of an insufficient amount of renal cortex.

  g. Avoid the renal hilus and major vessels when directing the biopsy instrument. It is recommended to direct the biopsy needle along the long axis of the kidney, solely through cortical tissue (Figure 2-3). Due to the small size of feline kidneys, it is common to obtain relatively large amounts of medullary tissue and this has been associated with infarction and fibrosis. The goal is to obtain sufficient renal cortex so that at least 5 glomeruli are present in the biopsy sample. Ideally, 8 to 12 glomeruli will be available for histopathologic interpretation.

  h. After using the open approach or keyhole technique, the kidney should be digitally compressed for 5 minutes and, after release, the abdomen inspected for hemorrhage.

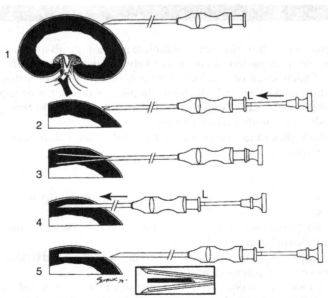

FIGURE 2-3 ■ Recommended technique for directing the renal biopsy needle. The ideal path for the needle is along the renal cortex where there is likely to be a higher density of glomeruli. Penetration of the needle into the medulla should be avoided because injury to vessels at the corticomedullary junction may occur and lead to renal infarction or serious hemorrhage. The needle should never be directed toward the renal hilus because damage to the renal pelvis with leakage of urine could occur or life-threatening hemorrhage could occur as a consequence of damage to the renal artery or vein.

---

c. Bard Biopty Biopsy System C.R. Bard Inc., Covington Ga.

i. Dislodge the biopsy sample from the biopsy instrument using a stream of sterile saline from a syringe or, alternatively, the biopsy instrument may be immersed directly in fixative.

j. For routine histopathology, the sample should be fixed in buffered 10% formalin for at least 3 to 4 hours.

k. For immunofluorescence studies helpful in the evaluation of immune-mediated glomerular injury (immune complexes), the sample can be preserved in Michel's transport medium. Immunopathology studies also may be performed by a peroxidase-antiperoxidase method using formalin-fixed samples without need for special preservation of the sample.

l. In special circumstances (e.g., early familial nephropathy, glomerulonephritis), samples processed in glutaraldehyde may be submitted for electron microscopy.

m. After renal biopsy, a brisk fluid diuresis should be initiated to prevent clot formation in the renal pelvis. Monitor hematocrit and plasma proteins over the next 12 to 24 hours to detect serious hemorrhage. Doppler blood flow at the biopsy site should be evaluated shortly after the biopsies, and then again at 1 and 3 hours to ensure that active bleeding from the site is not a problem. Patients that undergo early morning renal biopsy without complication often can be released to go home in the early evening.

Complications

Hemorrhage

a. The most common complication of renal biopsy is hemorrhage.

b. Subcapsular hemorrhage commonly occurs at the site of biopsy, and many patients experience microscopic hematuria during the first 48 hours after biopsy. Macroscopic hematuria is less common.

c. Severe hemorrhage into the peritoneal cavity is rare and usually associated with improper technique. Such hemorrhage must be treated aggressively by compression bandage of the abdomen, fresh whole blood transfusion, and exploratory surgery if necessary.

Linear Infarcts

a. Linear infarcts in the path of the biopsy needle are observed commonly after renal biopsy. These are small and superficial when the biopsy is limited to renal cortex. If, however, an arcuate artery is damaged by passage of the biopsy needle through the corticomedullary junction, a wedge-shaped infarct may occur.

b. This complication is more common in cats because of the small size of the kidneys in relation to the length of the biopsy needle.

Hydronephrosis

a. If the renal pelvis is penetrated by the biopsy needle, bleeding may occur and clot formation can lead to obstruction of the kidney and hydronephrosis.

b. This complication should be considered if the biopsy report indicates the presence of transitional epithelium at one end of the biopsy or if progressive renal enlargement is detected after renal biopsy.

c. The risk of this complication is minimized by limiting the biopsy site to the renal cortex and instituting a fluid diuresis afterward.

BLADDER AND URETHRAL BIOPSY

A. Urethral or bladder masses may be biopsied at the time of surgery, cystoscopy, or using catheter aspiration techniques (blind or with ultrasound guidance).

B. Samples obtained by cystoscopy may be very small when using smaller cystoscopes.

C. Tissue samples may be obtained by passing a urinary catheter to the site of the lesion, aspirating against the mass using a 6- or 12-mL syringe containing saline, and agitating the catheter gently while suction is applied. The sample then is expelled into 10% formalin for preservation and histopathologic evaluation. Tissue samples adequate for diagnosis often can be obtained using this technique, especially for the diagnosis of transitional cell carcinoma.

D. Ultrasound guidance can be used to direct the biopsy instrument to the lesion after it has been introduced into the bladder.

E. Bacterial culture of biopsy samples is indicated if chronic or recurrent UTI is suspected.

WHAT DO WE DO?

- Evaluate BUN and serum creatinine concentrations concurrently.
- Evaluate urine specific gravity in conjunction with BUN and serum creatinine concentrations before administering fluid therapy.
- Carefully differentiate prerenal, primary renal, and postrenal azotemia using all diagnostic information available.
- Use clearance methods to estimate GFR in nonazotemic patients with polyuria and polydipsia whenever the cause of these clinical signs is not apparent after evaluation of routine diagnostic test results.
- Use fractional clearance to resolve the pathophysiology of otherwise unexplained serum electrolyte abnormalities (e.g., unexplained hypokalemia).
- Use the urine protein-creatinine ratio and microalbuminuria test to investigate unexplained proteinuria taking into account the advantages and limitations of these tests.
- Interpret microbiology results taking into consideration the method of urine collection employed.
- Recognize that radiology and ultrasonography are not mutually exclusive imaging modalities and that each provides different but potentially valuable diagnostic information.
- Use uroendoscopy to diagnose and sometimes treat (e.g., collagen injections) lower urinary tract disorders.

THOUGHTS FOR THE FUTURE

- Practical tests to estimate GFR (e.g., iohexol clearance, cystatin C) will become more widely available to practitioners.
- Uroendoscopy and interventional radiology will become more widely employed in the diagnosis and treatment of urinary tract disease.
- Veterinarians will develop a better understanding of the prognostic value of the microalbuminuria test in the diagnosis and prognosis of animals with mild asymptomatic proteinuria.

COMMON MISCONCEPTIONS

- Patients with normal BUN or serum creatinine concentrations must have normal renal function. Certainly, this statement could be true, but more specifically normal BUN and serum creatinine concentrations mean only that 25% or more of its nephrons are functioning normally. It takes loss of function of 75% or more of the nephrons before BUN and serum creatinine concentration increase above the upper limit of their normal reference range.
- Determination of GFR to more precisely evaluate renal function is best left to secondary or tertiary referral centers and not primary care practices. With commercial availability of iohexol measurement, it is reasonable for practitioners to administer iohexol, collect 3 timed plasma samples after

injection, and submit plasma samples to a reference laboratory for determination of iohexol clearance as an estimate of GFR.

- Detection of proteinuria signifies serious renal disease. Although the protein in the urine may be originating from the kidneys and indicate cause for concern, it also may have originated from the lower urinary tract in response to inflammation or infection. Whenever evaluating proteinuria, the method of urine collection, urine specific gravity, and urine sediment changes must all be taken into consideration.

- Water deprivation test results are used in the evaluation of dogs and cats thought to have underlying chronic renal disease. Actually, a water deprivation test should not be performed in an animal suspected to have underlying renal disease because dehydration that arises may pose a risk to the remaining nephrons if renal ischemia occurs. The risk of renal damage from ischemia is greater in patients with diseased kidneys than in those with normal kidneys. In some instances, it is not clear in the nonazotemic patient if the cause of low urine specific gravity is chronic renal disease or some other underlying disease associated with polyuria and polydipsia. In such instances, careful monitoring during water deprivation is crucial.

FREQUENTLY ASKED QUESTIONS

Q: A 5-year-old dog with chronic renal disease has a serum phosphorus concentration of 7.1 mg/dL. This result is not cause for concern because it falls within my diagnostic laboratory's normal reference range for phosphorus (i.e., 3.5-8.5 mg/dL), right?

A: Unfortunately, many diagnostic laboratories have reference ranges for serum phosphorus concentration that go up to 8 mg/dL or even slightly higher. The reason is because young growing animals have been included in the population used to determine the normal reference range. A normal mature dog or cat should have a serum phosphorus concentration no greater than 5.5 mg/dL.

Q: Which is better in the evaluation of patients with suspected renal disease, BUN or serum creatinine concentration?

A: Neither one is better than the other. Both BUN and serum creatinine concentration are insensitive tests for evaluation of renal function during the early stages of nephron loss. Both BUN and serum creatinine concentration begin to increase when 75% or more of the nephrons are non-functional. BUN, however, is affected by more nonrenal factors than is the serum creatinine concentration, but both have pitfalls in their interpretation. Hence it is recommended that clinicians evaluate both BUN and serum creatinine concentration at the same time.

Q: On preoperative screening, a seemingly healthy dog has a BUN of 40 mg/dL and a serum creatinine concentration of 1.2 mg/dL. I thought both of these tests increased together in the presence of renal disease.

A: The most likely cause for such results is that the blood samples were taken within a few (4 to 8) hours after a protein-rich meal, which can result in an increased BUN without a corresponding increase in serum creatinine concentration. A blood sample should be collected after a 12-hour fast and resubmitted to the laboratory. Dehydration also can result in an increased BUN concentration relative to serum creatinine concentration because urea can be passively reabsorbed into the blood from the renal tubules during decreased tubular flow whereas creatinine cannot. In this instance, the urine specific gravity is expected to be high due to renal conservation of water if renal function is normal. Gastrointestinal hemorrhage is another possible reason why the BUN concentration could be increased disproportionately because bacteria in the intestinal tract hydrolyze urea to carbon dioxide and ammonia, and the ammonia is converted to urea in the liver. Alternatively, the increased BUN concentration may accurately reflect poor renal function while the lower serum creatinine concentration reflects reduced muscle mass in a cachectic animal.

Q: Is there any reason to order a U_{Pr}/U_{Cr} or microalbuminuria test if the dipstick for protein is negative or only shows only a trace?

A: In animals with suspected renal disease, systemic hypertension, hyperadrenocorticism, or hyperthyroidism, the U_{Pr}/U_{Cr} or microalbuminuria test may detect proteinuria indicative of early renal damage because these tests detect much lower concentrations of protein than does the dipstick methodology.

Q: Is there any reason to order a U_{Pr}/U_{Cr} or microalbuminuria test if the dipstick for protein is 1+ or 2+ on a urine sample with a specific gravity of 1.050 and negative urine sediment examination?

A: This magnitude of proteinuria on dipstick evaluation could be pathologic or could be a consequence of the concentrated nature of the urine sample. The microalbuminuria test corrects the sample to a standard 1.010 specific gravity and thus removes this variable from consideration. Similarly, dividing the urine protein concentration by the urine creatinine concentration corrects for the concentrated nature of the urine sample.

Q: Urinalysis on a voided urine sample from a dog with stranguria shows pink color, 50 to 60 red blood cells per high-power field (RBCs/hpf), 10 to 15 WBCs/hpf, and 3+ proteinuria on dipstick analysis. The urine U_{Pr}/U_{Cr} was 8.5 (normal, <0.5) and the microalbuminuria test result was 12 mg/dL (normal, <1 mg/dL). Are these results of concern?

A: There are abnormal amounts of protein in the urine sample, but the urine U_{Pr}/U_{Cr} and microalbuminuria test results are not helpful because the urine sediment is active (i.e., many RBC and WBC are present) which can explain the abnormal results. The presence of inflammation and bleeding anywhere along the urinary tract can add protein to the urine. The urine U_{Pr}/U_{Cr} and microalbuminuria tests are most useful to indicate renal origin proteinuria when the urine sediment is inactive. It is of no value to perform a urine U_{Pr}/U_{Cr} or microalbuminuria test on a urine sample that has gross hematuria or pyuria on sediment examination.

Q: I am trying to decide whether to perform ultrasound examination of the urinary tract or contrast urography in an older male cat with persistent stranguria. Which procedure is preferable?

A: These methods are not mutually exclusive and both may identify underlying bladder lesions. Ultrasonography requires specialized equipment and considerable technical expertise to derive maximal value, but it is less invasive than contrast urography, which necessitates sedation and passage of a urinary catheter. Ultrasonography does not provide much information about the urethra because of its primarily intra-pelvic location. Contrast urethrocystography allows more complete evaluation of the urethra and may provide more definitive information about small lesions in the bladder and urethra than can be obtained during ultrasound examination. Ultrasonography also is very dependent on how full the bladder is during the study, and over interpretation of bladder wall thickness may occur if the bladder is minimally distended during the examination. The extent of bladder filling can be controlled during cystography.

Q: Should we be recommending renal biopsy more often? If so, what protocol should we use?

A: Renal biopsy should not be approached lightly because complications are possible. You should only biopsy the kidney if you believe the results are likely to change how you treat the patient. Examples of situations in which the information obtained from renal biopsy may change your approach to management include: differentiating acute from chronic renal failure when this distinction is not apparent after thorough clinical evaluation, establishing a prognosis in ARF when the clinical course has been protracted, and differentiating glomerulonephritis from glomerular amyloidosis. It seldom is helpful to perform renal biopsy in patients with stage 3 or 4 chronic kidney disease. In these instances, the primary renal lesion may not be apparent due to extensive tubular atrophy, glomerular sclerosis and interstitial fibrosis. Whether or not biopsy earlier in the course of disease would be helpful is not clear. Clinical outcome after therapeutic intervention in animals with stage 1 or 2 chronic kidney disease is not well studied, although it is commonly thought that treatment at this early stage has the potential to limit progression.

Q: A 12-year-old female dog has had stranguria and recurrent UTI. Urine cultures have sometimes been positive; antibiotic treatment helps, but the clinical signs never completely resolve. The dog seems otherwise healthy. Ultrasound examination was normal except for a mildly thickened bladder wall. A double contrast cystogram was normal. What now?

A: The dog described would be a good candidate for urethrocystoscopy. This procedure provides excellent direct visualization of the vestibule, urethra, and bladder. Lesions not readily identified on ultrasonography or contrast cystography often are identified during uroendoscopy.

SUGGESTED READINGS

Adams LG, Polzin DJ, Osborne CA, et al: Correlation of urine protein/creatinine ratio and twenty-four-hour urinary protein excretion in normal cats and cats with surgically induced chronic renal failure, *J Vet Intern Med* 6:36–40, 1992.

Adams WH, Toal RL, Breider MA: Ultrasonographic findings in dogs and cats with oxalate nephrosis attributed to ethylene glycol intoxication: 15 cases (1984-1988), *J Am Vet Med Assoc* 199:492–496, 1991.

Adams WH, Toal RL, Walker MA, et al: Early renal ultrasonographic findings in dogs with experimentally induced ethylene glycol nephrosis, *Am J Vet Res* 50:1370–1375, 1989.

Barr FJ: Evaluation of ultrasound as a method of assessing renal size in the dog, *J Small Anim Pract* 31:174–179, 1990.

Barr FJ, Holt PE, Gibbs C: Ultrasonographic measurement of normal renal parameters, *J Small Anim Pract* 31:180–184, 1990.

Borjesson DL, Christopher MM, Ling GV: Detection of canine transitional cell carcinoma using a bladder tumor antigen urine dipstick test, *Vet Clin Pathol* 28:33–38, 1999.

Brown SA, Finco DR, Boudinot FD, et al: Evaluation of a single injection method, using iohexol for estimating glomerular filtration rate in cats and dogs, *Am J Vet Res* 57:105–110, 1996.

Cannizzo KL, McLoughlin MA, Chew DJ, DiBartola SP: Uroendoscopy: Evaluation of the lower urinary tract, *Vet Clin North Am Small Anim Pract* 31:789–807, 2001.

Drost WT, Couto CG, Fischetti AJ, et al: Comparison of glomerular filtration rate between Greyhounds and non-Greyhound dogs, *J Vet Intern Med* 20:544–546, 2006.

Feeman WE 3rd, Couto CG, Gray TL: Serum creatinine concentrations in retired racing Greyhounds, *Vet Clin Pathol* 32:40–42, 2003.

Finco DR, Braselton WE, Cooper TA: Relationship between plasma iohexol clearance and urinary exogenous creatinine clearance in dogs, *J Vet Intern Med* 15:368–373, 2001.

Finco DR, Brown SA, Crowell WA, et al: Exogenous creatinine clearance as a measure of glomerular filtration rate in dogs with reduced renal mass, *Am J Vet Res* 52:1029–1032, 1991.

Finco DR, Tabaru H, Brown SA, et al: Endogenous creatinine clearance measurement of glomerular filtration rate in dogs, *Am J Vet Res* 54:1575–1578, 1993.

Goy-Thollot I, Chafotte C, Besse S, et al: Iohexol plasma clearance in healthy dogs and cats, *Vet Radiol Ultrasound* 47:168–173, 2006.

Grimm JB, Grimm KA, Kneller SK, et al: The effect of a combination of medetomidine-butorphanol and medetomidine, butorphanol, atropine on glomerular filtration rate in dogs, *Vet Radiol Ultrasound* 42:458–462, 2001.

Heiene R, Moe L: Pharmacokinetic aspects of measurement of glomerular filtration rate in the dog: A review, *J Vet Intern Med* 12:401–414, 1998.

Newell SM, Ko JC, Ginn PE, et al: Effects of three sedative protocols on glomerular filtration rate in clinically normal dogs, *Am J Vet Res* 58:446–450, 1997.

Pressler BM, Vaden SL, Jensen WA, et al: Detection of canine microalbuminuria using semiquantitative test strips designed for use with human urine, *Vet Clin Pathol* 31:56–60, 2002.

Rogers KS, Komkow A, Brown SA, et al: Comparison of four methods of estimating glomerular filtration rate in cats, *Am J Vet Res* 52:961–964, 1991.

Van Vonderen IK, Kooistra HS, Rijnberk A: Intra- and interindividual variation in urine osmolality and urine specific gravity in healthy pet dogs of various ages, *J Vet Intern Med* 11:30–35, 1997.

Walter PA, Feeney DA, Johnston GR, et al: Feline renal ultrasonography: Quantitative analyses of imaged anatomy, *Am J Vet Res* 48:596–599, 1987.

Walter PA, Feeney DA, Johnston GR, et al: Ultrasonographic evaluation of renal parenchymal diseases in dogs: 32 cases (1981-1986), *J Am Vet Med Assoc* 191:999–1007, 1987.

Walter PA, Johnston GR, Feeney DA, et al: Applications of ultrasonography in the diagnosis of parenchymal kidney disease in cats: 24 cases (1981-1986), *J Am Vet Med Assoc* 192:92–98, 1988.

Walter PA, Johnston GR, Feeney DA, et al: Renal ultrasonography in healthy cats, *Am J Vet Res* 48:600–607, 1987.

Waters CB, Adams LG, Scott-Moncrieff JC, et al: Effects of glucocorticoid therapy on urine protein-to-creatinine ratios and renal morphology in dogs, *J Vet Intern Med* 11:172–177, 1997.

Wise LA, Allen TA, Cartwright M: Comparison of renal biopsy techniques in dogs, *J Am Vet Med Assoc* 195:935–939, 1989.

Yeager AE, Anderson WI: Study of association between histologic features and echogenicity of architecturally normal cat kidneys, *Am J Vet Res* 50:860–863, 1989.

3 Acute Renal Failure

INTRODUCTION

A. Acute renal failure (ARF) is a clinical syndrome characterized by an abrupt increase in serum creatinine and blood urea nitrogen (BUN) concentrations to above normal (azotemia).
   1. ARF also may be associated with abnormal regulation of electrolytes, acid-base, and fluid balances.
   2. ARF may be catastrophic for renal function or patient survival if resolution does not occur within a reasonable time period.
B. Acute renal failure can be prerenal, intrinsic (primary), or postrenal in origin.

> ❗ Acute renal failure is characterized by an abrupt increase in serum creatinine and blood urea nitrogen concentrations.

   1. The term *acute renal failure* is commonly used to refer to acute intrinsic renal failure (AIRF), but prerenal and postrenal causes also should be considered.
   2. Prerenal azotemia is the most important differential diagnosis to consider along with intrinsic causes of azotemia.
   3. Postrenal causes of ARF usually are easily excluded from consideration after complete physical examination and appropriate diagnostic imaging.
C. Early recognition of AIRF is crucial because it can be reversed in patients with enough surviving nephrons when treatment is instituted early on in the course of the disease.
D. AIRF probably occurs more frequently than appreciated and may go undiagnosed or be confused with chronic renal failure. Although AIRF can sometimes be successfully treated, many affected patients do not survive. Recognizing situations in which AIRF is likely to develop and taking appropriate preventive measures are preferable to treating established AIRF.
E. The frequency of underlying conditions associated with AIRF varies with the location and nature of veterinary practice.
   1. Nephrotoxicity is the most common cause of AIRF at The Ohio State University Veterinary Hospital, followed by nephritis (e.g., leptospirosis) and ischemia.
   2. The aggressive use of potentially nephrotoxic antibiotics, especially aminoglycosides, contributes to the frequency of nephrotoxic AIRF.
   3. Indiscriminate use of or accidental exposure to nonsteroidal anti-inflammatory drugs (NSAIDs) and exposure of veterinary patients to extensive surgical procedures and aggressive posttraumatic resuscitative maneuvers also may contribute to an increased frequency of ischemic AIRF.

PATHOGENESIS AND PATHOPHYSIOLOGY OF ACUTE RENAL FAILURE

Prerenal Acute Renal Failure (Figure 3-1)

1. Reduced perfusion of the kidneys results in retention of nitrogenous wastes. A substantial decrease in hydrostatic pressure in the glomeruli results in decreased glomerular filtration rate (GFR) and solute retention.
2. Early in the process of volume depletion, renal autoregulation preserves excretory function and continued excretion of waste products. Autoregulation eventually is overcome and azotemia develops.
3. The most common causes of reduced renal perfusion are dehydration, hypotension, shock, and reduced cardiac output.
4. Early prerenal ARF is associated with physiologic oliguria (assuming normal kidneys initially), which is a normal response to decreased renal perfusion.
5. Decreased renal perfusion is detected in the kidney and by peripheral baroreceptors, and results in increased reabsorption of salt and water from the glomerular filtrate.
6. Severe and prolonged hypoperfusion of the kidneys can produce primary lesions in the kidneys (ischemic nephrosis or ischemic acute tubular necrosis).
7. Prerenal azotemia readily resolves after correction of decreased cardiac output and circulating blood volume.
8. A component of prerenal azotemia often contributes to the total magnitude of azotemia in patients with primary renal or postrenal disease.

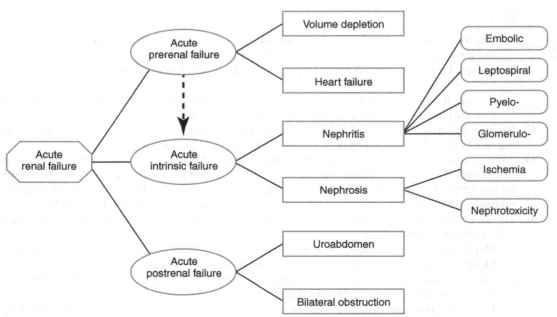

FIGURE 3-1 ■ Classification of acute renal failure: Prerenal, intrinsic renal, and postrenal causes must be considered.

Postrenal Acute Renal Failure (See Chapter 11, Obstruction Uropathy and Nephropathy, and Chapter 12, Urinary Tract Trauma and Uroperitoneum)

Causes

a. Bilateral renal obstruction.
   (1) Urolithiasis.
   (2) Bilateral ureteral or urethral obstruction.
   (3) Urethral plugs in cats.
b. Uroabdomen (rupture of urinary tract with accumulation of urine).

Pathogenesis

a. Obstruction results in failure to filter waste products due to back pressure in the nephron.
b. Uroabdomen results in recycling of waste products across the peritoneum.

Acute Intrinsic Renal Failure (primary ARF)

Causes of Acute Intrinsic Renal Failure (see Chapter 4, Specific Syndromes Causing Acute Intrinsic Renal Failure)

NEPHROTOXICITY
   (1) Ethylene glycol (EG).
   (2) Antimicrobials.
      (a) Aminoglycosides.
      (b) Amphotericin-B.
      (c) Sulfonamides administered to a dehydrated patient.
      (d) Tetracyclines administered IV.
      (e) Nafcillin administered intraoperatively.
   (3) Easter lily (cats).
   (4) Grape or raisin toxicity (dogs).
   (5) Hypercalcemia and hypercalciuria.
      (a) Cholecalciferol rodenticide (Quintox, Rampage).
      (b) Calcipotriene (Dovonex).
   (6) Anticancer drugs.
      (a) Cisplatin.
      (b) High dose doxorubicin (Adriamycin).
   (7) Radiocontrast agents administered IV.
   (8) Heavy metals (e.g., zinc, arsenic, lead).
   (9) Hydrocarbons.
   (10) Fluorinated inhalation anesthetics.
   (11) Calcium ethylenediaminetetraacetic acid (EDTA).
   (12) Mycotoxins (e.g., ochratoxin, citrinin).
   (13) Tainted food (melamine and cyanuric acid).
RENAL ISCHEMIA
   (1) Dehydration.
   (2) Trauma.
   (3) Anesthesia.
   (4) Sepsis.
   (5) Heat stroke.
   (6) Pigment nephropathy.
      (a) Hemolysis.
         (i) Immune-mediated hemolytic anemia.
         (ii) Envenomation.

(•) Coral snake.

(•) Hymenoptera (bee sting).

(b) Myoglobinuria.

(7) Angiotensin-converting enzyme (ACE) inhibitors.

(8) Shock.

(9) Hemorrhage.

(10) Surgery.

(11) Burns.

(12) Hypothermia.

(13) NSAIDs.

(14) Acute papillary necrosis (e.g., medullary renal amyloidosis, Fanconi syndrome).

NEPHRITIS

(1) Leptospirosis — acute tubulointerstitial nephritis.

(2) Borrelia — rapidly progressive glomerulonephritis.

(3) Acute bacterial pyelonephritis.

(4) Embolic nephritis.

(5) Allergic interstitial nephritis.

ACUTE HYPERPHOSPHATEMIA

(1) Tumor lysis syndrome.

(2) Phosphate enema.

(3) Phosphate acidifier.

(4) Massive soft tissue trauma.

Pathophysiology of Acute Intrinsic Renal Failure Due to Nephrosis

a. Exposure to nephrotoxins or ischemia causes tubular injury along a spectrum from degeneration to necrosis and is referred to as nephrosis or acute tubular necrosis (ATN) (Figure 3-2). Some patients have minimal to no light microscopic lesions but experience severe renal excretory failure.

(1) Early lesions may be distributed preferentially in tubules of the outer medulla, an area that is not easily biopsied.

(2) Renal tubular lesions may be subtle in nature and patchy in distribution making them easy to overlook on routine microscopy.

(3) Subtle tubular lesions can cause decreased sodium reabsorption proximally which can promote sustained vasoconstriction in parent glomeruli as sensed at the macula densa (so-called vasomotor nephropathy).

b. Factors that contribute to azotemia and oliguria during AIRF (Figure 3-3, *A-E*).

(1) Tubular backleak (across or between damaged tubules).

(2) Intraluminal tubular obstruction by casts, debris, or tubular swelling.

(3) Extraluminal tubular obstruction by interstitial edema or cellular infiltrates.

(a) Increased pressure inside tubular lumen.

(b) Decreased interstitial blood supply (i.e., as a consequence of edema).

(4) Primary filtration failure.

(a) Vasomotor nephropathy.

(i) Afferent arteriolar vasoconstriction.

(ii) Efferent arteriolar vasodilatation.

(b) Decrease in glomerular permeability.

(i) Decreased size or number of endothelial pores.

(ii) Decreased surface area of glomerular membranes.

c. The mechanism(s) that initiates AIRF may not be the same one(s) that maintains AIRF. A combination of mechanisms likely is operative in clinical patients.

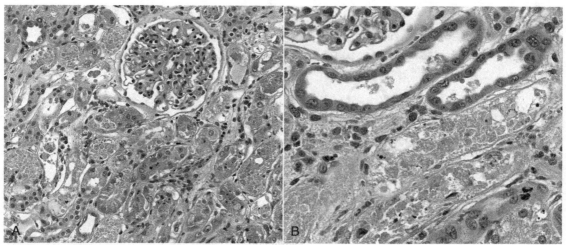

FIGURE 3-2 ■ Photomicrograph of acute tubular necrosis. **A,** Normal glomerulus with areas of tubular necrosis. Note some tubules with loss of tubular epithelium, some with flattened epithelium (suggesting restitution), and tubular lumens filled with necrotic debris. **B,** Note relatively normal tubules in upper left field (focal areas of attenuation exist here). Just below the normal tubules are several tubules with complete loss of epithelium and abundant intraluminal detritus (hematoxylin and eosin stain, ×200). (Courtesy of Dr. Steve Weisbrode, Columbus, Ohio.)

    d. Renal ischemia consists of a spectrum from prerenal azotemia to acute tubular necrosis and in its most devastating form, bilateral cortical necrosis.
      (1) The renal cortex is richly supplied with adrenergic innervation, which results in vasoconstriction during renal ischemia. Due to a large reserve of blood supply, temporary or mild reductions in renal blood flow do not result in tubular necrosis.
      (2) Deprivation of blood supply, if severe and prolonged, results in loss of cellular energy production and loss of cell integrity. Tubules with high metabolic activity are at greatest risk of injury during reduced oxygen supply.
        (a) It is not necessary for systemic hypotension to occur for the kidneys to experience intrarenal hypotension.

> **!** NSAIDs do not directly damage the kidney. Acute renal injury only occurs if mediators of vasoconstriction have been activated by the body's perception of volume depletion.

        (b) The outer medullary region of the kidney is the most metabolically active and is supplied with the lowest amount of oxygen. The last part of the proximal tubule (pars recta, P3) and the medullary thick ascending limb of the loop of Henle are located here and these areas are at increased risk for early injury during hypoxia. The medulla already is an area of low blood supply that is at increased risk when blood flow is further reduced.
    e. NSAIDs block renal production of vasodilatory prostaglandins that maintain renal blood flow during dehydration resulting in renal ischemia (Figure 3-4).
    f. True nephrotoxins exert their deleterious effects directly on the kidney after binding to tubular cell membranes. Reduced energy production and cell death follow. Some nephrotoxins also cause renal vasoconstriction, but the major effect is direct cell injury rather than ischemia.

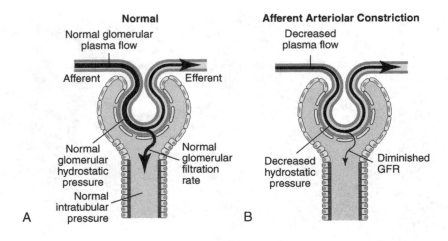

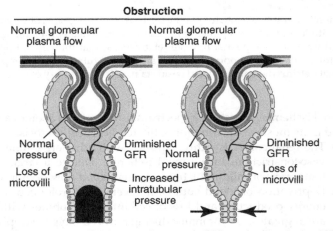

FIGURE 3-3 ■ General mechanisms contributing to decreased GFR and oliguria in AIRF. The illustration represents all nephrons in the kidneys. The mechanism or mechanisms that initiate the injury may differ from those that cause ongoing injury and maintain the state of AIRF. Multiple mechanisms may be operative simultaneously. It is almost never clinically possible to identify the specific operative mechanism in an individual patient. **A,** Normal nephron. Normally, about 30% of the blood entering the glomerulus is filtered into the Bowman's space. Glomerular filtration pressure normally is not impeded to any appreciable extent by the normally low intratubular pressure. The healthy renal tubular epithelium prevents tubular fluid from leaking between or across tubular cells. No obstructing material is present within the tubular lumen, and the lumen is completely patent. **B,** Afferent arteriolar constriction (vasomotor nephropathy). Glomerular filtration is severely decreased by constriction of the afferent arteriole. Decreased intraglomerular pressure can result in azotemia and decreased urine production. Sympathetically mediated vasoconstriction may result from systemic hypotension, pain, tissue handling during surgery, and anesthesia. Damaged afferent arteriolar myocytes perpetuate vasoconstriction as calcium enters the cells and results in contraction. Sustained vasoconstriction not only decreases GFR but also impairs oxygen delivery to the tubular cells via the post glomerular vessels, which can result in acute tubular necrosis. **C,** Obstruction, increased intratubular pressure. Increased intratubular pressure occurs proximal to the obstructed segment of the nephron. The obstruction can be intraluminal or extraluminal, and the resultant increase in pressure opposes glomerular filtration. The obstructing material can be cellular debris (e.g., sloughed brush border cell membranes, regurgitated organelles), precipitated proteins, or, occasionally, crystalline precipitates. Interstitial edema or cellular infiltrates can cause extraluminal obstruction and decrease renal blood flow by compressing interstitial blood vessels. Tubular swelling can also contribute to increased intraluminal pressure.

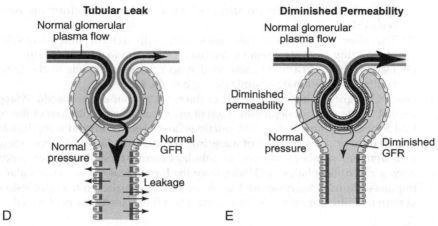

FIGURE 3-3, cont'd ■ **D,** Tubular backleak. In this situation, the filtration pressure may be normal, but filtered fluid leaks back across the damaged tubular epithelium into the interstitium. Some fluid also may accumulate within the damaged tubule. Tubular backleak occurs in patients with more severe tubular injury. Backleak is increased by any concurrent increase in tubular pressure. **E,** Decreased glomerular permeability. In this example, the disease process has decreased the surface area available for glomerular filtration. Decreased glomerular permeability can arise as a consequence of mesangial cell contraction and decreases in the number or diameter of the glomerular fenestrae. (Drawn by Tim Vojt.)

    g. The term *nephrotoxicant* refers to a chemical or drug that can result in renal injury regardless of whether it is by direct nephrotoxic injury (e.g., aminoglycosides) or by renal ischemia (e.g., NSAIDs, myoglobin).

    h. Patients with underlying renal disease develop episodes of AIRF more readily than patients that had normal kidneys before the insult.

        (1) The ability of diseased kidneys to autoregulate blood flow and GFR is decreased, placing them at greater risk for renal ischemia. They cannot undergo compensatory vasodilatation to compensate for systemic hypotension.

        (2) The ability to synthesize renal vasodilatory prostaglandins is reduced, placing them at risk for renal ischemia.

> **!** Animals with pre-existing renal disease develop AIRF more readily than do normal animals.

        (3) The increased tubular metabolic rate of remnant nephrons places them at risk due to their increased workload. They are more readily injured during ischemia and exposure to toxins.

        (4) Increased single nephron GFR in remnant nephrons provides an increased filtered load of potential toxins per remaining nephron.

        (5) Hypertrophy of tubular membranes in remnant nephrons provides increased surfaces for exposure to potential nephrotoxins.

    i. Dehydration magnifies the propensity for and severity of AIRF after exposure to renal ischemia or nephrotoxins.

> **!** Simultaneous exposure to nephrotoxins and renal ischemia dramatically increases the risk of renal injury.

        (1) Dehydration promotes maximal water and solute reabsorption along the nephron. Toxins that are filtered across the glomeruli progressively increase in concentration

along the course of the proximal tubule as water and sodium are iso-osmotically reabsorbed.

(2) The slow tubular flow rate associated with dehydration favors formation of obstructing casts after renal ischemia or exposure to a nephrotoxin.

(3) Dehydration already has activated vasoconstrictor signals to the kidneys, which facilitates additional ischemic damage to the kidneys.

j. Loss of integrity of the cytoskeleton of the renal tubular cell and actin dysregulation are pivotal early events in nephrosis. Loss of microvilli occurs with loss of the cytoskeleton. Cell adhesion is impaired at tight junctions (loss of occludin) and along basolateral membranes (loss or redistribution of integrin). These events facilitate detachment of tubular cells from one another and from the tubular basement membrane. Relocation of Na^+-K^+ adenosine triphosphatase (ATPase) from the basolateral to luminal cellular membranes impairs sodium reabsorption and results in activation of the renin-angiotensin-aldosterone system and afferent arteriolar vasoconstriction (i.e., vasomotor nephropathy). Depletion

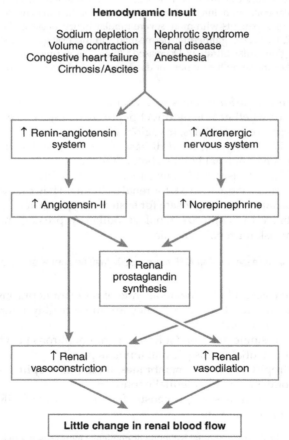

FIGURE 3-4 ■ Renal blood flow during times of hemodynamic insult. Normal renal vascular resistance and renal blood flow are relatively well maintained during times of vasoconstriction if synthesis of renal vasodilator substances is normal. Renal vasoconstriction, however, proceeds unopposed if the synthesis of renal vasodilatory prostaglandins has been blocked by NSAID administration. Progression to AIRF may occur.

of intracellular adenosine triphosphate (ATP) triggers a cascade of events that alters cell membrane permeability, increases calcium influx, and impairs cell function ultimately causing in cell death. The balance between nitric oxide and endothelin, which maintains normal renal blood flow, is altered (decreased nitric oxide and increased endothelin) favoring renal vasoconstriction. Damaged myocytes of afferent arterioles allow calcium influx which potentiates vasoconstriction. Growth factors (e.g., epidermal growth factor, hepatocyte growth factor, insulin-like growth factor, transforming growth factor) and heat shock proteins appear to be important in recovery from AIRF.

k. Phases for AIRF (Figure 3-5).

(1) The latent phase represents the time after exposure to a nephrotoxin or renal ischemia but before the onset of azotemia. It is associated with increasing number and severity of renal tubular lesions over time if the renal insult is not stopped.

(a) Lethal and sublethal renal tubular injury occurs.

(b) The latent phase usually is not detected because clinical signs are absent or minimal.

(c) Early removal of the inciting cause of injury will result in rapid return to normal renal function.

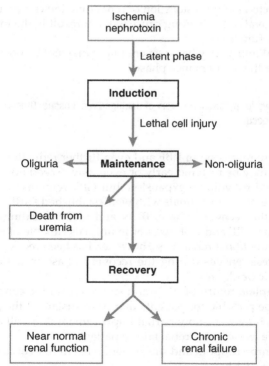

FIGURE 3-5 ■ Phases of AIRF. The progression from the latent to the fixed renal failure of the maintenance phase can be halted if the ischemic or toxic injury is corrected before azotemia has developed. Oliguria occurs in patients with more severe acute renal injury. Many patients do not survive without dialysis due to the metabolic effects of uremia. Recovery is possible, however, but often with substantial reduction in functional renal mass. Some patients survive and go on to develop chronic renal failure. Recovery is facilitated by the onset of diuresis in patients that initially were oligoanuric.

(d) The latent phase is most likely to be detected in closely monitored hospitalized patients with critical illness.

> **!** It's not the *quantity* of urine, but rather the *quality* of urine produced that matters most.

(e) Older definitions of AIRF required that oliguria be documented during the clinical course, but this is no longer a requirement. Oliguria, normal urine production, or polyuria all may occur depending on the specific cause and severity of renal injury and the phase of AIRF.

(f) Physiological oliguria is common during the latent phase and early maintenance phase.

(2) The maintenance phase of AIRF is characterized by a persistently increased serum creatinine concentration despite correction of all prerenal factors (i.e., restoration of extracellular fluid volume and cardiac output).

(a) Oligo-anuria occurs in patients with the most severe intrarenal injury (e.g., those with EG or lily toxicity).

(b) Nonoliguria is typical of AIRF caused by exposure to aminoglycosides.

(c) Entry into the maintenance phase signifies that a critical amount of lethal injury has occurred in the renal tubules and a course of 1 to 3 weeks of AIRF is expected before restoration of renal function can occur.

(d) Removal of the inciting cause will not result in the immediate return of normal renal function.

(e) Renal injury may be so severe that it may not be possible for the patient to ever leave the maintenance phase.

> **!** Preservation of some RBF allows for potential recovery of damaged renal tissue. Otherwise, complete necrosis of renal tissue would occur.

(f) Severe reduction in RBF and even further reduction in GFR characterize AIRF. RBF may be restored early or even may exceed normal in some patients when treated by volume expansion, but GFR remains very low during the maintenance phase in animals with well-established AIRF.

(3) During the recovery phase, BUN and serum creatinine concentration return to normal as GRF and RBF recover in animals capable of surviving the maintenance phase. Functional renal mass, however, has been reduced.

(a) Diuresis ensues during the recovery phase in patients that were previously anuric or oliguric.

(b) Complete return of BUN and serum creatinine concentrations to normal may not be possible for patients that have sustained the greatest renal injury. They may, however, show partial improvement that will allow a reasonable quality of life as a chronic renal failure patient.

(c) Nephron dropout and subsequent renal fibrosis occur, resulting in chronic renal failure (CRF).

(d) Remaining renal tissue is not completely normal even when BUN and serum creatinine concentrations have returned to normal. Some nephrons invariably have been lost and replaced with fibrous tissue. Renal hypertrophy and hyperplasia have enabled the kidney to restore some RBF and GFR with fewer remaining surviving nephrons.

(e) Maximal urinary concentrating ability and urinary acidification do not return entirely to normal, but these limitations are not usually of clinical consequence.

HISTORY AND CLINICAL SIGNS

Prerenal Acute Renal Failure

1. Oliguria is the most common sign of prerenal acute renal failure.
2. Patients with prerenal ARF usually have supporting historical or physical findings of dehydration, shock, hypotension, or reduced cardiac output.

Postrenal Acute Renal Failure (see Chapter 11, Obstructive Uropathy and Nephropathy, and Chapter 12, Urinary Tract Trauma and Uroperitoneum)

1. Patients with postrenal ARF usually have obvious supporting historical, physical, and diagnostic imaging findings.
2. Urinary outflow obstruction or urine accumulation in the peritoneum must be promptly ruled out as potential causes of ARF.

Acute Intrinsic Renal Failure

1. Clinical signs are those of uremia, including anorexia, lethargy, vomiting, and diarrhea. These signs are not specific for AIRF.
2. Signs will be of recent onset, and a longstanding history of polyuria or polydipsia should not be present.
3. Based on clinical studies, approximately 18% of affected patients are expected to have anuria, 43% to have oliguria (urine output of 0.1-1 mL/kg/hr), 25% to have normal urine output (1-2 mL/kg/hr), and 14% to have polyuria (urine output >2 mL/kg/hr).
4. Lack of urinations may be noted in animals with oliguric AIRF or polyuria may be noticed in those with nonoliguric ARF.
5. Recent trauma, shock, surgery, or anesthetic procedures suggests the possibility of ischemic nephropathy.
6. Recent administration of known nephrotoxins (e.g., aminoglycosides) should lead to a suspicion of nephrotoxic AIRF.
7. Recent administration or accidental ingestion of NSAIDs should lead to a suspicion of ischemic AIRF.
8. Access to EG or actual observation of EG consumption indicates nephrotoxic AIRF, but often a positive history cannot be obtained.
9. Postural changes (e.g., hunching of the back) or reluctance to move may be indicative of renal pain.
10. Lack of food and water intake associated with systemic illness arouses suspicion of ischemic nephropathy or nephritis (e.g., leptospirosis).

PHYSICAL EXAMINATION

Prerenal Acute Renal Failure

1. Dehydration often is detected by assessment of skin turgor and observation of dryness of the mucous membranes.
2. Poor quality femoral pulses may be detected.
3. Kidneys are normal-sized and nonpainful.
4. The lower urinary tract is normal.

Postrenal Acute Renal Failure (see Chapter 11, Obstructive Uropathy and Nephropathy, and Chapter 12, Urinary Tract Trauma and Uroperitoneum)

Acute Intrinsic Renal Failure

   a. Signs of uremia tend to be more severe than those observed with prerenal azotemia, and include uremic breath and oral ulceration.
   b. Mucous membrane pallor should not be observed (as may be the case with CRF).
   c. Fever may be present in animals with intra renal ARF due to nephritis (e.g., leptospirosis).
   d. Hypothermia is commonly encountered in animals with ARF due to nephrosis, but hypothermia can be encountered in any animal near death, regardless of the cause of azotemia.
   e. Dehydration frequently is present in animals with primary AIRF due to fluid losses from vomiting, diarrhea, and lack of food and water intake. Dehydration may be exacerbated by excessive urinary loss of fluid in animals with nonoliguric or polyuric AIRF.

> ! Dehydration is frequently present in animals with primary AIRF due to fluid losses from vomiting, diarrhea, and lack of food and water intake.

   f. Overhydration may be present in animals with severe oliguria that have received excessive amounts of intravenous fluids.
   g. Abdominal palpation.
      (1) Renal swelling and pain may be identified when palpating the costovertebral angles in patients with nephritis and nephrosis, but is not a consistent finding.
      (2) Kidneys are normal or enlarged with normal contour and not small and irregular as commonly encountered in animals with CRF.
      (3) The bladder may be very small if the animal is oliguric, or it may be normal or large if the animal is in nonoliguric AIRF.
      (4) No evidence for urinary obstruction is found.
   h. Bradycardia or other arrhythmia may be auscultated or pulse deficits palpated when hyperkalemia is present.

DIAGNOSIS

Prerenal Acute Renal Failure

1. Confirmation that azotemia is renal.
   a. Highly concentrated urine is expected from normal kidneys. Urine specific gravity should be ≥ 1.030 or more and often is >1.040.
   b. Results of urinalysis are normal.
      (1) Small numbers of hyaline casts may be seen because of an increased concentration of urinary mucoprotein.
      (2) During severe dehydration, a small amount of protein may leak across the glomeruli temporarily.
   c. Renal size, shape, and texture are normal on radiography and ultrasound examination.
   d. Restoration of effective circulating blood volume results in increased urine volume and improved renal function. If oliguria and poor renal function persist, suspect primary renal failure.
2. Confirmation of prerenal azotemia obligates the clinician to search for a nonrenal cause for dehydration and renal hypoperfusion. Historical, physical examination, radiographic,

ultrasonographic, or laboratory test results may help identify the system responsible for prerenal azotemia:
a. Severe vomiting of any cause.
b. Hypoadrenocorticism.
c. Severe diarrhea of any cause.
d. Obstructive gastrointestinal disease with sequestration of fluid in lumen of the bowel.
e. Hypovolemic shock of any cause.
f. Heart failure.
g. Any other cause of dehydration.

Postrenal Acute Renal Failure (see Chapter 11, Obstructive Uropathy and Nephropathy, and Chapter 12, Urinary Tract Trauma and Uroperitoneum)
Acute Intrinsic Renal Failure
a. No single test reliably differentiates AIRF from other forms of renal failure, and the diagnosis usually is established after information from the history and physical examination are integrated with results of urinalysis, renal imaging, serum chemistry and hematology (e.g., hematocrit).
b. Blood and urine samples should be collected before therapy because fluids and drugs can alter laboratory results and confuse interpretation. Serial evaluation of renal function during fluid therapy is necessary to determine an accurate diagnosis and prognosis.
c. Hemogram.
   (1) Anemia should not be present early in the course of AIRF, but occult hemorrhage can occur early in the course of AIRF as a consequence of uremic gastrointestinal ulceration.
   (2) A mild to moderate regenerative red cell response can be seen early in AIRF if acute blood loss occurs.
   (3) Total protein concentration may be normal or high, depending on degree of dehydration, and may be decreased if iatrogenic overhydration is present.
   (4) The leukogram may be normal or show a stress response with mature neutrophilia and lymphopenia. Leukocytosis with left shift may be seen in patients with nephritis.
d. Urinalysis.
   (1) Urine becomes dilute very early in the clinical course, regardless of whether the animal is oliguric or nonoliguric. Urine specific gravity often is fixed in the isosthenuric range (1.007-1.017).

! Dilute urine is typical in early AIRF, but also in CRF and consequently does not distinguish AIRF from CRF.

   (2) Dipstrip tests may show proteinuria, hematuria, glucosuria, or some combination of these findings.
   (3) The urine sediment may be very active in nephritis and nephrosis with many casts seen.
      (a) Fine and coarse granular casts.
      (b) Cellular casts.
         (i) Renal tubular epithelial casts.
         (ii) White blood cell casts are more likely to be seen in nephritis, especially pyelonephritis.
         (iii) Rarely, red blood cell casts will be observed. If seen, suspect acute glomerulonephritis.
         (iv) Mixed cellular casts.
         (v) Degenerating cellular casts.
      (c) Hyaline and waxy casts.

(4) The absence of casts does not exclude a diagnosis of AIRF.

(5) Excessive numbers of red blood cells, white blood cells, and small renal tubular epithelial cells can be seen due to non-specific release of these cells into the urine after renal injury.

(6) Excessive numbers of white blood cells may be seen in association with visible bacteria in animals with pyelonephritis.

(7) Presence of oxalate or *hippurate-like* crystals in the urinary sediment of animals with AIRF supports a diagnosis of EG poisoning.

e. Urine culture usually is submitted to exclude a role for active bacterial urinary infection in the course of AIRF.

f. Serum biochemistry.

(1) BUN and serum creatinine concentrations are high and continue to increase until a plateau is established, when the decline in renal function has reached its maximum (maintenance phase).

(a) It may take days to reach a steady-state serum creatinine concentration after a single massive renal insult.

(b) Serum creatinine concentration may continue to increase episodically as additional lethal renal cell injury occurs (i.e., ongoing undetected ischemia or nephrotoxic insult).

! Rapid increases in BUN, serum creatinine, and serum phosphorus concentrations may be observed during AIRF.

(2) The magnitude of increase in BUN or serum creatinine concentration is not helpful in the differentiation of AIRF from CRF or in the differentiation of prerenal, intrinsic renal, and postrenal azotemia.

(3) Rapid increases in BUN, serum creatinine, and serum phosphorus concentrations may be observed during AIRF. This finding is particularly helpful to document AIRF in the absence of recent serum biochemistry results for comparison. For example, sequential serum creatinine concentrations of 4.3 mg/dL, 6.0 mg/dL, and 7.5 mg/dL over 3 consecutive days support a diagnosis of AIRF. Serum creatinine and BUN concentrations would not increase this dramatically over a short time period in a hydrated patient with CRF.

(4) Serum potassium concentrations can be high (>5.5 mEq/L) or at the high end of the reference range due to a reduction in renal excretory function (normal or low concentrations generally are found in CRF patients). Serum potassium concentration was <5.0 mEq/L in 75% of dogs with AIRF in one large study despite the presence of oligoanuria in more than 60% of these dogs. Severe hyperkalemia is more likely in dogs with urethral obstruction, uroabdomen, or hypoadrenocorticism.

(5) Serum phosphorus concentration usually is high (>6.0 mg/dL) and may be disproportionately high during the earlier phases of AIRF. In CRF, renal secondary hyperparathyroidism maintains phosphorus balance despite a slow progressive decrease in GFR as a result of the effect of parathyroid hormone (PTH) on renal tubular cells, an effect that does not have sufficient time to develop in AIRF patients with severely injured renal tubular cells.

(6) Serum total calcium concentration usually is normal or low.

(7) Blood gas analysis during the maintenance phase usually shows moderate to severe metabolic acidosis. The acidosis in ARF is more severe than that seen in compensated CRF.

(8) Other less commonly used tests to distinguish ARF from CRF include plasma carbamylated hemoglobin concentration and nail creatinine content. A diagnosis of ARF is supported when these tests are within normal limits; a diagnosis of CRF is supported when test results are high.

g. Urine enzymology.

(1) Small amounts of enzymes are found in the urine of normal animals and finding increased amounts may support a diagnosis of AIRF.

(2) Urine gamma glutamyl transferase (GGT) arises from the brush border of the tubular cells and increased urinary GGT is very sensitive for developing renal injury. It may signal impending tubular necrosis or initially may arise from displacement of enzymes from the brush border.

(3) The use of urinary enzymes has been evaluated in experimental studies in animals, but clinical use has been limited. Measurement of urinary enzymes could facilitate early diagnosis of acute renal injury in clinical patients.

(4) Urine GGT may be measured or urine GGT-to-creatinine ratio calculated.

(5) Other urinary enzymes that arise from the cytoplasm of tubular cells include N-acetyl-glucosamine (NAG) and β-glucuronidase.

h. Renal imaging studies.

(1) Kidneys are normal-sized or enlarged and have normal shape in patients with AIRF. Assessment of kidney size based on length is insensitive because enlarging kidneys in AIRF tend to become plump before length increases.

(2) Intravenous pyelography (IVP) is contraindicated due to the potential for contrast-associated nephrotoxicity in kidneys with underlying damage.

(3) Renal ultrasonography.

(a) Increased cortical or medullary echogenicity may be seen.

(b) Normal ultrasound findings do not exclude AIRF.

(c) AIRF and CRF cannot be differentiated if normal-sized kidneys are seen.

(d) No specific cause of AIRF can be inferred from ultrasound, with the possible exception of EG toxicosis (extremely hyperechoic kidneys).

i. Serology.

(1) Submit acute and convalescent serum samples for leptospirosis titers if nephritis is a possible cause for AIRF.

(2) Submit serum samples for *Borrelia* titers if rapidly progressive glomerulonephritis is suspected as cause for AIRF.

> **!** Renal biopsy may be helpful to confirm that azotemia is due to primary renal lesions and to characterize the changes as acute or chronic.

j. Renal biopsy.

(1) Renal biopsy may be helpful to confirm that azotemia is due to primary renal lesions and to characterize the changes as acute or chronic.

(2) Renal biopsy may be necessary to confirm a diagnosis of AIRF in some animals or to evaluate the healing process in animals that have a protracted course of AIRF.

(3) Renal lesions compatible with AIRF include degenerative tubular changes, tubular necrosis, desquamation of renal tubules, denuding of tubular basement membranes, disruption of tubular basement membranes, and intrarenal cast formation. In ARF caused by nephrosis, interstitial inflammation is minimal, but in ARF due to nephritis, it is substantial. Lack of fibrosis and nephron loss is supportive of AIRF in its early clinical course rather than CRF.

    (4) Few or no obvious changes are seen by light microscopy in some animals with established primary AIRF. In these instances, ultrastructural changes may be responsible for renal dysfunction or the lesions may be deeper within the kidney than the site at which the biopsy sample was taken (i.e., medullary versus cortical).

    (5) Renal biopsy during a protracted recovery phase can be helpful to evaluate whether healing is occurring by fibrosis and nephron drop-out or by tubular regeneration and repopulation of the basement membranes with new tubular cells.

TREATMENT

A. The ultimate goal of management of the maintenance phase of AIRF is to provide adequate supportive care and allow time for healing to occur (Box 3-1).

> **!** The management goal of the maintenance phase of AIRF is to provide adequate supportive care and allow time for renal healing to occur.

    1. Treatment takes considerable time and effort.

    2. No treatment presently available can change the lesions already present in the kidney.

    3. Prevention of conversion from sublethally injured cells to lethally injured cells is a major goal of treatment.

    4. Prevention of additional renal cell injury is another important goal of treatment, and one that requires conscientious fluid therapy to provide optimal renal perfusion while at the same time avoiding overhydration.

B. It may take as long as 3 weeks of supportive care to determine if adequate renal function is likely to return.

    1. Ideally, BUN, serum creatinine concentration, serum phosphorus concentration and urinary concentrating ability will return to normal or nearly normal.

    2. When renal injury is more severe, permanent nephron loss and residual azotemia result. The magnitude of residual azotemia will determine whether or not the animal can be managed successfully as a CRF patient.

C. Initially, identify and correct the most life-threatening disturbances while searching for the underlying cause of AIRF.

    1. Stop administration of any nephrotoxin and do not prescribe any drugs with nephrotoxic potential.

■ BOX 3-1
■ **GOALS FOR MANAGEMENT OF THE MAINTENANCE PHASE OF ACUTE INTRINSIC RENAL FAILURE**

- Manage uremic crisis—initial stabilization.
- Attempt to convert oliguria to nonoliguria.
- Prevent overhydration.
- Optimize excretory renal function—minimize azotemia.
- Optimize environment for renal healing.
- Minimize additional renal damage.
- Manage the internal milieu to allow survival for 1 to 3 weeks.
- Consider dialysis early rather than late.
- Perform renal biopsy if clinical course is protracted or diagnosis is uncertain.

   2. Avoid hypotension, anesthesia, and surgery. Due to loss of renal autoregulation, the post-ischemic or post-nephrotoxic kidney may be unable to protect itself against ongoing episodes of reduced renal perfusion. Additional renal injury may result if hypotension occurs systemically or locally within the kidney.
   D. Initial stabilization.
      1. Place an indwelling intravenous catheter to administer fluids and drugs necessary to manage AIRF.
         a. Initially, a jugular catheter is preferred so that central venous pressure (CVP) can be monitored during aggressive fluid administration.
         b. Fluid administration should be decreased or discontinued temporarily if CVP exceeds 13 cm H_2O or increases rapidly by 2 cm or more H_2O in any 10 minute period.
         c. A volume challenge of 22 mL/kg administered over 10 minutes can be given to assess the likelihood of impending volume overload. CVP should not increase more than 2 cm H_2O if the heart is normal.
         d. Measurement of pulmonary capillary wedge pressure (although not commonly feasible) can provide earlier information about the development of overhydration.
      2. Rapidly correct dehydration, ideally within 6 to 8 hours to prevent additional renal injury as a result of ongoing ischemia.
         a. Dehydration can be calculated by the formula: Estimated dehydration (%) × Body Weight (kg) = dehydration (L).
         b. Alternatively, 2 to 3 times maintenance fluid needs (130 to 200 mL/kg/day) can be given.
         c. Hypovolemic shock should be reversed with fluids at 88 mL/kg/hr with or without monitoring of CVP until cardiovascular status has been stabilized.
         d. Additional fluids are given to match sensible (urinary volume), insensible (respiratory losses at approximately 22 mL/kg/day) and contemporary (estimated volume from vomiting and diarrhea) fluid losses.
      3. Place an indwelling urinary catheter to monitor urine output and facilitate fluid therapy in the initial 24 to 48 hours.
      4. Prompt recognition of oliguria is important because it limits the volume of intravenous fluids that can be given safely.
         a. Oliguria at initial evaluation may be due to hypovolemia arising from lack of food and water intake, vomiting, and diarrhea, severe intrarenal lesions or both.

❗ Prompt recognition of oliguria is important because it limits the volume of intravenous fluids that can be given safely.

         b. Oliguria occasionally develops later during the maintenance phase of AIRF.
         c. Oliguria at any time requires meticulous attention to additional fluid infusion to prevent overhydration.
         d. Normal urine output is 1 to 2 mL/kg/hr for animals that are eating and drinking.
         e. Absolute oliguria is urine production of <1.0 mL/kg/hr.
         f. Dehydrated animals are expected to have physiologic oliguria that is transient (i.e., responds to IV fluid infusion).
         g. Urine production of <2 mL/kg/hr in an adequately hydrated animal receiving fluid therapy is considered relative oliguria. Urine output of 2 to 5 mL/kg/hr is expected of normal dogs and cats receiving adequate fluid volume expansion.
         h. Oliguria most commonly is encountered in AIRF. Normal urine volume, anuria, and polyuria are encountered in decreasing order of frequency. Nonoliguric AIRF has been increasingly recognized in veterinary medicine, often with aminoglycoside nephrotoxicity.

5. Choice of fluid for rehydration.
   a. Normal saline (0.9% NaCl) usually is the initial fluid of choice for intravascular rehydration because it contains abundant sodium (154 mEq/L) and is devoid of potassium.
   b. When rehydration has been accomplished, hypotonic fluids (0.45% sodium chloride in 2.5% dextrose) usually are provided for maintenance needs in order to prevent hypernatremia.
   c. Potassium supplementation, if required, must be adjusted frequently based on serum potassium concentration.
      (1) Serum potassium concentration depends on urine output, renal excretory function, degree of metabolic acidosis, and oral intake.
      (2) Potassium usually is not supplemented during the initial days of stabilization until renal excretory function has been maximized unless otherwise indicated based on serum potassium concentration.
6. Treatment of hyperkalemia may be necessary.
   a. Electrocardiography (ECG) can be useful in detecting the physiologic effects of hyperkalemia, including bradycardia, prolongation of the P-R interval, widening of the QRS complexes, blunting or absence of P waves (atrial standstill), tenting of T waves, biphasic T waves, sinoventricular rhythm, ventricular fibrillation, and asystole (Figure 3-6).
      (1) ECG abnormalities usually are present when serum potassium concentration exceeds 8 mEq/L, but may be present with potassium concentration of 6 to 8 mEq/L when hyponatremia, hypocalcemia, or severe acidemia also are present.

> **!** Treatment of hyperkalemia may be necessary. ECG can be useful in detecting physiologic effects of hyperkalemia.

      (2) Serum potassium concentrations of 8 to 10 mEq/L are considered dangerous for cardiac function, and concentrations of 10 mEq/L or more are incompatible with life.

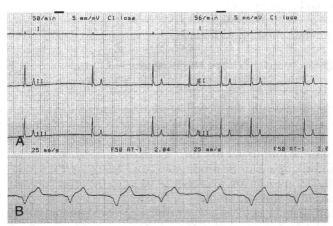

FIGURE 3-6 ■ Manifestations of hyperkalemia on the electrocardiogram. **A,** Note the slow heart rate, absence of P waves, and tall tented T waves typical of advanced hyperkalemia. This ECG was recorded from a dog with a serum potassium concentration of 8.2 mEq/L. **B,** Sinoventricular rhythm indicative of advanced, life-threatening hyperkalemia. The serum potassium concentration in this patient was 8.8 mEq/L. (Courtesy of Dr. Karsten Schober, Columbus, Ohio.)

b. If ECG changes associated with hyperkalemia are present, treatment should be instituted to stabilize cardiac abnormalities.
(1) Sodium bicarbonate at a dosage of 0.5 to 1.0 mEq/kg IV usually is infused first, especially if metabolic acidosis is present.
(2) Alternatively, infusion of 20% to 30% hypertonic glucose can stimulate endogenous release of insulin and translocation of potassium into cells. Glucose infusion may be selected over sodium bicarbonate when total or ionized calcium concentration is low, if seizures are a problem, or if metabolic alkalosis is present. Administration of insulin in combination with hypertonic glucose infusion is controversial.
(3) A 10% calcium gluconate solution (0.5-1.0 mL/kg) can be infused to counteract the effects of potassium on the heart, but does not lower serum potassium concentration. Calcium salts may be beneficial in patients with hypocalcemia, but also may promote mineralization of soft tissues when serum phosphorus concentration is high.
c. The ECG should become normal within minutes of these treatments, but they only provide temporary relief from the effects of hyperkalemia.
d. Maximizing renal excretory function and maintaining serum pH and bicarbonate concentration in the normal range will bring about more prolonged decreases in serum potassium concentration.
e. Chronic hyperkalemia may be treated with an ion exchange resin (sodium polystyrene sulfate, 2 g/kg divided into 3 doses per day and administered orally or as a retention enema) or may require dialysis.
7. Metabolic acidosis may be severe and require treatment during the maintenance phase of AIRF.

❗ Metabolic acidosis may be severe and require treatment during the maintenance phase of AIRF.

a. If blood gas analysis is not available, total CO_2 concentration (<15 mEq/L) can be used to identify metabolic acidosis. Additional alkali should be provided if total CO_2 is <15 mEq/L.
b. To correct metabolic acidosis, sodium bicarbonate (1-6 mEq/kg depending on the severity of acidosis) is added to maintenance fluids that do not contain calcium.
c. The bicarbonate deficit can be calculated from blood gas analysis using the following formula: Bicarbonate required (mEq) = 0.3 × Body weight (kg) × base deficit. This method requires use of serial measurements of blood gases and additional alkali are administered as needed.
d. Hypernatremia, hyperosmolality, metabolic alkalosis, ionized hypocalcemia with resultant seizures, and paradoxical cerebrospinal fluid acidosis are potential complications of alkali therapy.
8. Hyponatremia or hypocalcemia may require specific treatment during the maintenance phase, especially if accompanied by seizures or progressive dementia.
9. Control of serum phosphorus concentration.
a. Hyperphosphatemia frequently occurs and may be severe during the maintenance phase of AIRF.
b. Hyperphosphatemia may contribute to worsening of renal lesions and excretory function by several mechanisms including renal mineralization, direct nephrotoxicity, and vasoconstriction.
c. Hyperphosphatemia contributes to metabolic acidosis and serum ionized hypocalcemia.
d. Intestinal phosphate binders may be used in patients with AIRF.

(1) Phosphate binders should be given with food if possible.

(2) Intestinal phosphate binders may lower serum phosphorus concentration to some degree even in anorexic patients by binding with phosphorus in gastrointestinal secretions.

(3) Aluminum hydroxide gel and aluminum carbonate gel at 30 to 90 mg/kg/day in divided doses most often are recommended. The dosage should be modified according to the results of serial serum phosphorus measurements.

(4) Excessive administration of aluminum-containing phosphate binders may result in aluminum toxicity, which is manifested as dementia that may be difficult to distinguish from the effects of uremia.

10. Conversion from oliguria to nonoliguria.

   a. In some reports in the human medical literature, AIRF patients who received diuretics faired more poorly than those not treated with diuretics.

   b. Diuretics are recommended to convert oliguria to nonoliguria after rehydration and body weight gain.

   c. It is easier to manage nonoliguric patients because hyperkalemia and overhydration are less likely to occur, and the severity of retention of nitrogenous waste products may be less.

   d. Patients that remain oliguric despite diuretic therapy have a poor prognosis because of limited access to dialysis in veterinary practice.

   e. Decreased renin release and inhibition of glomerulotubular feedback are desirable effects of some diuretics used for treatment of AIRF.

   f. Reduced transport of sodium across damaged tubules after diuretic therapy may limit damage to sublethally injured tubular cells, especially those located in areas of relative hypoxia (e.g., outer medulla, pars recta, thick ascending limb of Henle's loop).

   g. Most often, conversion to nonoliguria occurs without a detectable increase in glomerular filtration, as typified by an increase in urine volume with no concomitant decrease in BUN and serum creatinine concentrations.

   h. To prevent dehydration and additional renal injury, it is important to replace excessive fluid losses in patients that respond vigorously with increased urine volume after diuretic administration.

   i. Types of diuretics and sites of action.

      (1) Osmotic diuretics. Osmotic diuretics are freely filtered, low–molecular-weight substances that undergo little or no reabsorption (i.e., nonreabsorbable solute). The increased osmolality of plasma, glomerular filtrate, and tubular fluid obligates water excretion and lowering of the concentration gradient for luminal sodium entry.

        (a) Mannitol.

❗ Do not administer mannitol if the patient is already overhydrated.

          (i) 10%, 15%, and 20% solutions are available commercially.

          (ii) Administered intravenously at a dosage of 0.25 to 0.50 g/kg and repeated once if no increase in urine volume is observed within 30 to 60 minutes. Do not exceed a total daily dose of 2 g/kg due to possible adverse effects on the nervous system and possible development of renal lesions.

          (iii) Once filtered, exerts its osmotic effect throughout the nephron.

          (iv) Effects exceed those observed with isotonic volume expansion (e.g., 0.9% NaCl) and are more potent than those achieved with hypertonic dextrose.

(•) Free radical scavenging.
(•) Attenuation of renal tubular mitochondrial calcium accumulation.
(•) Reduction of renal edema.
(•) Enhanced atrial natriuretic peptide (ANP) release.
(•) Decreased renin release.
(v) Adverse effects include volume overload and hyperosmolality, especially if not immediately filtered (e.g., congestive heart failure, primary renal disease).
(b) Glucose.
(i) A 10% or 20% solution is administered intravenously.
(ii) As its reabsorptive T_{Max} is exceeded, glucose acts as a nonreabsorbable solute.
(2) Benzothiadiazides and related agents (i.e., thiazides) generally are not potent enough for use in AIRF patients.
(3) Loop diuretics.
(a) Most important and most widely used diuretics in AIRF patients (e.g., furosemide).

> ! The most widely used diuretics in AIRF patients are loop diuretics (e.g., furosemide). Potassium-sparing diuretics are contraindicated because of the development of hyperkalemia.

(b) Used intravenously at a dosage of 1 to 2 mg/kg IV followed by an infusion of 1 mg/kg/hr for up to 6 hours in an attempt to convert oliguria to non-oliguria.
(c) If urine output increases, administer a constant rate infusion of 0.1 mg/kg/hr furosemide or administer higher intermittent doses as necessary to maintain urine output.
(d) If urine output does not increase, discontinue furosemide or consider adding dopamine.
(e) Peak diuresis is much greater than that achieved with other diuretics in normal animals.
(f) Major site of action is the thick ascending limb of Henle's loop.
(i) Inhibits co-transport of sodium along luminal surfaces.
(ii) Reduces renal vascular resistance and increases renal blood flow, but not as much as it increases GFR.
(iii) Impairment of tubuloglomerular feedback by furosemide may be beneficial if impaired sodium reabsorption has activated renal vasoconstriction.
(g) Furosemide must be secreted by the proximal tubular cells to enter tubular fluid and exert its effect in the thick ascending limb Henle's loop.
(h) Severe proximal tubular injury may limit secretion of furosemide into tubular fluid. Toxicity may include:
(i) Metabolic alkalosis.
(ii) Dehydration.
(iii) Deafness (ototoxicity).
(iv) Potentiation of aminoglycoside toxicity (contraindicated in this setting).
(4) Potassium-sparing diuretics are contraindicated in AIRF patients due to their propensity to cause hyperkalemia.
(5) Dopamine.
(a) Dopaminergic receptors are found in renal cortical vasculature and renal tubules. Cats originally were thought to lack dopaminergic receptors in their renal vasculature but recent reports have documented their presence. Diuresis in normal cats previously had been attributed to effects on tubular receptors and increased

cardiac output. RBF is increased in dogs due primarily to efferent arteriolar dilatation.
- (b) Only available for intravenous use.
- (c) Increases RBF and occasionally GFR in normal animals.
  - (i) This effect is seen only at low dosages (<10 µg/kg/min).
  - (ii) At high dosages, dopamine causes vasoconstriction which reduces GFR and RBF.
- (d) Causes natriuresis by blocking sodium reabsorption in the proximal tubules.
- (e) "Renal-dose dopamine" usually is defined as 2-5 µg/kg/min. The effectiveness of "renal-dose dopamine" has never been proven in human or veterinary medicine to be superior to supportive care. Intravenous administration requires dilution of dopamine and an infusion pump to provide accurate delivery of the calculated dose.
- (f) Newer dopaminergic drugs have specific DA-2 receptor effects and do not activate vasoconstrictor receptors and require less constraint of dosage.
  - (i) Fenoldopam and zelandopam are more potent and selective dopamine DA-1 receptor agonists that cause little activation of alpha or beta adrenoreceptors. Much higher doses of these agents can be used to create renal vasodilatation compared with dopamine without the activation of beta or alpha adrenoreceptors that limits the usefulness of higher doses of dopamine.
  - (ii) The use of these dopaminergic agents has not been reported in veterinary patients with AIRF.
- (g) Perform a baseline ECG, and monitor ECG during infusion because dopamine can be arrhythmogenic, especially during dose escalation.
- (h) Serial measurement of blood pressure should be performed to detect activation of adrenoreceptors at higher doses of dopamine.
- (6) Combination diuretic treatment.
  - (a) Mannitol and furosemide.
    - (i) Not specifically studied in veterinary medicine.
    - (ii) Some patients respond to this combination when they have failed both drugs when used separately.
  - (b) Furosemide and dopamine.
    - (i) Potent conversion to from oliguria to nonoliguria in experimental studies in dogs with severe nephrotoxicity.
    - (ii) Our experience indicates this combination may be most effective when other treatments have failed.
11. Atrial natriuretic peptide (ANP).
    - a. ANP causes diuresis, natriuresis, increased GFR, and maintenance of RBF during periods of increased vasoconstriction.
    - b. ANP promotes both vasodilatation of the afferent arteriole and vasoconstriction of the efferent arteriole, which increases GFR independently of RBF.
    - c. ANP also may protect the kidneys independently of its hemodynamic effects because renal tubular cell exfoliation, necrosis, and cast formation are reduced and ATP regeneration is enhanced.
    - d. ANP exerts beneficial effects immediately after ischemia and also during established postischemic ARF in which sustained increases in GFR and tubular function may occur.
    - e. ANP prevented radiocontrast-induced renal vasoconstriction in a study of dogs and proved beneficial in models of ischemic and nephrotoxic ARF. ANP also has been shown to ameliorate the effects of ischemic injury in dogs.

f. ANP has been used to treat human patients with oliguric AIRF, and it was most beneficial when administered early in the course of the disease.

g. High doses of ANP cause peripheral vasodilatation which can result in systemic hypotension as a limiting factor. A combination of ANP and dopamine may provide the
beneficial effects of ANP without the hypotension.

h. Use of ANP has not been reported in the treatment of dogs or cats with AIRF. Additional study of ANP appears to be warranted based on its potential benefits.

12. Nutritional support.

a. Not proven in veterinary medicine to make a difference in survival of AIRF patients,
but strongly suspected to have a beneficial effect.

b. Provides nutrients and energy for renal healing.

c. Increased insulin release promotes anabolism and decreases catabolism.

d. Initially, nutrition may be provided by a nasogastric tube, but parenteral nutrition may
be necessary in patients with severe uremia and vomiting.

e. Nutritional support should be started as early as possible in the course of AIRF.

13. Control of systemic blood pressure.

a. Control of hypotension is important because the damaged kidneys have lost their
autoregulatory ability, which normally lessens the impact of low renal perfusion pressure. Systemic hypotension may result in additional lethal injury to cells.

b. Systemic hypertension can contribute to worsening of intrarenal lesions and also cause
end-organ damage to the eyes and brain.

c. Hypertension occurs in the majority of dogs with AIRF. In one study, the incidence of
systolic and diastolic hypertension was reported to be 78% and 84%, respectively, in
dogs with AIRF at presentation.

d. Hypertension is defined as systolic blood pressure >150 to 160 mm Hg, diastolic blood
pressure >80 to 90 mm Hg, or both.

e. The presence of hypertension does not appear to be affected by etiology of AIRF,
hydration status, or urine production.

f. Physical examination and clinical monitoring are no substitute for direct or indirect
blood pressure measurements.

g. Some animals with AIRF may have normal systolic blood pressure at presentation, but
progressive increases in blood pressure may occur during intravenous fluid therapy.

h. Hypertensive crisis (i.e., systolic pressure >200 mm Hg, retinal hemorrhage, brain hemorrhage, deterioration in brain function) occurs in some patients with AIRF and requires
immediate and aggressive management (see Chapter 16, Miscellaneous Syndromes).

E. Success of therapy. Improvement in renal function and clinical status is the desired endpoint
of treatment.

1. Decreased BUN, serum creatinine, and serum phosphorus concentrations.
2. Serum potassium concentration stabilized within the normal range.
3. Return of serum bicarbonate concentration into the normal range.
4. Decreased signs of uremia (e.g., less vomiting, increased food intake).
5. Improved body condition score.
6. Return of urine output into the normal range from previous oligoanuria or polyuria.

F. Therapeutic failure.

1. BUN, serum creatinine, and serum phosphorus concentrations fail to decrease despite
adequate fluid therapy and supportive care.
2. Severe hyperkalemia or metabolic acidosis persists during treatment.
3. Severe uremic signs do not resolve to an acceptable level during aggressive treatment.
4. Overhydration develops during fluid therapy.

5. Uremic encephalopathy develops and is unresponsive to treatment.
6. Uremic pneumonitis develops during treatment (rare).
7. Thromboembolism develops as a consequence of multiple intravenous catheters and prolonged recumbency.
8. Severe malnutrition develops.
9. Sepsis develops as a consequence of long-term use of intravenous catheters, urinary catheters, and prolonged recumbency.
10. Aspiration pneumonia develops.
11. Severe anemia develops due to blood loss from gastrointestinal ulcerations.
12. Gastrointestinal ulcers perforate.
13. Bacterial urinary tract infection develops.

G. Dialysis treatment for AIRF.
  1. A discussion of hemodialysis and peritoneal dialysis is beyond the scope of this book.
  2. Dialysis treatment may be the only way for a dog or cat with AIRF to survive the metabolic consequences of advanced uremia, especially in the presence of oliguria or anuria.
  3. The availability of dialysis treatment for dogs and cats is limited to a few treatment centers.
  4. Hemodialysis removes uremic waste products and retained water very efficiently. It is technically demanding, very expensive, and available for dogs and cats only at a limited number of treatment facilities.
  5. Peritoneal dialysis requires less technical expertise, is less expensive, and more widely available than hemodialysis. Peritoneal dialysis is less efficient than hemodialysis for removal of most solutes but still can be very effective in removal of uremic waste products and retained water.
  6. At The Ohio State University Veterinary Teaching Hospital, Columbus, Ohio, peritoneal dialysis (rather than hemodialysis) has been used to perform dialysis treatments of AIRF patients. The Ash Advantage T-Fluted peritoneal dialysis catheter (Medigroup, Inc., Naperville, Ill.) allows more complete drainage of the peritoneal cavity and facilitates performance of peritoneal dialysis (Figure 3-7).

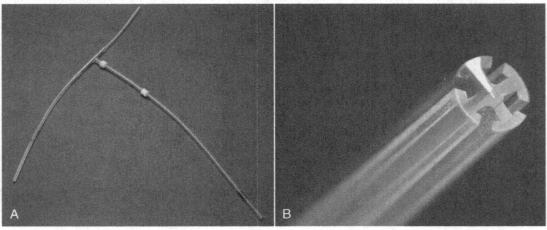

FIGURE 3-7 ■ **A,** Ash Advantage T-Fluted peritoneal dialysis catheter. **B,** Close-up showing troughs in catheter that facilitate fluid outflow.

7. Dialysis should be considered earlier in the clinical course for patients with AIRF in attempts to improve survival. Historically, dialysis has been attempted late in the clinical course of dogs and cats with AIRF when fluid, acid base and electrolyte abnormalities, and azotemia are advanced. Early institution of dialysis in severe AIRF provides greater opportunity for survival and recovery for affected patients.

8. Dialysis should be considered for dogs and cats that have missed the early window of opportunity for antidote treatment of EG intoxication (See Chapter 4, Specific Syndromes Causing Acute Intrinsic Renal Failure) because EG and its metabolites can be removed with short-term dialysis.

9. Short-term dialysis also may be helpful in the management of dogs with AIRF caused leptospirosis that do not improve adequately with standard medical treatment.

PROGNOSIS

Prerenal Acute Renal Failure

1. Prognosis is excellent if the extrarenal cause of renal hypoperfusion is recognized and corrected early enough.

Postrenal Acute Renal Failure

1. Ruptured bladder. Prognosis is good to excellent if recognized and repaired early.
2. Ruptured kidney or ureter. Prognosis is guarded to good.
3. Ruptured urethra. Prognosis is guarded.
4. Urethral obstruction. Prognosis is good if the cause of obstruction can be identified and removed.
5. Ureteral obstruction. Prognosis is guarded.

Acute Intrinsic Renal Failure

1. Oliguria or anuria that persists or develops during treatment is associated with poor to grave prognosis.
2. The underlying cause of AIRF affects prognosis because some causes of AIRF are worse than others.
   a. EG carries a grave prognosis without long-term dialysis.
   b. Leptospirosis carries a fair to good prognosis with appropriate antibiotic treatment and supportive care.
   c. Bacterial pyelonephritis carries a fair prognosis with appropriate long-term antibiotic treatment.
   d. Aminoglycoside nephrotoxicity generally carries a poor prognosis.
   e. NSAID-induced AIRF carries a guarded to poor prognosis.
   f. Easter lily-induced AIRF in cats generally carries a poor to grave prognosis.
   g. Acorn intoxication is reported to carry a grave prognosis.
3. Severity of stable azotemia. Patients with severe unresponsive azotemia are more difficult to manage with conservative medical treatment.
4. Severity of intrarenal damage.

❗ Patients with severe stable azotemia during the maintenance phase of AIRF often are not successfully managed without dialysis.

   a. Renal biopsy can help determine if tubular basement membranes are intact. Intact basement membranes are required as scaffolding for tubular cell repopulation.

b. Renal biopsy can help determine the extent of tubular necrosis and degeneration of renal tubules. Patients with severe necrosis involving all examined tissue have little chance for renal repair and survival.

5. Severity of associated biochemical or hematologic abnormalities and presence of other organ system diseases.
   a. Patients with major alterations in acid-base balance, electrolytes, or hematology are less likely to be successfully managed.
   b. Other organ system disease or failure also detracts from the prognosis (e.g., heart failure, diabetes mellitus, liver disease, pancreatitis, disseminated intravascular coagulation, neoplasia, sepsis).

6. Level of medical care available.
   a. AIRF patients require intensive care and major surveillance. The prognosis is worse if such support is not available.
   b. Availability of dialysis.
      (1) Early institution of hemodialysis has improved survival of AIRF patients at some referral centers.
      (2) Newer peritoneal dialysis techniques may improve survival in AIRF patients.
      (3) Dialysis may be needed for several months in patients with severe AIRF.

7. Severity of initial azotemia predicts survival in some, but not all, studies of AIRF.
   a. In one large series of dogs, death or euthanasia occurred in more than 50%, 24% survived with chronic renal failure, and 19% returned to normal as evaluated by serum creatinine concentration.
   b. In another series, 69% of the dogs died, another 11% were euthanized, and 20% survived.
   c. Chances for survival in dogs were less with varying combinations of serum creatinine >10.0 mg/dL, serum calcium concentration <8.6 mg/dL, packed cell volume (PCV) <33%, proteinuria, EG ingestion, and multiple organ system disorders.
   d. Hyperphosphatemia is associated with decreased survival in some studies but not in others.
   e. In a study of 25 cats with AIRF (most with nephrotoxicity), azotemia did not affect outcome but urine output was a crucial determinant. Mortality was 56% and all of the non-oliguric cats survived whereas none of the oliguric or anuric cats survived.
   f. In a series of dogs with hospital-acquired AIRF, 24% died, 38% were euthanized, and 38% survived.

8. Why are death and euthanasia common outcomes in animals with AIRF?
   a. Many animals are euthanized due to the severity of clinical signs of uremia that do not rapidly improve during initial treatment.
   b. Electrolyte imbalances, acid-base disturbances, uremic solute retention, hormonal dysfunction, and hematologic abnormalities can be severe and difficult to manage simultaneously.
   c. The attending veterinarian and client often have unrealistic expectations for immediate improvement after treatment. In some cases, the maintenance phase of AIRF persists for weeks before renal repair occurs and adequate renal function returns. In other cases, adequate renal function never returns.
   d. The most common causes for death or euthanasia during initial management of AIRF in the maintenance phase are hyperkalemia, metabolic acidosis, and severe azotemia.
   e. Overhydration with resultant pulmonary edema as a consequence of aggressive fluid therapy is another important cause of death or euthanasia.

WHAT DO WE DO?

- Make sure the diagnosis is accurate — definitive diagnosis and treatment must proceed simultaneously.
- Collect serum and urine samples before any treatments are administered.
- Submit serology for infectious diseases such as leptospirosis or borreliosis if appropriate.
- Perform a test for EG or measure serum osmolality, and calculate the osmolal gap to promptly identify and appropriately treat cases of EG poisoning. If there is a reasonable chance there has been exposure to EG within the past 12 to 24 hours, administer 4-methylpyrazole or ethanol as a potential antidote even in absence of definitive information.
- Place an intravenous catheter and rehydrate the patient rapidly (within 6 to 8 hours).
- Place a urinary catheter for the first 24 to 48 hours to measure urine output.
- Adjust fluid prescription orders based on urine output and serum electrolyte concentrations.
- Administer ampicillin initially if AIRF is thought to be associated with leptospirosis.
- Provide optimal fluid volume replacement and mild volume expansion.
- Monitor the patient carefully to avoid overhydration. Adjust fluid volume accordingly.
- Measure arterial blood pressure frequently. Fluctuations between hypotension and severe hypertension may occur.
- Perform renal biopsy early to differentiate AIRF from CRF if necessary, to differentiate nephritis and nephrosis, and to provide a prognosis by determining the extent of intrarenal damage.
- In patients with urine output of <2.0 mL/kg/hr, start diuretics in an attempt to convert oliguria to nonoliguria. If the attempt is successful, continue maintenance diuretics. If the attempt is not successful, discontinue diuretics and closely monitor fluid volume infused.
- Place a peritoneal dialysis catheter if severe azotemia is present and AIRF is likely. Also consider placement of a dialysis catheter if azotemia is increasing markedly despite adequate fluid volume replacement. To improve efficiency, combine renal biopsy with peritoneal dialysis catheter placement.
- Start dialysis early rather than waiting for more advanced uremia to develop.
- Start total parenteral nutrition (TPN) for the first week of hospitalization. It may be needed for 3 to 4 weeks.
- Try to maintain serum phosphorus concentration within the normal range by a combination of fluid therapy and oral phosphate binders to minimize additional renal cell injury.
- Monitor renal function and serum electrolyte concentrations daily for first the several days and then every other day if the patient is relatively stable.
- Remember that, if they occur at all, renal healing and return of normal renal function may take several weeks.
- Treat appropriately for CRF if azotemia resolves to a level compatible with survival. Surviving nephrons may be able to increase their excretory function over time to further minimize retention of nitrogenous wastes.

THOUGHTS FOR THE FUTURE

- Evidence continues to emerge that early hemodialysis improves the chance for survival in veterinary patients with AIRF and regional dialysis centers are becoming available. Even some anuric dogs with EG poisoning can survive with return of nearly normal renal function after 6 to 9 months of hemodialysis.
- Selective dopaminergic agonists that stimulate only DA-2 receptors may provide a potent method to increase renal blood flow and perhaps increase GFR in patients with AIRF.
- ANP may provide potent renoprotective effects in human patients with AIRF. Clinical trials with ANP are warranted in veterinary patients with AIRF.

- Felodopine and other calcium channel blockers may allow greater survival during AIRF.
- More selective and potent dopaminergic agents such as fenoldopam and zelandopam may prove useful in management of AIRF patients.
- Increased use of the Ash Advantage T-fluted peritoneal dialysis catheter appears warranted in veterinary medicine.

SUMMARY TIPS

- Make sure all prerenal azotemia has been resolved by correcting dehydration and optimizing renal perfusion.
- Make sure any postrenal azotemia has been identified and eliminated from consideration.
- Always consider nephritis due to leptospirosis as a treatable cause for AIRF and treat with penicillins early in the course of AIRF.
- If rapid improvement does not occur during the first several hours of fluid therapy or if adequate urine output cannot be determined, place an indwelling urinary catheter. Measurement of urine output provides pivotal information in the decision-making process.
- Weigh the animal at least twice daily during the first few days of treatment to avoid overhydration due to excessive fluid administration or worsening of dehydration due to under-appreciated ongoing losses.
- Consider early referral for renal biopsy and dialysis if substantial improvement does not occur after 2 to 3 days of conventional treatment.

COMMON MISCONCEPTIONS

- Three to 5 days of fluid therapy is enough time to make a decision about the likelihood that AIRF will resolve. This is often not enough time—it may actually take 1 to 3 weeks and, in some instances, months.
- Hyperkalemia only develops in patients with oligoanuria. It is true that hyperkalemia develops more readily in those with oligoanuria, but it can also develop in those with nonoliguria when the GFR has been severely reduced.
- The prognosis for all animals with AIRF is guarded to poor in general. Although the prognosis is guarded to poor in general for those with high level azotemia, surprisingly, some animals will survive.
- It really isn't important to measure urine output. Actually, it is vital to measure urine output especially during the first 48 hours of therapy as this can dramatically change the IV fluid therapy prescription. Without the knowledge of urine output it is easy to underestimate or overestimate the amount of fluids that the patient really needs.
- Diuretic use frequently changes the course of AIRF. There are no placebo-controlled studies to show that any diuretic therapy improves outcome for survival or level of renal function that is achieved. Diuretic therapy can convert patients from oligoanuria to higher levels of urine output. Despite lack of evidence for a salutary effect, we continue to use diuretics for those with severe oliguria or anuria, because patients that produce little urine have a poor chance for survival.
- Nutritional support is needed only after every other option has failed. We do not have any evidence-based outcome studies to show the impact of early or late nutritional support. Despite this, it makes sense to consider early nutritional intervention to provide nutrients that will be needed for renal healing.
- Dialysis does not make a difference in the outcome. Studies in veterinary medicine have shown that early intervention with dialysis improves survival and level of recovery for renal function.
- AIRF is relatively straightforward and predictable. Actually, AIRF is not predictable from one patient to the next, even in those with the same level of initial azotemia. The prognosis can be better established if the cause for the AIRF is known.

FREQUENTLY ASKED QUESTIONS

Q: How long should I wait to see if renal function will return in my patient with AIRF?

A: In patients with reversible AIRF, it may take 1 to 3 weeks of supportive care to allow for sufficient renal healing. The conventional wisdom has been to treat the patient for 3 to 5 days and then to make a decision regarding outcome – this often is not enough time to allow an accurate assessment for the likelihood of renal healing.

Q: Is the prognosis for AIRF in veterinary patients the same regardless of cause?

A: No. Prognosis varies depending on the underlying cause of AIRF as well as the severity of azotemia in the maintenance phase. In patients with EG poisoning, return of adequate renal function frequently does not occur in severely azotemic, oligoanuric animals. Some animals with severe AIRF caused by EG poisoning can survive for many months when treated by hemodialysis. Dogs with leptospirosis and AIRF usually have a good prognosis if treatment is started early.

Q: When should I consider renal biopsy in patients with suspected AIRF?

A: If the diagnosis of AIRF is readily apparent, renal biopsy may be unnecessary. If the diagnosis of AIRF is not clear, renal biopsy is helpful to rule out underlying chronic renal lesions and to document the presence of the acute lesions responsible for AIRF. Sometimes, renal biopsy is useful in providing a prognosis for patients with AIRF that do not improve as quickly as expected. The extent of renal tubular regeneration and fibrosis due to nephron loss are helpful histopathologic features. Distinguishing between AIRF caused by nephrosis or that caused by nephritis can be helpful, especially for patients suspected to have leptospirosis.

Q: When should I consider dialysis in patients with AIRF?

A: Patients with AIRF and rapidly escalating azotemia are more likely to survive and regain renal function when dialysis is started early. Too often, dialysis is not considered until supportive treatment with fluids and diuretics has failed. Dialysis may be the only hope for survival in dogs and cats with AIRF and severe azotemia, anuria, overhydration, hyperkalemia, and metabolic acidosis. Correcting the metabolic derangements of uremia however does not guarantee renal recovery or patient survival.

Q: I measured urine output in a patient with AIRF and it is 0.6 mL/kg/hr despite aggressive intravenous fluid therapy. What should I do now?

A: Normal animals (not receiving intravenous fluids) produce urine at a rate of 1.0 to 2.0 mL/kg/hr. Normal animals on intravenous fluids usually produce urine at a rate of 2.0 to 5.0 mL/kg/hr. Animals with AIRF receiving intravenous fluids that produce urine at rates <2.0 mL/kg/hr are said to have *relative* oliguria whereas those that produce <1.0 mL/kg/hr have *absolute* oliguria. If the patient has been adequately hydrated, a challenge with diuretics can be considered to see if urine output can be increased. Patients that do not produce an adequate volume of urine are more difficult to manage than those that have more urine production. If urine volume remains low despite proper fluid therapy and diuretic challenge, it is important to decrease the daily volume of intravenous fluids to reduce the risk of serious overhydration.

Q: The serum potassium concentration in my AIRF patient has increased from 5.5 to 6.5 mEq/L and then to 7.8 mEq/L over the course of 3 days. The cardiotoxic effects of hyperkalemia are apparent on an electrocardiogram. What should I do now?

A: Potassium supplementation of intravenous fluids should be discontinued immediately. Hyperkalemia can be treated acutely using infusions of alkali, glucose (with or without insulin), or calcium salts, but the effects of these treatments are short-lived if renal excretory function cannot be improved.

Exchange resins administered orally or rectally can be considered for sub-acute management of hyperkalemia with the hope that renal function will return. Ultimately, dialysis may be necessary to prevent death from hyperkalemia. Progressive hyperkalemia unresponsive to treatment is an ominous prognostic sign.

Q: I am concerned about giving gentamicin to a dog that has a resistant urinary tract infection. How should I monitor this patient to detect early renal injury so the drug can be discontinued before development of AIRF?

A: Aminoglycosides can put the patient at risk for development of AIRF, especially if underlying chronic renal disease is present or if the patient is dehydrated. Unfortunately, when AIRF develops, it often does so after the aminoglycoside has been discontinued. Patients given aminoglycosides once daily suffer less renal injury than those treated several times per day. Early signs of toxicity are the appearance of granular or cellular casts in the urine sediment, a finding that can occur before azotemia or other changes on the urinalysis. Measurement of urinary γ-glutamyl transferase (GGT) to urinary creatinine ratio has been shown to be sensitive for recognition of renal injury arising as a consequence of aminoglycoside administration in dogs.

Q: What usually results in the euthanasia of an animal with AIRF?

A: The primary reason for euthanasia of dogs and cats with AIRF is the poor prognosis for survival and high cost of the prolonged care needed to treat these animals. Overhydration, hyperkalemia, and severe metabolic acidosis contribute to death as do sepsis associated with prolonged use of intravenous and urinary catheters.

Suggested Readings

Behrend EN, Grauer GF, Mani I, et al: Hospital-acquired acute renal failure in dogs: 29 cases (1983-1992), *J Am Vet Med Assoc* 208:537–541, 1996.

Chew DJ, Gieg J: Fluid therapy during intrinsic renal failure. In DiBartola SP, editor: *Fluid, electrolyte, and acid-base disorders*, ed 3, St Louis, 2006, Elsevier, pp 518–540.

Grauer GF: Early detection of renal damage and disease in dogs and cats, *Vet Clin North Am Small Anim Pract* 35:581–596, 2005.

Labato MA: Strategies for management of acute renal failure, *Vet Clin North Am Small Anim Pract* 31:1265–1287, 2001.

Stokes JE, Forrester SD: New and unusual causes of acute renal failure in dogs and cats, *Vet Clin North Am Small Anim Pract* 34:909–922, 2004.

Vaden SL: Renal biopsy: Methods and interpretation, *Vet Clin North Am Small Anim Pract* 34:887–908, 2004.

Vaden SL, Levine J, Breitschwerdt EB: A retrospective case-control of acute renal failure in 99 dogs, *J Vet Intern Med* 11:58–64, 1997.

4 Specific Syndromes Causing Acute Intrinsic Renal Failure

Ethylene Glycol (EG) Toxicity

INTRODUCTION AND PATHOPHYSIOLOGY

A. Consumption of EG is an important cause of acute intrinsic renal failure (AIRF) in dogs and cats, and should always be considered in geographic regions and during times of the year in which antifreeze is used. Ingestion usually occurs as a consequence of improper storage or disposal of radiator fluid. It is the most common cause of AIRF in most veterinary practices, depending on the region.

B. EG toxicity is dose dependent.
   1. The minimal lethal dose in dogs is 4.4 to 13.2 mL/kg. Dogs that rapidly ingest large doses of EG frequently vomit, which may limit exposure.
   2. The minimal lethal dose in cats is 1.5 mL/kg.

> **!** Ethylene glycol by itself is not very toxic, but its metabolites are toxic. Toxicity is time- and dose-dependent.

C. Some brands of antifreeze contain propylene glycol as a replacement for EG. Propylene glycol does not cause nephrotoxicity, but its ingestion can be confused with EG intoxication because both increase the osmolal gap, result in positive reactions on the EG Test Kit (PRN Laboratories, Pensacola, Fla.) as well as cause central nervous system (CNS) depression, osmotic diuresis, and metabolic acidosis with increased anion gap.

D. EG is readily ingested by dogs and cats because it is viscid and sweet.

E. EG is readily absorbed from the gastrointestinal (GI) tract within 1 hour after ingestion and achieves peak serum concentrations in dogs and cats 3 hours later. EG remains detectable in the circulation for at least 12 hours, but usually cannot be detected 48 hours after ingestion.
   1. EG rapidly disappears from the circulation due to a combination of renal clearance and metabolism.
   2. EG is rapidly biotransformed into intermediary metabolites (Figure 4-1).
   3. About 50% of EG is excreted unchanged into the urine in animals with normal renal function. Peak concentrations of EG in urine occur approximately 6 hours after ingestion in dogs. Delayed renal clearance may occur in animals with pre-existing renal dysfunction, which may magnify EG toxicity because more conversion to cytotoxic metabolites may occur.

F. Dogs and cats of any age can be poisoned by EG but animals younger than 6 months of age may be less susceptible to permanent renal injury.

G. Unmetabolized EG is not very toxic. CNS depression can arise from hyperosmolality as EG is absorbed from the GI tract. Vomiting, which frequently occurs soon after EG ingestion, may be

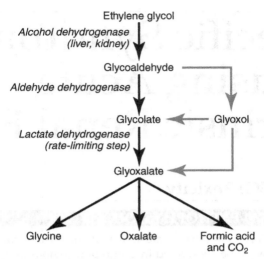

FIGURE 4-1 ■ Metabolic pathways for ethylene glycol conversion to cytotoxic metabolites. The intermediary metabolites cause nearly all of the clinical signs, rather than ethylene glycol or oxalate.

    caused by direct mucosal irritation or may be a due to the rapid increase in plasma osmolality. The polyuria that occurs soon after ingestion of EG is a result of osmotic diuresis.

H. Hepatic metabolism of EG rapidly produces circulating metabolites that are extremely toxic (see Figure 4-1). Renal metabolism of EG may result in local accumulation of nephrotoxic metabolites. The toxic metabolites of EG (in order of decreasing toxicity) are:
1. Glyoxylate.
2. Glycoaldehyde.
3. Glycolate.
4. EG.
5. Oxalate (the direct toxicity of oxalate is limited).

I. Large quantities of acid are produced as EG is metabolized. The resultant metabolic acidosis can be life-threatening.

J. Oxalate crystal accumulation in tissues is a marker of EG poisoning and not a major cause of tissue damage or organ failure.

K. All of the hallmark findings of EG poisoning can be reproduced by the metabolites of EG without oxalate accumulation.

L. The half-life of EG is <12 hours in dogs and <2 to 5 hours in cats; soon after ingestion it metabolizes to its very harmful end products.

M. Cats develop EG toxicity at lower dosages and develop crystalluria and renal failure earlier than do dogs. The metabolism of EG may be more rapid in cats than in dogs, and feline renal tubular cells may be more sensitive to the cytotoxic effects of EG metabolites.

N. The enzyme alcohol dehydrogenase (primarily in the liver) is important in the initial degradation of EG. This enzyme can be inhibited pharmacologically in an attempt to reduce production of toxic metabolites. Alcohol dehydrogenase also is located in the kidney, which may account for local generation of cytotoxic metabolites.

O. Clinically, the syndrome occurs in three phases each affecting a different body system: CNS, cardiopulmonary, and renal. Death can occur during any of these phases.
1. Central nervous system signs can be seen within 30 minutes of ingestion and persist for 12 hours.

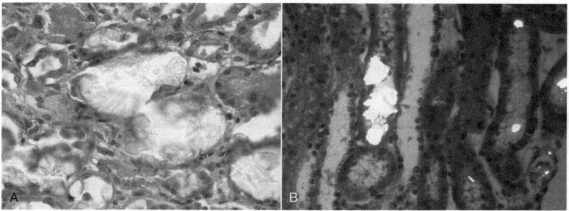

FIGURE 4-2 ■ **A,** Renal histopathology following ethylene glycol poisoning in a dog. **B,** Note the presence of intraluminal crystals that are easily seen under polarizing light (hematoxylin and eosin stain, ×400). (Courtesy of Dr. Steven Weisbrode, The Ohio State University, Columbus, Ohio.)

   a. Clinical signs are attributed to cytotoxic metabolites. Hyperkalemia, hypocalcemia, and metabolic acidosis also may contribute.
   b. Histopathology includes:
      (1) Brain edema and petechiae.
      (2) Vascular engorgement.
      (3) Sterile meningoencephalitis.
      (4) Calcium oxalate crystal accumulation in the brain.
2. Cardiopulmonary signs can develop at a variable time after EG ingestion depending on how much was ingested.
   a. Cardiopulmonary involvement may not be seen as a separate phase and may be obscured by initially severe CNS involvement and developing renal failure.
   b. The mechanisms for development of cardiopulmonary failure are obscure.
   c. Histopathology includes:
      (1) Petechiae of the lungs, pleura, and heart.
      (2) Degenerative changes in the myocardium.
      (3) Pulmonary edema.
      (4) Sterile bronchopneumonia.
      (5) Congestive heart failure.
3. Renal involvement can be detected within hours of EG ingestion, but confirmation of renal failure based on increased serum creatinine and blood urea nitrogen (BUN) concentrations is not apparent until 24 hours after ingestion.
   a. Lack of urinary concentrating ability occurs within 4 to 6 hours after ingestion.
   b. Obvious light microscopic lesions in the kidney are not identified until after 72 hours in some patients (evidence for ultrastructural damage occurs within hours) (Figure 4-2):
      (1) Dilated proximal tubules, due to downstream obstruction of the nephron by calcium oxalate crystals.
      (2) Tubular degeneration and necrosis.
      (3) Intracellular oxalate crystal accumulation.
      (4) Interstitial inflammation.
      (5) Edema.

    c. Nephrotoxicity is largely due to the metabolites of EG. Crystals contribute to tubular obstruction and may disrupt cellular function when deposited intracellularly. Severe pathology and renal dysfunction, however, can occur without any contribution from calcium oxalate crystals.

4. Calcium oxalate crystals may be deposited in blood vessels anywhere and may contribute to clinical signs.

DIAGNOSIS OF ETHYLENE GLYCOL POISONING

Signalment
1. Occurs in both dogs and cats, but is more easily recognized and diagnosed earlier in dogs.
2. Animals of any age may ingest EG.
3. Animals that roam free are more likely to ingest EG, but indoor pets sometimes gain access to it in the house.

History
1. Direct observation of consumption of the toxin may be made before the onset of any clinical signs, but this is not common. When exposure to EG is described by the owner, try to estimate the volume consumed and the time interval from consumption until presentation to your office, because the outcome for EG intoxication is both dose- and time-dependent. Prognosis is directly affected by this knowledge.
2. Owners should specifically be asked about access to EG when an acutely and severely ill dog or cat is presented in late fall or spring in geographical regions in which radiator fluid is used. Questions such as, "Did you or your neighbors recently change radiator fluid?" and "Are open containers of EG kept anywhere on the premises, such as in the garage?" are appropriate.
3. History will vary according to the stage of poisoning observed by the owner and the amount of EG ingested.
   a. Early effects after ingestion (within 6-8 hours).
      (1) CNS effects.
         (a) Inebriation may be the earliest finding. The animal may suddenly appear confused or depressed, with staggering and incoordination due to the direct effects of unmetabolized EG.
         (b) Severe depression or rapid progression to coma ("acute collapse") may occur due to the metabolic effects of EG and the metabolic acidosis associated with its metabolism.
         (c) Seizures may be due to rapid onset of hypocalcemia as the oxalates generated by metabolism of EG chelate calcium.
         (d) Vomiting at this stage may be due directly to CNS effects.
         (e) Sudden death may occur.
      (2) Cardiopulmonary effects.
         (a) Very variable.
         (b) Owners may notice rapid or difficult breathing.
      (3) Urinary effects.
         (a) Polyuria may be noted soon after ingestion of EG due to the osmotic effects of rapid GI absorption of EG and its subsequent filtration through the kidneys, which results in osmotic diuresis. EG (similar to ethanol) also may inhibit antidiuretic hormone, which may contribute to diuresis.

❗ Rapid progression from polyuria to oligoanuria is typical of EG poisoning.

(b) Polyuria may not be observed by the owner if sufficient time has elapsed since ingestion.

(c) Polydipsia can result from a sudden increase in serum osmolality after rapid absorption of EG and stimulation of osmoreceptors in the hypothalamus, an effect that is pronounced in dogs during the first hour after ingestion. Polydipsia can persist beyond this stage because dehydration and volume depletion stimulate water consumption until the animal becomes severely depressed.

b. Later effects after ingestion (12-24 hours or longer) are largely attributable to renal failure and include vomiting, diarrhea, and depression. The animal may appear in pain when picked up or may be reluctant to move because of pain arising from swollen muscles or kidneys.

(1) The initial phase of polyuria may not have been observed.

(2) Urine volume at this later stage usually is severely decreased, often nearly to the point of anuria.

(3) If the renal insult has been mild, normal urine volume or polyuria may continue, but this manifestation is rare.

PHYSICAL EXAMINATION

A. CNS depression to coma.

B. Hypothermia may be severe.

C. Dehydration is common due to polyuria accompanied by anorexia and vomiting, especially if the animal is presented 24 hours or more after ingestion of EG.

D. Signs of cardiopulmonary failure may be present in severely affected animals.

1. Tachypnea, increased bronchovesicular sounds or crackles associated with pulmonary edema or sterile bronchopneumonia.

2. Signs consistent with congestive heart failure, including tachycardia and venous distension.

3. Cyanosis.

E. Palpation of the costovertebral angles may disclose painful kidneys or muscle pain. The kidneys may be swollen or normal in size.

F. Uremic oral ulcers and foul oral odor may be present. A sweet oral odor may be detected immediately after consumption of EG.

G. Seizures may be observed.

H. Occasionally, vomitus and diarrhea may have a metallic, green sheen compatible with ingestion of radiator fluid.

LABORATORY FINDINGS IN ETHYLENE GLYCOL POISONING

A. Abnormalities will be present on urinalysis soon after ingestion of EG (as early as 4 to 6 hours after ingestion).

1. Urine specific gravity is decreased into the isosthenuric range regardless of urine volume.

2. Dipstrip analysis may show positive reactions for protein, blood, and sometimes glucose.

3. Calcium oxalate crystals may be seen on urinary sediment examination.

a. Often noted in experimental studies in animals but reported in <50% of naturally occurring cases.

b. Crystals may be present in the kidneys even if they are not seen in the urine.

c. Oxalate crystals may be observed in the urine of normal dogs and cats as a result of diet, and their presence therefore is not pathognomonic for EG poisoning. Their presence however is supportive of the diagnosis in the appropriate clinical setting.

      d. The physical appearance of oxalate crystals varies from the commonly recognized rectangular or square envelope or "Maltese Cross" configuration (calcium oxalate dihydrate) to the many morphologic forms of calcium oxalate monohydrate that can be more difficult to identify.

    4. Unidentified crystals often are reported from the laboratory in animals with EG poisoning.

      a. These unidentified crystals initially were thought to be hippurate, an alternative pathway metabolite.

      b. These hippurate-like crystals are now known to be forms of calcium oxalate monohydrate.

        (1) They often assume a picket fence appearance.

        (2) They may be observed to have small budding structures on them when examined carefully.

      c. Calcium oxalate monohydrate crystals form more frequently in EG poisoning than do calcium oxalate dihydrate crystals.

    5. Cylindruria may be present.

      a. The presence of epithelial cell casts, mixed cell casts, and granular casts supports a diagnosis of nephrosis from any cause.

      b. Casts also may be absent from the urinary sediment because anuria or severe oliguria may prevent their appearance in urine. Showers of casts may be seen if the patient converts from oliguria to diuresis.

B. Measured urine output.

    1. Very small urine volume is a hallmark of EG poisoning 12 to 24 hours after ingestion of a toxic dose.

    2. Transient polyuria may be observed in peracute cases.

    3. A return to normal urine volume or polyuria can be observed in animals that survive.

    4. Animals that initially had normal urine volume or polyuria can convert to oligoanuria days later.

C. Serum biochemistry.

    1. BUN and serum creatinine concentrations usually are increased by the time clinical signs have developed and the animal is presented to the veterinarian for evaluation.

      a. Some of the azotemia may be prerenal as a consequence of dehydration, but most of it is primary renal azotemia by 12 hours after EG ingestion.

      b. BUN and serum creatinine concentrations are normal in animals that are presented very soon after EG ingestion (within 8 to 12 hours).

      c. Initially normal BUN and serum creatinine concentrations do not accurately reflect the severity of renal injury. Typically, 24 to 48 hours are required before they increase to new steady state abnormal concentrations.

    2. Serum phosphorus concentrations may be disproportionately high compared with BUN and serum creatinine concentrations, possibly due to absorption from the GI tract of phosphate-containing rust inhibitors that are added to some antifreeze formulations. Later, hyperphosphatemia is primarily a consequence of renal failure.

    3. Serum osmolality may be dramatically increased soon after EG ingestion due to the presence of unmetabolized EG.

      a. Measured serum osmolality must be determined by an osmometer and should not be confused with the calculated osmolality that is supplied with serum biochemistry results by many commercial laboratories.

      b. Calculated osmolality (mOsm/kg) may be determined by the following formula: $2(Na + K) + glucose/18 + BUN/2.8$.

c. The difference between measured and calculated serum osmolality has been referred to as the osmolal gap. Normally, calculated serum osmolality is similar to measured serum osmolality and the normal osmolal gap is <10 mOsm/kg.

d. EG is rapidly absorbed from the GI tract into the blood and increases measured serum osmolality. Calculated serum osmolality, however, is unchanged because EG is not a component of the equation for calculated osmolality. Thus, EG ingestion increases the osmolal gap.

e. A high osmolal gap (often >50 mOsm/kg) is common in early EG poisoning in dogs and cats. Values of >100 mOsm/kg are not observed in any other disease in veterinary medicine.

f. In animals treated with ethyl alcohol, this solute also will contribute to serum osmolality measured by freezing point depression osmometry and will contribute to the increased osmolal gap. Ethyl alcohol is a volatile solute and will not contribute to osmolality measured by vapor point elevation osmometry.

g. Treatment with mannitol will increase the osmolal gap.

4. Serum potassium concentration may be increased, and hyperkalemia, if severe, can be life-threatening.

   a. Early in the course of the intoxication, hyperkalemia may occur as a consequence of severe metabolic acidosis associated with EG metabolism.

   b. Hyperkalemia is further exacerbated as renal potassium and net acid excretion are curtailed by AIRF and development of oligoanuria. Hyperkalemia will persist until urine output increases.

5. Serum calcium concentration often is decreased as a result of several factors:

   a. Chelation of calcium from plasma by oxalates.

   b. Deposition of calcium oxalate crystals in tissues (e.g., kidneys, blood vessels).

   c. Loss of calcium oxalate in urine.

   d. As renal failure becomes established, hyperphosphatemia contributes to a reciprocal fall in serum calcium concentration.

   e. Seizures may result from rapid severe decreases in serum ionized calcium concentration.

6. Detection of EG.

   a. Measurements of serum and urine EG concentration are not available from most commercial diagnostic laboratories.

   b. High concentrations of EG in either serum or urine will confirm poisoning. EG however does not persist long, and concentrations may fall below detectable levels before clinical samples are obtained for analysis.

   c. The EGTest Kit is an in-house test kit designed for veterinarians to allow rapid detection of unmetabolized EG.

      (1) A colorimetric reaction based on generation of formaldehyde in the presence of EG will identify concentrations as low as 50 mg/dL.

      (2) False-negative reactions can occur with patient samples obtained <30 minutes or more than 12 hours after ingestion.

      (3) False-positive reactions may occur in the presence of propylene glycol (present in some antifreeze preparations), metaldehyde (present in snail bait), or pharmaceutical products that contain glycerol (e.g., diazepam, phenobarbital, pentobarbital, dexamethasone, activated charcoal).

   d. Samples of urine or vomitus may fluoresce under Wood's lamp illumination due to the presence of fluorescein added to antifreeze to facilitate detection of radiator leaks.

7. Measurement of EG metabolites by chromatography.

    a. Increased concentrations of EG metabolites may be detectable for days after EG has disappeared.

    b. Results of such tests are unlikely to be available quickly enough to allow treatment decisions to be made.

  8. Blood gas analysis may support a diagnosis of EG poisoning.

> **!** The combination of high anion gap and high osmolal gap in a patient with severe metabolic acidosis supports a diagnosis of EG poisoning.

    a. The metabolites of EG result in severe metabolic acidosis early in the course of intoxication (within hours).

    b. Later, as renal failure becomes established, decreased excretion of acid by the kidneys contributes to the acidosis.

    c. Respiratory compensation (hyperventilation) and decreased pCO_2 are expected unless cardiopulmonary complications are present or the animal is comatose.

    d. A high anion gap is supportive of EG intoxication.

      (1) The increased anion gap occurs due to titration of bicarbonate by acid metabolites of EG and accumulation of the associated unmeasured anions (e.g., glycoaldehyde, glyoxylate).

      (2) The largest increase in anion gap occurs early, before renal failure develops. Phosphates and sulfates contribute to the anion gap after renal failure has been established.

      (3) The combination of high anion gap and high osmolal gap in a patient with severe metabolic acidosis supports a diagnosis of acute EG poisoning.

 D. Plain radiographs show normal to slightly enlarged kidneys. Excretory urography is contraindicated.

 E. Ultrasonography may disclose abnormalities soon after EG ingestion (Figure 4-3).

  1. Renal cortical echogenicity is increased by 3 to 4 hours after ingestion in experimental studies in dogs.

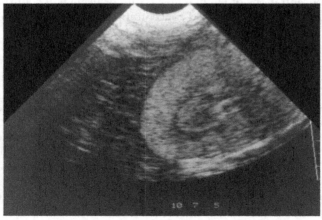

FIGURE 4-3 ■ Renal ultrasonography of dog with ethylene glycol poisoning. Note the extreme hyperechogenicity of the renal cortex which is nearly pathognomonic for this intoxication.

2. Renal medullary echogenicity is increased by 5 hours after ingestion and continues to increase until 8 to 10 hours after ingestion.
3. A *halo* sign at the corticomedullary junction may be associated with anuria.

> **!** An extreme increase in renal cortical echogenicity in normal-sized or enlarged kidneys is typical of EG toxicity.

4. An extreme increase in renal cortical echogenicity in normal-sized or enlarged kidneys is nearly pathognomonic for EG ingestion.
F. Renal biopsy findings vary according to the time interval after ingestion of EG.
   1. Lesions typical of nephrosis are seen.
   2. Intraluminal and intracellular calcium oxalate crystals may be observed under polarized light.
   3. Histologic features of renal tubular regeneration indicate the possibility of renal healing.
   4. When biopsied <72 hours after ingestion, renal lesions may be minimal. Interstitial edema may be noted in some cases.
   5. When biopsied more than 7-10 days after ingestion signs of healing by regeneration or healing by fibrosis and mononuclear cell infiltration may be observed.
   6. Some animals have minimal lesions even when biopsied late in the course of the disease and despite severe excretory failure, suggesting the possibility of an ultrastructural defect.

TREATMENT

> **!** 4-MP is the antidote of choice for EG poisoning in dogs. New protocols for use of 4-MP in cats show promise that it will also become the antidote of choice in cats.

A. The time interval for starting treatment is extremely critical because the half-life of EG is very short.
   1. The prognosis for survival is best when treatment is initiated within 3 hours of ingestion.
   2. Treatment initiated more than 24 hours after ingestion is associated with a grave prognosis.
   3. Treatment for presumptive EG poisoning should be instituted immediately in patients with compatible clinical signs if exposure is possible and ingestion suspected.
      a. If suspicion is high, do not wait for confirmatory evidence that EG has been ingested.
      b. A delay of even a few hours may make the difference between survival and death or euthanasia.
B. Therapy differs according the time that has elapsed between ingestion of EG and presentation to the veterinarian.
   1. Induction of vomiting and gastric lavage should be considered in animals presented within 1 to 2 hours after EG ingestion. These procedures are not considered if the animal is severely depressed or comatose because of increased risk for aspiration. Administration of activated charcoal is of questionable value because EG is not well adsorbed by charcoal. The effect of activated charcoal on adsorption of intermediary metabolites in the intestinal lumen after enterohepatic recirculation is not well known.
   2. Animals presented within 24 hours of probable ingestion should have therapy directed against any further metabolism of EG, measures taken to enhance EG excretion or removal from the body, and supportive measures to help combat metabolic abnormalities already present.

    3. Animals presented more than 24 hours after ingestion are not likely to benefit from therapy aimed at reducing metabolism of EG because most of the parent compound will have already been metabolized. If however EG is still detectable in body fluids, antidote treatment should be employed. Alternatively, supportive measures to combat metabolic disturbances should be carried out.

    4. Comatose or severely obtunded patients may require endotracheal intubation and ventilatory support.

C. Multiple approaches to treatment should be employed to increase the likelihood of survival, especially in animals in the early phases of EG poisoning.

D. Place an indwelling IV catheter. Even if the animal is presented early and does not appear critically ill, an IV line still should be placed because these patients can deteriorate rapidly and an IV catheter is the only reliable way to provide proper management for patients with complicated metabolic disturbances.

E. Administer fluid therapy.

    1. Correct dehydration.

    2. Provide fluids for maintenance needs but be very careful not to overhydrate the animal, because oliguria or anuria often is present or will develop soon after presentation.

F. Monitor urine output using an indwelling urinary catheter.

G. Correct hypocalcemia, as necessary to control tetany or seizures, with infusions of calcium gluconate or calcium chloride.

H. Correct metabolic acidosis immediately.

    1. Severe metabolic acidosis occurs early in the course of EG poisoning and can result in death.

    2. Infuse sodium bicarbonate as needed to correct acidemia, ideally by monitoring serial blood gas determinations.

    3. Ongoing acid production from continued metabolism of EG and acid retention as a consequence of developing renal failure can make the management of metabolic acidosis challenging.

    4. Overzealous alkali administration may contribute to the occurrence of seizures or tetany, especially if the animal is already hypocalcemic due to chelation of calcium by metabolites or as a result of developing uremia.

I. Decrease breakdown of EG to toxic metabolites.

    1. Increased survival of dogs and cats poisoned with EG in experimental studies was demonstrated when early treatment with ethanol was provided. Similar results were demonstrated with 4-methylpyrazole (4-MP; fomepizole) in experimental studies of dogs poisoned with EG.

    2. Both ethanol and 4-MP compete with EG as a substrate for the enzyme alcohol dehydrogenase, thus decreasing its metabolism to toxic compounds. This treatment results in higher plasma concentrations of EG and increased excretion of unchanged EG into urine when renal function is normal. Treatment with ethanol or 4-MP within 24 hours of ingestion is warranted.

    3. Ethanol therapy.

        a. The goal of treatment is to maintain ethanol concentrations high enough to effectively compete with EG as a substrate for alcohol dehydrogenase. The required ethanol concentration will vary with the individual patient and amount of EG ingested. Ethanol concentrations of 100 mg/dL are recommended for efficacy in human medicine but commercial veterinary diagnostic laboratories do not routinely provide this measurement. Ethanol concentrations >60 mg/dL are necessary for effective treatment of cats whereas concentrations as low as 35 mg/dL may provide effective inhibition of EG metabolism in dogs.

b. Never give undiluted ethanol IV because death can occur from acute myocardial depression.

c. The traditional high dose protocol for dogs consists of 5.5 mL/kg of a 20% ethanol solution IV every 4 hours for 5 treatments and then every 6 hours for 4 treatments. This protocol is equivalent to 1.1 g/kg of ethanol given intermittently.

d. Constant rate infusion (CRI) of ethanol after administration of a loading dose is likely to be superior pharmacologically. This method has not been reported in the veterinary literature but it has been used successfully in our hospital:
   (1) 1.1 g/kg loading dose using 20% ethanol.
   (2) 0.30 g/kg/hr ethanol for the first 20 hours.
   (3) 0.20 g/kg/hr ethanol for next 24 hours.

e. The following low dose CRI protocol for dogs is designed to maintain ethanol concentrations of 50 mg/dL using 30% ethanol:
   (1) 1.31 mL/kg loading bolus (300 mg/kg).
   (2) 0.42 mL/kg/hr for 48 hours (100 mg/kg/hr).

f. The dosage of ethanol for cats is 5 mL/kg intraperitoneally using a 20% ethanol solution and given every 6 hours for 4 treatments and then every 8 hours for 4 treatments. Although this regimen was developed in experimental studies of cats, it has been modified for IV use in cats:
   (1) 1.0 g/kg loading bolus.
   (2) 0.17 g/kg/hr for 24 hours.
   (3) 0.12 g/kg/hr for 32 hours.

g. Ethanol can be given orally by the owner in an emergency before departing for a veterinary hospital if the evidence for EG ingestion is conclusive. The dose is 1.0 to 1.4 mL/kg of a 40% (i.e., 80 proof) alcoholic beverage (e.g., vodka). Vomiting may occur after rapid administration of this dose.

h. Disadvantages of ethanol therapy.
   (1) Depressed or comatose animals are given another CNS depressant.
   (2) The ethanol infusion can produce a nearly comatose state for 72 hours.
   (3) Respiratory arrest is common with intermittent bolus treatments.
   (4) Obligatory polyuria follows ethanol treatments and can cause or worsen dehydration.
   (5) Animals that have ingested large quantities of EG may not be completely protected from EG metabolism by this regimen.

4. 4-Methylpyrazole therapy.
   a. Marketed commercially as Antizol-Vet, 4-MP is a specific antidote for EG poisoning if given early enough after ingestion.
   b. Rescue with 4-MP is superior to that achieved with ethanol in dogs and it does not produce CNS depression.
   c. Dosage of 4-MP (the following protocol provides a total dosage of 50 mg/kg):
      (1) 20 mg/kg given at admission.
      (2) 15 mg/kg given 12 hours after admission.
      (3) 10 mg/kg given 24 hours after admission.
      (4) 5 mg/kg given 36 hours after admission if necessary.
   d. 4-MP is less effective in cats than in dogs when at standard dosages. Neither 4-MP nor ethanol rescue is very effective 3 hours after a lethal dose of EG in cats, but ethanol appears to be superior to 4-MP.
   e. Preliminary studies indicate that higher dosages of 4-MP can be given to safely and effectively inhibit alcohol dehydrogenase in cats:
      (1) 125 mg/kg initially, followed by 31 mg/kg 12, 24, and 36 hours later.

             (2) Mild sedation is an adverse effect.

             (3) AIRF was prevented in cats when 4-MP was given within 3 hours of EG ingestion.

      f. Provide supplemental thiamine and pyridoxine to encourage metabolism to less harmful intermediates by alternate metabolic pathways. The value of this theoretical treatment has not been proven.

      g. Administer ethanol or 4-MP until EG is no longer detectable (negative EG TestKit result or normal osmolal gap).

J. Induce diuresis with IV fluids and some combination of furosemide, mannitol, and dopamine.

  1. Increasing or maintaining glomerular filtration rate (GFR) will facilitate renal excretion of EG and its metabolites.

  2. Mannitol may be the diuretic of choice before anuria has become established because of its superior effects on renal edema. Mannitol will be detected when serum osmolality is measured using either freezing point depression or vapor point elevation osmometry.

  3. If oxalate crystalluria was present initially, diuresis should be continued until it disappears.

  4. Diuresis should be attempted even if the animal has been presented long after ingestion of EG.

      a. Diuresis at this time does nothing to enhance excretion of EG because it has already been metabolized but may enhance excretion of metabolites.

      b. Successful conversion of oligoanuria to polyuria will facilitate patient management including fluid therapy and treatment of hyperkalemia and metabolic acidosis.

K. Eliminate EG from the body.

  1. Maintain diuresis to promote excretion in urine.

  2. Induce emesis if ingestion of EG has occurred recently and the patient does not have CNS depression or coma (i.e., high risk of aspiration).

  3. Administer an aqueous slurry of activated charcoal (5 g/kg) via stomach tube if the animal is not severely depressed. Otherwise the risk for aspiration increases.

      a. Some EG still in the lumen of the GI tract may be adsorbed and no longer available for absorption.

      b. EG may undergo some enterohepatic circulation and be bound by charcoal even after it was initially absorbed into the body.

      c. Improved survival has been reported in dogs with experimental EG poisoning when activated charcoal was added to standard therapy consisting of bicarbonate, ethanol, and fluids.

      d. Commercially available activated charcoal may contain propylene glycol and glycerol. Absorption of these vehicles can increase measured serum osmolality and osmolal gap, and cause confusion in the diagnosis of EG intoxication. A positive test result on the EG test kit can result from the propylene glycol.

  4. Dialysis is beneficial in removing EG and its toxic metabolites.

      a. Consider temporary peritoneal dialysis for several exchanges of peritoneal fluid. Dialysis may be necessary for <24 hours if started early enough.

      b. Long-term dialysis may be helpful or necessary if severe oliguria or anuria is present.

      c. Long-term dialysis can result in recovery from EG nephrotoxicity but dialysis may be necessary for an inordinately long period of time (6 to 9 months).

      d. Short-term hemodialysis removes both EG and toxic metabolites and may allow survival by decreasing nephrotoxicity after EG metabolism.

e. Long-term dialysis may be helpful or necessary to adequately manage animals with EG intoxication. Overhydration, hyperkalemia, severe metabolic acidosis, and retention of uremic toxins not manageable by conventional medical therapy will require dialysis if the patient is to have a chance for survival.

PROGNOSIS FOR PREVENTION OF ACUTE INTRINSIC RENAL FAILURE FROM ETHYLENE GLYCOL POISONING

A. Ultimately depends on the amount of EG consumed and the time from ingestion until definitive therapy is started.
B. Survival was 12% in one large study of dogs and cats with EG poisoning. Half of the survivors were nonazotemic animals treated <12 hours after EG ingestion whereas the other half were in renal failure but all were younger than 6 months of age. Thus, young age may be a factor favoring survival.
C. Prognosis for dogs after ingestion of a toxic dose of EG:
1. Excellent if treatment initiated <1 to 5 hours after ingestion.
2. Good if treatment initiated 5 to 8 hours after ingestion.
3. Fair if treatment initiated 8 to 10 hours after ingestion.
4. Poor to grave if treatment initiated more than 10 but <24 hours after ingestion.
5. Grave if treatment initiated more than 24 hours after ingestion.
D. Prognosis for cats after ingestion of a toxic dose of EG:
1. Excellent if treatment initiated up to 1 hour after ingestion.
2. Fair to good if treatment initiated more than 1 but <3 hours after ingestion.
3. Poor if treatment initiated more than 3 hours after ingestion.
E. Prognosis for recovery from intrinsic renal failure.
1. Prognosis should be considered grave if persistent oliguria or anuria characterizes the initial course after IV fluids.
2. Prognosis is grave for animals presented with established AIRF and more than 24 hours after ingestion of EG.
3. Prognosis is grave for any animal that develops progressive azotemia and severe oliguria despite adequate medical therapy, especially if complicated by hyperkalemia, severe metabolic acidosis, or overhydration.
4. Rarely, some dogs will recover from nonoliguric AIRF due to EG intoxication.
5. Survival after EG-induced AIRF is more likely in puppies than in adult dogs.

Leptospirosis

INTRODUCTION

A. Leptospirosis is a common infection in dogs based on serologic evidence of exposure of dogs. Infection in cats does not result in recognized clinical disease, but serologic evidence of exposure exists in cats.
1. Many infected animals do not develop clinical disease.
2. Leptospiral organisms are thin, coil-shaped, gram-negative, aerobic, and microaerophilic. Pathogenic strains are classified as *Leptospira interrogans* or *L. kirschneri* with at least 8 serovars in dogs and cats.
3. Classically, clinically relevant infections have been attributed to serovars *L. canicola* and *L. icterohemorrhagiae*.

4. Recently, clinical cases have most often been associated with infection by serovars *L. pomona* or *L. grippotyphosa*. Serovars *L. bratislava*, *L. australis*, and others may be the causative agent depending on locale.
5. Diagnosis of leptospirosis has been increasingly made at veterinary teaching hospitals and diagnostic laboratories throughout the world over the past two decades.
6. Infection with specific serovars varies by geographic location:
   a. In California, *L. pomona* and *L. bratislava* are most common.
   b. In New Jersey and Michigan, *L. pomona*, *L. grippotyphosa*, and *L. autumnalis* are most common and *L. bratislava* is not reported.
   c. In Massachusetts, *L. pomona* and *L. grippotyphosa* are most common.
   d. In upstate New York, *L. pomona* and *L. grippotyphosa* are most common.
   e. In Illinois, *L. grippotyphosa* is most common.
   f. In Ontario, Canada, *L. autumnalis* is most common, but *L. bratislava*, *L. grippotyphosa*, and *L. pomona* also occur.
   g. In Italy, *L. bratislava* and *L. icterohaemorrhagiae* have been most common but *L. australis* has been recently described.
B. Hosts that have adapted to leptospiral serovars act as a reservoir for maintenance of the infection. Clinical signs either are mild or inapparent in adapted hosts. Clinical signs are more severe in animals that are not adapted to the infecting serovar (Table 4-1).
C. Source of leptospiral transmission and pathogenesis.
   1. Sources of leptospiral organisms.
      a. Leptospiral organisms don't replicate outside of the host.
      b. The urine of infected animals can contain 10^5 organisms/mL.
      c. Shedding occurs in the urine of asymptomatic carriers and convalescent patients.
      d. Greater shedding of organisms occurs in hosts that have been adapted to the organism.
      e. Leptospiral organisms that are shed into water can survive for extended periods of time.
   2. Initially, the organism enters the host by:
      a. Conjunctival, nasopharyngeal, oral, esophageal, or genital mucous membranes.
      b. Physical contact, ingestion, venereal, or transplacental transmission.
      c. Urinary contamination of water, sewage, or food.
   3. The virulence of the various leptospiral serovars is influenced by several factors.
      a. Type of toxin elaborated (e.g., hemolysins, lipases).
      b. Severity of vasculitis that develops.
      c. Degree of immunologic injury elicited (i.e., the response will be less severe in an adapted host).

■ TABLE 4-1
■ ■ **Leptospiral Organisms and Their Associated Domestic or Wildlife Host**

Serovar	Domestic (Wildlife) Host
L. icterohaemorrhagiae	Dog (rat)
L. canicola	Dog
L. pomona	Cattle, pig (deer, skunk, opossum)
L. hardjo	Cattle
L. grippotyphosa	Cattle, (raccoon, opossum)
L. autumnalis	Mice
L. bratislava	Horse, swine (rat, raccoon, opossum, skunk, vole)
L. bataviae	Dog (rat, mouse)

   4. A seasonal distribution (late summer to fall) occurs and increased rainfall is a risk factor.
D. Clinical manifestations of leptospirosis depend on several factors.
   1. The infecting serovar.
   2. Potency of the strain of serovar.
   3. Age of the dog.
      a. Puppies younger than 3 months of age are particularly susceptible.
   4. Serologic response to previous vaccination (if any). Vaccination against serovars *L. canicola* and *L. icterohaemorrhagiae* decreases the likelihood of clinical disease with these serovars.
   5. Severity of specific organ dysfunction after leptospiremia.
E. Syndromes.
   1. The peracute syndrome is a fulminant form of the disease, most often seen in puppies, that causes septicemia and death.

> ❗ Leptospirosis is the most important inflammatory cause of AIRF in dogs. It is underdiagnosed and often undiagnosed.

   2. The acute systemic syndrome causes septicemia and severe illness with localization of organisms to various organs resulting in:
      a. Vasculitis.
      b. Myositis.
      c. Acute nephritis resulting in azotemia and oliguric AIRF.
      d. Hepatitis.
   3. The subacute syndrome is a less severe form of the disease in which renal failure may be the only obvious clinical manifestation.
      a. Easily confused with chronic renal failure (CRF).
      b. Polydipsia and polyuria may be the only clinical signs.
   4. The chronic renal syndrome is characterized by chronic shedding of organisms in urine after recovery, and its contribution to development of CRF is controversial. Most veterinary nephrologists do not believe infection with leptospiral organisms is a major cause of CRF.

PATHOPHYSIOLOGY

A. Clinical signs are either inapparent or mild in animals that already have high or intermediate titers from previous vaccination against the infecting strain.
B. Organisms initially penetrate mucous membranes, often after the animal drinks contaminated water. (Figure 4-4).
C. Organisms multiply in the bloodstream for up to 7 days after exposure (leptospiremic phase).
D. Organisms are distributed to the tissues after achieving critical numbers in the bloodstream.
E. By 1 week after exposure, organisms often are shed into the urine (leptospiruric phase).
F. Damage to vascular endothelium, liver, and kidney occur. The severity of this damage depends on the virulence of the infecting serovar.
   1. Variably severe vasculitis, hepatitis, and nephritis occur during this stage.
   2. Organisms penetrate blood vessels to enter the renal interstitium and then renal tubular cells and tubular fluid. Mononuclear interstitial inflammation occurs in response to the invading organisms. Interstitial hemorrhage and edema as well as multifocal tubular necrosis may occur as a consequence of ischemia and toxins from the organisms. Defects in excretory renal function and urinary concentrating ability develop at this time.
   3. Chronic hepatitis is a rare complication.

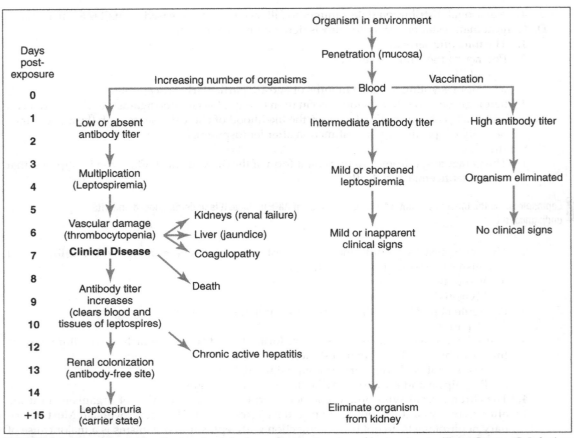

FIGURE 4-4 ■ Pathogenesis of leptospirosis in dogs—leptospiremia and leptospiruria. (From Greene, C: *Infectious disease of the dog and cat,* ed 3, St Louis, 2006, Elsevier, p 405.)

G. During the second week after exposure, antibodies against the infecting serovar are produced and the organisms are cleared from the bloodstream and most tissues except for the kidneys and eyes.
H. Death may occur before an adequate antibody response develops.
I. Due to the absence of antibodies in the kidneys, organisms are not rapidly cleared from the kidneys and a carrier state develops in which the organisms live in the kidneys after recovery from initial nephritis.
J. The carrier state may last for months to years and is much more common than previously appreciated based on recent polymerase chain reaction (PCR) data. The carrier state may arise after clinically obvious illness or after recovery from an inapparent infection.
K. Recovery from leptospiral nephritis may be complete with resolution of azotemia, may progress to CRF due to substantial nephron loss, or may result in death from AIRF.

SIGNALMENT

A. Puppies are more susceptible to experimental infections than are adult dogs.
B. No age predisposition to natural infection is observed when unvaccinated dogs are exposed to a virulent strain of leptospiral organisms.

C. Peak age at diagnosis is very variable and has ranged from 4 to 10 years.
D. German shepherd dogs and German shepherd mixed breeds were over-represented in some studies of infection with serovars *L. pomona* and *L. grippotyphosa*.
E. Increased incidence in male dogs (i.e., male:female ratio of 2:1 to 10:1).

HISTORY

A. Working and herding breeds had increased risk in some studies, whereas companion animals showed decreased risk.
B. Living near or having exposure to wildlife (e.g., recently urbanized areas, exposure to raccoons and opossums) increases risk of exposure.
C. Clinical signs may be non-specific.
   1. Anorexia.
   2. Lethargy.
   3. Vomiting (sepsis and azotemia may be contributory factors).
   4. Diarrhea with or without blood (constipation may precede diarrhea).
   5. Icterus in animals with severe hepatic involvement.
   6. Acholic stools may precede diarrhea in animals with icterus.
   7. Occasional polydipsia and polyuria.
   8. In many cases, clinical signs are minimal and most dogs have mild or inapparent infection.

PHYSICAL EXAMINATION FINDINGS IN SEVERELY AFFECTED DOGS

A. Sepsis-associated findings.
   1. High fever (105° F to 107° F) may progress to hypothermia within 48 hours.
   2. Lethargy.
   3. Weakness.
   4. Congested oral mucous membranes and injected sclera.
B. Normal-sized or enlarged kidneys.
C. Pain.
   1. Renal.
   2. Muscle.
   3. Abdominal pain may be difficult to differentiate from renal pain.
D. Tonsillitis and pharyngitis (petechiae may be seen on tonsils).
E. Icteric mucous membranes (e.g., oral, scleral, penile, vulvar).
F. Findings associated with uremia (e.g., oral ulcers, uremic breath).
G. Urine volume.
   1. Initially, physiologic oliguria (i.e., prerenal) due to dehydration.
   2. Pathologic oliguria due to severe nephritis.
   3. Polyuria during recovery from nephritis.

LABORATORY EVALUATION

A. Hematology findings are compatible with a response to sepsis.
   1. Leukocytosis with left shift.
   2. Absence of anemia early in the course of the disease.
   3. Hemoconcentration as a result of dehydration.
   4. Thrombocytopenia.

B. Coagulation studies.
1. Dogs with severe leptospirosis have been observed to have a tendency to bleed excessively.
2. Thrombocytopenia is noted in some patients early in the course of the disease.
3. Disseminated intravascular coagulation (DIC) is suspected in some patients by the presence of fibrin degradation products. Some serovars (e.g., *L. australis*) are more likely than others to be associated with DIC.
4. One stage prothrombin time (OSPT) and activated partial thromboplastin time (APTT) are normal, and serum fibrinogen concentration is increased.
C. Serum chemistry.
1. Increased BUN and serum creatinine concentrations.
    a. Early increases are due to prerenal azotemia and later increases to both prerenal and primary (intrinsic) renal azotemia.
    b. Hyperphosphatemia occurs with severe decreases in renal function.
2. Hyperkalemia occurs when pathologic oliguria is present.
3. Serum alkaline phosphatase (ALP) activity usually is increased, even in milder cases without icterus.
4. Alanine aminotransferase (ALT) and aspartate aminotransferase (AST) activities are variably increased.
D. Urinalysis findings depend on the extent of renal involvement.
1. Urine specific gravity (USG).
    a. Urine is concentrated early in the clinical course or if renal involvement is minimal.
    b. Urine becomes progressively more dilute as the severity of intrarenal lesions increases.
        (1) Disruption of countercurrent mechanism by inflammatory infiltrates.
        (2) Increased osmotic load in surviving nephrons.
        (3) Decreased urine specific gravity is associated with oliguria during severe nephritis and with diuresis during recovery from nephritis.
        (4) USG is <1.030 in most affected dogs at the time of diagnosis.
2. Dipstrip chemistry.
    a. Proteinuria in most.
    b. Glucosuria in up to 50% or more of affected dogs.

❗ The combination of AIRF with icterus or increased liver enzyme activity suggests leptospirosis.

3. Urinary sediment often is active due to ongoing renal tubular necrosis and inflammation.
    a. Cylindruria occurs in many cases.
        (1) Epithelial cell casts.
        (2) Coarse and finely granular casts.
    b. Renal tubular epithelial cells.
    c. Hematuria.
    d. Pyuria.

DIAGNOSTIC IMAGING

A. Normal-sized to enlarged kidneys are observed on radiographs or ultrasound examination. Enlarged kidneys have been identified in 20% to 50% of affected dogs.
B. Other ultrasonographic findings include hyperechogenicity in 75% of cases, perinephric effusion in 20%, pyelectasia in 50%, and medullary rim sign in 33%. Evidence for renal mineralization occurs in 10% to 20% of cases.

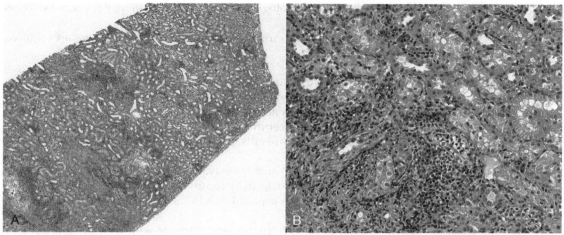

FIGURE 4-5 ■ Renal histopathology—leptospiral nephritis in a dog. Note the intense interstitial infiltration with lymphocytes and plasma cells. **A,** A punch biopsy specimen, magnified 40×. **B,** Image magnified 200×. (Hematoxylin and eosin stain). (Courtesy of Dr. Steven Weisbrode, The Ohio State University, Columbus, Ohio.)

RENAL BIOPSY RESULTS

A. Renal biopsy is useful to ensure the acute nature of the disease process, differentiate nephritis from nephrosis, and evaluate the extent of healing in patients with a protracted clinical course. (Figure 4-5).
B. Variable acute tubular cell degeneration and necrosis.
C. Acute inflammation characterized by lymphoplasmacytic, neutrophilic, and occasionally eosinophilic cellular infiltrates.
D. Rarely, leptospiral organisms can be demonstrated using special stains (e.g., Warthin-Starry silver stain).

LIVER BIOPSY

A. Often not necessary unless clinical (e.g., icterus) and laboratory findings (e.g., increased liver enzyme activity) of liver disease are predominant.
B. A cholestatic pattern with "dissociation of hepatocytes" often is described.

CONFIRMATORY TESTS

A. Demonstration of increasing antibody titer on the microscopic agglutination test using acute and convalescent serum presently is considered the gold standard for diagnosis of leptospirosis.
   1. A fourfold increase in titer is considered diagnostic.
   2. A single very high titer (>1:400, >1:800, or >1:3200 depending on the study) has been considered supportive for the diagnosis of active leptospirosis.
   3. Leptospiral serovar *L. hardjo* is less immunogenic than other strains and lower antibody titers against this serovar may indicate active infection.
   4. Titers against more than one serovar occur commonly because of some cross reactivity of antibodies. The infection typically is attributed to the serovar against which the patient has the highest antibody titer.

B. Demonstration of leptospires by histopathologic evaluation of renal biopsy specimens occurs infrequently.
C. Isolation of leptospires from blood or urine rarely is successful. Special techniques are required and cultures usually are not successful.
D. PCR using urine.
   1. Positive results have been obtained in some but not other studies.
   2. Positive results may occur before seroconversion and thus may be useful in early diagnosis.
   3. The negative predictive value of PCR is nearly 100%.
   4. Based on PCR results, shedding of leptospires in urine may be more common than previously suspected on the basis of serology results, regardless of the animal's apparent health status.
   5. A positive PCR result using currently available assays verifies presence of leptospires, but does not identify the responsible serovar. Quality control for laboratories performing PCR is crucial because contamination by leptospiral DNA in the laboratory can result in false-positive test results.
   6. The potential ability of PCR to identify pathogenic serovars without cross-reactions by nonpathogenic serovars or other bacterial organisms holds promise for early identification of leptospirosis.

TREATMENT

A. Leptospiremia is readily resolved by administration of penicillins (e.g., ampicillin, amoxicillin).
B. Penicillins readily clear leptospires from all organs except the kidney and occasionally the eye.
C. Doxycycline is used to clear the organism from the kidneys and eliminate the carrier state.
D. Traditionally, streptomycin has been used to clear the organism from the kidney and eliminate the carrier state, but it is nephrotoxic (see aminoglycoside nephrotoxicity below) and is no longer available.
E. Supportive treatment with IV fluids to correct dehydration, maintain hydration, and support renal perfusion is essential.
F. Diltiazem administered intravenously, in addition to standard therapy, may improve renal recovery by more rapidly reducing the serum creatinine concentration.
G. Dialysis support may be needed for survival of some patients with severe azotemia and oliguria. Often, <2 weeks of dialysis is required before renal function adequate for survival returns.

❗ Many dogs with AIRF due to leptospirosis recover if promptly treated with penicillins and supportive fluid therapy.

CLINICAL COURSE AND PROGNOSIS

❗ Short-term dialysis may be needed to support some dogs with oliguric AIRF due to leptospirosis.

A. Death may occur from the cumulative effects of systemic disease including nephritis and major damage to other organs.
B. Death also may result from uremia as well as fluid (e.g., overhydration) and electrolyte (e.g., hyperkalemia) imbalances that develop before and during treatment, especially in patients with pathologic oliguria.
C. Prognosis for survival depends on the severity of the systemic illness and whether or not severe liver and renal failure coexist.

D. Acute hepatic and renal lesions can resolve after treatment with penicillins and supportive care (e.g., fluids, peritoneal dialysis).
E. In one large study, more than 80% of dogs with leptospirosis survived.
   1. More than 85% of dogs with severe azotemia treated with hemodialysis survived.
   2. More than 80% of dogs with mild to moderate azotemia survived with conservative medical management.
F. In other studies, 78% to 88% of treated dogs were released from the hospital.
G. In one study, infection with serovar *L. pomona* was associated with more severe azotemia, hyperphosphatemia, and failure to survive.
H. The chronic prognosis for survival and recovery of renal function in dogs with leptospirosis is less clear.
   1. For decades, veterinary clinicians have suspected that some dogs can recover from acute nephritis caused by leptospirosis only to die from CRF a few years later. This suspicion has neither been substantiated nor refuted in the veterinary literature.
   2. In one study, 3 of 15 dogs that survived an acute episode of AIRF caused by leptospirosis died from CRF 10 to 22 months later.
   3. In another study, 8 of 10 of dogs survived AIRF. Two of the 8 had no evidence of renal insufficiency after recovery whereas 6 had varying degree of CRF.
   4. In yet another study, dogs with experimental infections caused by serovars *L. canicola* and *L. icterohemorrhagiae* were followed over a 3-year period. No differences in renal function or renal histopathology were identified between infected and control dogs.
   5. Yet another group of investigators concluded that experimental infection of dogs with serovar *canicola* led to development of CRF over a period of 2 years.
I. Possible reasons dogs that have recovered from leptospiral nephritis may develop CRF include:
   1. Persistence of the organisms in the kidney may elicit a chronic disease response (i.e., inflammation, fibrosis).
   2. Healing of nephritis may have caused permanent loss of many nephrons with subsequent development of hyperfiltration in remnant nephrons and development of progressive renal injury.
J. The prognosis for complete recovery of liver function appears to be excellent for most dogs that survive although chronic active hepatitis has been reported in a kennel of dogs where leptospirosis occurred.

PUBLIC HEALTH SIGNIFICANCE

A. Leptospirosis is a zoonotic disease, and many individuals must be considered.
   1. The owners and their family members.
   2. The veterinarian and the veterinary staff.
B. Good personal hygiene and appropriate precautions (e.g., gloves, masks, goggles) when handling urine are necessary to reduce risk of infection.
C. Risk for transmission of live leptospires in urine is reduced or eliminated after penicillin treatment.

VACCINATION

! Most recent reports attribute canine leptospirosis to serovars *L. pomona* and *L. grippotyphosa.*

A. Traditional bacterins provide protection for a maximal period of 6 months.
B. Protective titers may only last 1 to 3 months in some dogs but cell-mediated immunity lasts longer.

C. The bacterin available for many years was only directed against serovars *L. canicola* and *L. icterohemorrhagiae*.

D. Newer vaccines using subunit technology to isolate antigens protect against serovars *L. canicola, L. grippotyphosa, L. icterohemorrhagiae*, and *L. pomona*.

E. More frequent vaccination should be considered for working or herding dogs, show dogs, and dogs living in environments exposed to raccoons and opossums.

Aminoglycoside (AG) Toxicity

INTRODUCTION

A. Aminoglycoside nephrotoxicity (AGNT) is occasionally reported in dogs and cats, almost always after parenteral use of these drugs, but systemic absorption and nephrotoxicity after topical treatment of open wounds and otitis externa have been suspected in rare cases.

! **All aminoglycosides potentially are nephrotoxic.**

B. The incidence of AGNT is decreasing due to availability of newer potent antibiotics that are not nephrotoxic. Increased awareness and surveillance also have allowed earlier diagnosis and treatment.

C. AGs traditionally have been used to treat resistant gram-negative infections.

D. All AGs potentially are nephrotoxic, the risk of nephrotoxicity varies among different AGs.
1. Neomycin is the most nephrotoxic AG and should never be given systemically.
2. Streptomycin is the least nephrotoxic AG.
3. Tobramycin, netilmicin, and amikacin are less toxic than gentamicin. Gentamicin actually represents a group of compounds, consisting of gentamicins C1, C1a, and C2. Gentamicin C2 has greater nephrotoxicity than the other gentamicins, and gentamicin lots may vary in their nephrotoxic potential depending on how much C2 is present.

PATHOPHYSIOLOGY

A. AGs undergo little metabolism after parenteral administration.

B. They are distributed in the extracellular water with little protein binding.

C. AGs are eliminated from the body predominantly by glomerular filtration with a small but clinically important amount of AG reabsorbed by the tubules.

D. AGs accumulate in renal tissue, especially the renal cortex.

E. After glomerular filtration, AGs are concentrated in the proximal tubular fluid as water and solutes are reabsorbed. Injury to the luminal membranes occurs as AGs bind to the brush border (i.e., microvilli) of the proximal tubular cells.

F. Membrane binding leads to permeability changes that alter transport of solutes and water across the tubular cell membranes.

G. Adsorptive pinocytosis of the bound AG then occurs with subsequent lysosomal processing and resultant intracellular injury (i.e., myeloid body formation and lysosomal enzyme release).

H. AG also can bind to membranes of the distal and collecting duct cells with the potential for nephrogenic diabetes insipidus to develop.

I. In the glomeruli, AG may decrease the size of endothelial fenestrations and decrease glomerular surface area, which may reduce GFR directly, independent of tubular damage.

J. Neonatal puppies (<7 days old) are less susceptible to AG-induced tubular toxicity (i.e., no increases in serum creatinine concentration despite histopathologic evidence of tubular necrosis) compared with older puppies and adult dogs.

K. Fever can increase the volume of distribution of AG throughout the body, which in turn may increase delivery and deposition of AG to renal tissue.

RISK FACTORS

Patient Factors

1. Age (i.e., older animals more susceptible).
2. Obesity.
3. Dehydration increases serum AG concentration by volume contraction and decreased renal clearance. Although GRF is decreased, the higher plasma concentration of AG enables AG entry into tubular fluid and the concentration of AG is further increased in tubular fluid as water is reabsorbed.
4. Hypokalemia and potassium depletion.
5. Pre-existing renal disease increases plasma peak and trough AG concentrations and decreases renal clearance of AG.
6. Liver disease.
7. Metabolic acidosis.

Aminoglycoside Factors

1. Specific AG used.
2. Excessive dose.
3. High plasma trough concentrations of AG.
4. High plasma peak concentrations of AG.
5. More frequent administration of AG during a given day.
6. Longer duration of AG administration over time (e.g., weeks).
7. Prior administration of AG (i.e., AGs persist in renal cortex for months).

Concurrent Medications

1. Other AGs.
2. Cephalosporins, especially cephaloridine.
3. Amphotericin B.
4. Furosemide (especially with volume depletion) enhances renal cortical accumulation of AG.
5. Thiacetarsemide.
6. Cisplatin.
7. Cytotoxic drugs.
8. Nonsteroidal anti-inflammatory drugs.

The Typical Veterinary Patient with Aminoglycoside Nephrotoxicity

1. Has an increased number of risk factors.
2. Has not been monitored closely while receiving AG (or has been monitored only by determination of BUN or serum creatinine concentrations).
3. Develops progressive azotemia (often after the medication has been discontinued).
4. Can be oliguric, nonoliguric or polyuric.
   a. The prognosis is grave for dogs with oliguric AGNT.
   b. Nonoliguric renal failure is expected in 50% to 70% of patients with AGNT and more than 50% fail to survive despite a lack of oliguria.

    c. Humans often recover from AGNT with intense medical support but mean hospitalization is more than one month.

DIAGNOSIS

A. AGNT is characterized by a sudden increase in serum creatinine concentration some time after administration of AG.

B. Serum creatinine concentration continues to increase for several days after initial detection. Mean peak serum creatinine concentration was 10.0 mg/dL (6.2 mg/dL to 21.0 mg/dL) in one clinical study.

C. Hypokalemia may be a prominent feature (60% of dogs in one study had serum potassium concentrations <2.5 mEq/L) but hyperkalemia also may develop (in up to 50% of affected dogs).

> ! AG nephrotoxicity is characterized by a sudden increase in serum creatinine concentration after administration of AG.

D. Urine becomes dilute early in the course of AGNT as a consequence of nephrogenic diabetes insipidus and before the onset of renal failure. The presence of dilute urine does not necessarily mean that renal failure will develop.

E. Casts, small epithelial cells (presumably renal in origin), glucosuria, hematuria, and proteinuria are other urinalysis findings seen in AGNT that can occur before increases in BUN or serum creatinine concentrations occur.

F. The urinary enzyme γ-glutamyl transferase (GGT) is very sensitive in the detection of AG injury to the brush border of the proximal tubular cells.

    1. The ability of urinary enzyme measurements to predict development of renal failure after exposure to AG has yet to be demonstrated in clinical patients.

    2. Urinary enzymes may be excessively sensitive to the effects of AG on the tubular cells (i.e., their appearance in the urine may merely indicate displacement of brush border enzymes as opposed to lethal cellular injury).

    3. The GGT-to-creatinine ratio increased twofold during exposure to normal doses of gentamicin in dogs and a threefold increase in this ratio preceded increases in serum creatinine concentration.

    4. Measurement of other urinary enzymes such as N-acetyl-glucuronidase (NAG) can be useful to determine further extent of acute renal tubular cell injury. NAG is present in tubular cell cytoplasm, and its presence in urine indicates more severe injury.

G. Normal to enlarged kidneys are expected on radiography during early AGNT if the kidneys were normal before exposure to AG.

H. Renal biopsy shows changes typical of nephrosis, predominantly affecting the proximal tubules and no specific findings are pathognomonic for AGNT at the level of light microscopy.

    1. Loss of brush border staining early in AGNT can be demonstrated with periodic acid-Schiff (PAS) staining.

    2. Electron microscopy may show increased numbers of myeloid bodies, but these also are observed in AG-treated animals that do not develop renal failure.

    3. Renal biopsy can be helpful to evaluate the extent of tubular injury and the nature of the healing process. Healing by fibrosis and failure of glomerular filtration to return to an adequate level warrants a poor prognosis.

PREVENTION OF AMINOGLYCOSIDE NEPHROTOXICITY

A. Aminoglycosides should be chosen for antibacterial therapy only when specifically necessary.
B. Rapid correction of volume depletion and maintenance of normal hydration by fluid therapy are essential when AGs are to be administered.
C. Concurrent use of cephalosporins is thought by some to be a risk factor for AGNT and is not recommended, but this is controversial.
D. If at all possible, do not administer any other drug with nephrotoxic potential concurrently with AG.
E. Do not concurrently administer diuretic therapy during AG treatment because furosemide use has been shown to increase gentamicin nephrotoxicity in dogs.
F. Consider administering the total daily dose of AG as a single dose because this approach has been shown to be less nephrotoxic than administering the total daily dose divided into two or three doses throughout the day.

! AG should be used only when specifically indicated.

G. Although limiting duration of treatment will not necessarily prevent AGNT, consider using AG for fewer than 10 days.
H. Consider avoiding AG entirely if the animal is known to have major risk factors for AGNT. As an alternative, choose a third-generation cephalosporin, antipseudomonal penicillin (e.g., ticarcillin, piperacillin), or a carbapenem (e.g., imipenem, meropenem) if indicated.
I. Monitor the animal's serum potassium concentration carefully during AG treatment. Hypokalemia and potassium depletion can develop as a consequence of AG toxicity, but they also can aggravate AG toxicity.
J. Monitor urinalysis frequently and do not depend solely on BUN and serum creatinine concentrations to identify early AGNT. Loss of urinary concentrating ability and appearance of renal tubular or granular casts are early findings that predict progression to renal failure if AG treatment is continued.
K. Adjust the dosage of AG in animals known to have decreased GFR. Dose reduction should be accomplished by interval extension rather than dose reduction. Remember that cachectic animals may have lower serum creatinine concentrations that can lead to overestimation of their level of glomerular filtration.
L. Obese animals should be dosed with AG according to their estimated lean body mass to avoid overdosage.
M. Other experimental methods of renoprotection include dietary protein conditioning (high dietary protein intake before and during administration of AG increases clearance of the drug and reduces nephrotoxicity) as well as supplementation with calcium, magnesium, potassium, and thyroxine. Administration of a thromboxane synthetase inhibitor reduced AGNT in dogs exposed to gentamicin.

! The dosage of AG to be administered to obese dogs should be determined according to estimated lean body weight.

N. AGNT is partially mediated by generation of angiotensin II in some species. Experimentally, inhibition of angiotensin II production may prevent decreases in GFR during AG administration. The clinical usefulness of this approach has not been investigated.
O. AG and verapamil compete for transport across the brush border of the proximal tubular cells via the organic cation transport system. Verapamil or other calcium channel blockers could provide renal protection by this mechanism, but this approach has not been investigated.

Grape or Raisin Toxicity

INTRODUCTION

A. Since 1999, reports of AIRF in dogs after ingestion of grapes or raisins have emerged from various regions of the United States and Great Britain. Toxicity has not been reported in cats, but cats are considered far less likely to eat grapes or raisins than are dogs.

B. Vomiting after ingestion of variable quantities of raisins or grapes (sometimes trivial quantities) occurs in some dogs and is followed by development of AIRF within 48 hours (range 24-72 hours). Lethargy, anorexia, and diarrhea also are common findings.

! Ingestion of small quantities of grapes or raisins can result in AIRF in dogs.

C. Not all dogs that consume grapes or raisins develop clinical signs or AIRF. Some dogs have been observed to consume large quantities of grapes or raisins without ill effects. About 33% of dogs have no clinical signs or azotemia after ingestion of grapes or raisins, 15% develop clinical signs but no azotemia, and 50% develop clinical signs and AIRF.

D. The effect on development of AIRF of chronic ingestion of small numbers of grapes or raisins as compared to acute ingestion of larger quantities has not been studied.

PATHOPHYSIOLOGY

A. Many toxic principles have been proposed to explain grape- or raisin-induced AIRF in dogs including fungicides, herbicides, pesticides, heavy metals, vitamin D, fungus or mold, but thus far no specific cause has been identified. Ochratoxin has been associated with renal failure and may be present in grapes and raisins.

B. The dosages of grapes and raisins known to have caused AIRF range from 3 to 36 g/kg of raisins and from as few as 4 or 5 grapes to 148 g/kg. In a recent study, no association was identified between survival and ingested dose (g/kg).

C. Exposure to a nephrotoxin in the grapes or raisins, renal ischemia (e.g., arising from dehydration), and hypercalcemia are potential factors that could contribute to AIRF.

D. Tubular degeneration and necrosis of varying severity are consistently described, and are most pronounced in the proximal tubules. Tubular basement membranes usually are intact and tubular regeneration is apparent in about 50% of cases.

E. Mild to severe hypercalcemia either is present initially or develops during treatment in more than 50% of affected dogs with AIRF. Why hypercalcemia develops after ingestion of grapes or raisins remains to be determined. Whether hypercalcemia is associated with ionized hypercalcemia, which could damage the kidneys, or with changes in calcium regulatory hormones has not been determined. Other factors that may contribute to changes in serum calcium concentration include changes in extracellular fluid volume and presence of severe hyperphosphatemia (i.e., complexing of calcium with phosphate).

RISK FACTORS

A. Labrador retrievers comprise approximately 40% of reported cases. The reason for this observation is unknown and may reflect breed popularity, a genetic predisposition to a specific nephrotoxicity, or a tendency to eat more grapes and raisins than other breeds of dog.

DIAGNOSIS

A. Affected dogs have a history of recently ingesting grapes (e.g., fresh red or white grapes from stores or vineyards, fermented grapes from wineries) or raisins.

B. Partially digested grapes or raisins may be observed in the dog's vomitus or diarrhea.

C. The typical history is one of acute onset of vomiting with azotemia and AIRF. Median reported initial and peak serum creatinine concentrations have been approximately 10 mg/dL.

D. Median initial and peak serum calcium concentrations typically are only mildly increased, but severe hypercalcemia may occur (i.e., serum total calcium concentration >20 mg/dL).

E. Median initial and peak serum phosphorus concentrations have been >10 mg/dL and sometimes >20 mg/dL.

F. Urine specific gravity is <1.030 in most affected dogs. About half of the affected dogs have mild proteinuria and variable glucosuria. Cylindruria is found in approximately 20% of affected dogs within 72 hours of ingestion.

G. In one study, renal ultrasonography was abnormal in 7 of 13 affected dogs (e.g., renal hyper-echogenicity, renal pelvic dilatation, renomegaly).

H. Moderate to severe renal tubular degeneration is present in renal biopsy specimens, especially affecting the proximal tubules. Mineralization of necrotic epithelial cells or tubular basement membranes is observed in more than 50% of cases. Rarely, an affected dog will lack obvious tubular lesions. Mineralized tubular debris and granular or proteinaceous casts typically are present. Tubular basement membranes are intact, and regeneration of tubular epithelium is observed in 50% of cases. More than 50% of the cases exhibit a golden-brown globular intra-cellular pigment that varies in amount, size, and staining with Prussian blue. The significance of this pigment is unknown.

TREATMENT AND PREVENTION

A. Because of the unpredictability and severity of this toxicity, aggressive treatment is recommended for any dog suspected of having ingested grapes or raisins. Treatment as soon as possible after exposure should include induction of emesis, gastric lavage and administration of activated charcoal, and intravenous fluid therapy for a minimum of 48 hours. Induction of diuresis by fluid therapy and diuretic treatment provides renoprotection by reducing the time renal tubules are exposed to the putative nephrotoxin, dilutes the concentration of the nephrotoxin in tubular fluid, and maintains adequate urine output.

! Aggressive treatment is recommended for any dog suspected of having ingested grapes or raisins.

B. Dialysis may be helpful for dogs with intractable uremia but it does not guarantee survival.

C. Until more is known, clients should be advised not to allow their dogs to eat grapes or raisins.

PROGNOSIS

A. Approximately 50% of dogs with AIRF after grape or raisin ingestion can be expected to survive with treatment. In about two thirds of these survivors, complete resolution of azotemia and full clinical recovery occur. Several weeks of hospitalization with intensive treatment may be needed in those dogs that survive AIRF associated with grape or raisin ingestion.

B. Approximately 50% of dogs with grape- or raisin-associated AIRF will develop persistent oliguria or anuria. At least 75% of these dogs will not survive.

    C. Oligoanuria, ataxia, and weakness were negative prognostic indicators, and dogs that did not survive had higher serum total calcium and potassium concentrations and calcium-phosphorus products at presentation than did dogs that survived.

Lily Toxicity

INTRODUCTION

    A. Ingestion of lilies is highly toxic to cats. The specific toxic principle is unknown but all parts of the lily are toxic to cats. Prognosis for recovery often is poor after lily-induced AIRF.

> **!** Ingestion of lilies is highly toxic to cats.

    B. Three *Lilium* species have caused nephrotoxicosis in cats: Easter lilies, Tiger lilies, and Asiatic hybrid lilies. Other related plants suspected of causing nephrotoxicity include the day lily (*Hemerocallis* spp), early day lily, orange day lily, red lily, rubrum lily, stargazer lily, western lily, and wood lily. The *Lilium* genus contains nearly 100 species and hundreds of hybrids that often are maintained indoors but some are maintained outdoors. The *Hemerocallis* genus has fewer species but thousands of cultivars usually planted outdoors. Fresh cuttings (e.g., stems, leaves, flowers) are also a source for ingestion, and all should be considered potentially toxic.

    C. Calla lily and peace lily are not real lilies and are not associated with AIRF in cats. They do contain oxalates, but stomatitis from the ingestion limits intake so that oxalate nephrosis does not occur. Lily of the valley does not contain a nephrotoxin, but does contain a digitalis-like toxin.

PATHOPHYSIOLOGY

    A. Ingestion of a nephrotoxin present in lilies results in AIRF in cats. Nephrotoxicity has been observed in cats that have chewed only a small portion of a single lily leaf. Aqueous extracts of the flower and leaf from the Easter lily contain the toxic principle, with the flower being more potent. Very small doses of aqueous extracts from the flower portion of the plant are needed to induce clinical signs. The toxic fraction can be identified in urine by high performance liquid chromatography but the actual toxic principle remains unknown.

    B. Lilies are not reported to be toxic for dogs, but it is uncertain if lilies are not toxic to them, as lilies have not been fed to dogs in experimental studies as they have to cats. Dogs do not commonly eat houseplants as do cats. We have observed two dogs that developed AIRF following the ingestion of lily bulbs–both recovered with aggressive treatment.

    C. Between 33% and 50% of cats that ingest lilies will develop AIRF.

        1. Anuric renal failure frequently occurs 18 to 24 hours after exposure.

        2. Experimentally, cats vomit within 3 hours of lily ingestion. Anorexia, lethargy, and polydipsia occur, followed by polyuria that progresses to oliguria and, occasionally, seizures.

        3. Histopathologic changes are seen in the proximal tubules but glomeruli are unaffected. Pyknotic nuclei, swollen mitochondria with disrupted cristae, lipid infiltration, and edema have been described. Ultrastructurally, the most distinctive lesion was the presence of enlarged mitochondria along with loss of apical microvilli, disruption of basement membrane, and interstitial edema. Disruption of the basement membranes was described and may account for failure to recovery in many affected cats.

4. Pancreatic histopathology is observed in some cats and includes moderate, diffuse cytoplasmic vacuolation affecting most cells in the acini. No inflammatory cells are seen, and no changes have been described in the pancreatic islet cells except for the presence of enlarged mitochondria. Pancreatitis has been described in two clinically affected cats at necropsy.

DIAGNOSIS

A. The cat may be observed chewing on lily plants or fragments of the plant may be observed in the cat's vomitus.
B. Hypersalivation and vomiting may occur soon after ingestion of lilies due to local irritant effects on the GI tract.
C. Common clinical findings include vomiting and lethargy 1 to 5 days after plant ingestion.
D. Renomegaly and abdominal pain may be detected on physical examination.
E. Laboratory findings include severe azotemia, isosthenuria, and cylindruria. Serum creatinine concentration often is in the range of 15 to 20 mg/dL when AIRF is diagnosed. Some clinical reports have described a disproportionate increase in serum creatinine concentration as compared with BUN, but BUN and serum creatinine concentrations have increased proportionately in other instances. Occasionally, increases in creatine kinase (CK) are noted.
F. On urinalysis, isosthenuria, proteinuria, glucosuria, cylindruria, and occasionally ketonuria are present but crystalluria is notably absent.
G. Oliguria or anuria may persist despite intravenous fluid therapy.
H. Renal biopsy shows moderate to severe tubular nephrosis characterized by proximal tubular epithelial cell degeneration and necrosis with some interstitial edema. Occasional birefringent crystals that resemble calcium oxalate may be found in the renal tubules. Oxalate crystal accumulation can be a nonspecific finding in cats with either AIRF or CRF. In one clinical study, basement membranes were reported to be intact as compared with an experimental study in which disrupted basement membranes were observed. Mitotic figures also have been observed in renal tubular epithelium, an observation that suggests the possibility of tubular regeneration and recovery from AIRF.

TREATMENT

A. Decontamination combined with fluid diuresis for 48 hours prevents development of AIRF for up to 6 hours after ingestion of lilies. Decontamination 18 hours or more after lily ingestion does not prevent development of AIRF.
B. Induction of vomiting followed by administration of activated charcoal and a cathartic is recommended by the Animal Poison Control Center. Vomiting should not be induced in cats that already are vomiting as a consequence of lily ingestion.
C. No antidote is available to counteract effects of the absorbed nephrotoxin.
D. Aggressive supportive therapy with IV fluids and attempts to maintain or increase urine output with diuretics are recommended in affected cats with AIRF.

! Cats that survive AIRF after lily ingestion typically go on to develop CRF.

E. Dialysis may be necessary to manage complications of uremia or fluid overload. Some cats have survived severe lily-induced AIRF with peritoneal dialysis or hemodialysis.

PROGNOSIS

A. Mortality rate for cats presented in AIRF is 50% to 100%, depending on when treatment is started.
B. Nearly all cats presented early with GI signs alone survive after decontamination and induction of diuresis.
C. Magnitude of azotemia does not predict survival, but urine output does.
   1. Cats with AIRF that are polyuric are more likely to survive.
   2. Cats with AIRF and persistent oliguria or anuria are unlikely to survive.
D. Cats that survive severe AIRF after lily ingestion tend to have substantial permanent loss of renal mass and go on to develop CRF.
E. Pancreatitis may complicate the clinical course in some cats.

Nonsteroidal Anti-Inflammatory Drug (NSAID) Toxicity

INTRODUCTION

A. Accidental ingestion or therapeutic use of NSAID is the most common poisoning by a therapeutic product in dogs and cats. GI upset is the most common effect of NSAID exposure, but AIRF occasionally may occur, and an idiosyncratic hepatotoxicity also may occur in dogs.
B. Cats do not metabolize NSAID as well as dogs due to low glucuronyl transferase activity and are at greater risk to develop adverse reactions to NSAIDs.
C. Clearance rates for NSAIDs vary considerably in normal dogs, and this effect is greater in cats. Some animals demonstrate accelerated clearance and others slow clearance depending on the individual animal or the specific NSAID used.

! Accidental ingestion or therapeutic use of NSAIDs is the most common poisoning by a therapeutic product in dogs and cats.

D. Most cases of AIRF after NSAID ingestion occur as a consequence of improper drug storage. Dogs are more likely than cats to find and consume such medications. Also, some owners administer NSAIDs designated for human use to their dogs or cats without veterinary advice.
E. For unknown reasons, AIRF occasionally results after NSAID administration despite proper usage according to recommended dosages. This outcome is more common in cats than dogs.
F. NSAIDs are increasingly used for treatment of pain before and after surgery. Increased use of NSAIDs is expected to result in increased occurrence of AIRF, especially in animals with specific risk factors.
G. NSAIDs cause AIRF as a result of intrarenal ischemia rather than by direct nephrotoxicity. AIRF can sometimes occur after chronic NSAID exposure if sufficient necrosis of medullary interstitial cells occurs.
H. Nonselective NSAIDs (i.e., no preferential inhibition of cyclooxygenase-2 [COX-2]) include acetaminophen, aspirin, indomethacin, phenylbutazone, banamine, ibuprofen, naproxen, piroxicam, and ketoprofen. COX-2-selective NSAIDs include carprofen, etodolac, meloxicam, deracoxib, and firocoxib.

PATHOPHYSIOLOGY

A. Two well-studied isoforms of cyclooxygenase (COX-1 and COX-2) generate prostanoids and other COX classes also exist. COX-1 historically has been considered the isoform produced by tissues for normal physiological (so-called *housekeeping*) functions (i.e., "constitutive" isoform). Excessive inhibition of COX-1 is associated with gastric ulceration, hepatotoxicity, impaired platelet function, and decreased renal function. COX-2 also functions constitutively in some tissues, and its expression is upregulated in many disease states (i.e., it is inducible), especially inflammatory disease states. Inhibition of COX-2 provides desirable analgesic, anti-inflammatory, and antipyretic effects. COX-2-specific NSAIDs (i.e., COX-1 sparing NSAIDs) have been developed to minimize the adverse effects associated with COX-1 inhibition. The degree of COX-2 selectivity depends on species being treated, dose, and target tissue. The administration of COX-2-selective NSAIDs has decreased the GI adverse effects associated with NSAID use. Presumably, less AIRF also should occur, because fewer animals will experience hypotension from GI bleeding.

B. Local production of prostaglandins in the kidney affects renal blood flow (RBF), intraglomerular pressure, and tubular handling of electrolytes and water as well as providing cytoprotection to medullary interstitial cells. Renal prostaglandins also affect the renin-angiotensin-aldosterone system (RAAS) because they promote renal renin release, especially in patients with volume depletion. Historically, COX-1 was thought to be constitutively expressed and COX-2 to be induced by the presence of inflammation. The production of counter-protective vasodilatory prostaglandins that maintain RBF and GFR when vasoconstrictor signals are present (i.e., effective extracellular volume depletion activates angiotensin-II, epinephrine, and vasopressin) is under control of COX-1. It is now known that both COX-1 and COX-2 are constitutively expressed in the kidney in several locations. In addition to inflammation, COX-2 expression is increased in high renin states (e.g., extracellular fluid volume contraction, systemic hypotension, salt restriction, chronic renal disease, anesthesia, and during administration of angiotensin-converting enzyme [ACE] inhibitors and calcium channel blockers). Whether COX-2-selective NSAIDs exert fewer deleterious effects on the kidney has not yet been established. Because COX-2 is expressed in normal renal tissue, it is likely that any NSAID has the potential to result in AIRF.

C. Most of the dangerous acute effects of NSAIDs on the kidney occur as a result of hemodynamic changes in special circumstances. Either effective extracellular fluid volume depletion or systemic hypotension is necessary to produce AIRF associated with NSAID exposure. In this setting, signals for renal vasoconstriction predominate at a time when the kidney's ability to synthesize protective vasodilatory prostaglandins has been impaired by NSAIDs. NSAIDs can be toxic to medullary interstitial cells, but the relative importance of this toxicity to acute as compared with chronic renal disease is uncertain.

D. GI erosions commonly occur after NSAID use in some dogs. Anorexia, hypodipsia, and bleeding from GI ulcers can lead to decreased effective circulating volume and activation of the RAAS. Thus, renal vasoconstriction can occur at the same time administered NSAIDs are decreasing production of vasodilatory prostaglandins and limiting the kidney's ability to maintain intrarenal perfusion. NSAIDs have minimal effects on intrarenal hemodynamics when effective circulating volume and systemic blood pressure are normal.

E. Short-term administration of NSAIDs to normal dogs for 7 days has no deleterious effect on GFR. Some NSAIDs (e.g., ibuprofen), however, have a narrow margin of safety in dogs with repeated dosing.

F. Administration of meloxicam or carprofen just before or during anesthesia has minimal to no effect on GFR in healthy dogs. Transient azotemia has been observed in some dogs that received ketorolac or ketoprofen during anesthesia for routine ovariohysterectomy.

G. Less is known about the specific effects of NSAIDs on renal function in cats as compared with dogs, but meloxicam or carprofen can be administered safely to most cats during anesthetic induction or in the immediate postoperative period to prevent pain after ovariohysterectomy or onychectomy. Safe protocols for long-term use of NSAIDs in cats have not been developed, but use of meloxicam or ketoprofen for up to 5 days has been reported.

H. Some normal young cats undergoing routine surgery for neutering without administration of IV fluids or monitoring of blood pressure developed AIRF in association with use of NSAIDs (e.g., carprofen, meloxicam, ketoprofen) given at the time of or shortly after surgery. Half of the affected cats survived with return of normal BUN and serum creatinine concentrations after hospitalization and IV fluids for 1 to 5 days.

I. Administration of an NSAID concurrently with furosemide can decrease GFR in dogs by as much as 30%.

J. Based on calls to the Animal Poison Control Center concerning dogs with ibuprofen ingestion, approximately 45% of affected dogs can be expected to develop GI ulceration with hematemesis or melena without progression to AIRF whereas approximately 28% of dogs with ibuprofen exposures developed AIRF.

K. A precise relationship between dose of NSAID and development of AIRF does not exist, but lower doses of ibuprofen result in AIRF in clinical experience in dogs as compared with experimental studies in dogs.

L. Higher dosages of ibuprofen are required to produce AIRF in dogs as compared to dosages that cause GI ulceration.

M. Papillary necrosis was observed in experimental studies in dogs treated with ibuprofen at 50 mg/kg/day for 5 weeks.

RISK FACTORS

! **Avoid NSAIDs in animals with pre-existing chronic renal disease.**

A. NSAID use is most likely to be associated with development of AIRF when the animal is in a clinical situation characterized by dependence on vasodilatory prostaglandins to maintain intrarenal perfusion. Specific risk factors include:
   1. Dehydration and hypotension of any cause.
   2. Anesthesia and relative hypovolemia, especially without IV fluid support.
   3. Pre-existing renal disease.
   4. Overdosage of NSAID.
   5. Access to NSAID prescribed for human or veterinary use.
   6. Chronic NSAID use with sudden development of GI bleeding.
   7. Chronic NSAID use with sudden development of medullary interstitial cell necrosis.
   8. Breed predilection: German shepherd dogs are at increased risk for GI ulceration and AIRF associated with ibuprofen ingestion whereas Labrador retrievers are at decreased risk.
   9. Combination of NSAID with other drugs such as cisplatin, furosemide, ACE inhibitors, or calcium channel blockers. The risk of combining NSAIDs with antihypertensive drugs is not as well known in veterinary medicine as in geriatric human medicine, and in one study there was no change in GFR in dogs treated with enalapril and tepoxalin for 28 days.

DIAGNOSIS

A. Any animal that develops AIRF soon after treatment with or accidental consumption of an NSAID should be considered to have NSAID-associated AIRF until proven otherwise.

B. Some combination of anorexia, vomiting, hematemesis, and melena is likely to be seen early during NSAID toxicity leading to AIRF.

   C. About half of dogs with ibuprofen toxicity are 1 year of age or younger.

   D. No specific laboratory markers predict development of AIRF during chronic NSAID treatment and no specific urinary markers of NSAID-associated AIRF have been evaluated in veterinary patients.

TREATMENT

   A. Induce emesis and administer activated charcoal to prevent further GI absorption if accidental ingestion or acute oral overdosage is recognized within 2 hours.

   B. Administer IV fluids for 48 to 72 hours after acute exposure to NSAID (regardless of dose ingested) if anorexia or vomiting is present.

   C. Vomiting animals should receive nothing per os for 24 to 72 hours.

   D. Sucralfate and the prostaglandin analogue misoprostol should be administered to provide gastroprotection.

PROGNOSIS

   A. The longer the delay between NSAID exposure and treatment, the more unfavorable the outcome for recovery from AIRF.

PREVENTION

   A. High risk patients should be screened by baseline laboratory tests (e.g., complete blood count, serum biochemistry, urinalysis) in addition to routine history and physical examination before NSAID treatment.

   B. Avoid use of NSAIDs in animals known to have pre-existing chronic renal disease because such animals may have impaired ability to synthesize renal vasodilatory prostaglandins. The risk may be greater in patients with established azotemia.

   C. Use the lowest effective dosage of an NSAID.

   D. Do not prescribe more than one NSAID at a time and provide at least one week of washout time after the last dose of one NSAID before beginning treatment with another one.

   E. Do not prescribe NSAIDs concurrently with corticosteroids because of increased risk of GI ulceration and hemorrhage.

   F. Do not prescribe NSAIDs with other potentially nephrotoxic drugs.

   G. Educate clients that over-the-counter NSAIDs can be toxic to dogs and cats. Discuss early signs of NSAID toxicity (e.g., anorexia, vomiting, hematemesis, melena) so that early intervention and treatment can be sought.

   H. Provide IV fluid support intraoperatively when NSAIDs are administered in the peri-operative setting.

   I. Avoid prolonged anesthetic periods for animals being treated with NSAIDs.

   J. Detect and correct dehydration promptly in any patient being treated with NSAIDs.

   K. COX-2-selective NSAIDs may have less association with AIRF, possibly as a result of less GI toxicity. However, use of highly COX-2-selective NSAIDs may be dangerous to the kidney because constitutive functions of COX-2 are excessively inhibited in some patients.

   L. In the future, use of dual cyclooxygenase and lipoxygenase inhibitors such as tepoxalin may decrease the incidence of AIRF as a result of decreased GI toxicity.

Hypercalcemia

INTRODUCTION

A. Hypercalcemia is more likely to be associated with chronic renal injury than AIRF.
B. The toxic effects of calcium on the kidney only occur when serum ionized calcium concentration is increased. Serum ionized calcium concentration is not predictable based on serum total calcium concentration, especially in animals with azotemia.

> **!** The toxic effects of calcium on the kidney only occur when serum ionized calcium concentration is increased.

C. When hypercalcemia is associated with AIRF, hypercalcemia has developed rapidly and serum ionized calcium concentrations usually are very high.
D. The functional effects of hypercalcemia on the kidneys usually are readily reversible, but structural lesions are not completely reversible when advanced (Figure 4-6).
E. Acute azotemia may occur as a result of any cause of ionized hypercalcemia, but is more frequent in patients with hypervitaminosis D (e.g., exposure to cholecalciferol, calcitriol, or calcipotriene).

PATHOPHYSIOLOGY

A. Azotemia caused by hypercalcemia may be due to a combination of factors.
  1. Prerenal azotemia due to decreased extracellular fluid volume (e.g., anorexia, hypodipsia, vomiting, polyuria).
  2. Renal vasoconstriction as a consequence of ionized hypercalcemia.
  3. Decreased glomerular permeability coefficient (i.e., altered ultrafiltration coefficient [Kf]).

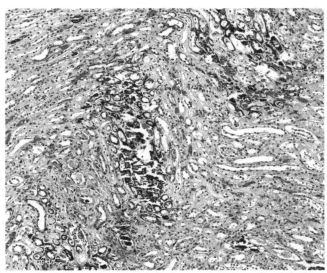

FIGURE 4-6 ■ Renal histopathology– severe mineralization (dark staining of tubules) from acute hypercalcemia and AIRF in medulla (×100). (Courtesy of Dr. Steven Weisbrode, The Ohio State University, Columbus, Ohio.)

  4. Acute tubular necrosis from ischemic and toxic effects of ionized hypercalcemia.
  5. CRF due to nephron loss, nephrocalcinosis, tubulointerstitial inflammation, and interstitial fibrosis.
B. Defective urinary concentrating ability results from a combination of reduced tubular reabsorption of sodium and impaired action of antidiuretic hormone (ADH) on tubular cells of the collecting duct in dogs.
  1. The effect of hypercalcemia on the kidney is a form of nephrogenic diabetes insipidus characterized by hyposthenuria if the diluting segment of the nephron (i.e., medullary thick ascending limb of Henle's loop) is unaffected.
  2. These effects arise from the intrinsic response of the kidney to hypercalcemia and are mediated by calcium-sensing receptors on the renal epithelial cells.
  3. Many cats with ionized hypercalcemia still are able to concentrate to specific gravities of more than 1.030. Why cats differ from dogs and experimentally treated animals in this regard is unknown.
C. Additional direct effects of hypercalcemia on the kidney include reduced tubular calcium reabsorption and antagonism of the actions of parathyroid hormone (PTH). These responses facilitate calcium excretion and ameliorate the clinical effects of hypercalcemia.
D. Renal medullary blood flow is increased in dogs with hypercalcemia and can result in medullary washout, which represents another mechanism contributing to hyposthenuria.
E. Tubular degeneration, interstitial fibrosis, and mineralization of renal tubules, basement membranes, and interstitium may occur secondary to hypercalcemia and contribute to impaired urinary concentrating ability.
F. Renal azotemia during hypercalcemia can be due to functional or structural changes in the kidney.
  1. Hypercalcemia can induce renal vasoconstriction resulting in decreased RBF and GFR.
  2. Reduced RBF and GFR are observed consistently when serum total calcium concentration exceeds 20 mg/dL. More than 50% of dogs have significant reductions in RBF and GFR when serum total calcium concentration is between 15 and 20 mg/dL.
  3. The effects of chronic hypercalcemia on RBF and GFR have not been studied.
G. Hypercalcemia may impair renal autoregulation and result in azotemia early in dehydration because the afferent arteriolar vasodilatation that would normally maintain GFR is inhibited.
H. The toxic effects of ionized hypercalcemia are enhanced by high PTH concentrations in animals with CRF because PTH increases calcium entry into cells.
  1. The ascending limb of Henle's loop and distal convoluted tubule show the earliest structural lesions, but lesions in the collecting ducts ultimately are the most pronounced.
  2. Thickening and mineralization of tubular basement membranes are most apparent in the proximal tubule.
  3. Tubular atrophy, mononuclear cell infiltration, and interstitial fibrosis occur chronically.
  4. Granular and tubular cell casts contribute to intrarenal obstruction.
I. Hypervitaminosis D (cholecalciferol or ergocalciferol) refers to poisoning from vitamin D (e.g., cholecalciferol, ergocalciferol) or its metabolites (e.g., calcitriol, calcipotriene). Vitamin D and its metabolites create hypercalcemia by increasing GI absorption of calcium, increasing bone resorption, and decreasing renal excretion of calcium. Both cholecalciferol and ergocalciferol are metabolized similarly in the dog and cat.
  1. Cholecalciferol poisoning in dogs and cats occurs after accidental ingestion of specific types of rat bait. Toxicity can be observed with ingestion of as little as 10 mg/kg. High risk groups include dogs younger than 9 months and weighing 12 kg or less. Cats appear to be more resistant to the toxic effects of cholecalciferol than are dogs. Recovery from previous cholecalciferol rat bait toxicity can be a risk factor for subsequent occurrence, because removal of the source from the premises may be difficult or impossible. Bluish

discoloration of feces or vomitus may be reported by owners or observed during hospitalization of animals that have ingested formulations of rat bait containing a dye commonly used in cholecalciferol-containing products.

> ❗ **Hypervitaminosis D is a common cause of hypercalcemia-induced AIRF.**

2. Rarely, dietary misformulation can result in hypervitaminosis D and hypercalcemia, but chronic renal injury is more common in these instances.
3. Overdosage with cholecalciferol or ergocalciferol and development of hypercalcemia during treatment of dogs and cats with primary hypoparathyroidism is common because these compounds have a narrow margin of safety and long half-lives that make accurate dosing difficult. AIRF or more commonly CRF may occur as a consequence of excessive vitamin D administration in patients with primary hypoparathyroidism.
4. Excessive use of vitamin supplements that contain vitamin D also may cause hypercalcemia and CRF.

J. Toxicity follows transformation of cholecalciferol to 25(OH)-cholecalciferol, that is 25-hydroxyvitamin D or 25(OH)-D. 25(OH)-D creates hypercalcemia by interacting with vitamin D receptors at pharmacological doses (physiologic concentrations have low binding affinity for the vitamin D receptor). 25(OH)-D is converted to 1,25-dihydroxycholecalciferol (1,25(OH)$_2$-vitamin D or calcitriol). In some instances, calcitriol is generated at higher than normal concentrations and contributes to genesis of hypercalcemia.

1. Cholecalciferol and ergocalciferol are rapidly transformed to 25(OH)-D, which is very lipid soluble. 25(OH)-D can be slowly released from fat depots into the circulation over weeks to months.
2. Activation of vitamin D receptors in the intestine and bone can result in increased serum phosphorus concentrations as well as hypercalcemia.
3. Hypercalcemia develops 24 hours after ingestion and often is severe (i.e., serum total calcium concentrations of 15 to 20 mg/dL). Mild hyperphosphatemia (7 to 8 mg/dL) often also is found simultaneously.
4. Azotemia develops later, usually serum creatinine concentration is < 3 mg/dL unless treatment has been delayed, in which case azotemia may be marked. It may take as long as 72 hours for azotemia to develop as a consequence of renal lesions caused by hypercalcemia.
5. Measurement of serum 25(OH)-D concentration provides conclusive evidence of hypervitaminosis D after exposure to cholecalciferol or ergocalciferol.
   a. Serum concentrations of 25(OH)-D are increased to at least twice the upper limit of normal, sometimes as high as 10 times normal. Serum 25(OH)-D concentration is increased for weeks to months in some cases because the half-life of cholecalciferol is approximately 1 month in dogs (based on experimental studies in dogs).
   b. Serum calcitriol concentration also is increased early in the course of the disorder in some dogs.
6. Death occurs in nearly 50% of dogs after development of hypercalcemia and renal failure in association with hypervitaminosis D if early treatment is not provided. The survival rate is approximately 80% when aggressive treatment is instituted soon after ingestion of a toxic dose. Approximately 80% of the survivors return to normal renal function, whereas 20% survive with development of CRF.

> ❗ **Death occurs in up to 50% of dogs with hypercalcemia-induced AIRF associated with hypervitaminosis D if treatment is not instituted early.**

7. Aggressive treatment with IV fluids (e.g., 0.9% NaCl) and some combination of furosemide, corticosteroids, and calcitonin often is needed for initial control of hypercalcemia. Hypercalcemia can be severe and protracted, and treatment with bisphosphonates often is needed along with a low calcium diet to limit vitamin D-mediated GI absorption of calcium.

K. Acute hypercalcemia can occur if inappropriately high doses of calcitriol are used to control renal secondary hyperparathyroidism in the management of CRF. At recommended dosages of 2.5 to 3.5 ng/kg daily, mild hypercalcemia occasionally may develop, but usually does not result in superimposition of AIRF on underlying CRF. Rarely, severe hypercalcemia can occur after seemingly normal doses of calcitriol because of calcitriol formulation errors.

L. Overdosage with calcitriol sometimes occurs during treatment of primary hypoparathyroidism as attempts are made to increase serum calcium concentrations.

M. Measured serum calcitriol concentration is sometimes normal when excessive administration of calcitriol is the underlying cause of hypercalcemia because, although its biological effects last days, the circulating half-life of calcitriol is hours. Thus, serum calcitriol concentration may or may not be increased, depending on the timing of the sample. Return of serum calcium concentration to normal within 5 to 7 days after discontinuation of calcitriol confirms excessive calcitriol administration as the cause of the hypercalcemia.

N. Ingestion of the toxic house plant *Cestrum diurnum* or day blooming jessamine (which contains calcitriol-like glycosides) is another potential cause of hypercalcemia.

O. Accidental ingestion of topical antipsoriasis creams containing the calcitriol analogue calcipotriol or calcipotriene (e.g., Dovonex) can result in rapid development of severe hypercalcemia, AIRF, and death (even before development of AIRF) in dogs.

1. Dovonex contains 0.005% calcipotriene. It is available in 30, 60, and 100 gram tubes that may be accidentally ingested when stored improperly.

2. In dogs, the estimated minimal toxic dose of calcipotriene is 10 μg/kg, the minimal lethal dose is 65 μg/kg, and the oral median lethal dose (LD50) is between 100 and 150 μg/kg. Ingestion of more than 1.3 grams of Dovonex cream per kg body weight (which represents 65 μg calcipotriene per kg body weight) is considered potentially life threatening. Consequently, it is important to approximate the ingested dose so as to determine an accurate prognosis and provide aggressive treatment.

> ❗ Accidental ingestion of topical antipsoriasis creams containing calcipotriene can rapidly result in hypercalcemia, AIRF, and death.

3. Exposure is more common during months when psoriasis is more severe (i.e., fall and winter in North America).

4. Toxicity is more likely in young and very small dogs because ingestion will be greater on a per-kilogram basis.

5. Approximately 30% of dogs that ingest calcipotriene die and 50% develop AIRF.

6. Hypercalcemia usually does not develop in the first 8 to 12 hours after exposure. Hypercalcemia does develop by 24 hours in all dogs that have ingested a toxic dose. Serum calcium concentration peaks within 48 hours and then begins to decline by 72 hours with appropriate treatment. Depending on when in the course of the toxicity it is measured, serum calcium concentration may have returned to normal and only evidence of AIRF will be present.

7. Serum calcium concentration often is >15 mg/dL at the time of diagnosis and may exceed 20 mg/dL.

8. Hyperphosphatemia is present in more than 75% of affected dogs at the time hypercalcemia is identified. Severe soft tissue mineralization can occur as a consequence of a very high calcium-phosphorus product.

9. The affinity of calcipotriene for the vitamin D receptor is similar to that of calcitriol. Calcipotriene binding to circulating vitamin D binding protein, however, is minimal and considerably more unbound calcipotriene is available for vitamin D receptor binding. This fact accounts for the rapid onset of hypercalcemia and hyperphosphatemia. Limited protein binding in plasma also accounts for the rapid catabolism and short duration of calcemic effect of calcipotriene. The hypercalcemic effect of calcipotriene diminishes after several days similar to what is observed with calcitriol and dissimilar to the prolonged calcemic effect of cholecalciferol (i.e., a week to months).

10. 25(OH)-cholecalciferol concentrations should be normal in dogs that have ingested calcipotriene. Currently, it is unknown if assays for calcitriol cross-react with calcipotriene. If not, serum calcitriol concentrations would be expected to be normal or low in dogs with calcipotriene intoxication.

CLINICAL SIGNS INITIALLY ARE CAUSED BY HYPERCALCEMIA AND LATER BY DEVELOPMENT OF AIRF

A. In dogs, decreased concentrating ability and polyuria are early functional effects of hypercalcemia on the kidneys.
  1. The concentrating defect often is out of proportion to the observed reduction in GFR and increase in BUN and serum creatinine concentrations.
  2. Urine specific gravity consistently is <1.030.
  3. Isosthenuria occurs if the diluting segments have been structurally altered by long-standing hypercalcemia.

! Polyuria and polydipsia are common in dogs with hypercalcemia.

B. Polydipsia develops as compensation for the obligatory polyuria, but there is some evidence that polydipsia can occur as a result of direct stimulation of the thirst center by hypercalcemia.
C. Dehydration is common due to increased fluid losses from vomiting and polyuria.
  1. Initially, extracellular fluid volume contraction decreases GFR and increases BUN and serum creatinine concentrations (i.e., prerenal azotemia).
  2. The clinical principle that dilute urine in association with azotemia indicates primary parenchymal renal disease is not necessarily true in animals with hypercalcemia because the urinary concentrating defect can occur without structural renal lesions. Thus, not all dogs with hypercalcemia, dilute urine, and azotemia have renal parenchymal disease, at least initially.
  3. If hypercalcemia and volume depletion persist, AIRF and renal azotemia develop.
D. Lethargy, weakness, anorexia, and GI signs can occur as a direct consequence of hypercalcemia or secondary to development of AIRF. Systemic signs of AIRF may be difficult or impossible to differentiate from those of hypercalcemia.

DIAGNOSIS

A. Documentation of an acute, moderate to severe increase in serum total calcium concentration before onset of azotemia is evidence that hypercalcemic nephropathy is the cause of AIRF. Serum ionized calcium concentration should be measured. Dogs and cats with CRF often have

increased serum total calcium concentration without an increase in ionized calcium because other calcium fractions (e.g., complexed, protein-bound) account for the increase in serum total calcium concentration.
- B. A potential source of vitamin D intoxication should be carefully sought from the history (e.g., rat bait, vitamin D products, antipsoriasis cream).
- C. Hypervitaminosis D caused by cholecalciferol or ergocalciferol can be confirmed by measurement of serum 25(OH)-D concentration.

TREATMENT

- A. Aggressive IV fluid therapy to correct dehydration, maintain hydration, and enhance renal perfusion and urine output. (Figure 4-7).
- B. Specific measures to lower serum ionized calcium concentration should be provided:
  1. Furosemide enhances calciuresis and has a rapid onset of action.
  2. Corticosteroids reduce serum calcium concentration by effects on bone, intestine, and kidney and they have a relatively prompt onset of action.
  3. Calcitonin decreases the activity of osteoclasts. It has a rapid onset of action but its duration of effect is limited to a few days due to development of tachyphylaxis.
  4. Bisphosphonates (e.g., pamidronate) may not be necessary if hypercalcemia abates with the first few days of treatment. Their use may be indicated if hypercalcemia is severe and persistent.
  5. A low-calcium diet is effective only in hypercalcemia caused by excessive amounts of vitamin D metabolites.

Rapidly Progressive Glomerulonephritis (RPGN) Associated With Borreliosis (Lyme Nephritis)

INTRODUCTION

- A. Glomerulonephritis usually is chronic in domestic animals, and acute glomerulonephritis is rarely recognized.
- B. Borreliosis (Lyme disease) can be associated with chronic glomerulonephritis.
- C. Less commonly, Lyme nephritis can be an acute disease. What appears to be a form of RPGN in dogs has been observed in areas of New Jersey, Pennsylvania, Maryland, Delaware, Connecticut, Vermont, and Minnesota that are endemic for borreliosis.
- D. Nearly all dogs reported to have RPGN have been serologically positive for *Borrelia burgdorferi*, the causative agent of Lyme disease.
- E. The disease has been uniformly progressive and fatal.

! Lyme nephritis is characterized by acute glomerulonephritis and renal tubular necrosis. It is rapidly progressive and fatal.

PATHOPHYSIOLOGY AND RENAL PATHOLOGY

- A. The relationship of positive serology for *B. burgdorferi* to development of RPGN is not clear.
- B. A relationship between vaccination for Lyme disease and development of RPGN has been suggested but not conclusively established.
- C. The cut surface of the kidneys at necropsy often shows pronounced bulging of the medulla. The cortex is smooth and sometimes contains pinpoint red foci.

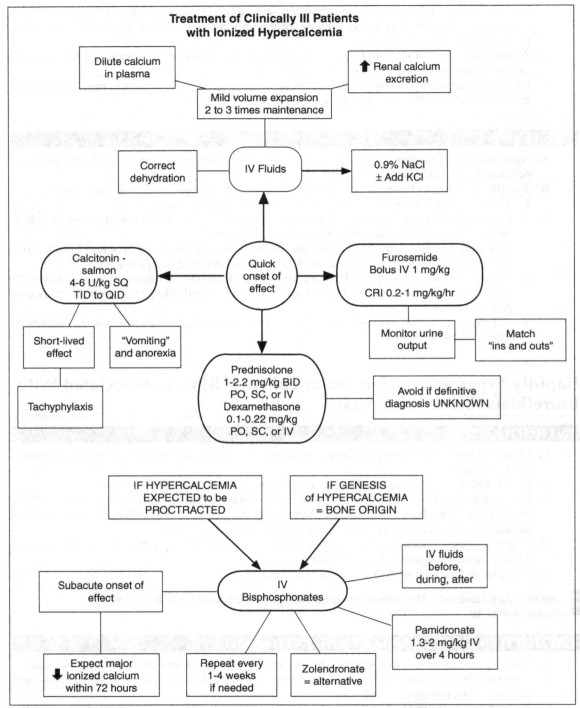

FIGURE 4-7 ■ Algorithm for treatment of severe hypercalcemia.

D. In affected dogs, more than 80% of cortical tubules are affected by severe dilataion, scattered necrosis, and evidence of active epithelial regeneration. Tubular atrophy, interstitial inflammation, and interstitial fibrosis are present but not prominent (Figure 4-8).

E. Membranoproliferative glomerulonephritis with subendothelial deposits of immunoglobulins IgG, IgM, and C3 is observed in more than 80% of cases. Deposits of IgA have not been detected. Membranous glomerulonephritis occurs in approximately 10% of cases and amyloidosis has been reported in an isolated case.

F. Silver staining of renal tissue may identify the presence of small numbers of spirochetes, but this finding is uncommon.

G. Necrosis of the glomerular tuft with influx of neutrophils is observed in some cases and glomerular crescents are seen in about 30% of cases.

H. Periglomerular fibrosis with a lamellar pattern is commonly identified.

I. Fibrinoid necrosis of small to medium-sized renal vessels may develop in some cases.

J. The combination of acute glomerulonephritis and severe cortical tubular necrosis with lack of interstitial inflammation or fibrosis is typical.

HISTORY

A. Clusters of cases occur from early spring through late fall.

B. Young dogs are affected (glomerulonephritis usually affects older dogs).

C. Labrador retrievers and golden retrievers are more commonly affected by *Borrelia*-associated RPGN but also by other forms of glomerulonephritis.

D. Lameness within the past few months is reported in approximately 25% of affected dogs.

E. The acute illness is characterized by a sudden onset of vomiting, anorexia, and polyuria associated with azotemia that increases in magnitude relatively rapidly. A prior history of polyuria and polydipsia usually is not documented.

F. The 6 to 8 week clinical course characterized by sudden onset of systemic illness may be followed by weight loss.

G. Peripheral edema may develop due to vasculitis and hypoproteinemia. Peripheral edema is very common at presentation or develops soon after IV fluid administration. Edema cannot be attributed to the hypoalbuminemia alone in most affected dogs.

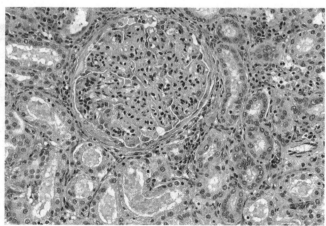

FIGURE 4-8 ■ Renal histopathology—acute Lyme nephritis in a dog. Notice membranoproliferative glomerulonephritis and areas of focal tubular necrosis.

DIAGNOSIS

A. Affected dogs have severe azotemia and hyperphosphatemia due to primary renal disease.
B. Hyperkalemia, hyperglobulinemia, and hyperbilirubinemia may be observed in some cases.
C. Hypoalbuminemia and hypercholesterolemia are present in association with glomerulonephritis.
D. Evidence for hypercoagulability and thromboembolic disease may be documented in some affected dogs.

> **!** Prognosis is poor in Lyme nephritis, and no treatment is known to be effective.

E. Urinalysis shows moderate to severe proteinuria, and may also show hematuria, glucosuria, and cylindruria.
F. Urine protein/creatinine ratio is increased.
G. Urine culture is negative.
H. Renal biopsy reveals the distinctive lesions of RPGN.
I. Systemic hypertension is present in most cases.

TREATMENT

A. No treatment is known to be effective.
B. Azotemia and hypoalbuminemia progressively become worse despite treatment.

PROGNOSIS

A. Affected animals typically die or are euthanized within 1 week of treatment.
B. Some affected dogs survive for up to 3 weeks.

Heatstroke

INTRODUCTION

A. Failure to dissipate heat, increased generation of heat, or both may contribute to rising core body temperature.
B. Clinically, heatstroke may be exercised-induced or may be from exposure to a hot environment.
  1. Extremely high temperatures are not required, and relatively short periods of exercise can create heatstroke in some dogs.
  2. In other dogs, heatstroke may occur due to lack of acclimation to warm temperatures or due to poor ability to dissipate heat.

> **!** Major organ damage occurs when core body temperature exceeds 106° F and is sustained.

C. Multiple organ damage and failure occurs with progressive heat damage. Affected organs and systems include bone marrow, liver, GI tract, brain, coagulation system, heart, muscles, and kidneys. Organ damage is proportional to both the peak core temperature and time that increased body temperature is maintained.

D. In dogs, sustained core body temperatures above 106° F cause major organ damage and death results at core body temperature of 109° F.

E. The temperature inside of vehicles with closed windows and no air conditioning can easily reach or exceed 120° F on hot summer days. Animals should never be left unattended in vehicles on hot days. Other enclosures with poor ventilation and high humidity may also promote development of heatstroke.

F. Dogs confined outside on hot, humid days without access to adequate shade or water also are at increased risk.

G. Approximately 33% of dogs with heatstroke develop AIRF despite aggressive treatment within 2 hours of presentation.

PATHOPHYSIOLOGY

A. More common in dogs than cats; cats have the same risk as do dogs when left unattended in hot vehicles.

B. Most common during hot days with high humidity. Increased humidity reduces the animal's ability to dissipate heat.

C. Belgian Malinois may be especially susceptible to develop heat stroke. Golden retrievers, Labrador retrievers, and brachycephalic breeds (especially English bulldogs) also are at increased risk. Small breed dogs may have decreased risk.

D. Injury from excessive heat occurs as a consequence of direct thermal cytotoxicity as well as a complex cascade of responses to endotoxins, inflammatory cytokines and chemokines, endothelial cell activation, and altered coagulation with microvascular thrombosis.

E. Exposure to heat causes vasodilatation. Decreased cardiac output and poor tissue perfusion arise from effective circulating volume contraction as well as decreased myocardial function and ventricular premature contractions due to heat damage. Fluid losses from hyperventilation, vomiting, and diarrhea also contribute to dehydration and poor renal perfusion.

F. Poor renal perfusion results in ischemic AIRF. The body's attempts to correct systemic vasodilatation may result in intrarenal vasoconstriction and myoglobinuria also may contribute.

G. Tubular necrosis may occur as a direct cytotoxic effect of heat injury.

H. Obesity, long hair coat, laryngeal paralysis, cardiovascular disease, and neurologic disease may not allow for control of adequate heat dissipation and thus increase risk for heatstroke.

CLINICAL SIGNS

A. Panting.

B. Hypersalivation (increases evaporative loss).

> **!** Approximately 33% of dogs with heatstroke develop acute renal failure.

C. Severe thirst.

D. Vomiting.

E. Collapse with inability to rise.

F. Neurologic signs.
   1. Mental dullness.
   2. Confusion.
   3. Stupor.
   4. Coma.
   5. Seizures (rarely).

G. Mucous membranes may be dark or bright red due to systemic vasodilatation.
H. Occasionally, red or brown urine due to myoglobinuria as a consequence of rhabdomyolysis.
I. Hyperthermia. The patient may be normothermic or even hypothermic at the time of clinical examination if the owners have made attempts to cool the animal and sufficient time has elapsed before presentation.

DIAGNOSIS

A. History of exposure to high temperature and compatible acute clinical signs are highly suggestive.
B. A history of vigorous exercise is suggestive, but minimal exercise can induce heatstroke in some individuals on hot, humid days.
C. Rectal temperature of >106° F but hypothermia (<100° F) may occur if attempts have been made to cool the patient before presentation.
D. Increased numbers of nucleated red cells are observed on complete blood count in more than 50% of cases likely as a result of premature release from damaged bone marrow.
E. Mild, moderate, or severe increase in serum CK activity in all affected dogs due to muscle damage.
F. Increased liver enzyme activity (e.g., AST, ALT, ALP) in most affected animals.
G. Hyperbilirubinemia in some patients.
H. Thrombocytopenia occurs in more than 80% of affected dogs, probably as a result of endothelial cell damage. Increased OSPT and partial thromboplastin time (PTT) and evidence of DIC (fibrin degradation products) are present in some patients.
I. Serum creatinine concentration initially may be mildly increased due to release of creatinine from damaged muscles or from dehydration and prerenal azotemia. Serum creatinine concentration increases much more in affected animals that go on to develop AIRF. Serum creatinine concentration is increased in approximately 50% of affected animals at initial examination, usually due to decreased renal perfusion and prerenal azotemia.
J. Hypoglycemia (blood glucose concentration <50 mg/dL) is observed in about 40% of affected dogs.
K. Urinalysis may show a positive reaction for occult blood, which may really be reacting to the presence of myoglobin released from damaged muscles. The presence of renal tubular casts may be observed from tubular damage. The presence of hyaline casts may be seen due to high body temperature, which increases movement of plasma protein across glomeruli.

TREATMENT

A. Place an IV catheter and provide supportive fluid therapy to correct dehydration and support perfusion of damaged organs.
B. Patients with high core body temperatures should be sprayed with cool water, and a fan should be directed at the wet hair coat. This approach increases evaporative loss and can effectively cool patients safely.
C. Ice water baths are not very efficient because the resultant cutaneous vasoconstriction and shivering limit the ability of the animal to dissipate heat.
D. Discontinue cooling efforts when core temperature has decreased to <104° F to prevent excessive correction and hypothermia.
E. Administer bolus doses of lidocaine to control ventricular arrhythmias and follow with a constant rate infusion (CRI) of lidocaine as needed. Lidocaine also may function as a free radical scavenger.

F. Monitor urine output during the initial 48 hours after presentation.
G. Provide symptomatic treatment as necessary for multisystemic organ system failure.

PROGNOSIS

A. Overall, a 50% to 65% survival rate is expected.

> **!** Survival in heatstroke is 50% to 65% if AIRF is not present.

1. Survival rate decreases to approximately 20% in animals with AIRF.
2. DIC alone also lowers the survival rate.
3. Only 10% of patients with both AIRF and DIC are expected to survive.
B. Ventricular premature contractions and hypoglycemia are more common in patients that don't survive.
C. Other predictors of failure to survive include hypocholesterolemia, hypoalbuminemia, hypoproteinemia, hyperbilirubinemia, and increased serum creatinine concentration.
D. Mild to moderate increases in serum creatinine concentration are common in survivors. More severe increases in serum creatinine concentration present 24 hours after initial treatment often are found in nonsurvivors.
E. Oliguria or anuria after adequate volume replacement with IV fluids also is a negative predictor for survival.
F. Patients treated within 90 minutes of heat exposure are more likely to survive than those treated later.
G. Death often occurs in the first 24 hours of hospitalization. Patients surviving for 48 hours or more are more likely to survive to discharge.
H. Additional factors that are correlated with mortality include coma, hypothermia, hypoglycemia, prolonged APTT and OSPT, seizures, and obesity.

Food-Associated Toxicity (Melamine/Cyanuric Acid-Associated Renal Failure; MCARF)

INTRODUCTION

A. Outbreaks of renal failure associated with the ingestion of toxin-containing pet foods occurred in 2004 and 2007.
B. In 2007, renal failure resulted in animals that consumed pet foods containing melamine and cyanuric acid, which were present in wheat gluten, rice protein, and corn gluten that had been imported from China. These pet foods were primarily canned food products.
C. In 2004, renal failure was initially reported to be caused by mycotoxins, but retrospectively has been shown to have been caused by melamine and cyanuric acid. This outbreak affected primarily dogs and a few cats in Asia.
D. Melamine is a nitrogen-rich compound that is used in the manufacture of plastics and as a fertilizer. Cyanuric acid is also nitrogen-rich, and is a chemical stabilizer. Melamine and cyanuric acid were intentionally added to feed ingredients in China to increase the nitrogen content. Increasing the nitrogen gives the appearance of a product with a higher protein content, which has more monetary value.

PATHOPHYSIOLOGY

A. Melamine alone does not cause renal failure, but in combination with cyanuric acid, insoluble crystals form that obstruct and damage renal tubules.
B. Crystals are present in the distal tubules and collecting ducts. Crystals are polarizable, light green to slightly basophilic, with radiating striations.
C. Renal distal tubular necrosis is present, and some have interstitial fibrosis and lymphoplasma-cytic inflammation, indicating a more chronic stage.
  1. Inflammation surrounding crystal-containing tubules is more prominent in chronic stages.
  2. Large crystals in the medulla are more common in chronic cases, with occasional tubular rupture.

CLINICAL SIGNS

A. Acute anorexia, vomiting, lethargy, polyuria, and polydipsia are common.
B. Oral ulcers, mineralization of the gastric mucosa, and mineralization of pulmonary smooth muscle and alveolar walls have occurred in some patients.
C. Some animals may have a more chronic onset after ingesting contaminated food for 1 month or more.
D. Cats appear to be more sensitive to developing MCARF, though this may be related to a higher percentage of cats being fed canned food products.

DIAGNOSIS

A. Azotemia and hyperphosphatemia are consistent findings. Serum hepatic enzyme activities are typically not increased.
B. Polarizable crystals may be identified in urine (Figure 4-9). These crystals appear similar to oxalate crystals observed in ethylene glycol (EG) poisoning, but are more brown in color, and have a radiating linear pattern.
C. A dietary history of consuming affected foods, along with clinical signs of acute renal failure is diagnostic.

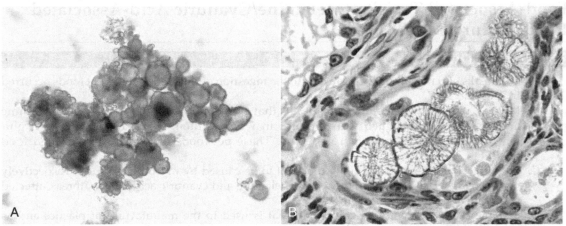

FIGURE 4-9 ■ **A,** Crystals in the urine of a cat with melamine/cyanuric acid-associated renal failure (MCARF) **B,** Renal histopathology showing acute distal renal tubular necrosis with distinctive intratubular polarizable crystals (**A,** Courtesy of Clinical Pathology, The Ohio State University College of Veterinary Medicine, Columbus, Ohio. **B,** Courtesy of Dr. Cathy Brown, University of Georgia, Athens, Ga.)

TREATMENT

A. Aggressive treatment of the acute renal failure is necessary.
B. Treatment is mainly supportive.

PROGNOSIS

A. Many affected animals die or are euthanized due to the severity of the renal failure.
B. If an affected animal survives the acute episode with aggressive medical therapy, long-term treatment of CRF is necessary.

WHAT DO WE DO?

- Monitor urine output in all patients with AIRF to facilitate optimal fluid therapy and establish a prognosis for patients without access to dialysis.
- Provide definitive antidote therapy with 4-MP or ethanol in dogs (or ethanol in cats) suspected to have EG intoxication until a definitive diagnosis is established.
- When dialysis is not feasible, provide a realistic prognosis (i.e., grave) early in the disease process for owners of animals with AIRF caused by EG, especially those patients with severe oliguria or anuria.
- Always consider leptospirosis as a cause for AIRF in dogs, unless specific evidence indicates otherwise.
- Aggressively treat dogs with leptospirosis-induced AIRF because most of them will survive if prompt treatment is provided.
- Do not use AGs unless no other effective antibiotics are available.
- Provide fluid therapy for any dog or cat that has been receiving NSAIDs and becomes suddenly ill. Appropriate fluid therapy will prevent activation of vasoconstrictor signals that could otherwise cause severe renal ischemia in NSAID-treated patients due to synthetic blockade of renoprotective vasodilatory prostaglandins.
- Treat all cats known to have ingested any amount of lily as potential AIRF patients.
- Don't abandon treatment prematurely in cats with lily-induced AIRF because some survive despite severe azotemia and oliguria.
- Provide IV fluids for any suddenly ill dog that has recently ingested any quantity of raisins or grapes.
- Provide 3 to 5 days of fluid therapy for dogs that have ingested calcipotriene (Dovonex) until hypercalcemia abates.
- Measure serum ionized calcium concentration in all patients with increased serum total calcium concentration.
- Biopsy the kidney when it is not clear clinically if the diagnosis is nephritis or nephrosis or to differentiate AIRF from CRF.
- Use bisphosphonates to treat severe and prolonged hypercalcemia in patients with hypervitaminosis D.
- Use calcitonin to treat severe hypercalcemia in patients that have not responded adequately to fluid therapy and furosemide.

THOUGHTS FOR THE FUTURE

- Regimens to optimize the use of 4-MP as a treatment for EG toxicity in cats are on the horizon.
- Early dialysis, including short-term peritoneal dialysis by primary care practitioners or emergency services, may find increased use in efforts to decrease circulating EG and its toxic metabolites and to improve survival in patients with EG ingestion.

- Addition of nontoxic substances that decrease palatability to antifreeze products could decrease the risk of EG toxicity in dogs and cats.
- Use of PCR may become more routine in the diagnosis of leptospirosis in dogs.
- Additional epidemiological studies are needed to determine the association of *Borrelia* with rapidly progressive glomerulonephritis in dogs.

FREQUENTLY ASKED QUESTIONS

Q: A dog is determined to have ingested EG at least 24 hours ago and now is semi-comatose with BUN concentration of >100 mg/dL and serum creatinine concentration of >10 mg/dL. What is the chance of saving this dog?

A: The odds are very low. If the owner wishes to proceed, resuscitative efforts with fluids and management of acid-base and electrolyte disturbances should be undertaken. The prognosis (without dialysis) is grave if urine output is minimal despite rehydration, administration of a fluid volume challenge, and treatment with diuretics. Even with dialysis, months may elapse before it can be determined if recovery of renal function is possible.

Q: Is there any role for dialysis early in the course of EG intoxication even if azotemia is minimal?

A: Dialysis can remove both EG and its toxic metabolites and consequently there is a role for dialysis even if azotemia is not yet severe. Even in animals with renal azotemia, dialysis may be useful to prevent additional renal toxicity caused by retention of toxic metabolites. Early peritoneal dialysis for 1 to 2 days is feasible for primary care veterinarians. This method of treatment has the potential to improve clinical outcome.

Q: What is the best way in primary care practice to identify EG intoxication?

A: The combination of a high osmolal gap and high anion gap is very suggestive of EG intoxication. Measured osmolality is not readily available in primary care practice, but is available from most commercial diagnostic laboratories. Most laboratories provide a calculated osmolality on the serum biochemical profile. The osmolal gap is the difference between the measured and calculated serum osmolality and normally is <10 mOsm/kg. Other clinical features that suggest the presence of EG include hyperphosphatemia that is out of proportion to observed increases in BUN and serum creatinine concentrations (due to the presence of phosphorus-containing rust inhibitors in antifreeze preparations). Hypocalcemia also may occur in affected animals when EG has been rapidly metabolized to toxic intermediates. The EGTest Kit may identify unmetabolized EG in whole blood soon after ingestion.

Q: What is the best way to definitively diagnose leptospirosis as the cause for AIRF?

A: Documentation of increasing serologic titers based on microscopic agglutination testing is presently the standard method. A titer that rises between the acute and convalescent serum samples by a factor of at least 4 is considered diagnostic. An single titer of >1:800 also can be very suggestive in a dog that has not been vaccinated in the past 6 to 12 months against the serovar identified by serology. Some dogs have no measurable titer in serum samples collected during the acute phase, but have diagnostic titers a few weeks later. Depending on the phase of the disease, PCR of blood or urine likely will become the gold standard for diagnosis in the future.

Q: Why is it clinically relevant to know that AIRF is caused by leptospirosis rather than some cause of acute tubular necrosis (e.g., toxins or ischemia)?

A: The prognosis for leptospirosis is considerably better than that of most other causes of AIRF. Thus, if the diagnosis of leptospirosis is certain, aggressive treatment is warranted because successful outcome is very possible. Also, antibiotic treatment to eliminate the carrier state is necessary in AIRF caused by leptospirosis.

Q: How can I know for sure that a dog recently treated with gentamicin for 9 days has AIRF caused by AGNT?
A: No definitive laboratory, imaging, or histopathologic findings establish the diagnosis of AGNT with certainty. If renal function was normal before and severe azotemia has developed after administration of AGs (especially in a critically ill hospitalized animal), the diagnosis of AIRF caused by AGNT is quite likely.

Q: Which NSAID is least likely to produce AIRF?
A: All NSAIDs have the potential to cause AIRF if hypotension occurs while the NSAID is present in therapeutic concentrations. NSAIDs do not cause AIRF unless vasoconstriction has been activated, as is likely to occur during hypotension or shock. Unfortunately, GI bleeding is common with NSAID administration, and hypotension may occur as a result. Newer NSAIDs may be less likely to provoke GI bleeding and consequently may be less likely to result in AIRF.

Q: I have a 3-year-old dog in my practice that was normal until 2 days ago. Now, the dog is moribund. It is severely dehydrated and has a 1.010 urine specific gravity with several granular casts per low power microscopic field in the urinary sediment. Abnormal serum chemistry results include a serum creatinine concentration of 6.1 mg/dL, serum phosphorus concentration of 9.0 mg/dL, and serum total calcium concentration of 18.2 mg/dL. What is the prognosis for this dog?
A: The severe hypercalcemia and hyperphosphatemia suggest exposure to a vitamin D metabolite such as cholecalciferol in rat bait or calcipotriene in antipsoriasis cream. How much azotemia is primary and how much is prerenal cannot be determined at the time of presentation because hypercalcemia interferes with urinary concentrating ability. Repeated measurement of serum creatinine concentration after IV fluid therapy has corrected dehydration will allow you to determine how much, if any, of the azotemia was prerenal in origin. Assuming the history is correct, ionized hypercalcemia is likely to be present and measurement of serum ionized calcium concentration would be useful. Persistence of ionized hypercalcemia in the face of azotemia increases the risk for development of additional primary renal lesions. Thus, ionized hypercalcemia should be treated promptly. IV fluids alone or furosemide usually do not decrease serum ionized calcium concentration adequately when hypervitaminosis D is the underlying cause. Adding calcitonin to rapidly decrease serum ionized calcium concentration is advisable, but its effect is limited in magnitude and duration. Intravenous administration of pamidronate is valuable in the rescue treatment of hypercalcemia caused by hypervitaminosis D. Rapid reversal of hypercalcemia is crucial to successful treatment of this dog.

Q: I have a 5-year-old female Labrador retriever in my clinic. She presented to our office with a sudden onset of anorexia, vomiting, and lethargy. Her physical examination was unremarkable. There was no history of previous polyuria or polydipsia. Her urine specific gravity is 1.015 with 3+ proteinuria and up to 4 granular casts per low power microscopic field and occasional epithelial cell casts are present. Her serum biochemistry results include a serum creatinine concentration of 9.3 mg/dL, serum phosphorus concentration of 8.5 mg/dL, and hypoalbuminemia (1.5 g/dL). Her serum creatinine concentration has not responded to an IV fluid challenge. Her kidneys are normal-sized with normal renal pelves but hyperechoic on ultrasonography. Her Lyme disease titer is positive. Is this AIRF or CRF, and what is the prognosis?
A: Hypoalbuminemia is not usually a feature of AIRF except in RPGN associated with *Borrelia* infection. Severe proteinuria is compatible with glomerular disease and is not common with other causes of AIRF. Differential diagnosis at this point should include leptospirosis, rapidly progressive

glomerulonephritis, amyloidosis with acute medullary necrosis, or a chronic glomerulopathy with acute exacerbation. Renal biopsy will be an important tool to establish a definitive diagnosis and offer a more realistic prognosis. Unfortunately, advanced azotemia associated with renal amyloidosis or RPGN has a grave prognosis. The positive Lyme titer is not necessarily helpful because many normal dogs in endemic regions have positive titers without obvious clinical disease. The positive titer could indicate exposure rather than active disease.

SUGGESTED READINGS

Ethylene Glycol Intoxication

Adams WH, Toal RL, Breider MA: Ultrasonographic findings in dogs and cats with oxalate nephrosis attributed to ethylene glycol intoxication: 15 cases (1984-1988), *J Am Vet Med Assoc* 199:492–496, 1991.

Adams WH, Toal RL, Walker MA, et al: Early renal ultrasonographic findings in dogs with experimentally induced ethylene glycol nephrosis, *Am J Vet Res* 50:1370–1376, 1989.

Connally HE, Thrall MA, Hamar DW: Safety and efficacy of high-dose fomepizole as therapy for ethylene glycol intoxication in cats, *J Vet Emerg Crit Care* 12:191, 2002.

Dial SM, Thrall MA, Hamar DW: 4-Methylpyrazole as treatment for naturally acquired ethylene glycol intoxication in dogs, *J Am Vet Med Assoc* 195:73–76, 1989.

Dial SM, Thrall MA, Hamar DW: Comparison of ethanol and 4-methylpyrazole as treatments for ethylene glycol intoxication in cats, *Am J Vet Res* 55:1771–1782, 1994.

Gaynor AR, Dhupa N: Acute ethylene glycol intoxication. Part I. Pathophysiology and clinical stages, *Compendium for Continuing Education* 21:1014–1023, 1999.

Gaynor AR, Dhupa N: Acute ethylene glycol intoxication. Part II. Diagnosis, treatment, prognosis, and prevention, *Compendium for Continuing Education* 21:1124–1133, 1999.

Grauer GF, Thrall MA, Henre BA, et al: Early clinicopathologic findings in dogs ingesting ethylene glycol, *Am J Vet Res* 45:2299–2303, 1984.

Lascelles BD, Court MH, Hardie EM, Robertson SA: Nonsteroidal anti-inflammatory drugs in cats: A review, *Vet Anaesth Analg* 34:228–250, 2007.

Tarr BD, Winters LJ, Moore MP, et al: Low-dose ethanol in the treatment of ethylene glycol poisoning, *J Vet Pharmacol Ther* 8:254–262, 1985.

Thrall MA, Grauer GF, Mero KN: Clinicopathologic findings in dogs and cats with ethylene glycol intoxication, *J Am Vet Med Assoc* 184:37–41, 1984.

Leptospirosis

Adin CA, Cowgill LD: Treatment and outcome of dogs with leptospirosis: 36 cases (1990-1998), *J Am Vet Med Assoc* 216:371–375, 2000.

Birnbaum N, Barr SC, Center SA, et al: Naturally-acquired leptospirosis in 36 dogs: Serological and clinicopathological features, *J Small Anim Pract* 39:231–236, 1998.

Brown CA, Roberts AW, Miller MA, et al: *Leptospira interrogans* serovar grippotyphosa infection in dogs, *J Am Vet Med Assoc* 209:1265–1267, 1996.

Forrest LJ, O'Brien RT, Tremelling MS, et al: Sonographic renal findings in 20 dogs with leptospirosis, *Vet Radiol Ultrasound* 39:337–340, 1998.

Goldstein RE, Lin RC, Langston CE, et al: Influence of infecting serogroup on clinical features of leptospirosis in dogs, *J Vet Intern Med* 20:489–494, 2006.

Klaasen HL, Molkenboer MJ, Vrijenhoek MP, Kaashoek MJ: Duration of immunity in dogs vaccinated against leptospirosis with a bivalent inactivated vaccine, *Vet Microbiol* 95:121–132, 2003.

Mastrorilli C, Dondi F, Agnoli C, et al: Clinicopathologic features and outcome predictors of *Leptospira interrogans* Australis serogroup infection in dogs: A retrospective study of 20 cases (2001-2004), *J Vet Intern Med* 21:3–10, 2007.

Rentko VT, Clark N, Ross LA, Schelling SH: Canine leptospirosis: A retrospective study of 17 cases, *J Vet Int Med* 6:235–244, 1992.

Ward MP, Glickman LT, Guptill LE: Prevalence of and risk factors for leptospirosis among dogs in the United States and Canada: 677 cases (1970-1998), *J Am Vet Med Assoc* 220:53–58, 2002.

Ward MP, Guptill LF, Prahl A, Wu CC: Serovar-specific prevalence and risk factors for leptospirosis among dogs: 90 cases (1997-2002), *J Am Vet Med Assoc* 224:1958–1963, 2004.

Ward MP, Guptill LF, Wu CC: Evaluation of environmental risk factors for leptospirosis in dogs: 36 cases (1997-2002), *J Am Vet Med Assoc* 225:72–77, 2004.

Aminoglycoside Nephrotoxicity
Albarellos G, Montoya L, Ambros L, et al: Multiple once-daily dose pharmacokinetics and renal safety of gentamicin in dogs, *J Vet Pharmacol Ther* 27:21–25, 2004.

Brown SA, Barsanti JA, Crowell WA: Gentamicin-associated acute renal failure in the dog, *J Am Vet Med Assoc* 186:686–690, 1985.

Cronin RE, Bulger RE, Southern P, Henrich WL: Natural history of aminoglycoside nephrotoxicity in the dog, *J Lab Clin Med* 95:463–474, 1980.

Frazier DL, Aucoin DP, Riviere JE: Gentamicin pharmacokinetics and nephrotoxicity in naturally acquired and experimentally induced disease in dogs, *J Am Vet Med Assoc* 192:57–63, 1988.

Greco DS, Turnwald GH, Adams R, et al: Urinary gamma-glutamyl transpeptidase activity in dogs with gentamicin-induced nephrotoxicity, *Am J Vet Res* 46:2332–2335, 1985.

Rivers BJ, Walter PA, O'Brien TD, et al: Evaluation of urine gamma-glutamyl transpeptidase-to-creatinine ratio as a diagnostic tool in an experimental model of aminoglycoside-induced acute renal failure in the dog, *J Am Anim Hosp Assoc* 32:323–336, 1996.

Spangler WL, Adelman RD, Conzelman GM Jr, Ishizaki G: Gentamicin nephrotoxicity in the dog: Sequential light and electron microscopy, *Vet Pathol* 17:206–217, 1980.

Grape and Raisin Nephrotoxicity in Dogs
Eubig PA, Brady MS, Gwaltney-Brant SM, et al: Acute renal failure in dogs after the ingestion of grapes or raisins: a retrospective evaluation of 43 dogs (1992-2002), *J Vet Intern Med* 19:663–674, 2005.

Mazzaferro EM, Eubig PA, Hackett TB, et al: Acute renal failure associated with raisin or grape ingestion in 4 dogs, *J Vet Emerg Crit Care* 14:203–212, 2004.

Morrow CM, Valli VE, Volmer PA, Eubig PA: Canine renal pathology associated with grape or raisin ingestion: 10 cases, *J Vet Diagn Invest* 17:223–231, 2005.

Lily Nephrotoxicity in Cats
Hadley RM, Richardson JA, Gwaltney-Brant SM: A retrospective study of day lily toxicosis in cats, *Vet Hum Toxicol* 45:38–39, 2003.

Langston CE: Acute renal failure caused by lily ingestion in six cats, *J Am Vet Med Assoc* 220:49–52, 2002.

Rumbeiha WK, Francis JA, Fitzgerald SD, et al: A comprehensive study of Easter lily poisoning in cats, *J Vet Diagn Invest* 16:527–541, 2004.

Tefft KM: Lily nephrotoxicity in cats, *Compend Contin Educ Pract Vet* 26:149–157, 2004.

Nonsteroidal Anti-inflammatory Drugs
Bergh MS, Budsberg SC: The coxib NSAIDs: Potential clinical and pharmacologic importance in veterinary medicine, *J Vet Intern Med* 19:633–643, 2005.

Forsyth SF, Guilford WG, Pfeiffer DU: Effect of NSAID administration on creatinine clearance in healthy dogs undergoing anaesthesia and surgery, *J Small Anim Pract* 41:547–550, 2000.

Jones RD, Baynes RE, Nimitz CT: Nonsteroidal anti-inflammatory drug toxicosis in dogs and cats: 240 cases (1989-1990), *J Am Vet Med Assoc* 201:475–477, 1992.

Jones CJ, Budsberg SC: Physiologic characteristics and clinical importance of the cyclooxygenase isoforms in dogs and cats, *J Am Vet Med Assoc* 217:721–729, 2000.

Lascelles BD, Court MH, Hardie E: Nonsteroidal anti-inflammatory drugs in cats: A review, *Vet Anesth Analg* 34:228–250, 2007.

Lascelles BD, McFarland JM, Swann H: Guidelines for safe and effective use of NSAIDs in dogs, *Vet Ther* 6:237–251, 2005.

Poortinga EW, Hungerford LL: A case-control study of acute ibuprofen toxicity in dogs, *Prev Vet Med* 35:115–124, 1998.

Robson MC, Chew D, van Aalst S: Intrinsic acute renal failure (ARF) associated with non-steroidal anti-inflammatory drug (NSAID) in juvenile cats undergoing routine desexing – 16 cases 1998-2005 (abstract), *J Vet Intern Med* 20:740, 2006.

Stichtenoth DO, Frolich JC: COX-2 and the kidneys, *Curr Pharm Des* 6:1737–1753, 2000.

Wilson JE, Chandrasekharan NV, Westover KD, et al: Determination of expression of cyclooxygenase-1 and -2 isozymes in canine tissues and their differential sensitivity to nonsteroidal anti-inflammatory drugs, *Am J Vet Res* 65:810–818, 2004.

Hypercalcemia

Dougherty SA, Center SA, Dzanis DA: Salmon calcitonin as adjunct treatment for vitamin D toxicosis in a dog, *J Am Vet Med Assoc* 196:1269–1272, 1990.

Fooshee SK, Forrester SD: Hypercalcemia secondary to cholecalciferol rodenticide toxicosis in two dogs, *J Am Vet Med Assoc* 196:1265–1268, 1990.

Gunther R, Felice LJ, Nelson RK, Franson AM: Toxicity of a vitamin D3 rodenticide to dogs, *J Am Vet Med Assoc* 193:211–214, 1988.

Hare WR, Dobbs CE, Slayman KA, Kingsborough BJ: Calcipotriene poisoning in dogs, *Vet Med* 95:771–778, 2000.

Hostutler RA, Chew DJ, Jaeger JQ, et al: Uses and effectiveness of pamidronate disodium for treatment of dogs and cats with hypercalcemia, *J Vet Intern Med* 19:29–33, 2005.

Kruger JM, Osborne CA, Nachreiner RF, Refsal KR: Hypercalcemia and renal failure. Etiology, pathophysiology, diagnosis, and treatment, *Vet Clin North Am Small Anim Pract* 26:1417–1445, 1996.

Rumbeiha WK, Fitzgerald SD, Kruger JM, et al: Use of pamidronate disodium to reduce cholecalciferol-induced toxicosis in dogs, *Am J Vet Res* 61:9–13, 2000.

Rumbeiha WK, Kruger JM, Fitzgerald SF, et al: Use of pamidronate to reverse vitamin D3-induced toxicosis in dogs, *Am J Vet Res* 60:1092–1097, 1999.

Spangler WL, Gribble DH, Lee TC: Vitamin D intoxication and the pathogenesis of vitamin D nephropathy in the dog, *Am J Vet Res* 40:73–83, 1979.

Rapidly Progressive Glomerulonephritis

Dambach DM, Smith CA, Lewis RM, Van Winkle TJ: Morphologic, immunohistochemical, and ultrastructural characterization of a distinctive renal lesion in dogs putatively associated with *Borrelia burgdorferi* infection: 49 cases (1987-1992), *Vet Pathol* 34:85–96, 1997.

Heat stroke

Bruchim Y, Klement E, Saragusty J, et al: Heat stroke in dogs: A retrospective study of 54 cases (1999-2004) and analysis of risk factors for death, *J Vet Intern Med* 20:38–46, 2006.

Drobatz KJ, Macintire DK: Heat-induced illness in dogs: 42 cases (1976-1993), *J Am Vet Med Assoc* 209:1894–1899, 1996.

Hanneman GD, Higgins EA, Price GT, et al: Transient and permanent effects of hyperthermia in dogs: A study of a simulated air transport environmental stress, *Am J Vet Res* 38:955–958, 1977.

Shapiro Y, Rosenthal T, Sohar E: Experimental heatstroke. A model in dogs, *Arch Intern Med* 131:688–692, 1973.

Food-Associated Toxicity

Brown CA, Jeong K-S, Poppenga RH, et al: Outbreaks of renal failure associated with melamine and cyanuric acid in dogs and cats in 2004 and 2007, *J Vet Diagn Invest* 19:527–531, 2007.

5 Chronic Renal Failure

■ ■ ■

INTRODUCTION

A. Chronic renal failure (CRF) occurs when the compensatory mechanisms of chronically diseased kidneys are no longer able to maintain adequate functions to excrete waste products; regulate electrolyte, water, and acid-base homeostasis, degrade hormones; and synthesize endocrine hormones. The resultant retention of nitrogenous solutes; derangements of fluid, electrolyte, and acid-base balance; and failure of hormone production constitute the syndrome of CRF.
   1. Azotemia does not develop until 75% or more of the nephron population has become nonfunctional. Isosthenuria occurs when greater than 66% of the nephron population has become nonfunctional; the ability to elaborate maximal urine concentration is lost earlier.
   2. CRF is thought to affect 0.5% to 1.0% of geriatric dogs and 1.0% to 3.0% of geriatric cats.

❗ CRF is the third most common cause of death in dogs and the second most common cause of death in cats with chronic disease.

B. Renal functions affected are:
   1. Excretory: Retention of solutes handled by glomerular filtration rate (GFR) (e.g., urea, creatinine).
   2. Regulatory: Derangements in solutes handled by GFR and some combination of reabsorption and secretion can result in abnormalities of water, electrolytes, and acid-base balance. Depending on the solute in question, retention or loss can result.
   3. Degradative: Many small peptides (e.g., gastrin) normally are filtered by the kidney, reabsorbed, and degraded in the proximal tubular cells. Loss of this clearance function can result in metabolic derangements because many of these small peptides are hormones.
   4. Endocrine: Diminished production of the hormones erythropoietin and calcitriol occurs in CRF.
C. International Renal Interest Society (IRIS) staging of chronic kidney disease (CKD).
   1. IRIS is an international special interest group seeking to identify and disseminate information on better methods for the diagnosis and treatment of dogs and cats with renal disease.
   2. The term CKD is recommended over chronic renal disease (CRD) or CRF to avoid confusion during conversations with pet owners.
   3. IRIS has proposed a staging system for CKD based on the serum creatinine concentration of the stable patient on at least two occasions (Table 5-1). A substage then is assigned based on whether or not the animal is proteinuric (Table 5-2) and the absence or presence (and extent) of hypertension (Table 5-3).

■ TABLE 5-1
■ ■ Serum Creatinine Concentrations for Assignment of International Renal Interest Society Stage of Chronic Kidney Disease in Dogs and Cats

Stage	Serum Creatinine Concentration (mg/dL)	Serum Creatinine Concentration (μmol/L)	Comments
1	<1.4 (dog) <1.6 (cat)	<125 (dog) <140 (cat)	Nonazotemic. Often discovered fortuitously during routine examination. May have evidence of decreased urinary concentrating ability or proteinuria. Usually no obvious clinical signs. May be polyuric.
2	1.4-2.0 (dog) 1.6-2.8 (cat)	125-179 (dog) 140-249 (cat)	Mildly azotemic. Decreased urinary concentrating capacity. May have proteinuria. Clinical signs minimal. May have polyuria and polydipsia.
3	2.1-5.0 (dog) 2.9-5.0 (cat)	180-439 (dog) 250-439 (cat)	Moderate azotemia. Decreased urinary concentrating capacity. May have proteinuria. Many systemic clinical signs may be present.
4	>5.0 (dog) >5.0 (cat)	>440 (dog) >440 (cat)	Severe azotemia. Decreased urinary concentrating capacity, proteinuria. Systemic clinical signs present and may be severe.

■ TABLE 5-2
■ ■ Proteinuria* for Assignment of International Renal Interest Society Substage of Chronic Kidney Disease in Dogs and Cats

Urine Protein/Creatinine Ratio	Classification
<0.2 (dogs) <0.2 (cats)	Nonproteinuric
0.2-0.5 (dogs) 0.2-0.4 (cats)	Borderline proteinuric
>0.5 (dogs) >0.4 (cats)	Proteinuric

*Assessed by urine protein/creatinine ratio.

■ TABLE 5-3
■ ■ Systemic Blood Pressure for Assignment of International Renal Interest Society Substage of Chronic Kidney Disease in Dogs and Cats

Systolic Blood Pressure (mm Hg)	Diastolic Blood Pressure (mm Hg)	Risk Level
<150	< 95	Minimal
150-159	95-99	Low
160-179	100-119	Moderate
≥180	≥ 120	High

        a. Serial measurements of serum creatinine concentration should be made by the same laboratory. Interassay variability for creatinine determinations is minimal within a given laboratory but not among laboratories.

        b. Serum creatinine concentration should be measured using standard automated methods (i.e., Jaffe colorimetric reaction). The serum creatinine concentrations proposed in the IRIS guidelines do not refer to creatinine determined by enzymatic methods.

4. Staging of CKD should allow more rational treatment strategies to be employed based on stage of disease. The goal of treatment is to slow or prevent progression of disease.

        a. Most studies of treatment for CKD have been reported for dogs and cats with overt azotemia and clinical signs (i.e., IRIS stages 3 and 4; see Table 5-1).

        b. More cats than dogs with CKD are identified in IRIS stages 1 and 2. Most dogs with CKD are not identified until IRIS stage 3 or 4.

5. The low cutoff values for maximal serum creatinine concentration considered to be normal will allow identification of more animals with CKD but also occasionally will include normal animals (see Table 5-1).

> **!** The use of a lower cutoff value for maximal normal serum creatinine concentration will allow identification of more patients with earlier CKD.

6. Many laboratories report reference ranges for serum creatinine concentration much wider than those proposed in the IRIS guidelines and some animals with serum creatinine concentrations at the upper end of such reference ranges likely have CKD.

7. Guidelines for serum creatinine concentrations are based on average-sized adult dogs. Extremely small or large dogs may have lower or higher normal serum creatinine concentrations. Breed-specific results for serum creatinine concentration are not addressed in the IRIS guidelines (e.g., normal Greyhounds tend to have higher serum creatinine concentrations than other breeds). Also, young dogs normally have lower serum creatinine concentrations than mature dogs.

8. Prerenal and postrenal conditions also must be excluded based on results of history, physical examination, urinalysis, and urinary tract imaging as necessary.

9. Complete IRIS classification requires assessment of proteinuria (see Table 5-2) and systemic blood pressure (see Table 5-3).

CAUSES OF CHRONIC RENAL FAILURE IN DOGS AND CATS

> **!** Most often, the underlying cause of CKD in dogs and cats is not determined.

Dog

1. Chronic tubulointerstitial nephritis of unknown cause (most common pathologic diagnosis).
2. Chronic pyelonephritis (can be difficult to distinguish histologically from chronic tubulointerstitial nephritis).
3. Chronic glomerulonephritis (can be difficult to distinguish histologically from chronic tubulointerstitial nephritis).
4. Amyloidosis (familial in Shar-pei dogs; see Chapter 6, Familial Renal Diseases of the Dog and Cat).
5. Hypercalcemic nephropathy.
6. Chronic obstructive uropathy (hydronephrosis).
7. Familial renal disease (see Chapter 6, Familial Renal Diseases of the Dog and Cat).

8. Progression after acute renal failure (ARF).
9. Chronic toxicity (e.g., food-associated, drugs, environmental toxins).
10. Neoplasia.
11. Primary systemic hypertension.

Cat

1. Chronic tubulointerstitial nephritis of unknown cause (most common pathologic diagnosis).
2. Chronic pyelonephritis (can be difficult to distinguish histologically from chronic tubulointerstitial nephritis).
3. Chronic glomerulonephritis (can be difficult to distinguish histologically from chronic tubulointerstitial nephritis).
4. Amyloidosis (familial in Abyssinian cats; see Chapter 6, Familial Renal Diseases of the Dog and Cat).
5. Polycystic kidney disease (familial in Persian cats; see Chapter 6, Familial Renal Diseases of the Dog and Cat).
6. Hypercalcemic nephropathy.
7. Progression after ARF.
8. Chronic obstructive uropathy (e.g., hydronephrosis as a consequence of ureteral urolithiasis).
9. Neoplasia (e.g., renal lymphoma).
10. Acromegaly (excessive growth hormone production) resulting in renomegaly.
11. Pyogranulomatous nephritis due to feline infectious peritonitis.
12. Hypokalemic (kaliopenic) nephropathy.
13. Chronic toxicity (food-associated, drugs, environmental toxins).
14. Primary systemic hypertension.

PATHOPHYSIOLOGY OF CHRONIC RENAL FAILURE

Uremia

1. Uremia is a syndrome that occurs after substantial reduction in renal function so that azotemia develops in conjunction with clinical signs. A variety of laboratory findings (hematologic, endocrine, serum biochemistry) usually accompany clinical signs recognized by the owner (lethargy, weight loss, decreased appetite, and vomiting).
2. A uremic toxin is any compound that accumulates in excess due to decreased renal function and contributes to the clinical signs of uremia.
   a. Urea, guanidine compounds, products of bacterial metabolism (e.g., polyamines, aliphatic amines, indoles), myoinositol, trace elements, and "middle molecules" (i.e., some hormones and other compounds with molecular weights of 500-3000) have been considered as potential uremic toxins.
   b. Many compounds are involved in the pathophysiology of uremia, and no single compound is likely to explain the diversity of uremic symptoms.

! Intraglomerular hypertension and hyperfiltration are compensatory mechanisms that likely contribute to the progression of CKD.

   c. Parathyroid hormone (PTH) is the best characterized uremic toxin. It exerts adverse effects on the brain, heart, bone marrow, and other tissues. Its role in the development of renal osteodystrophy (i.e., "rubber jaw") is well known (see "Renal Secondary Hyperparathyroidism").

Hyperfiltration

1. Hyperfiltration occurs as a result of an increase in single nephron GFR (SNGFR) above the normal range in surviving remnant nephrons. In most instances, increased SNGFR also is associated with increased transglomerular pressure (Figures 5-1 and 5-2).
   a. A fixed and dilated afferent glomerular arteriole allows delivery of increased pressure to the glomerular capillaries.
   b. Although not well documented, efferent arteriolar vasoconstriction could contribute to increased transglomerular pressure.
   c. Intraglomerular hypertension is a term used to describe increased hydrostatic pressure in remnant nephron glomerular capillaries. Intraglomerular hypertension is not necessarily related to the presence of systemic hypertension.

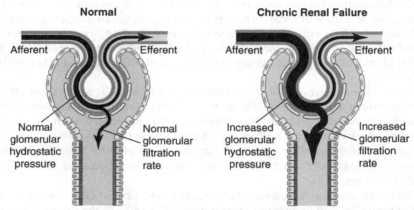

FIGURE 5-1 ■ Development of the *super nephron*—renal adaptation in the remnant kidney following substantial loss of renal mass. Increased single nephron GFR (SNGFR) is accomplished by vasodilation of the afferent arteriole. Some increase in GFR is also attributed to an increase in glomerular volume which increases surface area for filtration. (Drawn by Tim Vojt.)

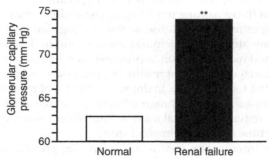

FIGURE 5-2 ■ Note the presence of intraglomerular hypertension in cats with substantial loss of nephron mass compared with normal cats (pressure measurements obtained by micropuncture). (Brown SA, Brown CA: Single nephron adaptations to partial renal ablation in cats. *Am J Physiol* 269: R1002-R1008, 1995.)

d. Increased glomerular volume in glomeruli of remnant nephrons also may contribute to hyperfiltration, but does not necessarily increase glomerular pressure. Increased glomerular volume itself may contribute to adverse consequences such as proteinuria.

e. Increased SNGFR facilitates excretion of waste products, but has adverse effects on the long-term survival of remnant nephrons.

2. Renal disease tends to be inexorably progressive once a critical number of nephrons has been destroyed, even when the initial cause of renal injury has been removed.

3. Total GFR represents the sum of the SNGFR for all nephrons of both kidneys. There are approximately 1,000,000 nephrons in a dog (500,000 per kidney) and 400,000 nephrons in a cat (200,000 per kidney). In a healthy animal, the range of SNGFR is fairly narrow.

4. During progressive renal disease, the decline in total GFR is offset by an increase in SNGFR in functional remnant nephrons (so-called *glomerular hyperfiltration*). Thus, the normally narrow range of SNGFR widens during development of CRF because diseased nephrons have low SNGFR and remnant nephrons have supra-normal SNGFR. Glomerular hyperfiltration has been incriminated as one important factor contributing to the progressive nature of renal disease based on experimental studies in animals.

5. Glomerular hyperfiltration has been demonstrated to occur experimentally in dogs and cats and in the few clinical dogs and cats it which it was measured. It is assumed that glomerular hyperfiltration is present in azotemic dogs and cats with primary renal disease.

6. The mechanisms responsible for this increase in SNGFR result from alterations in the normal determinants of SNGFR. In dogs, hyperfiltration results primarily from increases in the glomerular ultrafiltration coefficient (Kf) associated with increased glomerular volume by hypertrophy and increased glomerular capillary plasma flow and increased transglomerular capillary pressure largely due to afferent arteriolar dilatation. Experimentally, dogs and cats develop glomerular hyperfiltration after ablation of 75% or more of renal mass.

7. Following nephron loss, adaptation occurs to recoup lost GFR. This is to such an extent that total GFR will increase approximately 40% to 60% in the remnant renal tissue over a period of 4 weeks after renal ablation. For example, if one kidney is removed from a dog with GFR of 40 mL/min, GFR will immediately decline to 20 mL/min but within one month will stabilize at approximately 30 mL/min due to the effects of hyperfiltration in remnant nephrons.

8. Proteinuria and glomerular sclerosis in remnant nephrons are adverse functional and morphological consequences of glomerular hyperfiltration that may lead to progressive deterioration of the remaining renal tissue. These glomerular lesions are more prominent in rats with experimental renal disease than in dogs and cats in which tubulointerstitial lesions predominate. Also, proteinuria often is mild in dogs and cats with experimental renal disease and its contribution to progression is less certain than in rats.

9. The extent of renal damage that results in progressive deterioration of the remnant kidney is not known for all species. In dogs, 85% to 95% of renal tissue must be destroyed to result in progression, whereas progression occurs in rats after 75% to 80% renal ablation. Cats with 83% reduction in renal mass did not show evidence of progression over a one-year period of time in an experimental study.

10. In rats, dietary intervention (restriction of protein, phosphorus, and calories) can abrogate this maladaptive response by reducing glomerular hyperfiltration. Dietary restriction of protein to the same degree in dogs with experimental models of renal failure does not prevent hyperfiltration.

Factors Contributing to the Progression of Chronic Renal Disease

Species Differences

a. Clinical experience indicates that naturally occurring renal disease often is progressive in dogs. In experiments in dogs with subtotal nephrectomy, renal disease may not become progressive until 85% to 95% reduction in renal mass has occurred.

b. Limited information is available in cats. Naturally occurring renal disease often is progressive in cats, but it seems to progress much more slowly than in dogs. Cats with experimentally induced renal disease (5/6 nephrectomy) showed minimal evidence of progression over a 1-year period of time, but longer study may be needed to identify progression.

Functional and Morphologic Changes in Remnant Renal Tissue

a. Hyperfiltration increases movement of protein across the glomerular capillaries into Bowman's space and the mesangium, a process referred to as "protein trafficking."

> **!** Increased protein trafficking across glomeruli and protein processing by renal tubules cause adverse reactions in the mesangium, tubules, and interstitium contributing to tubulointerstitial nephritis and glomerulosclerosis.

b. Increased filtration of proteins through the glomeruli is toxic to the kidney and may contribute to renal disease progression (Figure 5-3). The magnitude of proteinuria correlates with rate of progression of renal disease in dogs and cats but whether or not proteinuria causes progression or is simply a marker of progression is not resolved.

   (1) The increased filtered load of protein may overload the proximal tubular cells leading ultimately to rupture of lysosomes and exposure of tubular cells and renal interstitium to damaging enzymes.

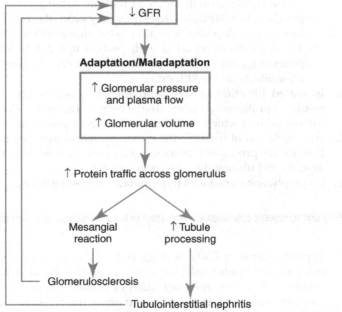

FIGURE 5-3 ■ A unifying hypothesis for the progressive loss of GFR and increased renal lesions in CRF. Protein leakage into the mesangium leading to glomerulosclerosis and protein leakage into the tubular lumens resulting in tubulointerstitial fibrosis are central to this hypothesis.

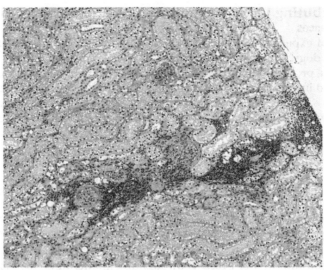

FIGURE 5-4 ■ Chronic renal disease histopathology–early lesions. (Hematolxyin and eosinstain, x600). (Courtesy of Dr. Steven Weisbrode, The Ohio State University, Columbus, Ohio.)

  (2) Tubular cells possess receptors for hormones and growth factors, some of which are small molecular weight proteins (e.g., insulin-like growth factor 1 [IGF-1], transforming growth factor β) that are filtered excessively and taken up by the proximal tubular cells where they may promote cellular proliferation and extracellular matrix deposition leading to tubulointerstitial damage.
  (3) Tubular cells overloaded with protein upregulate inflammatory and vasoactive genes (e.g., monocyte chemoattractant protein-1, endothelin), which have potential toxic effects on the kidney.
 c. Increased filtration of serum proteins also occurs into the mesangial space, which results in proliferation of mesangial cells and accumulation of increased mesangial cell matrix, both of which contribute to the development of glomerulosclerosis.
 d. Accumulation of lipids in the mesangium also may promote mesangial cell proliferation, excess production of mesangial matrix components such as collagen and proteoglycans and ultimately glomerular sclerosis.
 e. Hyperphosphatemia and hyperparathyroidism are associated with progression.

❗ Proinflammatory and fibrogenic cytokines are important in the pathophysiology of progression of CKD.

 f. Typical lesions of CKD in dogs and cats include a varying degree of lymphoplasmacytic tubulointerstitial nephritis, fibrosis, tubular dropout, hypertrophy of some tubular epithelium, mineralization of tubular basement membrane and interstitium, glomerulosclerosis, and obsolescent glomeruli (Figures 5-4 and 5-5).
Dietary Intake
 a. Dietary intake of varying levels of protein, phosphorus, calories, and lipids can have either protective or adverse effects on the progression of CRF (see "Treatment").

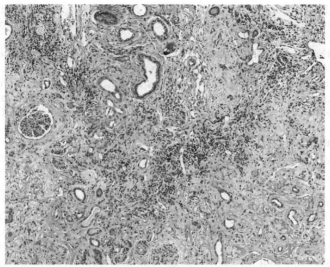

FIGURE 5-5 ■ Chronic renal disease histopathology—advanced lesions. (Hematolxyin and eosinstain, x600). (Courtesy of Dr. Steven Weisbrode, The Ohio State University, Columbus, Ohio.)

Systemic Complications
    a. Systemic complications of renal insufficiency may affect progression.
        (1) Systemic hypertension may have an impact on the extent of glomerular hypertension.
        (2) Urinary tract infection (UTI).
        (3) Fluid, electrolyte, and acid-base imbalances.
        (4) Unidentified uremic toxins likely contribute to renal disease progression because nonspecific adsorbent treatment ameliorates progression in rats with experimentally induced renal disease and humans with naturally occurring CRF.
        (5) Therapeutic interventions with modified dietary intake, phosphorus binders, angiotensin-converting enzyme (ACE) inhibitors and other antihypertensive agents, and treatment of secondary hyperparathyroidism with calcitriol also potentially can alter clinical signs and progression of CRF (see "Treatment").

Solute Balance
    1. Despite distortion of renal architecture by disease, glomerular and tubular functions in remaining functional nephrons are as closely integrated in diseased kidneys as in normal kidneys (i.e., glomerulotubular balance is maintained).
    2. For any given solute, the diseased kidney maintains glomerulotubular balance as GFR declines by decreasing the fraction of the filtered load of that solute that is reabsorbed and increasing the fraction of the filtered load of that solute that is excreted.
    3. In some instances, the mechanisms of the adaptive changes have adverse effects on the animal as explained by Neil Bricker's trade-off hypothesis: "The biological price to be paid for maintaining external solute balance for a given solute as renal disease progresses is the induction of one or more abnormalities of the uremic state." The classic example of the trade-off hypothesis is maintenance of normal calcium and phosphorus balance at the expense of renal secondary hyperparathyroidism and bone demineralization. Other examples include bone buffering by carbonate at the expense

of bone demineralization, and increasing SNGFR by glomerular hyperfiltration at the expense of proteinuria, glomerular sclerosis, and progressive destruction of remnant renal tissue.

4. Some of these ultimately maladaptive mechanisms and their consequences can be prevented by a proportional reduction in the intake of the responsible solute. This strategy will avoid the need for the kidneys to alter the fractional reabsorption and excretion of the solute in question. Using this approach with dietary phosphorus in patients with CRD has been shown to prevent or reverse renal secondary hyperparathyroidism.

Water Balance

1. Both the ability to produce concentrated urine (i.e., to conserve water) and the ability to excrete a water load are impaired in CRF.
2. The development of this concentrating defect is noted clinically by the onset of polyuria and compensatory polydipsia (more so in dogs than in cats).
3. Increased solute load per residual functioning nephron rather than architectural damage to the tubules and interstitium probably is the most important factor contributing to the concentrating defect (i.e., the remnant nephrons experience an osmotic diuresis).
4. Another contributing factor is the limited ability of the distal nephron to respond to antidiuretic hormone (ADH), possibly due to higher tubular flow rate in remnant nephrons.
5. In most instances, impairment of concentrating ability develops when 67% of the nephron population has become nonfunctional. This concentrating defect is recognized clinically by the presence of isosthenuria (urine osmolality of 300-600 mOsm/kg or urine specific gravity [USG] of 1.007-1.015) when obvious azotemia has developed.
6. For unknown reasons, some cats with CRF retain considerable concentrating ability even after development of azotemia. In one study, cats with 58% to 83% loss of functional nephrons could produce concentrated urine (USG 1.022-1.067). Thus, cats with azotemia and relatively concentrated urine do not necessarily have prerenal azotemia.
7. Urinary concentrating ability also may be preserved in the presence of renal azotemia in some dogs with CRD and early CRF. In these instances, GFR is decreased but postglomerular blood flow is thought to be sufficiently preserved so that concentrated urine still can be produced.
8. In some diseases, damage to the distal nephron or distortion of the normal architecture of the medullary interstitium may play a more important role in the concentrating defect and accounts for the early appearance of impaired concentrating ability (e.g., medullary amyloidosis in cats, pyelonephritis, polycystic renal disease, obstructive nephropathy, hypercalcemic nephropathy).
9. Animals with CRD usually retain the ability to produce dilute urine (i.e., to excrete solute-free water) but ability to excrete a sudden increase in water load may be impaired.

DIAGNOSIS OF CHRONIC RENAL FAILURE

Clinical History in Chronic Renal Failure
Polyuria and Polydipsia

a. Polyuria and polydipsia may be the first abnormalities noted by observant owners of dogs and cats. Nocturia may be the first thing noticed in dogs when they awaken their owners so as to be allowed outside to urinate during the night. Polydipsia and polyuria frequently are not noticed by owners of cats. Polyuria in cats may be identified if questions about the weight of the litter box are included in the history.

b. Some owners misinterpret polyuria as incontinence or pollakiuria because the animal is urinating in the house when it never did so in the past. The owner must be questioned to differentiate incontinence (lack of voluntary control; dribbling) from polyuria (normal voluntary control; increased volume of urine) and pollakiuria (normal control, urinating small volumes frequently and sometimes accompanied by straining or pain).

c. If polyuria and polydipsia are not recognized, nonspecific signs of uremia may be the first abnormalities the owner detects.

Gastrointestinal Signs

a. Vomiting: Common in uremic dogs but much less so in cats. Stimulation of the chemoreceptor trigger zone by a uremic toxin may be the cause. Gastrointestinal ulcers also may contribute, as may increased gastric hyperacidity.

b. Gastroenteritis with hemorrhage (especially in uremic dogs) can occur. Many factors may contribute to uremic gastropathy:
   (1) Uremic alterations in mucus layer may cause back diffusion of acid.
   (2) Bleeding due to platelet dysfunction.
   (3) Erosions or ulcers due to ammonia production from urea by bacteria in the gastrointestinal tract are less common in dogs and cats than in humans with CRF.
   (4) Ischemia due to vascular lesions (uremia induced vasculitis), but gastric necrosis is uncommon.
   (5) Edema and thickening of the gastric mucosa.
   (6) Increased concentration of circulating gastrin due to impaired renal degradation has been documented in both dogs and cats. Excess gastrin stimulates acid secretion in the stomach and contributes to uremic gastroenteritis.
   (7) Gastric mineralization.

c. Diarrhea: A relatively uncommon late finding in uremic dogs.

Anorexia

a. Centrally mediated impairment of appetite.

b. Oral erosions or ulcers and uremic gastroenteritis contribute.

Weight Loss

a. May be due to lack of adequate caloric intake but also can be associated with catabolic processes that are activated even when adequate calories are consumed.

b. Excess glucagon may contribute to negative nitrogen balance and increased tissue catabolism.

c. Metabolic acidosis can activate protein catabolic pathways in muscle.

Lethargy, Weakness, and Neurologic Signs

a. Centrally mediated mental dullness in uremic patients.

b. Loss of lean muscle mass.

c. Uremic encephalopathy.
   (1) Uremic encephalopathy may occur when GFR decreases to less than 10% of normal. Encephalopathy is more readily recognized when the onset of uremia is rapid (as in ARF) but it also can be severe in CRF.
   (2) Calcium influx in the brain mediated by high PTH concentration may play a role in uremic encephalopathy of CRF. Amino acid alterations due to malnutrition or accumulation of uremic toxins may alter neurotransmitter function. Electroencephalographic abnormalities in dogs with experimentally induced and naturally occurring renal failure have been noted that parallel the severity of the observed clinical signs.
      (a) Low serum ionized calcium concentration may contribute in some cases.
      (b) Systemic hypertension may contribute in some cases.

(c) Aluminum accumulation in the brain also may contribute, especially in patients treated with aluminum-containing intestinal phosphate binders for extended periods of time (poorly documented in veterinary medicine).

(3) Clinical signs reported in affected dogs include facial twitching, head bobbing, abnormal behavior, tremors, and seizures.

d. Uremic neuropathy is an insidious, distal, symmetrical polyneuropathy (i.e., "dying back neuropathy") indistinguishable from other metabolic neuropathies.

(1) Occurs when GFR decreases below 10% of normal.

(2) Decreased nerve conduction velocity may be present in the absence of any obvious clinical signs.

(3) Sometimes has been associated with high PTH concentrations.

Physical Findings in CRF
Weight Loss Including Loss of Lean Muscle Mass
Poor Hair Coat (i.e., Dull, Dry)
Oral Lesions (More Common in Dogs Than Cats)

a. Foul oral odor may be due to accumulation of ammonia and aliphatic amines.

b. Erosions and ulcers of the buccal mucosa and tongue (often the lateral margins of tongue) may be observed. Ulcers may be due to excretion of urea into saliva and breakdown to ammonia by oral bacteria.

c. Tongue tip necrosis may result from fibrinoid necrosis and arteritis with focal ischemia, necrosis, and ulceration. This lesion is much more common in dogs than in cats. It is more commonly described in patients with CRF but also can develop in those with ARF.

d. Pallor of mucous membranes due to anemia.

Dehydration with Loss of Skin Elasticity and Dryness of Mucous Membranes

a. Occurs as a result of the lack of fluid intake and increased fluid losses in urine and from the gastrointestinal tract (e.g., vomiting).

b. Extent of dehydration may be overestimated based on skin turgor when evaluating cachexic animals.

Abnormal Auscultation

a. Heart murmurs and gallop rhythms are relatively common.

(1) These may occur as a consequence of systemic hypertension.

(2) Anemia in patients with advanced CRF also may contribute to the development of a heart murmur.

(3) Heart failure usually is not present.

b. Crackles arising from pulmonary edema and congestive heart failure or uremic pneumonitis are very rare.

Abdominal Palpation

a. Small, normal, or enlarged kidneys may be identified, depending on the underlying disease process.

b. The kidneys in patients with CRF usually are not painful.

c. Small, hard, irregular kidneys are consistent with CRF, but normal to enlarged kidneys do not rule out CRF (especially in cats).

d. The presence of an enlarged bladder in a patient known to be urinating indicates polyuria of CRF. If an enlarged bladder is palpated, it is essential to ensure that urinary obstruction is not a contributing factor.

Osteodystrophy

a. Fibrous osteodystrophy is most dramatic in young growing dogs with uremia (so-called *rubber jaw*).

(1) Loose teeth and loss of lamina dura dentes in maxilla and mandible.

(2) Expansion of the maxillary bones is common.

b. Pathologic fractures are rare.

Subcutaneous Edema

a. Subcutaneous edema or ascites suggests the possibility of glomerular disease with severe loss of plasma proteins (see Chapter 7, Diseases of the Glomerulus).

Blindness

a. Blindness may occur as a consequence of systemic hypertension.

(1) Hypertension may not be identified by blood pressure measurement at presentation if severe volume depletion also is present.

(2) Retinal detachments occasionally may occur even with minimal hypertension and hypoalbuminemia.

(3) Fundic examination findings include:

(a) Retinal detachment.

(b) Retinal hemorrhages.

(c) Retinal vascular tortuosity.

(d) Optic disc cupping.

Systemic or Local Infections

a. Chemotaxis is impaired in uremia.

b. Cell-mediated immunity is impaired to a greater extent than humoral immunity.

Hemostasis Defects

a. Uremia is characterized by abnormal hemostasis and a predisposition to hemorrhage.

Systemic Hypertension

1. The prevalence of hypertension in dogs with CKD has been reported to be as low as 9% and as high as 93%, and in cats with CKD the prevalence of hypertension has been reported to range between 19% and 65%. Many factors including differences in the types of renal diseases present, methodological differences, differences in body size, and interaction with human beings, (so-called *white coat effect*) all likely have contributed to variability in the reported range of prevalence of hypertension in dogs and cats with CKD. We estimate that 20% to 30% of cats and dogs with CKD have systemic hypertension at the time of diagnosis in our hospital, and that another 10% to 20% develop hypertension within a year of the initial diagnosis. Standardization of blood pressure measurement methodology and longitudinal studies will be required to better understand the natural history of hypertension in dogs and cats with CKD.

2. Normal blood pressure in dogs and cats is similar to that of human beings (i.e., systolic 120 mm Hg, diastolic 80 mm Hg). The white coat effect can increase the blood pressure of dogs and cats.

3. Because of white coat artifact, it is difficult to diagnose hypertension in dogs and cats.

a. Some studies have used a systolic blood pressure of >175 mm Hg on 2 occasions or >175 mm Hg in the presence of ocular lesions as indicating hypertension in cats.

b. Dogs with CRF and in-hospital systolic blood pressures of 145 to 165 mm Hg are considered mildly to moderately hypertensive and those with systolic blood pressures of 165 to 200 mm Hg are considered moderately to severely hypertensive. Those with systolic blood pressures >200 mm Hg are considered to have severe hypertension.

c. Patients with CKD may be at greater risk for end organ damage from systemic hypertension because the normally protective autoregulatory mechanism is not operative in afferent arterioles of glomeruli of remnant nephrons.

4. Factors contributing to hypertension in CKD include:
   a. Sympathetic nervous system stimulation.
   b. Renal ischemia with activation of renin-angiotensin-aldosterone system (RAAS).
   c. Plasma volume expansion when sodium excretion is impaired at very low levels of GFR (i.e., <5% of normal).
   d. An intrarenal mechanism for sodium retention plays an important role in glomerular disease (see Chapter 7, Diseases of the Glomerulus).
5. Clinical and pathologic manifestations of systemic hypertension include adverse effects on the eyes, heart, nervous system, and kidneys.

Laboratory Findings in CRF
Hemogram

a. A nonregenerative (normochromic, normocytic; hypoproliferative) anemia is common in CRF but variable in severity. The severity of the anemia is roughly correlated with the severity of the CRF as judged by serum creatinine concentration. Anemia may be masked by dehydration, which causes hemoconcentration. Thus, the hematocrit should be evaluated in conjunction with the serum total protein concentration.
   (1) The primary cause of anemia in CRF is an absolute or relative deficit in the production of erythropoietin in diseased kidneys by peritubular interstitial cells so that the uremic patient cannot meet the demand for new red cells necessitated by loss from hemolysis, hemorrhage, and normal turnover. Erythropoietin stimulates the final differentiation of committed erythroid progenitor cells in the bone marrow into mature red blood cells.
   (2) The life span of red cells in uremic patients is approximately 50% that of healthy individuals. The decreased life span is thought to be due to a toxic factor (possibly PTH) in uremic plasma that promotes hemolysis.
   (3) Some uremic toxins may impair erythropoiesis (e.g., polyamines, ribonuclease, PTH).
   (4) Increased red blood cell (RBC) 2,3-diphosphoglycerate due to hyperphosphatemia lowers hemoglobin affinity for oxygen and enhances oxygen delivery to tissues. This partially compensates for the anemia but reduces the hypoxic stimulus for erythropoiesis.
   (5) Platelet dysfunction promotes insidious ongoing blood loss (e.g., gastrointestinal hemorrhage).
   (6) Some dogs and cats with CRF have microcytosis and iron deficiency based on evaluation of serum iron concentrations.
   (7) Serum erythropoietin concentrations are decreased or normal in dogs and cats with CRF. A normal concentration of erythropoietin in an anemic animal with CRF represents an inadequate response. Assays for erythropoietin in dogs and cats are not available from commercial diagnostic laboratories.
b. Mature neutrophilia and lymphopenia (i.e., stress of chronic disease).
c. Normal platelet numbers but platelet function may be abnormal.
   (1) The qualitative platelet function defect (platelet numbers are normal) is most important, and risk of hemorrhage is best correlated with the buccal mucosal bleeding time (normally <2-3 min). Other coagulation tests (e.g., one stage prothrombin time [OSPT], activated partial thromboplastin time [APTT], activated coagulation time [ACT]) usually are normal.
   (2) Abnormalities of platelet function include abnormal platelet aggregation, abnormal platelet factor 3 release, abnormal platelet adhesiveness, decreased clot retraction, and decreased thromboxane production by platelets.

(3) Platelet dysfunction is thought to be caused by a uremic toxin. Guanidines and PTH are suspected but not proved to be involved.

Routine Serum Biochemistry

BLOOD UREA NITROGEN (BUN) AND SERUM CREATININE CONCENTRATIONS

(1) By definition, to be in renal failure, BUN and serum creatinine concentrations are increased above normal. Usually, both are increased simultaneously.

    (a) Early in the course of CRF in some cats, the serum creatinine concentration may be increased while the BUN concentration remains normal. Anorexia or poor appetite may contribute to the lower BUN concentration in this situation.

    (b) In animals with substantial muscle wasting, serum creatinine concentration may not reflect the severity of CRF.

    (c) Gastrointestinal bleeding also may increase BUN concentration out of proportion to serum creatinine concentration.

SODIUM

(1) Serum sodium is normal in most patients with compensated CRF. Hypernatremia is observed in some patients with decompensated CRF due to dehydration or alternatively due to sodium retention with advanced loss of nephron mass and extremely low GFR (i.e., <5% of normal). Hyponatremia occurs sporadically in CRF if water retention has occurred (e.g., administration of hypotonic fluids and impaired renal excretion of an acute water load).

    (a) To maintain balance for sodium as renal disease progresses, the kidneys must reduce the fraction of filtered sodium that is reabsorbed (and increase the fraction that is excreted). Natriuretic hormones play an important role in this adaptive process. For example, a higher concentration of atrial natriuretic peptide enhances sodium excretion by the kidneys in CRF.

    (b) Patients with CRF are able to maintain sodium balance despite very low GFR but they are much less flexible than normal individuals in their response to abrupt changes in sodium intake (i.e., they take longer to excrete an abrupt sodium load). If sodium intake is gradually reduced over several months, patients with CRF can gradually reduce sodium excretion.

    (c) The fractional reabsorption of sodium can only be reduced so far. When GFR falls below 5% of normal, positive balance for sodium may develop with consequent expansion of extracellular fluid volume, hypernatremia, and rarely edema.

POTASSIUM

(1) Most animals with CRF have normal serum potassium concentrations. Hyperkalemia usually does not develop unless the animal becomes oliguric or anuric. Hypokalemia may occur in 10% to 30% of dogs and cats with chronic CRF due to some combination of anorexia, loss of muscle mass, vomiting, and polyuria.

    (a) A significant body deficit of potassium can exist without the development of hypokalemia. Serum potassium levels can underestimate total body potassium since most of the body's potassium lies within the cells. As potassium is lost excessively from the plasma, potassium leaches out of the cells down a concentration gradient masking the initial loss of potassium.

    (b) One study of cats with CRF and normokalemia revealed decreased potassium content (kaliopenia) of muscles.

(2) Potassium balance is maintained by an adaptive increase in the fractional excretion of potassium as renal disease advances. Increased secretion of potassium per functional remnant nephron occurs in the distal nephron. Adaptive changes include

increases in the activity of Na$^+$-K$^+$ adenosine triphosphatase (ATPase) and in the basolateral surface area of principal cells in the cortical collecting ducts. This adaptive response is facilitated by (but does not require) aldosterone.

(3) Patients with CRF are less flexible in their response to added potassium. They have a reduced ability to tolerate an acute potassium load and may require 1 to 3 days to reestablish potassium balance when the intake of potassium is abruptly increased.

(4) Hypokalemic (kaliopenic) nephropathy has been described as a specific syndrome in clinical cats either as a result of CKD or resulting in CKD.

> ! Hypokalemia can be a consequence of CKD but also can contribute to worsening of lesions in animals with pre-existing CKD.

(a) Whether kaliopenia without hypokalemia can result in CKD in cats has not been established.
   (i) In one experimental study of cats, the development of CRF and hypokalemia was discovered at the same time in cats fed a marginally replete urinary acidifying and magnesium restricted diet.

(b) Hypokalemia can contribute to anorexia, depression, and weakness independent of the effects of CRF. Severe muscle weakness (the "hanging-head" posture, truncal ataxia) is seen in many cats with serum potassium <2.5 mEq/L and in some with <3.0 mEq/L (Figure 5-6).

(c) The fractional excretion of potassium into urine is high despite the low serum potassium. Cats with normokalemic CKD also have high fractional excretion for potassium as part of the adaptive nephron response to maintain potassium balance.

(d) Hypokalemia can be associated with functional and or structural changes in the kidneys.
   (i) Reduced ability to concentrate the urine–initially functional, structural later.
   (ii) Decreased GFR initially can be a result of hemodynamic changes, later due to structural changes.

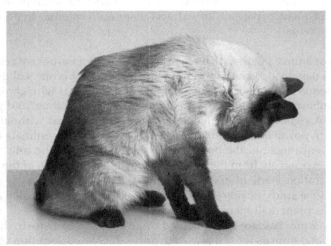

FIGURE 5-6 ■ "Hanging-head" posture typical of severe hypokalemia in a cat with hypokalemic nephropathy.

(iii) Structural lesions of tubulointerstitial inflammation and fibrosis associated with CRF have been reported to develop in cats fed marginally potassium replete diets that are highly acidifying and magnesium restricted.

(iv) Some cats with CRF and hypokalemia will improve their excretory renal function following correction of the hypokalemia. Whether this improvement is due to correction of prerenal factors, intrarenal hemodynamics, or resolution of some intrarenal lesions is not clear.

(v) Some cats with CRF periodically develop hypokalemia during the course of their disease.

PHOSPHORUS

(1) In early stages of CKD (i.e., IRIS stage 1 and early stage 2), serum phosphorus concentration often is normal due to the corrective effect of renal secondary hyperparathyroidism.

(2) Hyperphosphatemia develops with advancing CRF when 85% and more of the nephrons become nonfunctional. At this point, the corrective effect of high PTH concentration is overwhelmed.

(3) Serum phosphorus concentration in normal adult dogs and cats should be <5.5 mg/dL. Many laboratories report a higher upper end of the normal range for serum phosphorus concentration, presumably because young animals with active bone growth have been included in the population used to determine the normal reference range.

CALCIUM

(1) Serum total calcium concentrations are normal in the majority of CRF patients but can be low or high in some patients.

(2) Serum total, ionized, protein-bound, and complexed calcium concentrations vary considerably in dogs and cats with CRF. Differences in total calcium concentration tend to be attributable primarily to changes in the complexed calcium component. The complexed calcium fraction can vary from 6% to 39% of serum total calcium in dogs with CRF.

! Errors in interpretation of calcium status occur when serum total calcium concentration is evaluated instead of ionized calcium concentration. Serum ionized calcium concentration cannot be predicted from total calcium concentration or any other combined parameters.

(3) Serum total calcium concentrations are an unreliable predictor of ionized calcium status in CRF. Measurement of serum ionized calcium concentration is the method of choice for accurate assessment of calcium status in dogs with CRF.

(a) Dogs. In a recent study, 22% of 490 CRF dogs were classified as hypercalcemic and 19% were classified as hypocalcemic on the basis of serum total calcium concentrations. Using serum ionized calcium concentrations, however, 9% of the CRF dogs were classified as hypercalcemic and 36% were classified as hypocalcemic. Serum total calcium concentration incorrectly predicted serum ionized calcium concentration in 36% of dogs with CRF. Use of an adjustment formula based on serum albumin or total protein concentration only increased the amount of misdiagnosis.

(b) Cats. In 102 cats with CRF, 20% were classified as hypercalcemic, and 11% were classified as hypocalcemic based on serum total calcium concentration. Using serum ionized calcium concentrations, 29% were classified as hypercalcemic, and 10% were classified as hypocalcemic. Serum total calcium concentration incorrectly predicted serum ionized calcium concentration in 32% of cats with CRF.

(4) Hypocalcemia.
   (a) Dogs. The percentage of hypocalcemic CRF dogs is underestimated when using serum total calcium concentration to evaluate calcium status. Based on serum ionized calcium concentration, between 30% and 40% of CRF dogs can be expected to be hypocalcemic.
   (b) Between 8% and 15% of cats with CRF have been reported to be hypocalcemic based on serum or plasma total calcium concentration determinations. In a study of 102 cats with CRF, 10% were found to have ionized hypocalcemia.
   (c) The Mass Law Effect decreases serum calcium as a consequence of increased serum phosphorus concentration. The amounts of calcium and phosphorus that can remain in solution together are defined by the $[Ca(mg/dL)] \times [Pi(mg/dL)]$ product. When this value is greater than 60 to 70, soft tissue mineralization may occur. Decreased production of calcitriol by the diseased kidneys also results in impaired intestinal absorption of calcium.
   (d) Vitamin D_3 activation (conversion of 25-hydroxycholecalciferol to 1,25-dihydroxycholecalciferol) occurs primarily within mitochondria of the proximal tubules. This activation becomes limited with advanced loss of nephron mass and phosphorus retention.
   (e) Hypocalcemia in CRF usually is asymptomatic (i.e., tetany is not observed) because metabolic acidosis leads to an increase in the ionized component of total serum calcium. This occurs because of a decrease in net negative charge on plasma proteins that occurs during acidosis which reduces protein binding of calcium.
(5) Hypercalcemia.
   (a) Dogs. In 490 dogs with CRF, 22% were classified as hypercalcemic based on serum total calcium concentration. When ionized calcium concentration was evaluated, only 9% were hypercalcemic. Hypercalcemia was greatly overestimated in dogs with CRF when serum total calcium was measured.
   (b) Cats. In 102 cats with CRF, 20% were classified as hypercalcemic based on serum total calcium concentration. When ionized calcium concentration was evaluated, 29% were hypercalcemic. Hypercalcemia was underestimated in cats with CRF when serum total calcium was measured.

> **!** Hypercalcemia can contribute to CKD, and CKD can result in hypercalcemia. Measurement of serum ionized calcium concentration is helpful because only ionized hypercalcemia can cause CKD.

   (c) Hypercalcemia may further damage the kidney by causing renal vasoconstriction and mineralization of the interstitium and tubular basement membranes.
   (d) Possible mechanisms of ionized hypercalcemia in renal failure include reduced urinary excretion of calcium due to very low GFR, decreased renal degradation of PTH, unregulated parathyroid gland secretion of PTH, and increased PTH set point for calcium. Decreased numbers of calcium-sensing receptors due to loss of tubular mass or decreased receptor upregulation due to calcitriol deficits also could contribute to decreased urinary excretion of calcium.
   (e) In some hypercalcemic patients with renal failure it can be difficult to determine which occurred first, the renal failure or the hypercalcemia. Careful consideration of historical, physical, laboratory, and radiographic findings usually facilitates this decision. Measurement of serum ionized calcium concentration is essential in these instances. If the serum ionized calcium concentration is normal or low, then the noted increase in serum total calcium concentration was most likely a consequence of CRF and not the cause of CRF.

GLUCOSE
    (a) Peripheral insulin resistance and mild fasting hyperglycemia (<200 mg/dL) are common in uremia.
    (b) Very high PTH concentrations have been associated with insulin resistance and decreased insulin secretion.
    (c) This finding usually is not clinically relevant.

Acid-Base Balance

a. Mild metabolic acidosis (decreased pH) that is well compensated (decreased pCO_2) is common in patients with stable CRF.

    (1) The metabolic acidosis of CRF usually is not severe despite development of positive balance for H^+ ions. The relatively mild decrease in plasma HCO_3^- concentration observed in CRF is a consequence of the large reservoir of buffer (e.g., calcium carbonate) in bone. The metabolic acidosis of CRF contributes to renal osteodystrophy and represents yet another example of the trade-off hypothesis.

    (2) In a recent study, metabolic acidosis was documented in 53% of cats with advanced CRF but in only 15% of cats with mild CRF.

    (3) The metabolic acidosis of CRF is hyperchloremic (normal anion gap) early in its course and normochloremic (high anion gap) later in its course when acid metabolites that titrate HCO_3^- have accumulated as unmeasured anions (e.g., phosphate, sulfate, organic anions).

    (4) Effects of the metabolic acidosis of CRF that are "adaptive" include preservation of serum ionized calcium concentration by the effects of acidosis on the charge of plasma proteins and shifting of the hemoglobin-oxygen saturation curve to the right with improved tissue delivery of oxygen. The latter effect partially compensates for the anemia of CRF.

b. The main cause of metabolic acidosis in progressive renal disease is limitation of renal ammonium excretion.

    (1) The chronically diseased kidney maintains H^+ ion balance primarily by enhanced renal ammoniagenesis from glutamine. Absolute ammonium excretion falls during progressive CKD, but ammonium excretion is markedly increased when expressed per remnant nephron. On a per nephron basis, the diseased kidney can increase its ammonium excretion threefold to fivefold.

    (2) This adaptive mechanism is maximal when GFR falls to 10% to 20% of normal. At this point, the diseased kidneys can no longer effectively cope with the daily fixed acid load and a new steady state is established at a lower than normal plasma HCO_3^- concentration. Compensation may remain adequate until GFR falls to 5% of normal but such patients are in a precarious state of balance that easily may be disrupted by other disease states (e.g., acute diarrhea).

Hormonal Status

PARATHYROID HORMONE
    (1) Hyperparathyroidism is a consistent finding in progressive renal disease when sensitive and specific assays are used to detect PTH. PTH concentrations cannot be predicted from creatinine, calcium, or phosphorus concentrations, and must be measured for accurate assessment.

> **!** A single serum measurement of PTH in the normal range cannot rule out the possibility of an increase from the animal's own normal baseline concentration. Repeated measurements may be helpful in documenting renal secondary hyperparathyroidism.

(2) PTH is increased above the normal range in patients with more advanced CRF.

    (a) PTH may be increased in an individual animal but still be within the laboratory's reference range.

    (b) Small increases in PTH in dogs and cats with early renal disease may not be detectable unless the individual animal's baseline PTH concentration was determined previously.

    (c) Development of renal secondary hyperparathyroidism classically has been explained by the effect of phosphorus retention on serum ionized calcium concentration (Figure 5-7); in recent years the important role of impaired renal production of calcitriol in the pathogenesis of renal secondary hyperparathyroidism has been elucidated.

       (i) Reduction in GFR decreases phosphate excretion and results in hyperphosphatemia.

      (ii) Hyperphosphatemia causes a reciprocal decrease in serum ionized calcium concentration by the Mass Law Effect ($[Ca] \times [Pi]$ = constant). The contribution of the Mass Law Effect currently is thought to be small because a very large change in phosphorus concentration is required to produce a very small change in serum calcium concentration.

     (iii) Ionized hypocalcemia stimulates the parathyroid glands to synthesize and secrete PTH.

     (iv) The increase in PTH stimulates increased renal excretion of phosphate and increased release of calcium and phosphate from bone, which returns serum phosphorus and ionized calcium concentrations to normal. Some of the increased calcium is due to an indirect effect of PTH on the intestine from increased synthesis of calcitriol.

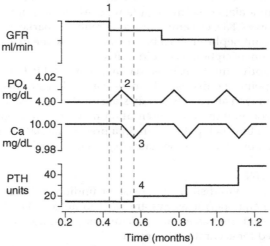

FIGURE 5-7 ■ Development of renal secondary hyperparathyroidism—classic theory. Step 1 is the loss of nephron mass by some chronic disease process. With every loss of nephron mass there is a small increase in circulating phosphorus (step 2). Ionized calcium decreases (step 3) as a consequence of the increase in the serum phosphorus. PTH increases (step 4) in response to the decreased ionized calcium. This theory ignores the important genomic effects of calcitriol required to inhibit PTH synthesis (shown in Figure 5-8).

(v) PTH decreases the fractional reabsorption of phosphate in the kidney by decreasing the tubular reabsorptive maximum (T_{max}) for phosphate. This effect initially decreases serum phosphorus concentration to within normal limits as more phosphorus is excreted into the urine. The limit of this compensatory response is reached when GFR declines to approximately 15% to 20% of normal. As GFR declines further, hyperphosphatemia occurs.

(d) The effect of phosphorus retention and loss of tubular mass on renal calcitriol production suggests an alternate explanation for development of renal secondary hyperparathyroidism called the calcitriol trade-off hypothesis in which the genomic effects of calcitriol on the synthesis of PTH are most important (Figure 5-8).

(i) Phosphorus retention and hyperphosphatemia inhibit renal 1α-hydroxylase, which impairs conversion of 25-hydroxycholecalciferol to 1,25-dihydroxycholecalciferol (calcitriol).

(ii) Calcitriol normally causes decreased synthesis and secretion of PTH by the parathyroid gland. This negative feedback loop is impaired in CRF due to decreased renal production of calcitriol. In addition, there are decreased numbers of parathyroid gland calcitriol receptors in uremia with a resultant decrease in the responsiveness of the parathyroid glands to the inhibitory effect of calcitriol on PTH synthesis and release.

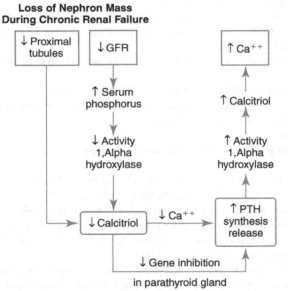

FIGURE 5-8 ■ Development of renal secondary hyperparathyroidism—calcitriol trade-off hypothesis. Chronic renal diseases result in the loss of tubular mass. Since calcitriol is synthesized within the renal tubules, deficits of calcitriol synthesis occur. Increases in phosphorus burden within the body also contribute to decreased calcitriol as activity of the 1-alpha-hydroxyalse system within the renal tubules is impaired. Circulating calcitriol provides an important negative effect on PTH synthesis by inhibition of gene transcription within the parathyroid gland cell nucleus. The combination of low calcitriol and low ionized calcium allows high levels of PTH to be synthesized and secreted. The higher levels of PTH upregulate the activity of the 1-alpha-hydroxylase system within the renal tubules, returning calcitriol production to normal (if there is sufficient residual renal tubular mass). The restored calcitriol concentrations in the circulation are maintained at the expense of a higher-than-normal PTH. There is a negative impact from chronically high PTH levels on a variety of organs including the kidneys.

(iii) The effects of calcitriol on PTH secretion normally arise, in part, from its ability to induce synthesis of the calcium receptor in parathyroid gland cells.

(iv) Thus, decreased calcitriol production, decreased numbers of parathyroid gland calcitriol receptors, and decreased numbers of calcium receptors all play roles in the development of renal secondary hyperparathyroidism.

CALCITRIOL

(1) Serum calcitriol concentrations are normal in most dogs and cats in the early stages of CRF due to the stimulatory effect of high PTH concentration on renal production of calcitriol. Given the high PTH concentration, however, even normal concentrations of calcitriol may be considered inappropriate. In fact, the high PTH concentration maintains relatively normal serum calcitriol concentration during early to moderate CRF.

(2) Serum calcitriol concentrations are low in patients with advanced CRF.

THYROID HORMONE CONCENTRATIONS

(1) Thyroid hormone concentrations may be decreased in patients with CRF.

(a) CRF is a nonthyroidal illness that results in lower measured concentrations of thyroid hormones.

(b) Lower thyroxine (T4) concentrations can cause confusion in the diagnosis of hyperthyroidism in older cats with CRF and hyperthyroidism (see Chapter 16, Miscellaneous Syndromes).

(c) Lower T4 concentrations in dogs with CRF can result in an erroneous diagnosis of hypothyroidism and inappropriate treatment with L-thyroxine.

PLASMA CORTISOL CONCENTRATIONS

(1) Plasma cortisol concentrations may be normal to slightly increased in patients with CRF.

RENIN-ANGIOTENSIN-ALDOSTERONE SYNDROME ACTIVATION (RAAS)

(1) RAAS activation contributes to systemic hypertension and to adverse effects in chronically diseased kidneys.

ERYTHROPOIETIN

(1) Erythropoietin is discussed below under endocrine replacement therapy.

Urinalysis

a. Isosthenuria develops when 67% of nephrons become nonfunctional (USG 1.007-1.015). Cats can retain concentrating ability after onset of azotemia (see above) especially when serum creatinine concentration is in the 2.0-3.0 mg/dL range.

b. Submaximally concentrated urine (USG <1.040 in cats and <1.030 in dogs) in association with azotemia suggests intrinsic renal disease. Some cats with intrinsic CKD still can concentrate urine to USG >1.045.

c. Proteinuria may indicate increased disease severity or progression in patients with CKD. Persistent severe proteinuria without active sediment suggests primary glomerular disease (see Chapter 7, Diseases of the Glomerulus).

d. Pyuria and bacteriuria suggest UTI but do not localize it.

(1) Bacterial UTI is common in cats with CRF.

(2) UTI may be present despite the presence of an inactive urinary sediment, especially in cats with CRF.

Diagnostic Imaging

a. Decreased renal size is compatible with CRF but normal renal size does not rule out CRF (Figure 5-9).

b. Irregularly shaped kidneys suggest CRF.

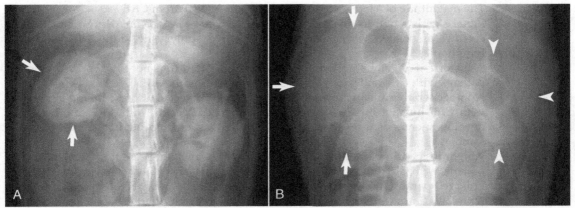

FIGURE 5-9 ■ Chronic renal disease radiology. Note small and irregular kidneys. **A,** Both kidneys are small compared with the length of L2. *Arrows* point to irregular flattened areas. **B,** Note disparity between left and right kidney sizes. The left kidney (*arrow heads*) is small compared with the length of L2, while the right kidney is slightly enlarged (*small arrows*). (Courtesy of Dr. Paul Barthez, Ghent, Belgium.)

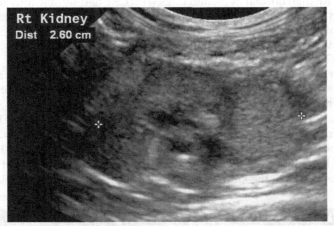

FIGURE 5-10 ■ Chronic renal disease ultrasonography of a cat. Note hyperechogenic and irregular renal cortex, loss of corticomedullary junction definition, and small size (2.6 cm length shown between + signs). (Courtesy of Dr. Valerie Samii, The Ohio State University, Columbus, Ohio.)

    c. Renal ultrasonography often shows increased echogenicity of renal tissue, but echogenicity can be normal despite advanced renal disease (Figure 5-10).

    d. Some CKD (especially in cats) can be associated with enlarged kidneys (e.g., polycystic renal disease, renal lymphoma).

    e. Enlargement of the left ventricle may be observed on thoracic radiographs or echocardiography as a consequence of systemic hypertension.

Differentiation of Acute Renal Failure from Chronic Renal Failure

    a. Sometimes it is difficult to determine whether the animal is suffering from ARF or CRF.

    b. Differentiation is essential because ARF is a potentially reversible disease process whereas CRF is not.

    c. The magnitude of azotemia does not differentiate ARF from CRF.

    d. Renal size is small to normal in CRF and normal to large in ARF. Some CRDs in cats are associated with enlarged kidneys (e.g., polycystic kidney disease, renal lymphoma).

    e. A history of previous polyuria and polydipsia often (but not always) is present in patients with CRF and should be absent in patients with ARF.

    f. Nonregenerative anemia often (but not always) is detected at presentation in patients with CRF but not initially in patients with ARF. Patients with ARF can, however, develop anemia as a result of ongoing blood loss and repeated collection of blood samples.

    g. Weight loss and poor hair coat often (but not always) are present at presentation in patients with CRF but usually (although not always) absent in patients with ARF.

    h. Enlarged parathyroid glands on ultrasound examination may be observed in patients with CRF. In one study, dogs with CRF had significantly larger (3.9-8.1 mm length) parathyroid glands than did normal dogs (2.0-4.6 mm length) and those with ARF (2.4-4.0 mm length). The size of parathyroid glands in dogs seems to be related to body weight.

    i. Increased carbamylated hemoglobin concentration or nail creatinine concentration. In one study, carbamylated hemoglobin concentrations were higher in dogs with ARF and CRF than normal dogs, and dogs with CRF had significantly higher concentrations than did dogs with ARF. Neither test is routinely performed by commercial diagnostic laboratories.

    j. Hypothermia occasionally is present in patients with ARF, but is absent in patients with CRF except terminally.

    k. Hyperkalemia may be observed with development of oliguria or anuria in patients with ARF or CRF. Hyperkalemia should be absent in patients with polyuric renal failure whether it is CRF or ARF.

    l. Blood pressure may be low in both decompensated CRF and ARF before treatment, presumably as a consequence of dehydration and volume depletion. Hypertension may be present after volume expansion in both patients with ARF and CRF.

    m. Renal biopsy may be the only way to differentiate CRF from ARF. Renal biopsy is not warranted when the kidneys are small and irregular and azotemia is advanced.

TREATMENT OF CHRONIC RENAL FAILURE

A. Box 5-1 provides a checklist of possible treatments for CRF, and Box 5-2 provides a status checklist to review during treatment of CRF.

General Principles of Management

1. Ideally, match treatment to the IRIS stage of renal disease. Most available studies of treatment have been performed in dogs and cats in IRIS stages 3 and 4 of CRD.

2. Search for potentially reversible causes of renal failure (e.g., pyelonephritis, hypercalcemia, obstructive nephropathy).

3. Eliminate reversible factors that may be aggravating renal failure.

    a. Do not pass judgment on the animal until it has been rehydrated. Appropriate intravenous fluid therapy should be provided to resolve prerenal azotemia. Complete rehydration may require 1 to 5 days.

    b. Concurrent systemic or urinary tract bacterial infections should be treated with appropriate antibiotics.

■ BOX 5-1
■ **CHECKLIST OF POSSIBLE TREATMENTS FOR COMPENSATED CHRONIC RENAL FAILURE**

First Level of Treatment

Change to renal therapeutic diet—reduced phosphorus intake is most important — commercially available or homemade—wet foods better than dry if possible

Fresh water available at all times

H_2 receptor or proton pump blocker—combat gastric hyperacidity

Use intestinal phosphate binders to effect of serum phosphorus concentration—aim for mid-normal range; aluminum or calcium salts used most often

Treat serious hypertension now (>180 mm Hg systolic)—get below 180 mm Hg soon

Treat urinary or systemic infection

Avoid anesthesia or exposure to nephrotoxicants when possible

Second Level of Treatment

Subcutaneous fluids if not maintaining hydration

Add in metoclopramide or other anti-emetic to reduce vomiting and nausea effects if needed

Potassium supplementation if hypokalemia is overt or borderline

Optimize phosphate restriction (diet or binders) based on PTH or serum Pi — consider dose or class change for phosphate binders

Further blood pressure control—minimal aim <165 mm Hg, optimal aim <145 mm Hg

Provide peri-operative renal protection with IV fluids for several hours before, during, and following anesthetic and surgical procedures

Anabolic steroids for DOGS ONLY when poor body condition persists—monitor liver parameters

Third Level of Treatment

Provide ACE inhibition for renoprotection and antiproteinuric effects, independent of normal systemic blood pressure

Blood pressure control optimized for renal patient—multiple drug therapy or dose escalation as needed to maintain systolic blood pressure at <145 mm Hg

Calcitriol—daily or intermittent dosing protocol to control PTH and prevent parathyroid gland hyperplasia—base doses on ionized calcium and PTH

PEG tube placement when patient will not consume adequate nutrition and body condition is poor

EPO if patient approaches transfusion dependency—not for minor anemia

Fourth Level of Treatment

Renal transplantation—consider for selected cats

Chronic dialysis—acute on chronic decompensation—temporary stabilization

Emerging or Unproven Treatments

Epakitin—chitosan & calcium carbonate powder for intestinal phosphate binding

Renalzin—lanthanum carbonate gel dispenser system for intestinal phosphate binding

Azodyl—probiotic to reduce azotemia following bacterial utilization

Kremezin (Covalzin or AST-120)—nonselective sorbent to remove uremic toxins from intestinal lumen

Spironolactone—anti-adverse remodeling and further antiproteinuric effects

Cinacalcet — calcimimetic to lower PTH, calcium, and phosphorus

■ BOX 5-2
■ **STATUS CHECKLIST DURING TREATMENT OF THE PATIENT WITH CHRONIC RENAL FAILURE**

Nutritional Status
Body weight
Body condition score
Muscle condition score
Serum albumin
Total protein
BUN
Cholesterol
Poor, acceptable, excellent; worse, stable, improving

Serum Phosphorus Control
Poor, acceptable, excellent; worse, stable, improving

Serum Calcium Control
Serum total calcium
Serum ionized calcium (preferred)
Poor, acceptable, excellent; worse, stable, improving

Serum Potassium Control
Poor, acceptable, excellent; worse, stable, improving

Acid-Base Control
Blood gas (preferred); HCO_3 on profile
Poor, acceptable, excellent; worse, stable, improving

Systemic Blood Pressure Control
Poor, acceptable, excellent; worse, stable, improving

Proteinuria Control
Urinary protein-to-creatinine ratio; microalbuminuria testing
Poor, acceptable, excellent; worse, stable, improving

PTH Control
Poor, acceptable, excellent; worse, stable, improving

CKD Progression Control
BUN
Creatinine
Phosphorus
Proteinuria
Renal size
Systemic blood pressure
Poor, acceptable, excellent; worse, stable, improving

4. Maintain fluid, electrolyte, acid base, and caloric balance while preventing accumulation of metabolic waste products.
5. Counteract the effects of the lost endocrine functions of the kidney.

Dietary Management

1. Provide free access to water at all times. Do not restrict water in patients with polyuria and polydipsia because dehydration will rapidly ensue.
2. Diets designed to be helpful in the management of CRF in dogs and cats are restricted in protein, phosphate, and sodium while containing supplemental potassium, alkali, and omega-3 fatty acids.
    a. Several pet food manufacturers (Hill's, Nestle-Purina, Royal-Canin, Iams) provide renal therapeutic diets for dogs and cats.
    b. Homemade diets may be preferred by some owners who wish to prepare food for their pets (Tables 5-4, 5-5, and 5-6). We recommend the purchase of an inexpensive diet scale that measures grams or ounces to facilitate preparation of these recipes.

■ TABLE 5-4
■ ■ **Homemade Diet for Dogs in Chronic Renal Failure**

Ingredients	Grams
Cooked white rice	
May substitute rice baby cereal	
Can flavor either above with meat broth during cooking	237
Regular cooked beef, retain the fat	78
Large boiled egg	20
White bread	50
Vegetable oil	3
Calcium carbonate	1.5
Iodized salt	0.5
Total	390
Also feed one human adult vitamin-mineral tablet daily	

Nutrient Analysis – Dry Matter Basis	
Dry matter %	41.0
Energy kcal/100g	445
Protein %	21.1
Fat %	13.7
Linoleic acid %	1.8
Crude fiber %	1.4
Calcium %	0.43
Phosphorus %	0.22
Potassium %	0.26
Sodium %	0.33
Magnesium %	0.091

Balanced reduced-protein/low-phosphorus homemade formula for an 18-kg adult dog. Daily food as fed.
(Remillard RL, Paragon BM, Crane SW, et al: Making pet foods at home. In Hand MS, Thatcher CD, Remillard RL, Roudebush P, editors: *Small animal clinical nutrition*, ed 4, Marceline Mo., 2000, Walsworth Publishing, p 169.)

■ TABLE 5-5
■ ■ **Homemade Diet for Cats with Chronic Renal Failure**

Ingredients	Grams
Cooked white rice	
May substitute rice baby cereal	
Flavor either with meat broth during cooking	98
Cooked chicken liver	21
Cooked white chicken	21
Vegetable oil	7
Calcium carbonate	0.7
Iodized salt	0.5
Salt substitute (KCl)	0.5
Total	149
Also feed one-half human adult vitamin-mineral tablet daily.	
Add one-half to one 500 mg taurine tablet	

Nutrient Analysis–Dry Matter Basis	
Dry matter %	37.8
Energy kcal/100g	458
Protein %	24.4
Fat %	17.5
Linoleic acid %	7.9
Crude fiber %	0.85
Calcium %	0.54
Phosphorus %	0.29
Potassium %	0.66
Sodium %	0.42
Magnesium %	0.09

Balanced reduced-protein/low-phosphorus formula for a 4.5 kg adult cat. Daily food as fed. (Remillard RL, Paragon BM, Crane SW, et al: Making pet foods at home . In Hand MS, Thatcher CD, Remillard RL, Roudebush P, editors: *Small animal clinical nutrition*, ed 4, Marceline Mo., 2000, Walsworth Publishing, p 169.)

3. Protein restriction.
   a. Although widely advocated, the ability of dietary protein restriction to ameliorate clinical signs in dogs and cats with CRF remains unclear.
   b. Potential benefits are a reduction in uremic symptomatology by decreasing the production of toxic metabolites of protein metabolism in patients with overt azotemia and decreasing hyperfiltration in remnant nephrons.
   c. Moderate protein restriction is indicated to relieve uremic symptomatology and promote patient well-being in patients with moderate to severe azotemia, but moderate protein restriction does not appear to prevent hyperfiltration in dogs and cats. Protein restriction as a single dietary change does not seem to provide protection against progression of renal disease in dogs and cats with advanced CRD. Low protein diets should only be used with caution in hypoproteinemic animals with protein-losing nephropathy (see Chapter 7, Diseases of the Glomerulus). Low protein diets also are restricted in phosphorus, which may provide benefits previously attributed to the protein restriction.

■ TABLE 5-6
■ ■ **Homemade Diet for Either Dogs or Cats with Chronic Renal Failure**

Ingredients	Amount
Cooked meat: beef, chicken, pork, eggs	1.5 cups
Substitute:	
2% Cottage cheese	2 cups
Salmon, tuna	1.5 cups
Peanut butter	12 tablespoons
Soybean curd (tofu)	3 cups
Cooked starch: rice, pasta, potato	4 cups
Vegetable oil	1 teaspoon
Calcium carbonate–Tums, 500 mg tablets	2
Children's complete vitamin-mineral supplement	1
For cats, taurine, 500 mg tablet	1
Small amounts of fruits, vegetables, fats (butter, margarine, mayonnaise, salad dressing), and desserts (cake, cookies, unsalted popcorn, sherbet) may be added to increase palatability as needed	

Approximate Nutritional Analysis	
Calories	1200 kcal (20% protein, 40% carbohydrate, 40% fat)
Protein	60 g
Calcium	600 mg
Phosphorus	400 mg
Potassium	500 mg
Sodium	140 mg

Reduced-phosphorus, reduced-protein diet for dogs and cats. This diet is designed to combine six servings of protein with four servings of carbohydrates. Servings are derived from standards of human nutrition that can be consulted for alternate sources.
(Buffington CA, Holloway C, Abood S: Clinical dietetics. In *Manual of veterinary dietetics.* St Louis, 2004, Elsevier, p 108).

    d. The development of protein-calorie malnutrition always is a concern in dogs and cats with CKD, but even more so when such patients are consuming low protein diets.

    e. When in the course of CKD protein restriction should be started is uncertain. It is not recommended early in the course of CKD before nitrogenous waste products accumulate. If there is evidence of progression (e.g., progressively less concentrated urine, increasing proteinuria, progressive changes in the kidneys on repeated ultrasound examinations) even in patients without overt azotemia, dietary intervention may be prescribed before the animal becomes systemically ill. Once the animal becomes systemically ill, it will be less likely to tolerate a change in diet.

    f. Original guidelines for protein restriction in dogs with CRF were introduced in 1972. At that time, 0.6 g/lb/day of high quality (biologic value 90-100) protein was recommended. Guidelines for institution of this diet were as follows:

        (1) BUN stable and >80 mg/dL.

        (2) Serum creatinine stable and >2.5 mg/dL.

        (3) Serum phosphorus stable and >6.0 mg/dL.

This degree of dietary protein restriction may lead to malnutrition in dogs and is currently not recommended. Today, a minimum protein intake of nearly twice this amount (i.e., 1 g/lb/day) is recommended for dogs with CRF.

    g. Current guidelines for instituting dietary therapy are BUN stable and >60 to 80 mg/dL and serum creatinine concentration stable and >2.0 to 2.5 mg/dL. There is no clear evidence that dietary intervention provides any benefits to dogs or cats that are not yet azotemic.

    h. Feeding moderately restricted protein diets (e.g., 15%-17% protein) to dogs with CRF is preferable to feeding extremely high or low protein diets. A gradual transition from the previous diet to the prescribed diet over 2 to 4 weeks is recommended.

    i. While consuming a low protein diet with adequate caloric intake, BUN will decrease due to dietary manipulation alone and will no longer be a good indicator of renal function. A decrease in BUN when the animal is on a low protein diet does not imply improved renal function, however. Serum creatinine concentration is not affected to any relevant extent by a change in dietary composition.

    j. The nutritional needs of cats differ from dogs. Dogs require that a minimum of approximately 4% to 5% of calories come from protein whereas cats require that a minimum of 20% of calories come from protein. These represent minimum requirements and do not provide for bodily nitrogen reserves. Cats also seem to prefer diets higher in fat and require a source of taurine in their diet. It has been recommended that cats with renal failure receive a minimum of approximately 2 g/lb/day protein.

    k. Stable body weight, stable serum albumin concentration, and decreased BUN are indications that a low protein diet is being used successfully.

    l. Some studies have supported the use of very low protein diets (0.3-0.6 g/kg/day) for slowing the rate of progression of renal disease whereas others have not found a beneficial effect of protein restriction.

        (1) A low protein diet may limit interstitial inflammation and fibrosis and glomerulosclerosis by decreasing proteinuria and its deleterious effects in rats with experimentally induced models of renal failure.

        (2) As a single dietary modification, however, protein restriction has not been determined to prevent progression of CRD.

        (3) Prevention of hyperfiltration by feeding an extremely low protein diet may not be feasible in dogs without induction of malnutrition.

    m. Low protein diets may ameliorate uremic symptomatology in patients with marked azotemia, but this effect has not been specifically studied in dogs and cats with naturally occurring CRF.

  4. Dietary phosphorus restriction.

    a. Dietary phosphorus restriction is the most valuable dietary modification for dogs and cats with CRF. The beneficial effect of phosphorus restriction is independent of protein restriction in dogs and cats with experimental CRF.

> **❗** Dietary phosphorus restriction alone or in conjunction with intestinal phosphate binders is the most important therapeutic intervention in dogs and cats with stable compensated CRF.

        (1) Dietary phosphorus restriction in CRF has been shown in cats and dogs to blunt or reverse renal secondary hyperparathyroidism. Renal lesions are less severe, GFR is better maintained and survival time is longer.

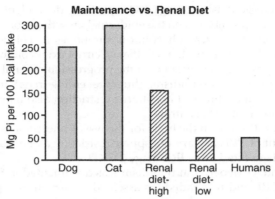

FIGURE 5-11 ■ Dietary phosphorus intake between dogs and cats eating commercial or renal therapeutic foods compared with average western diet of humans. Note that dogs and cats consume five and six times as much phosphorus as the average human, which makes it difficult to achieve adequate dietary phosphorus restriction. (Developed by Nutritional Support Services, The Ohio State University College of Veterinary Medicine, Dr. Tony Buffington, 2006.).

(2) Dogs consume five times more, and cats six times more phosphorus than humans consuming a typical Western diet. With such a high initial consumption of phosphorus, it is difficult to achieve the degree of phosphorus restriction in dogs and cats that is recommended for human patients with CKD (Figure 5-11).

b. Although the role of dietary protein restriction is less clear, diets restricted in protein are by nature also restricted in phosphorus and represent the only practical method to provide dietary phosphorus restriction.

(1) Extremely phosphorus-restricted diets are unpalatable because of the extent of protein restriction necessary to provide adequate phosphorus restriction.

c. A 0.44% phosphorus diet caused less renal disease progression than a 1.5% phosphorus diet in experimental studies with dogs, with 94% reduction in renal mass. Both groups were fed identical amounts of protein.

d. Hyperphosphatemia can be prevented or reversed in dogs with experimentally induced CRD by reducing dietary intake of phosphorus in proportion to the decrease in GFR.

e. Dogs with naturally occurring CRF managed with a diet that contained restricted phosphate (as well as restricted protein and sodium), however, did not show improvement in renal secondary hyperparathyroidism based on measurement of serum PTH concentrations. In a study of cats with naturally occurring CRF, treatment with a protein- and phosphorus-restricted diet and phosphate binders did correct renal secondary hyperparathyroidism based on serum PTH concentrations in most cats.

f. Dietary phosphate restriction relieves the inhibition of renal 1α-hydroxylase caused by phosphorus retention and results in increased calcitriol production by the kidneys. The increase in calcitriol enhances intestinal absorption of calcium, increases ionized calcium concentration, and results in decreased PTH synthesis and secretion as a result of the negative feedback effects of calcitriol on the parathyroid glands.

g. Later in the course of progressive CKD, the kidneys are unable to produce sufficient calcitriol to promote normal intestinal absorption of calcium or suppress PTH synthesis. Regardless, phosphorus restriction in advanced CKD still decreases PTH secretion by mechanisms that are independent of serum ionized calcium or calcitriol concentrations.

h. Parathyroid hyperplasia during CKD is partially dependent on action of transforming growth factor alpha (TGFα) on the epidermal growth factor receptor (EGFR). Calcitriol blocks this effect, whereas phosphorus stimulates it. This effect is thought to be the major antiproliferative mechanism that calcitriol exerts on the parathyroid glands.

i. Phosphorus restriction may prevent the progression of renal disease by blunting renal secondary hyperparathyroidism, thus preventing renal interstitial mineralization, inflammation, and fibrosis. Phosphorus restriction also may have direct benefits that are independent of PTH control.

j. These observations form the basis for the use of phosphorus restriction in the medical management of CRF. Dietary phosphate restriction alone may be adequate in patients with IRIS stage 1 and early IRIS stage 2 CKD.

k. Renal secondary hyperparathyroidism was documented in 84% of cats with naturally occurring CRF and responded (as assessed by serum phosphorus and PTH concentrations) to dietary phosphorus restriction in most cats. Some cats required intestinal phosphate binders to achieve adequate phosphate restriction.

l. Diets moderately restricted in phosphorus may be adequate (based on normal serum phosphorus and PTH concentrations) during the early stages of CKD. Diet alone, however, is unlikely to be successful in adequately controlling phosphorus as CRD becomes more advanced. In these instances, serum phosphorus concentration increases into or above the upper limit of the normal reference range.

m. Renal diets may successfully control serum phosphorus concentrations in dogs and cats with naturally occurring CRF, but serum PTH concentrations do not necessarily return to normal. In one study of dogs with naturally occurring CRF and another of cats with stage 2 or 3 CRF, feeding commercial veterinary renal diets did not result in decreases in serum PTH concentrations over a 2 year period in either species.

n. When CRF is diagnosed, phosphorus restriction is initiated by feeding a low phosphorus, low protein diet.

o. If necessary, orally administered phosphorus binding agents are added to the treatment regimen as necessary to maintain adequately decreased phosphorus and PTH concentrations (see below).

5. Reduction of intestinal phosphate absorption.

a. Phosphorus-binding agents trap phosphorus in the lumen of the intestinal tract and increase its excretion in feces (Figure 5-12). These products generally should be given with meals or within 2 hours of feeding to maximize their ability to bind dietary phosphorus.

! Dietary phosphorus binders work best when given with food or within 2 hours of feeding to maximize phosphorus binding in the gastrointestinal tract.

b. Aluminum hydroxide (Amphojel) initially is used at a dosage of 30 mg/kg every 8 hours or 45 mg/kg every 12 hours given with food. An attempt should be made to maintain serum phosphorus concentration of <6.0 mg/dL. Higher doses are employed as needed. Constipation is the most common adverse effect encountered during treatment with aluminum-containing phosphorus binders, especially in cats. Treatment with lactulose may alleviate constipation in affected cats.

(1) In human patients, chronic aluminum intoxication with resultant bone disease and encephalopathy has been recognized as an important complication of aluminum-containing phosphorus binders. In human medicine, it is felt that there is no safe dosage of aluminum-containing phosphorus binder that will provide sufficient phosphorus restriction without risk of aluminum intoxication. Consequently,

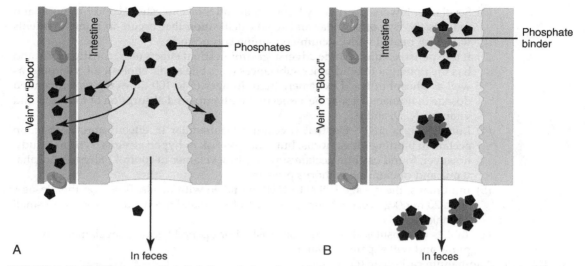

FIGURE 5-12 ■ Effect of orally administered phosphate binder to bind phosphate within the intestinal lumen, preventing its absorption across the intestinal tract. Some binders undergo absorption across the intestine and others do not. (Drawn by Tim Vojt.)

calcium-containing phosphorus binders replaced aluminum-containing phosphorus binders in human patients with CRF. It is not clear yet that aluminum intoxication is a problem in dogs and cats with CRF because they do not live as long with their disease as human patients do. Consequently, aluminum-containing phosphorus binders are still used by most veterinary clinicians. The use of aluminum-containing phosphorus binders in veterinary practice should be reassessed in the future as dogs and cats live longer with improved treatment of CRF.

c. Sucralfate contains 200 mg aluminum per gram and can help lower serum phosphorus in CRF.

d. Calcium carbonate (Tums: 500 mg $CaCO_3$ per tablet; Os Cal 500: 1.25 grams $CaCO_3$ per tablet) also may be used at a starting dosage of 30 mg/kg every 8 hours or 45 mg/kg every 12 hours given with food. Calcium-based intestinal phosphorus binders were developed for use in human medicine because of concerns about aluminum intoxication.

e. Calcium acetate is more effective than other calcium-containing phosphorus binders and may be used at a slightly lower dosage. It is available in 667 mg capsules (PhosLo) or tablets (Calphron). The recommended dosage in human patients is 20 to 40 mg/kg with each meal.

f. Animals should be monitored for development of hypercalcemia whenever calcium-containing phosphorus binders are used. Development of hypercalcemia is more likely when calcium-containing phosphorus binders are used simultaneously with calcitriol. Non-calcium-containing phosphorus binders are preferred when dogs and cats with CRF are also being treated with calcitriol.

g. Sevelamer HCl (Renagel) is a relatively new phosphorus binder used in human patients on dialysis. Its effects on dogs and cats with naturally occurring CRF have not been reported.

   (1) Sevelamer is a cross-linked polymeric resin that binds phosphorus and releases chloride. It does not contain aluminum or calcium and is not systemically absorbed.

(2) Sevelamer lowers low density lipoprotein and total cholesterol concentrations, and reduces the risk of vascular and renal calcification that occurs in human patients with CRF treated with calcium-containing compounds.

(3) It is expensive, causes some adverse gastrointestinal effects (e.g., constipation), and has the potential to bind other substances (e.g., bile acids, cholesterol, vitamins) as well as phosphorus. At extremely high dosages (6 to 100 times the recommended dosage in humans), it may be associated with impaired absorption of folic acid and vitamins K, D, and E.

(4) Initial reports suggested that sevelamer was similar in effectiveness to calcium acetate in binding phosphorus, but with less risk of hypercalcemia. A recent study, however, found calcium acetate superior to sevelamer in control of hyperphosphatemia and calcium-phosphorus product.

(5) In humans, the dosage is 800 to 1600 mg taken with meals. Based on this dosage, 10 to 20 mg/kg every 8 hours given with food may be considered for use in small animals.

(6) Tablets or capsules should not be crushed or opened because sevelamer is hydrophilic and will expand in water.

h. Lanthanum carbonate (Fosrenol).

(1) Contains no aluminum and no calcium, is not absorbed from the gastrointestinal tract, and acts as an efficient phosphorus binder. It is very expensive.

(2) Its effects are similar to those of calcium carbonate but without risk of hypercalcemia.

(3) Lanthanum is excreted primarily in bile and should not accumulate in patients with renal failure, but its long-term safety is unknown.

(4) Toxicity studies in dogs show that lanthanum accumulates in many tissues (especially gastrointestinal tract, bone, and liver) during treatment. Tissue concentrations remained high for longer than 6 months in dogs after treatment was discontinued.

(5) The use of lanthanum carbonate as a phosphorus binder has not been reported in dogs and cats with naturally occurring CRF, but its use could be considered in veterinary patients that fail to respond or experience adverse effects with other phosphorus binders.

(6) The starting dosage in human patients is 250 to 500 mg orally with each meal. The dosage is titrated every 2 to 3 weeks until an acceptable serum phosphorus concentration is obtained. Most humans require between 500 and 1000 mg with each meal to achieve serum phosphorus of <6.0 mg/dL. Thus, a starting dosage of 3 to 7 mg/kg every 8 hours with food could be considered in veterinary patients.

(7) The carbonate moiety of the salt also may be beneficial for control of metabolic acidosis.

(8) Lanthanum carbonate octahydrate (Lantharenol) has been recently approved in the European Union as a feed additive for all feline diets, serving to reduce the phosphorus availability.

i. Epakitin is a nutraceutical marketed to veterinarians for phosphorus control in CRF patients.

(1) Contains the adsorbent chitosan (8% crab and shrimp shell extract) and 10% calcium carbonate.

(2) Digestibility of dietary protein and phosphorus was decreased when it was administered to 10 normal cats and 6 cats with CRF.

(3) Its beneficial effects in dogs and cats with naturally occurring CRF have yet to be demonstrated.

j. Due to the possibility that intestinal phosphate binders could impair absorption of drugs, it is advisable to give other drugs 1 hour before or 3 hours after intestinal phosphate binders are administered.

k. If the patient is not hyperphosphatemic at the time of initial evaluation, phosphorus restriction still may be beneficial in reversing existing renal secondary hyperparathyroidism. Fractional excretion of phosphorus can be monitored but is not a very sensitive indicator of renal hyperparathyroidism. All serum phosphorus determinations should be made in the fasting state. Serial PTH determinations are an ideal but costly way to monitor treatment of renal hyperparathyroidism.

6. Caloric needs.

a. Adequate nonprotein calories to maintain body condition should be provided by carbohydrate and fat. Approximately 30 kcal/lb/day are recommended as a general guideline, but older animals may eat fewer calories normally (e.g., 20 kcal/lb/day).

b. One study of rats with the remnant kidney model indicated that improvement in proteinuria and renal morphologic changes was due to reduced caloric intake and not reduced protein intake. The mechanism of this effect is unknown, and its relevance for cats and dogs with naturally occurring CRF is unclear.

7. Lipids.

a. Supplementation of the diet with omega-6 polyunsaturated fatty acids (PUFA) may hasten progression of CRD whereas supplementation with omega-3 PUFA may be renoprotective.

b. The ideal ratio of omega-6 to omega-3 PUFA in the diet is not known. Studies demonstrating beneficial effects of omega-3 PUFA in dogs with renal ablation have employed very low ratios (e.g., 0.2:1) that are not commercially achievable. An omega-6 to omega-3 ratio of somewhere between 5:1 and 15:1 may be reasonable. Alternatively, the diet can be supplemented with 1 to 5 g/day of omega-3 PUFA. A minimum of 2 to 4 weeks is thought to be necessary for potential benefits to be observed and additional beneficial effects may occur over longer periods of time.

c. Increasing the amount of omega-3 PUFA relative to omega-6 PUFA in the diet decreases production of the pro-inflammatory, platelet aggregating, vasoconstrictive prostaglandin Thromboxane A2 (TXA2) and increases production of vasodilatory prostaglandins (PGE, PGI) that have the potential to increase GFR and renal blood flow (RBF). These effects may slow renal disease progression.

! The ratio of omega-3 to omega-6 fatty acids impacts diseased kidneys. Larger amounts of omega-3 fatty acids confer renoprotection to patients with CKD.

d. Studies of dogs with the remnant kidney model of CRF have demonstrated beneficial effects of omega-3 PUFA as opposed to omega-6 PUFA supplementation (e.g., decreased cholesterol and triglycerides, lower urinary eicosanoid excretion, reduction in proteinuria, preservation of GFR, less severe renal morphologic changes).

e. In a recent study of cats with CRF fed several different modified diets designed for cats in CRF, median survival was 16 months in cats fed the modified diets compared with 7 months in cats fed conventional diets. Survival on one of the modified diets with a very high content of eicosapentaenoic acid was 23 months, suggesting benefit from omega-3 PUFA supplementation.

8. Sodium chloride.

a. Increased fractional sodium excretion in CRF allows maintenance of sodium balance during the course of progressive renal disease.

  b. In dogs and cats with CRF and hypertension and in those with glomerular disease that have sodium retention and edema, sodium restriction is advisable.
  c. In the absence of edema, hypertension, primary glomerular disease, or congestive heart failure, no abrupt changes in sodium intake should be made.
  d. In one experimental study of cats with the remnant kidney model of CRF, sodium supplementation had minimal effects on blood pressure but low sodium intake was associated with decreased GFR, activation of RAAS, kaliuresis, and hypokalemia. These results suggest that sodium restriction in cats with CRF could contribute to progressive renal injury by predisposing to hypokalemic nephropathy. In this same study, systemic hypertension was not adequately controlled by dietary salt restriction alone.
  e. Patients with CRF are less able to adjust to changes in dietary sodium load. Any changes should be made slowly, beginning with a dietary intake of sodium similar to the animal's previous diet and changing gradually over the next month to the desired level of sodium intake. Many commercial pet foods provide more sodium than needed (often approximately 1%), and commercial products marketed for dogs and cats with CRF often provide approximately 0.2% to 0.3% sodium. Gradually switching an animal to one of these latter products will result in gradual sodium restriction.
9. Sodium bicarbonate.
  a. The metabolic acidosis of CRF often is well compensated, and routine treatment may not be necessary.
  b. If metabolic acidosis is severe (serum bicarbonate concentration 12 mEq/L or less), $NaHCO_3$ may be added to the treatment regimen. The dosage should be adjusted to maintain the serum bicarbonate concentration of 14 mEq/L or more. One teaspoon of $NaHCO_3$ contains approximately 5 g of $NaHCO_3$ and 1300 mg sodium. Potassium gluconate or potassium citrate are alternative sources of alkali that provide potassium and do not pose the potential problem of additional sodium.
  c. Consider adding sodium bicarbonate treatment only after a renal diet has been fed for several weeks, because these diets are usually supplemented with alkali precursors such as potassium citrate that may be sufficient to ameliorate the acidosis.
10. Potassium.
  a. Hyperkalemia usually is not a problem in CRF. The kidneys can maintain normal serum potassium concentrations even when GFR is approximately 5% of normal if urine volume is adequate.
  b. Hypokalemia in dogs and cats with CRF may be treated with oral potassium gluconate or citrate. The necessary dosage of potassium in cats usually is 2 to 4 mEq/day whereas dogs may require as little as 2 or as much as 40 mEq/day depending on their body size.
11. Water-soluble vitamins (B complex and C) should be supplied in the diet of dogs and cats with CRF because the ability of the diseased kidney to conserve these vitamins is diminished. Standard manufacturer-recommended dosages for multivitamin products can be used on a daily or alternate day basis. Caution should be exercised to avoid oversupplementation with fat-soluble vitamins A and D.
12. Several studies of dogs and cats with naturally occurring CRF have shown the benefits of feeding veterinary renal diets as compared to maintenance diets. Feeding veterinary renal diets was associated with increased survival time (up to as much as a twofold or more increase in survival) and decreased occurrence of uremic crises. Veterinary renal diets differ from maintenance diets in many nutrients and minerals including protein, fat, calcium, phosphorus, sodium, potassium, vitamin D, and omega-3 PUFA. It is unclear which

rgh stop.

nutrient or mineral or combination of nutrients and minerals is responsible for these beneficial effects.

Control of Vomiting and Inappetence
Suppression of Gastric Acid Production

a. H_2-receptor antagonists may have beneficial effects in CRF patients. Gastrin concentrations are increased in uremic dogs and cats. H_2-receptor antagonists block gastrin-mediated increases in gastric acid secretion and may be helpful in the treatment of hemorrhagic gastroenteritis in uremic dogs and cats. Although there are no studies to document the clinical efficacy of this treatment, H_2-receptor antagonists have been used in this setting for more than 20 years in our hospital and we subjectively feel they decrease episodes of vomiting and increase food intake in dogs and cats with CRF. We usually prescribe H_2-receptor antagonists initially in CRF patients that have a history of anorexia, vomiting, or weight loss. If serum gastrin is measured, the administration of H_2-receptor antagonists may cause an increase in circulating gastrin.
   (1) The dosage of cimetidine is 5 to 10 mg/kg every 12 hours followed by 5 mg/kg every 12 to 24 hours. Cimetidine inhibits hepatic metabolism of many drugs by interference with microsomal enzymes or decreased hepatic blood flow and caution should be exercised when using cimetidine with other drugs especially ketoconazole, theophylline, phenytoin, propranolol, lidocaine, quinidine, procainamide, metronidazole, warfarin, and meperidine.
   (2) Other H_2-blockers (e.g., ranitidine [Zantac], famotidine [Pepcid]) are less likely to result in adverse drug reactions when used in combination with other drugs. In addition, famotidine may be used every 24 hours at a dosage of 1 mg/kg in dogs and cats.
b. Proton pump inhibitors (e.g., omeprazole [Prilosec]).
   (1) These agents generally have been used when H_2-receptor antagonists have not been effective.
   (2) Reduction in cost now allows consideration for their more routine use in treatment of uremic gastroenteritis.
   (3) Proton pump inhibitors may be a preferred treatment for long-term control of acid production.

Anti-Emetics

a. Metoclopramide.
   (1) Some clinicians prefer metoclopramide as initial treatment for uremic gastroenteritis instead of an H_2-receptor antagonist.
   (2) Useful to decrease nausea and vomiting in patients with severe vomiting that is thought to be centrally mediated.
   (3) Can be used in conjunction with H_2-receptor antagonists if necessary.
   (4) The recommended starting dosage is 0.2-0.4 mg/kg subcutaneously every 6 hours, but a longer dosage interval (e.g., every 12 hours) may be necessary in CRF patients.
b. Chlorpromazine (0.5 mg/kg intramuscularly in dogs and cats) or promazine (2.2 mg/kg intramuscularly in dogs and cats) may be used as a centrally acting anti-emetic in hospitalized patients in uremic crisis. Central nervous system depression may be an adverse effect due to the sedative properties of these drugs.
c. Butorphanol (0.4 mg/kg intramuscularly in dogs and cats) or as a constant rate infusion (0.1 mg/kg/hr) may be effective for intractable vomiting in dogs.
d. Ondansetron is a serotonin antagonist that can be used as a very effective anti-emetic at a dosage of 0.1-0.2 mg/kg subcutaneously in dogs or cats.

Gastroprotectants
a. Sucralfate (0.25 to 1.0 g orally every 8-12 hours depending on the size of the animal) may provide gastroprotection for patients with gastrointestinal bleeding.
b. Zinc-carnosine (GastriCalm) adheres to the gastric mucosa and may provide additional gastrointestinal barrier protection.

Percutaneous Esophagostomy (PEG) or Esophagostomy Feeding Tubes
a. Long-term feeding with percutaneous esophagostomy (PEG) or esophagostomy feeding tubes may be considered when nutritional intake is inadequate and owners are frustrated because they cannot effectively administer medications to their pet (especially cats).

! Esophagostomy and PEG tube feedings improve the lives of some cats and dogs with CKD and should not be considered a treatment of last resort.

(1) PEG tube feedings can be used for months to years (especially in cats) and provide ready access for administration of medications and fluids.
(2) Consider esophagostomy tube feeding initially, and, if successful, a PEG tube can be considered for longer term care.
(3) Body weight and body condition score can be maintained or improved in many animals with CRF.
(4) Due to the common occurrence of anorexia in dogs and cats with serum creatinine concentrations of >5.0 to 6.0 mg/dL, feeding tubes may be the only effective method to maintain adequate nutrition in some CRF patients.
(5) Quality of life may be improved considerably after provision of PEG feedings in some animals.

Endocrine Replacement Therapy
Recombinant Human Erythropoietin (rhEPO; Epogen)
a. This drug has been successfully used to correct the nonregenerative anemia of CRF in some dogs and cats.
b. Dogs and cats treated with Epogen demonstrate resolution of anemia, weight gain, improved appetite, improved hair coat, and improved sociability with their owners within a few months of treatment (depending on the severity of anemia at the outset of treatment).

! Because of development of anti-human EPO antibodies, human recombinant EPO treatment should be reserved for CRF dogs and cats that have severe, transfusion-dependent anemia.

c. Epogen is not approved for use in animals and there is a 20% to 50% risk of anti-erythropoietin (EPO) antibody formation that may result in severe anemia and subsequent transfusion dependence. Antibodies tend to form 30 to 90 days after initiation of therapy and are heralded by a marked increase in the myeloid:erythroid (M:E) ratio of the bone marrow. In some cases, in addition to formation of antibodies against human EPO, autoantibodies may form against native erythropoietin. In this situation, an animal may develop a more serious anemia than before treatment and become transfusion dependent until autoantibodies are cleared which can take up to 6 months after stopping treatment. Darbepoetin (Aranesp) may be less likely to generate an antibody response in animals.
d. The starting dosage is 100 U/kg SC 3 times a week.

e. Hematocrit must be monitored closely during therapy and the dosage adjusted to achieve and maintain a target hematocrit of 30% to 40%. The frequency of administration is decreased to 2 times per week as soon as the animal's hematocrit enters the target range. Always measure the hematocrit by the same method, so that the values obtained can be compared with one another (i.e., do not compare packed cell volumes [PCVs] determined by table-top centrifuge to hematocrits calculated on a Coulter Counter). Small sequential decreases in hematocrit or PCV while an animal is being treated with Epogen are presumptive evidence of anti-EPO antibody formation.

f. Other adverse effects observed during treatment of dogs and cats with Epogen include vomiting, seizures, hypertension, uveitis, and mucocutaneous hypersensitivity-like reactions.

g. Because of adverse effects and expense, Epogen is reserved for animals with severe and symptomatic anemia (e.g., PCV <12% to 15%).

h. Iron supplementation should be provided during (and ideally before) Epogen treatment to ensure that the animal is iron replete.

i. Recombinant canine (rcEPO) and feline (rfEPO) erythropoietin has been produced and used to successfully correct the anemia in dogs and cats with CRF. These products also were somewhat successful in treating animals that had experienced red cell aplasia after treatment with recombinant human erythropoietin (rhEPO). Unexpectedly, some CRF cats that initially responded to rfEPO (including some that had previously been treated with rhEPO and some that had not) later developed anemia that was refractory to continued treatment with rfEPO. The mechanism for this effect is not known.

Calcitriol (activated vitamin D; 1,25-dihydroxyvitamin D) Therapy

a. In the kidney, 25 hydroxyvitamin D_3 is converted to the active form of vitamin D_3, 1,25 dihydroxyvitamin D_3 (calcitriol) by the enzyme 25 hydroxyvitamin D 1α-hydroxylase (1α-hydroxylase), which is found in the tubular cells (Figure 5-13). Do not confuse vitamin D_3 with the "triol" contained in calcitriol as there is no equivalence.

b. The quantity and activity of 1α-hydroxylase are closely regulated in the kidney.
   (1) The number and activity of enzyme molecules are increased by PTH.
   (2) Phosphorus genomically inhibits 1α-hydroxylase formation and inhibits its activity.
   (3) Its synthesis is repressed by its product (calcitriol).
   (4) There is an inverse relationship between dietary calcium intake and the activity of the enzyme. Hypercalcemia impairs and hypocalcemia stimulates calcitriol production.

c. The major effects of 1,25 dihydroxyvitamin D (calcitriol) are:
   (1) Increased intestinal absorption of calcium and phosphate.
   (2) A permissive effect on PTH-mediated bone resorption of calcium and phosphorus.
   (3) Negative feedback control on PTH synthesis by the parathyroid glands (relative lack of this effect plays an important role in the development of renal secondary hyperparathyroidism in patients with CRF) (Figure 5-14).
   (4) Increased renal tubular reabsorption of calcium and phosphate.

d. Serum calcitriol concentrations are decreased in dogs with renal failure as compared with normal dogs. Initially in CRF, calcitriol synthesis is impaired due to inhibition of 1α-hydroxylase by hyperphosphatemia. This may be relieved by dietary phosphorus restriction and, if necessary, administration of phosphorus binders. Later in CRF, there may be insufficient renal mass to produce adequate amounts of calcitriol. Calcitriol supplementation is indicated in management of CRF patients both before and after the amount of functional renal mass becomes insufficient to produce calcitriol, because

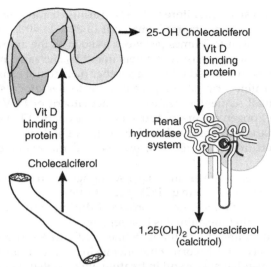

FIGURE 5-13 ■ Vitamin D metabolism in dogs and cats. Inactive vitamin D (cholecalciferol or D_3) is absorbed across the intestine and transported to the liver where a 25-alpha hydroxy group is added, 25-hydroxyvitamin D_3 is transported to the kidney where a tightly controlled hydroxylase system adds a 1-alpha hydroxy group resulting in the activated vitamin D compound 1,25(OH)$_2$-cholecaciferol (calcitriol). (Drawn by Tim Vojt.)

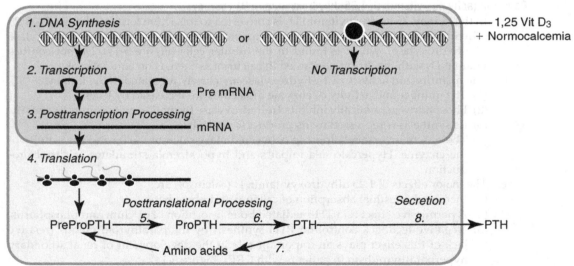

FIGURE 5-14 ■ Calcitriol's effect to genomically control the synthesis of PTH. Note that the basal condition in the parathyroid gland is to synthesize PTH unless adequate calcitriol and ionized calcium are present. Calcitriol in concert with ionized calcium and other transcription factors serves as an "off" switch by binding to a silencing region of the DNA. (Drawn by Tim Vojt.)

increased serum PTH concentration was maintaining calcitriol production before renal mass became inadequate to produce sufficient amounts of calcitriol, and PTH is known to be a uremic toxin. Calcitriol has intrinsic value by virtue of its ability to feed back to calcitriol receptors in the parathyroid glands and decrease PTH synthesis and secretion.

    e. Calcitriol must only be used after hyperphosphatemia has been adequately controlled by a low protein/phosphorus diet and oral phosphorus binding agents if necessary.

    f. If the Ca (mg/dL) × P (mg/dL) solubility product is > 60 to 70, calcitriol therapy should be decreased or discontinued because of the risk of soft tissue mineralization.

      (1) Intestinal phosphorus binders should be added if not presently being used, their dosage should be increased, or the type of phosphorus binder changed to provide optimal phosphorus control.

      (2) Calcitriol provides most efficient negative feedback on the parathyroid glands when serum phosphorus concentration is <6.0 mg/dL.

    g. Daily dosing method: A very low dosage of calcitriol (2.5 to 3.5 ng/kg/day) has been used in dogs and cats with CRF to prevent or reverse renal secondary hyperparathyroidism. Serial serum calcium concentrations are monitored to avoid development of hypercalcemia and measurement of serum ionized calcium is preferred for this purpose. Serum PTH concentrations either decrease or remain stable in dogs and cats with CRF treated with calcitriol.

    h. Intermittent dosing method: We have recently used calcitriol at a dosage of 9.0 ng/kg twice weekly for dogs and cats with CRF. The suppressive effects of calcitriol on PTH synthesis and secretion last up to 4 days, and this interval should not be exceeded. We recommend dosing calcitriol every 3.5 days such as on Sunday AM and Wednesday PM to stay within this time frame.

      (1) This regimen may be preferable to daily dosage with respect to client compliance.

      (2) This regimen may reduce the risk of hypercalcemia that accompanies daily dosing regimens.

      (3) Calcitriol programs enterocytes that are leaving the intestinal crypts for calcium absorption. Daily dosing of calcitriol programs more enterocytes than does intermittent dosing. Intermittent dosing allows continued use of calcitriol when the Ca × P solubility product is at its upper limit of normal.

    i. Pulse dosing method: Pulse dosing should not be confused with intermittent dosing.

      (1) The same time interval is used for both intermittent and pulse dosing.

      (2) The pulse dosage is 20 ng/kg twice weekly.

      (3) Pulse dosing is used if intermittent or daily dosing has failed to control serum PTH concentration.

      (4) The goal of pulse dosing is to induce more vitamin D receptors in the parathyroid glands and make them more responsive to lower doses of calcitriol that can be used in the future.

Angiotensin II and Angiotensin-Converting Enzyme Inhibitors

! Treatment with ACE inhibitors is considered standard care for dogs and cats with CKD and proteinuria. Beneficial effects also may occur in CKD patients without overt proteinuria.

    a. Potential detrimental effects of angiotensin II.

      (1) Increased efferent arteriolar vasoconstriction relative to afferent arteriolar vasoconstriction increases hydrostatic pressure within glomeruli and potentially causes intraglomerular hypertension.

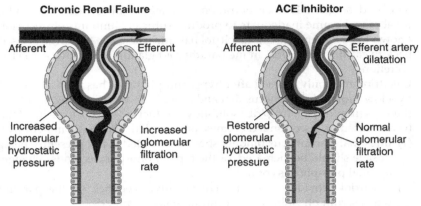

FIGURE 5-15 ■ ACE inhibition provides glomerular afterload reduction. High pressures of the super nephron (*left panel*) are created by dilatation of the afferent arteriole. In the right panel, intraglomerular pressure has been restored to normal during treatment with ACE inhibition. ACE inhibitors reduce the effect of angiotensin-II to cause intrarenal vasoconstriction but the effect is greater on the efferent arteriole, which lowers resistance to outflow from the glomerular beds. (Drawn by Tim Vojt.)

      (2) Contraction of mesangial cells decreases glomerular surface area available for filtration.

      (3) Increased protein traffic in the mesangium due to hyperfiltration of proteins.

      (4) Stimulation of mesangial cell proliferation leading to glomerular sclerosis.

  b. ACE inhibitors (e.g., enalapril, benazepril) may have protective effects in patients with CKD due to their ability to block adverse effects of angiotensin II.

      (1) Reduction in proteinuria.

      (2) Limitation of glomerular sclerosis and slower progression of renal disease.

      (3) Improvement in systemic blood pressure.

  c. The ability of ACE inhibitors to slow the progression of renal disease is independent of their effects on systemic blood pressure and may be related to their ability to decrease intraglomerular pressure and proteinuria (Figure 5-15).

  d. ACE inhibitors should not be used patient is well hydrated, and they should be discontinued during periods of uremic crisis.

> ❗ ACE inhibitors preferentially decrease efferent arteriolar tone, an effect that decreases transglomerular pressure. Relief from intraglomerular hypertension is beneficial for the long-term survival of diseased nephrons.

  e. In one study of dogs with biopsy-proven, naturally-occurring idiopathic glomerulonephritis, enalapril stabilized renal function (serum creatinine concentration), decreased proteinuria, and decreased systolic blood pressure compared to placebo over a period of 6 months. Similar results have been found in Samoyed dogs with X-linked hereditary nephritis treated with enalapril.

      (1) Enalapril was used at a dosage of 0.5 mg/kg orally once daily in most patients, and twice daily in some.

      (2) Dogs were included if the serum creatinine concentration was <3.0 mg/dL and urine protein-creatinine ratio (UPC) was >3.0.

      (3) An increase in serum creatinine concentration of 0.2 mg/dl or greater over baseline was seen at 6 months in 13 of 14 placebo-treated dogs and in 3 of 16 dogs treated with enalapril.

      (4) During treatment with enalapril, 9 dogs improved, 4 had no progression, and 3 had progression of their renal disease. With placebo treatment, 0 dogs improved, 4 had no progression, and 10 had progression of their renal disease. Two of the enalapril-treated dogs were euthanized due to severe decreases in their renal function.

  f. In another study of naturally-occurring CKD in dogs, significantly higher veterinarian-rated health scores, higher GFR and decreased proteinuria were seen at day 180 of treatment with benazepril compared to baseline, effects not seen with placebo treatment.

      (1) Benazepril was used at a dosage of 0.5 mg/kg once daily orally.

      (2) Dogs were included in the study if their serum creatinine concentration was >1.3 mg/dl and their GFR was <2.6 mL/min/kg. Dogs were not selected based on the severity of their proteinuria as in the study previously mentioned.

  g. In a study of 192 cats with naturally-occurring CKD, benazepril at a dosage of 0.5 to 1.0 mg/kg once daily orally was compared to treatment with placebo (BENRIC study).

      (1) Cats were included in the study if the initial serum creatinine concentration was stable and ≥2.0 mg/dl with urine specific gravity ≤1.025.

      (2) Survival time did not differ significantly between benazepril (mean, 637 days) and placebo treatments (mean, 520 days).

      (3) Survival time also did not differ by treatment in a sub-group of cats with proteinuria (UPC ≥1.0).

      (4) Cats with UPC ≥1.0 had improved appetite during benazepril treatment compared to placebo.

      (5) Plasma protein concentration was higher in cats with initial UPC <1.0 when treated with benazepril compared to placebo.

      (6) The magnitude of proteinuria was decreased in cats treated with benazepril compared to placebo. This effect was seen even in those cats with initial UPC <0.2.

  h. Benazepril treament demonstrated benefits compared to placebo for naturally-occurring CKD in 61 cats of another study.

      (1) Cats were included for study if the urine specific gravity was ≤1.025 in association with a serum creatinine concentration ≥2.0 mg/dl or urine protein concentration ≥ 2+ by dipstick.

      (2) Urine protein excretion based on UPC was lower at days 120 and 180 for cats treated with benazepril compared to placebo.

      (3) Rapid deterioration in renal function occurred in 3 cats receiving placebo treatment and in one cat receiving benazepril.

      (4) More cats stayed within IRIS stage 2 or 3 rather than progressing to IRIS stage 4 when treated with benazepril (93%) compared to placebo (73%) despite the short study period.

  i. Survival time of cats with CKD is associated with the severity of proteinuria, even mild proteinuria that previously has been considered trivial. Cats with CKD and UPC >0.4 lived for the shortest time, those with UPC 0.2 to 0.4 had intermediate survival times, and those with UPC <0.2 lived the longest. Whether targeted intervention with ACE inhibitors to lower their urinary protein excretion will increase survival times has yet to be proven.

  j. General guidelines for use of ACE inhibitors in CKD.

      (1) Recheck renal function 1 week after beginning ACE inhibitors to make sure GFR has not decreased too much. It is common to see a small increase in serum creatinine concentration at this time (20% to 30% increase over baseline). If serum

creatinine concentration has increased more than 20% to30%, decrease the dosage of the ACE inhibitor. Some dogs and cats are relatively intolerant of ACE inhibitors in that their renal function will be much worse during initial treatment and treatment must be discontinued.

(2) Recheck the UPC 1 and 3 months after the start of ACE inhibition. The goal is to achieve a 50% decrease in UPC in patients in which UPC initially was increased.

(3) There is minimal to no difference between benazepril and enalapril for clinical use in dogs and cats with CKD. Benazeprilat is cleared by both the kidney and liver compared to enalaprilat which is cleared only by the kidney.

Blood Pressure Detection and Control
Effect of Hypertension on Progression of Clinical Renal Disease

a. Dogs with naturally occurring CRF and hypertension have been reported to undergo more rapid progression of their renal disease and are more likely to develop uremic crises and die than those with lower blood pressure.

b. Experimentally, dogs with the remnant kidney model of CRF and high systolic blood pressure (165-170 mm Hg) tend to have lower GFR, higher urine protein/creatinine ratios, and higher scores for kidney lesions such as increased mesangial matrix, tubular damage, and fibrosis, than remnant kidney dogs with lower systolic blood pressure.

General Guidelines for Treatment of Hypertension in Dogs and Cats

a. Summarized from American College of Veterinary Internal Medicine (ACVIM) Consensus Statement of 2007:

(1) Blood pressure of <150/95 mm Hg: re-evaluate in 3 to 6 months.

(2) Blood pressure of 150/95 mm Hg or more and no evidence of target organ (e.g., ocular) damage.

(a) Re-evaluate blood pressure in 7 days. If blood pressure remains increased, antihypertensive therapy may be considered, depending on magnitude of increase.

(b) If <150/95 mm Hg: re-evaluate in 1 to 3 months.

(3) Blood pressure of 150/95 mm Hg or more and evidence of target organ (e.g., ocular) damage: initiate (or escalate) antihypertensive therapy.

b. Previous guidelines in cats with hypertension suggested initiating treatment (with amlodipine) if systolic blood pressure was >175 mm Hg on two separate occasions seven days apart or one reading of >175 mm Hg was obtained in a cat with ocular disease at presentation (i.e., acute onset blindness).

Treatment of Hypertension

a. A low-salt diet is not an effective treatment for persistent hypertension secondary to CRF. Feeding of a low-salt diet to cats with experimentally-induced renal failure led to kaliuresis, hypokalemia, and reduced GFR.

b. Diuretics such as furosemide and thiazides are not effective for control of hypertension secondary to CRF and potentially are associated with dehydration and superimposition of prerenal azotemia on an already azotemic patient.

c. ACE inhibitors (e.g., enalapril, benazepril) and amlodipine are the most commonly employed safe and effective antihypertensive medications for use in dogs and cats with CRF.

d. Benazepril and enalapril (0.5 mg/kg PO every 12 to 24 hours) can be used for initial management of hypertension in dogs with CRF. A mild increase in azotemia is expected due to decreased intraglomerular pressure associated with ACE inhibition and is not a reason to discontinue or change treatment as long as the animal is otherwise doing well.

   e. In cats with CRF and hypertension, treatment usually is begun with 0.625 to 1.25 mg amlodipine PO every 24 hours. Amlodipine is well tolerated by cats with minimal evidence of adverse effects.

Anabolic Steroids

1. Many products (e.g., methyltestosterone, stanozolol, oxymetholone, nandrolone decanoate) are available but there are no long-term studies demonstrating their efficacy in dogs and cats with CRF.
2. Stanozolol had equivocal effects in one short-term study of dogs with experimentally induced CRF. Total amount of food consumed, lean body mass, and nitrogen balance increased but there was no significant effect on body fat, bone mineral, or food consumption per kg of body weight.
3. Stanozolol has a narrow margin of safety in cats and is hepatotoxic. It resulted in increased liver enzyme activities and vitamin K-responsive coagulopathy. Hepatic lipidosis and cholestasis were observed histologically.
4. We do not recommend the use of anabolic steroids in cats with CRF. If used in dogs, pretreatment and posttreatment evaluation of liver enzymes and liver function should be carefully evaluated to ensue toxic hepatic effects are not developing.

Emerging Treatments

Azodyl (Vetoquinol)

   a. Azodyl is a probiotic designed as a daily treatment to alter colonic flora and promote degradation of urea and creatinine by colonic bacteria.
   b. BUN and serum creatinine concentrations were modestly reduced in a small study of CRF cats after 30 and 60 days of treatment.
   c. Decreased BUN and serum creatinine concentrations do not imply improved renal function, but rather suggest a reduction in production and accumulation of uremic waste products.
   d. The product must be kept refrigerated and the capsules not broken before administration to ensure that the living organisms in the product will survive.
   e. Transient diarrhea has been observed as an adverse effect of Azodyl.
   f. Beneficial effects on renal function, clinical signs, and survival have not been established in dogs and cats with CRF.

Kremezin (Covalzin)

   a. An orally administered, nonselective adsorbent that relies on carbon-based granules to remove uremic toxins from the gastrointestinal tract.
   b. Widely used in Japan to treat humans and cats with CRF.
   c. Studies in humans and experimental studies in rodents with renal failure suggest that kremezin may slow the progression of renal disease and additional benefits may be gained by use of kremezin in conjunction with ACE inhibitors.
   d. During 8 weeks of treatment, a reduction in signs of uremia was observed in more than 65% of CRF cats treated with kremezin at a daily dose of 400 or 800 mg compared to 15% of cats treated with placebo. The rate of disease progression also was reported by the manufacturer to have been decreased over this time period.

Spironolactone

   a. Aldosterone may contribute to the pathogenesis of progressive renal disease beyond its role in the RAAS.
   b. Aldosterone and angiotensin II both play roles in maintaining glomerular hypertension and contribute to glomerular sclerosis in the remnant kidney.

    c. Selective blockade of aldosterone decreases proteinuria and glomerular sclerosis in experimental studies in rats with remnant kidneys.

    d. No controlled studies of the use of aldosterone as a treatment for dogs and cats with CRF have been reported.

    e. Spironolactone often is considered as additional therapy to further decrease proteinuria in patients treated with ACE inhibitors. Hyperkalemia is a possible adverse effect of treatment with spironolactone in such patients. Serum potassium concentration should be monitored in all patients receiving spironolactone in conjunction with an ACE inhibitor.

Cinacalcet (Sensipar)

    a. Calcimimetic drug designed to increase the sensitivity of the calcium-sensing receptor in the parathyroid gland.

    b. Decreases PTH secretion as well as serum phosphorus and calcium concentrations.

    c. Approved for use in humans to control renal secondary hyperparathyroidism and usually used in conjunction with calcitriol to obtain better control of serum PTH concentration.

    d. Limited experience in veterinary medicine but may be considered when dietary phosphorus restriction, phosphorus binders and calcitriol are not sufficient for control of renal secondary hyperparathyroidism.

Chronic Dialysis

    a. Rarely performed in patients with CRF because of expense and long term complications.

    b. Occasionally performed during uremic crisis to give the patient time to recompensate.

Renal Transplantation

    a. Considered for some cats but not dogs with CRF.

    b. Expense and long-term complications presently limit its recommendation.

Stressful Situations

1. Situations that may be stressful to the animal (e.g., boarding, extensive absence of the owner) should be avoided if possible.

    a. The animal should be managed on an outpatient basis as much as possible. Uremic crises requiring intravenous fluid therapy represent an exception.

    b. Owners can be taught to administer subcutaneous fluids to their animal at home to prevent dehydration and facilitate excretory renal function during times of stress. This technique is particularly convenient in cats and small dogs. The additional fluid support can have important beneficial effects on the animal's quality of life.

COURSE AND PROGNOSIS

A. Ultimately, prognosis is poor if renal disease is documented to be progressive by serial evaluation of history, physical examination, and laboratory findings.

1. Rate of progression varies among individuals, but affected animal may live many months to several years. Plotting 1/serum creatinine versus time gives a crude indication of the rate of progression of CRF (i.e., the slope of the line is an indication of rate of progression).

2. In a study of dogs with naturally occurring CRF, urine protein/creatinine ratio >1.0 was associated with greater risk of uremic crisis, progression of renal disease, and death. Systolic hypertension may contribute to proteinuria and also is associated with increased risk of uremic crisis and decreased survival.

3. In cats with naturally occurring CRF, even mild proteinuria (urine protein/creatinine ratios <1.0) was associated with disease progression and decreased survival. It is unclear if disease progression is a consequence of the proteinuria or simply a marker of the underlying renal disease.
4. Increased proteinuria as a result of glomerular hyperfiltration has been identified as a contributing factor to renal disease progression in animal models of CRF.

B. Findings suggestive of a poor prognosis.
1. Extensive endstage lesions on renal biopsy.
2. Advanced osteodystrophy (rarely a problem in adult animals with CRF).
3. Progressive proteinuria despite treatment.
4. Progressive loss of lean muscle mass, with or without weight loss.
5. Progressive weight loss.
6. Severe intractable anemia that cannot be managed with rhEPO due to antibody formation.
7. Unmanageable systemic hypertension.
8. Progressive azotemia despite fluid therapy and conservative medical management.
9. Inability to maintain fluid and electrolyte balance despite supplementation with subcutaneously administered fluids.

WHAT DO WE DO?

- Classify patients with CKD using the IRIS scheme of classification (see Table 5-1).
- Collect blood from fasted CKD patients at the same time of day to facilitate comparison of results over time.
- Evaluate patients with CKD for proteinuria.
- Measure systolic blood pressure (usually by Doppler method) in all patients with CKD and determine their risk for end-organ damage including progressive renal injury.
- Serially evaluate patients with CKD using clinical tools such as body weight, body condition score, systemic blood pressure, and parameters of renal function.
- Closely monitor phosphorus control and aim to keep serum phosphorus concentration <5.5 mg/dL using a combination of dietary phosphorus restriction and phosphate binders.
- Measure serum PTH and serum ionized calcium concentration to evaluate renal secondary hyperparathyroidism and make therapeutic decisions.
- Consider therapeutic intervention whenever evidence for progression is present (progressive increase in serum creatinine concentration, progressive increase in urine protein/creatinine ratio, progressive loss of urinary concentrating ability, decreasing renal size, development of nephrocalcinosis) regardless of the presence or absence of overt azotemia.
- Consider renal transplantation as a therapeutic option in selected cats with CRF.

THOUGHTS FOR THE FUTURE

- Development of foods for patients with CKD that are markedly restricted in phosphorous but not in protein.
- Development of new phosphate binders that provide excellent phosphate control even when a nonrenal diet is fed.
- Development of methods to more accurately measure blood pressure in animals so that early onset of hypertension can be detected and treated.
- Development of balanced antihypertensive treatment protocols that include control of both systemic and intraglomerular hypertension.

- Development of antifibrotic protocols that can minimize progression.
- Development of better protocols to decrease renal proteinuria.
- Evaluation of aldosterone inhibitors (e.g., spironolactone, eplerenone) to decrease progression of renal disease.
- Evaluation of selective and nonselective gastrointestinal adsorbents to better manage uremic signs and to slow progression of renal disease.
- Development of long-acting ACE inhibitors that have selective renal effects.
- More common use of calcimimetics (e.g., cinacalcet) to provide optimal control of renal secondary hyperparathyroidism.
- Intermittent dosing of calcitriol will replace daily dosing for safer control of renal secondary hyperparathyroidism.
- Development of erythropoietin products that will not stimulate the immune system of dogs or cats.
- Development of antirejection medications that protect transplanted kidneys while not placing the host at major risk for systemic infection.
- Efficient temporary methods of dialysis will become more available as a means to periodically remove uremic waste products.
- Development of species-specific PTH assays that are sensitive and specific for dogs and cats.
- A greater understanding of the role of the calcium-sensing receptor in CKD will be achieved.

COMMON MISCONCEPTIONS

- Normal serum creatinine concentration means that renal disease is not present. Actually, serum creatinine concentration is not sensitive for the detection of CKD because more than 75% of nephrons must be nonfunctional before serum creatinine concentration is increased above normal. Other parameters must be evaluated to determine extent of renal disease before loss of 75% of renal mass (e.g., iohexol clearance, proteinuria, cylindruria, decreased renal concentrating ability, renal parenchymal changes on imaging).
- Stable serum creatinine concentration over a few months means that renal disease is not progressive. This could be true, but animals with severe muscle mass loss and otherwise stable renal function should experience a decrease in serum creatinine concentration. Stable serum creatinine concentration in the presence of severe muscle mass loss could mask progression of renal disease.
- A decrease in BUN while the patient is eating a renal diet means that renal function has improved. Actually, when the animal is eating a diet low in protein but adequate in calories, BUN concentration decreases because less nitrogenous waste products are generated. In such a situation, BUN concentration is not good indicator of renal function.
- Blood pressure monitoring is not that important in dogs and cats with CKD. False. Systemic hypertension has no outward clinical signs. Blood pressure must be measured to determine if hypertension is present and to monitor response to treatment. Good blood pressure control may prevent end-organ damage and slow progression of renal disease.
- Renal diets help all patients with CKD regardless of their stage of disease. Although studies have shown that feeding a renal diet, as compared with a maintenance diet, can help both dogs and cats with CKD, some patients may be harmed by this treatment. This outcome is especially likely in dogs and cats that are not eating well at the time of transition to the new diet. Continued anorexia will cause protein-calorie malnutrition and loss of lean muscle mass.
- A renal diet should be fed as soon as it has been documented that the patient has renal disease. Actually, there is no evidence to indicate that any dietary intervention is helpful in patients with nonazotemic renal disease (IRIS Stage 1). Evidence is strongest that renal diets are helpful in slowing progression of CKD when fed to moderately to severely azotemic patients (IRIS stage 3 and 4).

- Potassium supplementation is helpful in all cats with CKD. Actually, potassium supplementation is helpful in any CKD patient with hypokalemia. Hypokalemic nephropathy has been well documented in cats. The value of potassium supplementation in normokalemic patients with total body potassium deficits is more controversial. Given in small amounts with a gradual increase in dosage over time likely is not harmful to patients with CKD because the diseased kidney can adapt to handle the additional potassium.
- Anabolic steroids should be considered in all CKD patients, especially if they have poor appetite, loss of lean muscle mass, or progressive anemia. There is little evidence in dogs and cats with CKD to support the use of anabolic steroids. Stanozolol has been shown to increase lean muscle mass in dogs with experimental renal disease without a change in appetite. Stanozolol can be hepatotoxic in cats, and we do not recommend its use in cats with CKD.
- A normal serum phosphorus concentration indicates that renal secondary hyperparathyroidism is adequately controlled. False. Persistently high serum phosphorus concentration in a patient with CKD likely means that serum PTH concentration is abnormal, but a normal serum phosphorus concentration does not necessarily mean that serum PTH concentration is normal. There really is no way of knowing if serum PTH concentration is being adequately controlled without measuring it.
- Administration of fluids subcutaneously is helpful in all CKD patients. Subcutaneous administration of fluids is helpful only for patients that do not maintain optimal hydration on their own. Optimal hydration enhances renal excretory function and less uremic waste is retained. CKD patients do not benefit from subcutaneous administration of fluids if they maintain hydration on their own.
- Calcitriol treatment should only be considered for CKD patients if they have metabolic bone disease, hypocalcemia, or very high serum PTH concentrations. These advanced situations are indications for the use of calcitriol, but calcitriol has potential advantages when used earlier in the course CKD.

SUMMARY TIPS

- Serially measure BUN, serum creatinine, and serum phosphorus concentrations as surrogates of renal function and to monitor the effects of therapeutic interventions.
- Serially measure serum albumin, total protein, and cholesterol concentrations as indicators of the patient's nutritional state during feeding of protein-restricted renal diets.
- Serially monitor serum potassium concentration in patients (especially cats) with CKD. Provide potassium supplementation for patients with overt or marginal hypokalemia.
- Serially measure urine protein ratio to identify trends, and change therapy if necessary.
- Aim to maintain systolic blood pressure of <145 mm Hg in patients with CKD. CKD patients have limited ability to protect their kidneys against fluctuations in systemic blood pressure due to impaired renal autoregulation.
- Perform urine culture in cats with CKD every 3 to 6 months because many cats with CKD have bacterial UTI, often without clinical signs. UTI poses a threat of pyelonephritis to the already damaged kidney and any documented UTI should be treated with antibiotics.

FREQUENTLY ASKED QUESTIONS

Q: What is the value of probiotics in the treatment of azotemic dogs and cats with CKD? Should we be using these products?

A: There is little evidence on which to judge these products. The premise is that bacteria in the probiotic will populate the colon and decrease the BUN and creatinine concentrations as a consequence of their metabolism. This process has been called "enteric dialysis" but it really has nothing to do with dialysis.

Q: Chitosan-based products recently have been advocated as intestinal phosphate binders. How does this kind of product compare with other phosphate binders?

A: A small study in cats with CRD indicated that cats eating food supplemented with chitosan had decreased serum phosphorus concentrations as a consequence of decreased digestibility. No studies have compared chitosan to salts of aluminum, calcium, or lanthanum or to sevelamer as phosphate binders.

Q: I can't get many of my patients to eat phosphorus-restricted renal diets. Is it reasonable to recommend feeding the animal's regular diet with the addition of a phosphate binder?

A: This approach is not recommended because the large amount of phosphorus in regular foods makes it unlikely that the added phosphate binder will be effective.

Q: When should ACE inhibitors be used in patients with CKD? Should they only be used in patients with proteinuria, only in patients with CKD but not renal failure, or only in patients with renal failure regardless of the presence or absence of proteinuria?

A: ACE inhibitors are most likely to slow the progression of renal disease in dogs and cats with CKD and proteinuria. ACE inhibitors lower high intraglomerular pressure in dogs and cats with experimental renal failure. Assuming that most animals with naturally occurring renal disease also suffer from glomerular hypertension in remnant nephrons, it is logical to provide treatment designed to decrease the glomerular hypertension thought to be pivotal in the progression of CKD. Clinical studies in dogs and cats have been limited to patients with azotemia. ACE inhibitors also may provide renoprotection in nonazotemic dogs and cats with progressive renal disease.

Q: Doesn't treatment with ACE inhibitors aggravate azotemia?

A: Intraglomerular pressure will decrease during treatment with ACE inhibitors, and single nephron GFR will decline. Thus, BUN and serum creatinine concentrations can be expected to increase during treatment. In human patients, a 20% increase in serum creatinine concentration above baseline is considered acceptable. Interestingly, in cats with experimentally induced renal failure, benazepril lowered intraglomerular pressure without decreasing GFR, presumably because glomerular surface area increased as mesangial cells relaxed with blockade of angiotensin II.

Q: Is benazepril preferable to enalapril for treatment of CKD in dogs and cats?

A: Both benazepril and enalapril are pro-drugs. Benazeprilat and enalaprilat are the active forms of the drug, and both are cleared by the kidneys. Benazeprilat undergoes more clearance by the liver than enalaprilat, and less benazeprilat accumulates in the serum in patients with CKD. Both drugs have similar ability to inhibit ACE.

Q: Is calcitriol more useful in dogs with CRF than in cats with CRF?

A: Dogs with naturally occurring CRF fed renal diets and treated with calcitriol survived longer than those treated with placebo. Similar studies in CRF cats did not demonstrate a difference in survival after one year of treatment. CRD often progresses more slowly in dogs than in cats, and cats with CRF may need to be followed for 2 years or more to identify a beneficial effect of calcitriol treatment. We use calcitriol to treat both dogs and cats with progressive CKD.

Q: Do I need to measure both serum ionized calcium and PTH concentrations during treatment of CRF patients with calcitriol?

A: Doing so is the ideal way to monitor treatment of renal secondary hyperparathyroidism. Determination of serum PTH concentration is necessary to document the effectiveness of therapy. It also is important to determine if serum PTH concentrations previously within the normal range have increased. Serum ionized calcium concentrations also should be monitored to identify toxicity from ionized hypercalcemia. Trends in serum total calcium concentration may be useful, but serum ionized calcium concentrations are needed to accurately assess calcium status.

Q: Does routine vaccination in cats increase their risk for the development of CKD?
A: Recent studies have shown that vaccinated cats can develop antibodies against renal tubular antigens, presumably because the viruses used in vaccine development are grown in feline kidney cells. Although antibodies may develop, there is no evidence that CKD results as a consequence. At the present time, there is no evidence to support changing routine vaccination practices.

Q: Is calcitriol beneficial in dogs or cats with CKD and hypercalcemia?
A: Not usually, but if the diagnosis of hypercalcemia is based on serum total calcium concentration rather than serum ionized calcium concentration, it is possible that better control of renal secondary hyperparathyroidism by calcitriol treatment will result in decreased serum complexed calcium concentration with a corresponding decrease in serum total calcium concentration. If serum ionized calcium concentration is increased, all of the possible causes for hypercalcemia must be considered. It is very uncommon for high serum ionized calcium concentration to be a result of tertiary hyperparathyroidism. In these instances, very high serum PTH concentration is likely to be present, and calcitriol treatment may improve the ability of the parathyroid gland to decrease PTH secretion in response to hypercalcemia. Some cats with idiopathic hypercalcemia have CKD, and calcitriol treatment is not indicated in these cats because serum PTH concentration typically is normal or low.

Q: Is there one brand of renal veterinary diet that you consistently recommend over others?
A: Two pet food companies have reported evidence-based medicine outcomes studies of dogs and cats with CRF that were treated either with a renal diet or a maintenance diet. In one study of cats with CRF, all 7 of the studied renal therapeutic diets had resulted in prolonged survival compared with a maintenance diet. The most important factor is that the CRF patient actually consumes the diet, and switching from one brand of veterinary therapeutic diet to another is appropriate to maintain adequate nutrient intake based on palatability. It is advisable to switch to a diet with less phosphorus in patients in which serum phosphorus or PTH concentrations are not well controlled. Comparison of nutrient intake corrected for energy density for therapeutic foods is maintained by the OSU Nutrition Support Service and is available for review at http://vet.osu.edu/nssvet (select Diet Manual).

Suggested Readings

Adams LG, Polzin DJ, Osborne CA, et al: Effects of dietary protein and calorie restriction in clinically normal cats and in cats with surgically induced chronic renal failure, *Am J Vet Res* 54:1653–1662, 1993.

Barber PJ, Elliott J: Feline chronic renal failure: Calcium homeostasis in 80 cases diagnosed between 1992 and 1995, *J Small Anim Pract* 39:108–116, 1998.

Barber PJ, Rawlings JM, Markwell PJ, et al: Effect of dietary phosphate restriction on renal secondary hyperparathyroidism in the cat, *J Small Anim Pract* 40:62–70, 1999.

Bourgoignie JJ, Gavellas G, Martinez E, et al: Glomerular function and morphology after renal mass reduction in dogs, *J Lab Clin Med* 109:380–388, 1987.

Brenner BM, Meyer TW, Hostetter TH: Dietary protein intake and progressive nature of kidney disease: The role of hemodynamically mediated glomerular injury in the pathogenesis of progressive glomerular sclerosis in aging, renal ablation, and intrinsic renal disease, *N Engl J Med* 307:652–659, 1982.

Brown S, Atkins C, Bagley R, et al: Guidelines for the identification, evaluation, and management of systemic hypertension in dogs and cats, *J Vet Intern Med* 21:542–558, 2007.

Brown SA, Brown CA, Crowell WA, et al: Beneficial effects of chronic administration of dietary omega-3 polyunsaturated fatty acids in dogs with renal insufficiency, *J Lab Clin Med* 131:447–455, 1998.

Brown SA, Crowell WA, Barsanti JA, et al: Beneficial effects of dietary mineral restriction in dogs with marked reduction of functional renal mass, *J Am Soc Nephrol* 1:1169–1179, 1991.

Brown SA, Finco DR, Crowell WA, et al: Single nephron adaptations to partial renal ablation in the dog, *Am J Physiol* 258:F495–F503, 1990.

Buranakarl C, Mathur S, Brown SA: Effects of dietary sodium chloride intake on renal function and blood pressure in cats with normal and reduced renal function, *Am J Vet Res* 65:620–627, 2004.

Cowan LA, McLaughlin R, Toll PW, et al: Effect of stanozolol on body composition, nitrogen balance, and food consumption in castrated dogs with chronic renal failure, *J Am Vet Med Assoc* 211:719–722, 1997.

Cowgill LD, James KM, Levy JK, et al: Use of recombinant human erythropoietin for management of anemia in dogs and cats with renal failure, *J Am Vet Med Assoc* 212:521–528, 1998.

Elliott J, Barber PJ: Feline chronic renal failure: Clinical findings in 80 cases diagnosed between 1992 and 1995, *J Small Anim Pract* 39:78–85, 1998.

Elliott J, Barber PJ, Syme HM, et al: Feline hypertension: Clinical findings and response to antihypertensive treatment in 30 cases, *J Small Anim Pract* 42:122–129, 2001.

Elliott J, Rawlings JM, Markwell PJ, et al: Survival of cats with naturally occurring chronic renal failure: Effect of dietary management, *J Small Anim Pract* 41:235–242, 2000.

Elliott J, Syme HM, Markwell PJ: Acid-base balance of cats with chronic renal failure: Effect of deterioration in renal function, *J Small Anim Pract* 44:261–268, 2003.

Elliott J, Syme HM, Reubens E, et al: Assessment of acid-base status of cats with naturally occurring chronic renal failure, *J Small Anim Pract* 44:65–70, 2003.

Grauer GF, Greco DS, Getzy DM, et al: Effects of enalapril versus placebo as a treatment for canine idiopathic glomerulonephritis, *J Vet Intern Med* 14:526–533, 2000.

Harkin KR, Cowan LA, Andrews GA, et al: Hepatotoxicity of stanozolol in cats, *J Am Vet Med Assoc* 217:681–684, 2000.

Jacob F, Polzin DJ, Osborne CA, et al: Association between initial systolic blood pressure and risk of developing a uremic crisis or of dying in dogs with chronic renal failure, *J Am Vet Med Assoc* 222:322–329, 2003.

Jacob F, Polzin DJ, Osborne CA, et al: Clinical evaluation of dietary modification for treatment of spontaneous chronic renal failure in dogs, *J Am Vet Med Assoc* 220:1163–1170, 2002.

Jacob F, Polzin DJ, Osborne CA, et al: Evaluation of the association between initial proteinuria and morbidity rate or death in dogs with naturally occurring chronic renal failure, *J Am Vet Med Assoc* 226:393–400, 2005.

King LG, Giger U, Diserens D, et al: Anemia of chronic renal failure in dogs, *J Vet Intern Med* 6:264–270, 1992.

King JN, Gunn-Moore DA, Tasker S, et al: Tolerability and efficacy of benazepril in cats with chronic kidney disease, *J Vet Intern Med* 20:1054–1064, 2006.

Mizutani H, Koyama H, Watanabe T, et al: Evaluation of the clinical efficacy of benazepril in the treatment of chronic renal insufficiency in cats, *J Vet Intern Med* 20:1074–1079, 2006.

Plantinga EA, Everts H, Kastelein AM, et al: Retrospective study of the survival of cats with acquired chronic renal insufficiency offered different commercial diets, *Vet Rec* 157:185–187, 2005.

Polzin DJ, Osborne CA, Hayden DW, et al: Influence of reduced protein diets on morbidity, mortality, and renal function in dogs with induced chronic renal failure, *Am J Vet Res* 45:506–517, 1983.

Polzin DJ, Osborne CA, Stevens JB, et al: Influence of modified protein diets on the nutritional status of dogs with induced chronic renal failure, *Am Vet Res* 44:1694–1702, 1983.

Randolph JE, Scarlett JM, Stokol T, et al: Expression, bioactivity, and clinical assessment of recombinant feline erythropoietin, *Am J Vet Res* 65:1355–1366, 2004.

Reusch CE, Tomsa K, Zimmer C, et al: Ultrasonography of the parathyroid glands as an aid in differentiation of acute and chronic renal failure in dogs, *J Am Vet Med Assoc* 217:1849–1852, 2000.

Ross LA, Finco DR, Crowell WA: Effect of dietary phosphorus restriction on the kidneys of cats with reduced renal mass, *Am J Vet Res* 43:1023–1026, 1982.

Ross SJ, Osborne CA, Kirk CA, et al: Clinical evaluation of dietary modification for treatment of spontaneous chronic kidney disease in cats, *J Am Vet Med Assoc* 229:949–957, 2006.

Schenck PA, Chew DJ: Prediction of serum ionized calcium concentration by use of serum total calcium concentration in dogs, *Am J Vet Res* 66:1330–1336, 2005.

Schenck PA, Chew DJ: Calcium fractionation in dogs with chronic renal failure, *Am J Vet Res* 64:1181–1184, 2003.

Schenck PA, Chew DJ, Nagode LA, Rosol TJ: Disorders of calcium: Hypercalcemia and hypocalcemia. In Dibartola S, editor: *Fluid therapy in small animal practice*, ed 3, St. Louis, 2006, Elsevier, pp 122–194.

Syme HM, Markwell PJ, Pfeiffer D, Elliott J: Survival of cats with naturally occurring chronic renal failure is related to severity of proteinuria, *J Vet Intern Med* 20:528–535, 2006.

Tenhundfeld J, Wefstaedt P, Nolte IJ: A randomized controlled clincial trial of the use of benazepril and heparin for the treatmet of chronic kidney disease in dogs. *J AM Vet Med Assoc* 234(8): 1031-1037, 2009.

6 Familial Renal Diseases of Dogs and Cats

INTRODUCTION AND PATHOPHYSIOLOGY

A. Most familial renal diseases result in chronic renal failure (CRF) at a young age (<5 years) but some are characterized by renal tubular defects (e.g., Fanconi syndrome in the Basenji) or morphologic abnormalities that result in hematuria (e.g., renal telangiectasia in Pembroke Welsh corgi dogs).

B. A familial disease is one that occurs in related animals with a higher frequency than would be expected by chance.

C. Congenital diseases are present at birth and may be genetically determined or result from exposure to adverse environmental factors during development.

D. In many familial renal diseases of dogs, the kidneys are thought to be normal at birth but undergo structural and functional deterioration early in life.

E. Some familial renal diseases of dogs probably are examples of renal dysplasia.
   1. The term renal dysplasia refers to disorganized development of renal parenchyma due to abnormal differentiation and is characterized by the presence of structures in the kidney inappropriate for the stage of development of the animal.
   2. Lesions suggestive of renal dysplasia include asynchronous differentiation of nephrons (indicated by persistence of immature or "fetal" glomeruli; Figure 6-1) and persistent mesenchyme (usually in the medullary interstitium).
   3. Persistent metanephric ducts, atypical tubular epithelium, and dysontogenic metaplasia are observed less frequently.

F. Many familial renal diseases are very variable in severity and rate of progression among individual animals.

G. Most of these diseases are progressive and ultimately fatal, and therapy usually is limited to conservative medical management of CRF.

H. The mode of inheritance and specific pathogenesis for many of these diseases are unknown.

SIGNALMENT

A. Familial renal disease has been reported in many breeds of dog (Table 6-1) and may occur sporadically in mixed breed animals.

B. The clinician should consider the possibility of familial renal disease whenever CRF occurs in immature or young adult animals.

C. Most of these diseases have no clear sex predilection.

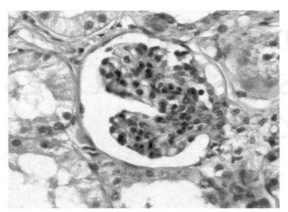

FIGURE 6-1 ■ Fetal glomerulus with decreased lobulation and closed capillary loops from a Standard poodle with familial renal disease (Hematoxylin and eosin stain, ×160.)

■ TABLE 6-1
■ ■ **Familial Renal Diseases of Dogs and Cats**

Breed	Disease Description	Age at Presentation	Inheritance; Mutation	Progressive Renal Failure?
Abyssinian cat	Amyloidosis	1-5 years	Autosomal dominant (incomplete penetrance)*	Yes
Beagle	Amyloidosis	5-11 years	Unknown	Yes
English foxhound	Amyloidosis	5-8 years	Unknown	Yes
Oriental shorthair cat	Amyloidosis	<5 years	Unknown	Variable; severe liver involvement
Shar pei	Amyloidosis	1-6 years	Unknown	Yes
Siamese cat	Amyloidosis	<5 years	Unknown	Variable; severe liver involvement
Bull terrier	Basement membrane disorder	<1-10 years	Autosomal dominant	Yes
Bullmastiff	Basement membrane disorder	2.5-11 years	Autosomal recessive	Yes
Dalmatian	Basement membrane disorder	<1-8 years	Autosomal dominant	Yes
Doberman pinscher	Basement membrane disorder	<1-6 years	Unknown	Yes
English Cocker spaniel	Basement membrane disorder	<2 years	Autosomal recessive; *COL4A4* mutation	Yes
Newfoundland	Basement membrane disorder	<1 year	Unknown	Yes
Rottweiler	Basement membrane disorder	≤1 year	Unknown	Yes
Samoyed	Basement membrane disorder	<1 year (males)	X-linked dominant	Yes (males)

■ TABLE 6-1
■ ■ **Familial Renal Diseases of Dogs and Cats—cont'd**

Breed	Disease Description	Age at Presentation	Inheritance; Mutation	Progressive Renal Failure?
Texas NAV dogs	Basement membrane disorder	<1 year (males) 1-3 years (females)	X-linked dominant	Yes (males)
Beagle	Glomerulopathy (basement membrane disorder?)	2-8 years	Unknown	Yes
Bernese mountain dog	Membranoproliferative glomerulonephritis	2-5 years	Autosomal recessive*	Yes
Brittany spaniel	Membranoproliferative glomerulonephritis (C3 deficiency)	4-9 years	Autosomal recessive	Variable
Soft-coated Wheaten terrier	Membranoproliferative glomerulonephritis	2-11 years	Unknown	Yes
German shepherd	Multiple renal cystadenocarcinomas	5-11 years	Autosomal dominant*	Variable
Norwegian elkhound	Periglomerular fibrosis	<1-5 years	Unknown	Yes
Bull terrier	Polycystic kidney disease	<1-2 years	Autosomal dominant	Yes; valvular heart disease
Cairn terrier	Polycystic kidney disease	6 weeks	Autosomal recessive*	Not reported
Persian cat	Polycystic kidney disease	3-10 years	Autosomal dominant; *polycystin I* mutation	Yes
West Highland white terrier	Polycystic kidney disease	5 weeks	Autosomal recessive*	Not reported
Alaskan malamute	Renal dysplasia	<1 year	Unknown	Yes
Chow	Renal dysplasia	<1-5 years	Unknown	Yes
Golden retriever	Renal dysplasia	<1-3 years	Unknown	Yes
Lhasa apso and Shih tzu	Renal dysplasia	<1-5 years	Unknown	Yes
Miniature Schnauzer	Renal dysplasia	<1-3 years	Unknown	Yes
Soft-coated Wheaten terrier	Renal dysplasia	<1-3 years	Unknown	Yes
Standard poodle	Renal dysplasia	<1-2 years	Unknown	Yes
Pembroke Welsh corgi	Renal telangiectasia	5-13 years	Unknown	No
Basenji	Tubular dysfunction (Fanconi syndrome)	1-5 years	Unknown	Variable
Norwegian elkhound	Tubular dysfunction (renal glucosuria)	Not reported	Unknown	No
Beagle	Unilateral renal agenesis	Incidental finding	Unknown	No

*Suspected.

D. The age of onset of familial renal disease usually is 6 months to 5 years, with many animals presented before 2 years of age.
   1. Renal amyloidosis in beagles and English foxhounds, suspected glomerular basement membrane disease in beagles, and telangiectasia of the Welsh corgi, however, occur in older dogs (>5 years).
   2. Polycystic kidney disease (PKD) in Cairn and West Highland white terriers is detected at a very young age (5 to 6 weeks).

HISTORY

A. Signs of CRF occur in many of these familial diseases:
   1. Anorexia.
   2. Lethargy.
   3. Stunted growth or weight loss.
   4. Polyuria, nocturia, polydipsia.
   5. Vomiting.
   6. Poor hair coat.
   7. Diarrhea (less common than vomiting).
   8. Foul breath.
B. Clinical findings in Basenji dogs with Fanconi syndrome may include polyuria, polydipsia, weight loss, dehydration, and weakness.
C. Hematuria, dysuria, and apparent abdominal pain may be reported by owners of Pembroke Welsh corgi dogs with renal telangiectasia.
D. Hematuria may be reported in German shepherd dogs with multifocal renal cystadenocarcinomas.

PHYSICAL FINDINGS

A. Poor body condition.
B. Dehydration.
C. Pallor of the mucous membranes.
D. Foul oral odor.
E. Uremic ulceration of the oral cavity.
F. Small, irregular kidneys (Cairn and West Highland white terriers and Persian cats with PKD are exceptions and have kidneys that often are markedly enlarged).
G. Signs of fibrous osteodystrophy (e.g., *rubber jaw*) can sometimes be detected on physical examination of young growing dogs with CRF. Signs of renal osteodystrophy rarely are apparent in older dogs with CRF.
H. Blood pressure should be measured and fundic examination performed to evaluate for complications of hypertension (e.g., retinal hemorrhages, retinal detachments).

LABORATORY FINDINGS

Hemogram
   1. Anemia.
      a. When present in animals with CRF due to familial renal disease, anemia usually is nonregenerative (normochromic, normocytic).
      b. Blood loss anemia may occur in Welsh corgi dogs with renal telangiectasia.
   2. Lymphopenia (indicative of chronic stress).

Serum Chemistry
1. Increased blood urea nitrogen (BUN) and serum creatinine concentrations.
2. Hyperphosphatemia.
3. Variable serum total calcium concentration (decreased, normal, increased).
   a. Hypercalcemia may be more common in young dogs with renal failure than in older ones according to some investigators.
4. Compensated metabolic acidosis.
5. Presence of hypoalbuminemia and hypercholesterolemia (along with proteinuria) should prompt suspicion of primary glomerular disease.

Urinalysis
1. Isosthenuria.
2. Proteinuria in animals with glomerular disease.
   a. Beagles with glomerular amyloidosis.
   b. Abyssinian cats and Shar pei dogs with familial amyloidosis if there is sufficient glomerular involvement.
   c. Bernese mountain dogs with membranoproliferative glomerulonephritis.
3. Glucosuria.
   a. Norwegian elkhounds with primary renal glucosuria.
   b. Basenji dogs with Fanconi syndrome (will also have proteinuria, isosthenuria, and aminoaciduria).
4. Hematuria in Welsh corgi dogs with renal telangiectasia or German shepherd dogs with multifocal renal cystadenocarcinomas.
5. Pyuria and other evidence of urinary tract infection (UTI) may occur (e.g., Welsh corgi dogs with renal telangiectasia).

IMAGING

A. In many dogs and cats with familial renal disease the kidneys are small on radiographs and show irregular contour, increased echogenicity, and decreased corticomedullary distinction on ultrasound examination.
B. Renal cysts in animals with PKD have a characteristic ultrasonographic appearance (i.e., multiple round anechoic lesions with distal acoustic enhancement in both kidneys).
C. Welsh corgi dogs with renal telangiectasia may have evidence of nephrocalcinosis or hydronephrosis if ureteral obstruction by a blood clot occurs.

PATHOLOGIC FINDINGS

A. Familial renal disease is characterized by the presence of primary dysplastic lesions, compensatory lesions, and degenerative lesions.
B. In many cases, the secondary degenerative lesions overshadow the underlying primary dysplastic lesions, making the correct diagnosis difficult.
C. Primary dysplastic lesions that have been observed in some familial renal disease of dogs include:
   1. Immature or "fetal" glomeruli (see Figure 6-1).
   2. Hyperplasia or adenomatoid proliferation of the medullary collecting ducts.
   3. Persistent mesenchyme in the renal medulla.
D. Primary dysplastic changes are most prominent in the Lhasa apso, Shih tzu, soft-coated Wheaten terriers with renal dysplasia, standard poodle, chow, and miniature Schnauzer.

E. Juvenile renal diseases in the Samoyed, English Cocker spaniel, and bull terrier result from abnormalities of type IV collagen in glomerular basement membranes and represent animal models of X-linked dominant, autosomal recessive, and autosomal dominant hereditary nephritis in humans, respectively.

F. Secondary degenerative lesions that are observed commonly in familial renal disease include interstitial fibrosis, interstitial infiltration by mononuclear inflammatory cells, dystrophic mineralization, and cystic glomerular atrophy.

Abyssinian Cat (Amyloidosis)

INTRODUCTION AND PATHOPHYSIOLOGY

A. Difficulty in determining the mode of inheritance arises from variability in severity and progression of amyloidosis among affected Abyssinian cats, but the disease appears to be inherited as an autosomal dominant trait with variable penetrance.

B. Amyloid deposits in the kidneys of affected Abyssinian cats contain amyloid protein AA.

C. The amino acid sequence of the amyloid AA protein in affected Siamese cats differs slightly from that found in affected Abyssinian cats and this difference may explain the predilection for hepatic deposition in affected Siamese cats (see later).

SIGNALMENT

A. Abyssinian cats with familial amyloidosis usually are presented between 1 and 5 years of age.

B. Male and female cats are equally affected.

CLINICAL COURSE

A. Amyloid deposits first appear in the kidneys between 9 and 24 months of age and, in many cats, amyloid deposition leads to CRF within the first 3 years of life.

B. Amyloid deposition in the kidney may be mild, and some affected cats may live to an advanced age without detection of their amyloid deposits.

C. Proteinuria is a variable clinical finding and reflects the severity of glomerular involvement.

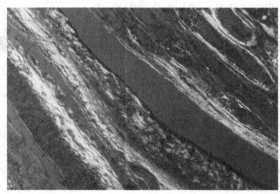

FIGURE 6-2 ■ Medullary amyloid deposits in an Abyssinian cat with familial amyloidosis (Congo red stain, polarized, ×100.)

PATHOLOGIC FINDINGS

A. The principal pathologic lesions in the kidneys of Abyssinian cats with familial amyloidosis are medullary amyloid deposits (Figure 6-2), papillary necrosis (Figure 6-3), chronic tubulointerstitial nephritis characterized by lymphoplasmacytic infiltration and fibrosis, and variable glomerular amyloid deposits.

B. Glomerular amyloidosis is mild and often difficult to detect in many affected cats, but occasionally it can be severe.

C. Medullary amyloid deposition was found in all affected Abyssinians whereas glomerular deposits were found in 75%.

D. Medullary interstitial amyloid deposits interfere with blood flow to the renal papilla, resulting in papillary necrosis and secondary interstitial medullary fibrosis and mononuclear inflammation.

E. Amyloid deposition is not restricted to the kidneys in Abyssinian cats with amyloidosis, and deposits frequently are found in other organs (e.g., adrenal glands, thyroid glands, spleen, stomach, small intestine, heart, liver, pancreas, colon).

   1. Amyloid deposits in these other organs generally do not appear to make an important contribution to the clinical syndrome, which is that of CRF.

   2. In Siamese cats (including the Oriental Shorthair cat, which is a color variant of the Siamese) severe deposition of amyloid in the liver can result in hepatic rupture and hemoabdomen.

Alaskan Malamute (Suspected Renal Dysplasia)

I. CRF in 3 sibling malamute pups (4 to 11 months of age) was associated with histologic evidence of renal dysplasia.

II. The lesions observed included immature ("fetal") glomeruli, cystic glomerular atrophy, glomerular sclerosis, periglomerular fibrosis, adenomatoid hyperplasia of tubules, and persistent mesenchymal tissue.

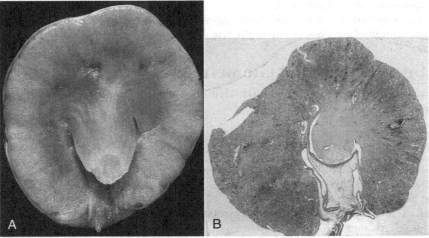

FIGURE 6-3 ■ Gross (**A**) and microsopic (**B**) appearance of papillary necrosis in an Abyssinian cat with familial amyloidosis (×4.25).

Basenji (Tubular Dysfunction)

I. Histologic findings in the kidneys of Basenji dogs with Fanconi syndrome are not consistent.
   A. Nonspecific findings include tubular atrophy and interstitial fibrosis.
   B. One morphologic marker for this disease may be enlarged, hyperchromatic nuclei in renal tubular cells (renal tubular cell karyomegaly).
II. Affected animals may deteriorate rapidly and die of acute renal failure with papillary necrosis or pyelonephritis.
III. See Chapter 17, Miscellaneous Syndromes, for more information about Fanconi syndrome in Basenji dogs.

Beagle (Amyloidosis, Suspected Basement Membrane Disorder)

I. A family of adult beagles developed glomerular amyloidosis and nephrotic syndrome characterized by proteinuria, hypercholesterolemia, and renal failure. Some dogs had mild medullary deposition of amyloid. The amyloid deposits were sensitive to permanganate oxidation, suggesting the presence of amyloid protein AA.
II. In another study, a family of beagles with proteinuria, late-onset renal failure, and multilaminar splitting of the glomerular basement membranes was described.

Bernese Mountain Dog (Familial Glomerulonephritis)

I. Membranoproliferative glomerulonephritis resembling membranoproliferative glomerulonephritis type I in human beings was described in young (2-to-5-year-old) male and female Bernese mountain dogs.
II. Affected dogs had typical laboratory abnormalities of renal failure as well as marked proteinuria, hypercholesterolemia, and hypoalbuminemia.
III. Pedigree analysis suggested an autosomal recessive mode of inheritance.
IV. Ultrastructural lesions included a double-layered glomerular basement membrane and electron-dense deposits, primarily in a subendothelial location.
V. Immunoglobulin M and the third component of complement were identified by immunofluorescence in glomeruli of affected dogs.
VI. Most of the dogs had high serologic titers against *Borrelia burgdorferi*, but the organism could not be detected immunohistochemically in the tissues of affected dogs.

Brittany Spaniel (Familial Glomerulonephritis)

I. Membranoproliferative glomerulonephritis has been reported in Brittany spaniels with deficiency of the third component of complement.

Bull Terrier Basement Membrane Disorder (Hereditary Nephritis)

I. Familial renal disease leading to CRF has been reported in bull terriers aged 1 to 8 years.
II. Both male and female dogs are affected.
III. Inherited as an autosomal dominant trait.
IV. Proteinuria is an early manifestation and correlates with underlying glomerular lesions in affected bull terriers. Repeated urine protein-to-creatinine ratios of >0.3 are considered to be supportive evidence of the disease in suspect bull terriers older than 2 years of age, but without overt evidence of renal failure.

V. Hematuria also may occur.
VI. Light microscopic lesions include glomerular sclerosis, periglomerular fibrosis, interstitial fibrosis with minimal inflammation, and cystic dilatation of Bowman's space.
VII. Characteristic ultrastructural lesions of the glomerular basement membranes included lamellations, subepithelial frilling, vacuolation, and intramembranous electron-dense deposits. Foot process effacement and mesangial matrix expansion also were observed in glomeruli of affected dogs.
VIII. Immunohistochemical staining demonstrated presence of type IV collagen in the kidneys of affected dogs.

Bull Terrier Polycystic Kidney Disease

I. Inherited as an autosomal dominant trait.
II. Multiple cysts occur in the cortex and medulla of both kidneys.
III. Affected dogs did not have hepatic cysts.
IV. The epithelial cysts are of nephron or collecting tubule origin and secondary renal lesions include atrophic glomeruli, dilatation of Bowman's space, tubular loss, tubular dilatation, interstitial fibrosis, and inflammation.
V. Renal failure does not occur until middle to owd age.
VI. There is evidence that PKD and hereditary nephritis can occur simultaneously in some bull terriers.

Bullmastiff (Suspected Basement Membrane Disorder)

I. A familial glomerulonephropathy characterized by segmental glomerular sclerosis has been described in bullmastiffs.
II. Pedigree analysis suggested autosomal recessive inheritance.
III. Both males and females were affected.
IV. Age at euthanasia or death ranged from 2.5 to 11 years.
V. Clinical signs were nonspecific and related to chronic renal failure.
VI. Onset was insidious, and several dogs appeared healthy until shortly before death.
VII. Severe proteinuria on urinalysis and increased urine protein-to-creatinine ratios were observed.
VIII. Glomerular lesions included segmental expansion of mesangial matrix by collagen (i.e., sclerosis), increased numbers of cells in the expanded areas, and marked dilatation of Bowman's space (cystic glomerular atrophy).
IX. Secondary lesions included interstitial fibrosis, tubular atrophy, and lymphoplasmacytic cellular infiltrates.
X. Immunoglobulin deposition was mild and thought to be a secondary lesion.
XI. Suspected to be a glomerular basement membrane disorder.
XII. Histologic findings resemble focal segmental glomerular sclerosis in humans.

Cairn and West Highland White Terrier (Polycystic Kidney Disease)

I. Autosomal recessive PKD in the young (6-week-old) Cairn terrier is characterized by the presence of multiple cysts in the liver and kidneys.
II. Autosomal recessive PKD also has been reported in young (5-week-old) West Highland white terriers.

Chow (Suspected Renal Dysplasia)

I. CRF in 6 young related chows (5 male and 1 female) was suggestive of renal dysplasia.

II. Renal failure developed in four dogs by 6 months of age and in two dogs after 1 year of age.

III. Renal dysplasia was suspected based on presence of immature ("fetal") glomeruli and pseudostratified columnar epithelium in renal tubules of some dogs.

English Cocker Spaniel (Basement Membrane Disorder)

I. Juvenile renal disease in the English Cocker spaniel is an animal model of autosomal recessive hereditary nephritis in human beings. Hereditary nephropathies can arise from mutations in any one of three genes that code for the type IV collagen heterotrimer component chains found in the glomerular basement membranes (i.e., *COL4A3, COL4A4, COL4A5*).

II. Autosomal recessive hereditary nephritis of the English Cocker spaniel is a type IV collagen defect caused by a mutation in exon 3 of the *COL4A4* gene.

III. Absence of the type IV collagen heterotrimers α3.α4.α5(IV) in the glomerular basement membranes of affected dogs accounts for the observed progressive ultrastructural renal pathology. This pathology is the same as described in Samoyeds and Navasota Texas (NAV) dogs with X-linked dominant hereditary nephritis that lack α3.α4.α5(IV) in their glomerular basement membranes as a consequence of mutations in the *COL4A5* gene (see later).

IV. The disease affects both male and female English Cocker spaniels and manifests itself between 6 and 24 months of age.

V. The earliest detectable abnormality (5 to 8 months of age) is proteinuria followed by reduced growth rate, impaired urinary concentrating ability, and azotemia (7 to 17 months of age).

VI. The primary lesion is thickening and multilaminar splitting of the glomerular basement membrane. This lesion is identical to that observed in Samoyeds with X-linked hereditary nephritis (Figure 6-4).

VII. The disease ultimately leads to diffuse glomerular sclerosis and periglomerular fibrosis with secondary tubulointerstitial disease and is invariably fatal.

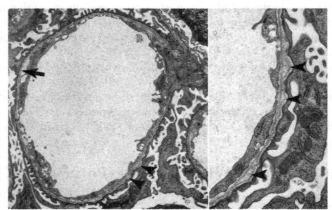

FIGURE 6-4 ■ Endothelial cell separation (*thin arrow, left panel, ×8000*) and bilaminar splitting of glomerular basement membrane (*thick arrowhead, right panel, ×17,300*) in a 1-month-old male Samoyed dog with hereditary nephritis. (From: Jansen B, Thorner P, Baumal R, et al: Samoyed hereditary glomerulopathy (SHG). Evolution of splitting of glomerular capillary basement membranes. *Am J Pathol* 125:536, 1986.)

Dalmatian (Basement Membrane Disorder)

   I. Autosomal dominant pattern of inheritance affecting males and females equally.
  II. Mean age of onset of renal failure was 18 months.
 III. May be identified initially by increased urine protein-to-creatinine ratios (>0.3).
  IV. Renal histopathology includes segmental glomerular sclerosis, tubulointerstitial inflammation, and interstitial fibrosis.
   V. Ultrastructural findings consist of lamellation of the glomerular basement membrane with sub-epithelial frilling, vacuolation, and occasional intramembranous deposits.
  VI. All α1(IV) to α5(IV) type IV collagen chains were identified in the kidneys of affected dogs by immunohistochemistry.

Doberman Pinscher (Suspected Basement Membrane Disorder)

   I. Diffuse thickening or multifocal irregular thickening with lamellation of the lamina densa has been observed in the glomerular basement membranes of Doberman pinschers with glomerulopathy.
  II. Occasionally, deposits of immunoglobulins have been detected in the glomerular capillary wall, but these are thought to result from nonspecific trapping of immune complexes in basement membranes with some underlying structural defect.
 III. Unilateral renal aplasia has been observed in some affected female Doberman pinschers.
  IV. Additional glomerular lesions include lobular accentuation of glomerular capillary loops, increased mesangial matrix, hypercellularity, intraglomerular adhesions, fibroepithelial crescent formation, and periglomerular fibrosis.

English Foxhound (Amyloidosis)

   I. Renal amyloidosis was reported in related adult English foxhounds.
  II. The disease had an acute presentation characterized by renomegaly and papillary necrosis in some affected dogs.
 III. Amyloid deposits were sensitive to permanganate oxidation, suggesting the presence of amyloid protein AA.

German Shepherd (Renal Cystadenocarcinoma)

   I. German shepherd dogs with bilateral multifocal renal cystadenocarcinomas are presented between 5 and 11 years of age for nonspecific signs such as anorexia, weight loss, polydipsia, and gastrointestinal disturbances.
  II. The renal lesions were accompanied by cutaneous and subcutaneous nodules (dermatofibrosis) and multiple uterine leiomyomas in affected female dogs.
 III. The disorder is thought to be inherited as an autosomal dominant trait.

Golden Retriever (Suspected Renal Dysplasia)

   I. CRF has been reported in young golden retrievers (<3 years of age).
  II. Hypercholesterolemia was a common finding despite lack of other evidence of primary glomerular disease in most affected dogs.
 III. Hypercalcemia also was common and attributed to increased serum complexed calcium concentration.

IV. Cystic glomerular atrophy and periglomerular fibrosis were common histologic lesions whereas immature ("fetal") glomeruli were uncommon.
V. Adenomatoid proliferation of the collecting ducts suggestive of primitive metanephric ducts was observed in several dogs and supports a diagnosis of renal dysplasia.
VI. Pyelonephritis occasionally complicated the disease in affected dogs.

Lhasa Apso and Shih Tzu (Suspected Renal Dysplasia)

I. In the Lhasa apso and Shih tzu, microscopic findings include a reduced number of glomeruli, glomerular atrophy, and small, immature ("fetal") glomeruli, which are hypercellular and have inconspicuous capillary lumens (see Figure 6-1).
II. Tubular changes include atrophy, dilatation, and epithelial hyperplasia.
III. Interstitial fibrosis is particularly severe in the renal medulla, whereas interstitial inflammation is minimal.
IV. To a certain extent, increased interstitial medullary tissue may represent persistent mesenchyme and, along with the immature glomeruli, is evidence of a primary renal dysplasia.

Miniature Schnauzer (Suspected Renal Dysplasia)

I. CRF suggestive of renal dysplasia was reported in eight related miniature Schnauzers ranging in age from 4 months to 3 years.
II. Immature ("fetal") glomeruli, glomerular sclerosis, and severe interstitial fibrosis were observed.

Newfoundland

I. A glomerulonephropathy characterized by expansion of the mesangium by collagen (glomerular sclerosis) was observed in three male and female Newfoundland dogs younger than 1 year of age from one litter of eight dogs.
II. Clinical findings included proteinuria, hypoalbuminemia, and severe renal failure at a very young age.

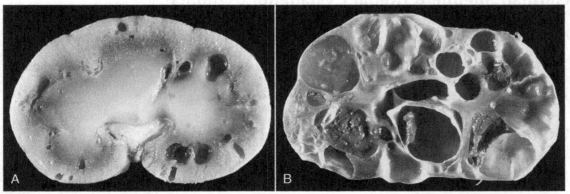

FIGURE 6-5 ■ Gross appearance of Persian cat kidneys with polycystic disease. **A,** Kidney from a younger affected cat. **B,** Kidney from an older affected cat with advanced disease (notice hemorrhage in some cysts).

Norwegian Elkhound (Suspected Renal Dysplasia, Renal Glucosuria)

I. In the Norwegian elkhound, periglomerular fibrosis is an early histologic lesion that may be detected in some dogs before the onset of azotemia.

II. Pathologic findings in dogs with more advanced disease consist of generalized interstitial fibrosis with glomerular sclerosis and atrophy.

III. Hyperplasia of the collecting ducts also has been observed and may represent a primary dysplastic change, but immature ("fetal") glomeruli have not been observed.

IV. Norwegian elkhounds may also develop primary renal glucosuria that is not associated with CRF.

Persian Cat (Polycystic Kidney Disease)

I. PKD is inherited as an autosomal dominant trait in Persian cats.

II. The prevalence of PKD in Persian cats in various countries has been observed to be between 35% and 57% as determined by ultrasonography. Worldwide, approximately one third of Persian cats appear to be affected.

III. Cysts originate from both the proximal and distal tubules, occur both in the renal cortex and medulla, and increase in number and size over time (Figure 6-5).

IV. Cysts can be detected by ultrasound examination of affected kittens as early as 6 to 8 weeks of age, but the absence of cysts at this early age does not preclude their development at a later age. In one study, ultrasound examination had a sensitivity of 75% and specificity of 100% when performed at 16 weeks of age and a sensitivity of 91% and specificity of 100% when performed at 36 weeks of age.

V. Although common in human patients with PKD, hypertension has been absent or mild in cats with PKD that have been evaluated.

VI. Affected Persian cats usually do not develop renal failure until later in adult life (average, 7 years), and renomegaly may be an incidental finding on physical examination.

VII. Occasionally, cysts may be found in the liver.

VIII. A mutation in exon 29 of the polycystin I gene has been identified in affected Persian cats. No cats homozygous for the mutation have been identified, suggesting that the mutation is lethal to the developing fetus. Genetic tests for the disease have been developed.

Rottweiler (Suspected Basement Membrane Disorder)

I. CRF was reported in 8 Rottweilers (five females and three males) ranging in age from 6 to 12 months. Several of the reported dogs were related to one another.

II. Affected dogs were azotemic, hyperphosphatemic, hypoproteinemic, and some had hypercholesterolemia.

III. Isosthenuria, proteinuria on dipstrip analysis, and high urine protein-to-creatinine ratios were observed.

IV. On light microscopy, dilated Bowman's spaces, mesangial hypercellularity and mesangial matrix expansion, irregular thickening of glomerular capillary loops, occasional crescents, glomerular sclerosis, tubular atrophy, and interstitial fibrosis were described.

V. On electron microscopy, glomerular basement membranes had extensive thickening and splitting of the lamina densa. Podocyte foot process effacement also was described. The ultrastructural findings were considered compatible with a primary basement membrane disorder.

Samoyed (Basement Membrane Disorder)

   I. Juvenile renal disease in this family is a hereditary glomerulopathy arising from a mutation in exon 35 of the COL4A5 gene for the 5(IV) collagen chain on the X chromosome.
  II. Male Samoyed dogs with hereditary nephritis develop proteinuria, glucosuria, and isosthenuria by 2 to 3 months of age, azotemia by 6 to 9 months of age, and die due to renal failure usually by 12 to 16 months of age.
 III. Because affected male dogs have a single mutated copy of the COL4A5 gene, they completely lack 3. 4. 5(IV) in their glomerular basement membranes.
  IV. Mesangial thickening, glomerular sclerosis, and periglomerular fibrosis are observed by light microscopy in affected males by 8 to 10 months of age.
   V. Carrier female dogs have two copies of the COL4A5 gene, one mutated and one normal. Because of normal random inactivation of one X chromosome in each cell of the female embryo during development, their glomerular basement membranes contain mosaic expression of α3.α4.α5(IV); that is, the normal collagen IV network is present in some areas and completely absent in others, at least initially.
  VI. Carrier female dogs develop proteinuria at 2 to 3 months of age but remain clinically normal as young adults (<5 years of age) other than sometimes failing to achieve normal adult body weight.
 VII. At birth, the glomerular basement membranes of affected male Samoyed dogs are morphologically normal, but reduplication and bilaminar splitting of the lamina densa are detected by electron microscopy at 1 month of age and progress to multilaminar splitting, thickening, and glomerular sclerosis by 8 to 10 months of age (see Figure 6-4). Carrier female dogs have only focal splitting of their glomerular basement membranes and generally do not develop juvenile-onset progressive disease.
VIII. Proteinuria and progressive renal disease presumably result from wear and tear on glomerular basement membranes weakened by abnormal cross-linking of type IV collagen.
  IX. Deterioration of basement membranes and onset of renal failure in affected male dogs can be delayed but not prevented by feeding a diet low in protein and phosphorus beginning at 1 month of age.
   X. Treatment of affected dogs with angiotensin-converting enzyme (ACE) inhibitors or cyclosporine A has slowed (but not prevented) progression of the disease.

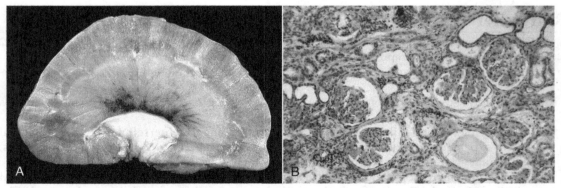

FIGURE 6-6 ■ Gross appearance (**A**) of Shar pei dog kidney with medullary amyloid deposition (stained dark blue with Lugol's iodine) and microscopic appearance (**B**) of glomerular amyloid deposition (Congo red stain, nonpolarized, ×40).

XI. Juvenile renal disease in the mixed breed (Navasota) dog kindred is a hereditary glomerulopathy arising from a mutation in exon 9 of the *COL4A5* gene for the α5(IV) collagen chain on the X chromosome. This family of dogs has been perpetuated in a research colony (at Texas A&M University) to study the disease. The clinical, histopathologic, ultrastructural, and immunohistologic features of this disease are basically the same as those described above for the Samoyed kindred.

Shar Pei (Amyloidosis)

I. Familial amyloidosis resulting in CRF at a young age (mean, 4 years) occurs in male and female Shar pei dogs.

II. Proteinuria and laboratory evidence of nephrotic syndrome (e.g., hypoalbuminemia, hypercholesterolemia) may be present, depending on the severity of glomerular involvement.

III. Some affected Shar pei dogs had a previous history of episodic joint swelling (usually the tibiotarsal joints) and high fever that resolves within a few days, regardless of treatment.

IV. Recurrent fever and joint swelling, culminating in CRF due to reactive systemic amyloidosis in young Shar pei dogs may represent an animal model of familial Mediterranean fever in man.

V. There is some evidence that amyloidosis in the Shar pei dog is inherited as an autosomal recessive trait.

VI. Affected Shar pei dogs have moderate to severe renal medullary deposition of amyloid, but only two thirds have glomerular involvement (Figure 6-6). These findings are similar to those observed in Abyssinian cats with familial amyloidosis.

VII. The remaining renal lesions are those of end-stage renal disease.

VIII. Amino acid sequence analysis has demonstrated that the amyloid deposits in affected Shar pei dogs contain amyloid A protein.

IX. In addition to the kidney, amyloid deposits may be observed in many other organs (e.g., liver, spleen, gastrointestinal tract, thyroid gland).

X. Icterus, hepatomegaly, and occasionally hepatic rupture with hemoabdomen may occur in Shar pei dogs with severe deposition of amyloid in the liver.

Familial Renal Disease in the Soft-Coated Wheaten Terrier (SCWT)

I. May Take the Form of Renal Dysplasia or Membranoproliferative Glomerulonephritis.

A. Pathologic findings in some SCWT with juvenile renal disease are suggestive of renal dysplasia.

1. Histologic lesions include interstitial fibrosis, periglomerular fibrosis, cystic glomerular atrophy, decreased numbers of glomeruli, and the presence of immature ("fetal") glomeruli (see Figure 6-1).

2. Adenomatous proliferation of the collecting duct epithelium also is a prominent feature.

3. Multiple small cysts, renal cortical hyperechogenicity, and decreased corticomedullary distinction may be observed on ultrasonography.

B. SCWT also are predisposed to protein-losing enteropathy (PLE), protein-losing nephropathy (PLN) or both.

1. Food hypersensitivity and increased gut permeability presumably lead to immune complex glomerulonephritis that progresses to end-stage renal disease.

2. Results of gastroscopic food sensitivity testing and dietary challenge support the hypothesis of food hypersensitivity, but gluten hypersensitivity does not seem to be involved.

3. The disease is thought to be present in 10% to 15% of SCWT and affects middle-aged to older dogs with a slight predilection for females.

4. The mode of inheritance is uncertain.

5. Clinical findings include polyuria, polydipsia, vomiting, and weight loss in dogs with PLN, and proteinuria, hypoalbuminemia, hypercholesterolemia, azotemia, hyperphosphatemia, and nonregenerative anemia are common laboratory findings.
6. Hypertension occasionally develops, and thromboembolism complicates the disease in 12% of SCWT with PLN.
7. Renal lesions consist of membranous to membranoproliferative glomerulonephritis that progresses to glomerular sclerosis, periglomerular fibrosis, and chronic interstitial nephritis.
8. Mesangial deposition of immunoglobulin A (IgA), immunoglobulin M (IgM), and complement has been detected by immunofluorescence, suggesting that renal disease in the SCWT may be an animal model of IgA nephropathy or IgM mesangial nephropathy.
9. The disease is progressive, treatment is palliative, and the prognosis is poor.
10. Treatment with sodium chromoglycate to stabilize mast cells and decrease intestinal permeability and a protein hydrolysate diet (if not contraindicated due to the presence of renal failure) has been tried in SCWT with PLE.
11. Dogs with CRF due to PLN should be fed an appropriate diet for renal failure patients. SCWT with PLN also should be treated with an ACE inhibitor (e.g., enalapril) to reduce the severity of proteinuria.

Standard Poodle (Suspected Renal Dysplasia)

I. In affected standard poodles, cystic glomerular atrophy and large numbers of immature ("fetal") glomeruli are observed, especially in dogs presented at 3 to 4 months of age (see Figure 6-1).
II. The cortical interstitium contains segmental areas of fibrosis, whereas more diffuse lesions occur in the medulla.

Welsh Corgi (Renal Telangiectasia)

I. Welsh corgi dogs with renal telangiectasia have red to black nodules in the kidneys, especially in the renal medulla adjacent to the corticomedullary junction.
II. Clotted blood often is identified in these lesions and in the renal pelvis.
III. Hydronephrosis (presumably due to ureteral obstruction) occurs in almost half of affected dogs.
IV. Similar nodular lesions may be identified in other tissues including the subcutis, spleen, duodenum, anterior mediastinum, thoracic wall, retroperitoneal space, and central nervous system.
V. Histologically, these lesions are cavernous, blood-filled spaces lined with endothelium, and thrombosis is a frequent finding in the sinuses.
VI. These sinuses with their simple endothelial linings may represent vascular malformations rather than benign tumors of vascular origin.

WHAT DO WE DO?

- Obtain renal biopsy specimens from young dogs and cats with clinical abnormalities suspicious of familial renal disease before azotemia develops.
- Submit renal biopsy specimens from affected animals for special stains (e.g., Masson's trichrome, periodic acid Schiff, Congo red), for immunohistochemistry to detect immunoglobulins, and for transmission electron microscopy to evaluate ultrastructural morphology in addition to samples for routine light microscopy. Samples should be submitted to a pathologist who is familiar with the light and electron microscopic features of familial renal disease.
- Avoid renal biopsy in affected animals with very small kidneys and advanced azotemia.

THOUGHTS FOR THE FUTURE

- The genes and mutations responsible for additional familial renal diseases of dogs and cats will be identified, and genetic tests to identify animals at risk will be developed.

FREQUENTLY ASKED QUESTIONS

Q: A 3-month-old dog of a specific breed is presented for evaluation of polyuria, polydipsia, dilute urine (urine specific gravity [USG] 1.012), and moderate azotemia (serum creatinine concentration, 3.7 mg/dL). Proteinuria (2+) is found on urine dipstrip evaluation. The health status of the other littermates cannot be determined. What is the chance that this dog has a familial nephropathy?

A: It is very possible that the dog indeed has a familial nephropathy. It is also possible, however, that renal disease was acquired in utero or soon after birth as a result of nongenetic factors. Information from diagnostic imaging and renal histopathology would allow an accurate diagnosis to be made.

Q: A 5-year-old dog of a specific breed is presented in what appears to be chronic renal failure. Could a genetic disease be responsible for chronic renal failure in this dog?

A: The age of onset of many familial renal diseases is very variable and clinical signs can be manifested later in life. Proving the underlying cause for chronic renal failure in middle-aged animals can be challenging. Some renal histopathologic findings may suggest familial renal disease (e.g., fetal glomeruli). Absence of such changes however does not necessarily exclude familial renal disease.

Q: What can be done to preserve renal structure and function as well as to prolong survival in dogs and cats with familial renal disease?

A: Dietary intervention using a veterinary renal diet and ACE inhibition have been shown to be beneficial in some forms of familial nephropathy (e.g., X-linked familial nephropathy in Samoyed dogs). ACE inhibition may be beneficial to decrease intraglomerular pressure and proteinuria in many animals with familial nephropathies characterized by proteinuria.

SUGGESTED READINGS

General
Picut CA, Lewis RM: Microscopic features of canine renal dysplasia, *Vet Pathol* 24:156–163, 1987.

Abyssinian Cats
Boyce JT, DiBartola SP, Chew DJ, et al: Familial renal amyloidosis in Abyssinian cats, *Vet Pathol* 21:33–38, 1984.
Chew DJ, DiBartola SP, Boyce JT, et al: Renal amyloidosis in related Abyssinian cats, *J Am Vet Med Assoc* 181:139–142, 1982.
DiBartola SP, Benson MD, Dwulet FE, et al: Isolation and characterization of amyloid protein AA in the Abyssinian cat, *Lab Invest* 52:485–489, 1985.
DiBartola SP, Tarr MJ, Benson MD: Tissue distribution of amyloid deposits in Abyssinian cats with familial amyloidosis, *J Comp Pathol* 96:387–398, 1986.
Godfrey DR, Day MJ: Generalised amyloidosis in two Siamese cats: Spontaneous liver haemorrhage and chronic renal failure, *J Small Anim Pract* 39:442–447, 1998.
Niewold TA, van der Linde-Sipman JS, Murphy C, et al: Familial amyloidosis in cats: Siamese and Abyssinian AA proteins differ in primary sequence and pattern of deposition, *Amyloid* 6:205–209, 1999.

Alaskan Malamutes
Vilafranca M, Ferrer L: Juvenile nephropathy in Alaskan Malamute littermates, *Vet Pathol* 31:375–377, 1994.

Basenji

Bovee KC, Joyce T, Blazer-Yost B, et al: Characterization of renal defects in dogs with a syndrome similar to the Fanconi syndrome in man, *J Am Vet Med Assoc* 174:1094–1099, 1979.

Hsu BY, McNamara PD, Mahoney SG, et al: Membrane fluidity and sodium transport by renal membranes from dogs with spontaneous idiopathic Fanconi syndrome, *Metabolism* 41, 1992:253–159.

Noonan CH, Kay JM: Prevalence and geographic distribution of Fanconi syndrome in Basenjis in the United States, *J Am Vet Med Assoc* 197:345–349, 1990.

Beagle

Bowles MH, Mosier DA: Renal amyloidosis in a family of beagles, *J Am Vet Med Assoc* 201:569–574, 1992.

Rha JY, Labato MA, Ross LA, et al: Familial glomerulonephropathy in a litter of beagles, *J Am Vet Med Assoc* 216:46–50, 32, 2000.

Bernese Mountain Dog

Minkus G, Breuer W, Wanke R, et al: Familial nephropathy in Bernese Mountain dogs, *Vet Pathol* 31:421–428, 1994.

Reusch C, Hoerauf A, Lechner J, et al: A new familial glomerulonephropathy in Bernese mountain dogs, *Vet Rec* 134: 411–415, 1994.

Brittany Spaniel

Cork LC, Morris JM, Olson JL, et al: Membranoproliferative glomerulonephritis in dogs with a genetically determined deficiency of the third component of complement, *Clin Immunol Immunopathol* 60:455–470, 1991.

Bull Terrier

Burrows AK, Malik R, Hunt GB, et al: Familial polycystic kidney disease in bull terriers, *J Small Anim Pract* 35:364–369, 1994.

Hood JC, Dowling J, Bertram JF, et al: Correlation of histopathological features and renal impairment in autosomal dominant Alport syndrome in Bull terriers, *Nephrol Dial Transplant* 17:1897–1908, 2002.

Hood JC, Robinson WF, Clark WT, et al: Proteinuria as an indicator of early renal disease in Bull terriers with hereditary nephritis, *J Small Anim Pract* 32:241–248, 1991.

Hood JC, Robinson WF, Huxtable CR, et al: Hereditary nephritis in the bull terrier: Evidence for inheritance by an autosomal dominant gene, *Vet Rec* 126:456–459, 1990.

Hood JC, Savige J, Hendtlass A, et al: Bull terrier hereditary nephritis: A model for autosomal dominant Alport syndrome, *Kidney Int* 47:758–765, 1995.

Hood JC, Savige J, Seymour AE, et al: Ultrastructural appearance of renal and other basement membranes in the Bull terrier model of autosomal dominant hereditary nephritis, *Am J Kidney Dis* 36:378–391, 2000.

Jones BR, Gethring MA, Badcoe LM, et al: Familial progressive nephropathy in young Bull terriers, *N Z Vet J* 37:79–82, 1989.

O'Leary CA, Ghoddusi M, Huxtable CR: Renal pathology of polycystic kidney disease and concurrent hereditary nephritis in Bull Terriers, *Aust Vet J* 80:353–361, 2002.

Robinson WF, Shaw SE, Stanley B, et al: Chronic renal disease in Bull terriers, *Aust Vet J* 66:193–195, 1989.

Bullmastiff

Casal ML, Dambach DM, Meister T, et al: Familial glomerulonephropathy in the Bullmastiff, *Vet Pathol* 41:319–325, 2004.

Cairn and West Highland White Terrier

McAloose D, Casal M, Patterson DF, et al: Polycystic kidney and liver disease in two related West Highland White Terrier litters, *Vet Pathol* 35:77–81, 1998.

McKenna SC, Carpenter JL: Polycystic disease of the kidney and liver in the Cairn terrier, *Vet Pathol* 17:436–442, 1980.

Chow

Brown CA, Crowell WA, Brown SA, et al: Suspected familial renal disease in Chow Chows, *J Am Vet Med Assoc* 196: 1279–1284, 1990.

English Cocker Spaniel

Davidson AG, Bell RJ, Lees GE, et al: Genetic cause of autosomal recessive hereditary nephropathy in the English Cocker spaniel, *J Vet Int Med* 21:394–401, 2007.

Lees GE, Helman RG, Homco LD, et al: Early diagnosis of familial nephropathy in English cocker spaniels, *J Am Anim Hosp Assoc* 34:189–195, 1998.

Lees GE, Helman RG, Kashtan CE, et al: A model of autosomal recessive Alport syndrome in English cocker spaniel dogs, *Kidney Int* 54:706–719, 1998.

Lees GE, Wilson PD, Helman RG, et al: Glomerular ultrastructural findings similar to hereditary nephritis in 4 English cocker spaniels, *J Vet Intern Med* 11:80–85, 1997.

Dalmatian

Hood JC, Huxtable CR, Naito I, et al: A novel model of autosomal dominant Alport syndrome in Dalmatian dogs, *Nephrol Dial Transplant* 17:2094–2098, 2002.

Doberman Pinscher

Chew DJ, DiBartola SP, Boyce JT, et al: Juvenile renal disease in Doberman pinscher dogs, *J Am Vet Med Assoc* 182:481–485, 1983.

Picut CA, Lewis RM: Juvenile renal disease in the Doberman pinscher: Ultrastructural changes of the glomerular basement membrane, *J Comp Pathol* 97:587–596, 1987.

Wilcock BP, Patterson JM: Familial glomerulonephritis in Doberman pinscher dogs, *Can Vet J* 20:244–249, 1979.

English Foxhound

Mason NJ, Day MJ: Renal amyloidosis in related English foxhounds, *J Small Anim Pract* 37:255–260, 1996.

German Shepherd

Lium B, Moe L: Hereditary multifocal renal cystadenocarcinomas and nodular dermatofibrosis in the German Shepherd dog: Macroscopic and histopathologic changes, *Vet Pathol* 22:447–455, 1985.

Moe L, Lium B: Computed tomography of hereditary multifocal renal cystadenocarcinomas in German shepherd dogs, *Vet Radiol Ultrasound* 38:335–343, 1997.

Moe L, Lium B: Hereditary multifocal renal cystadenocarcinomas and nodular dermatofibrosis in 51 German shepherd dogs, *J Small Anim Pract* 38:498–505, 1997.

Golden Retriever

De Morais HS, DiBartola SP, Chew DJ: Juvenile renal disease in golden retrievers: 12 cases (1984-1994), *J Am Vet Med Assoc* 209:792–797, 1996.

Kerlin RL, Van Winkle TJ: Renal dysplasia in golden retrievers, *Vet Pathol* 32:327–329, 1995.

Lhasa Apso and Shih Tzu

O'Brien TD, Osborne CA, Yano BL, et al: Clinicopathologic manifestations of progressive renal disease in Lhasa apso and Shih tzu dogs, *J Am Vet Med Assoc* 180:658–664, 1982.

Miniature Schnauzer

Morton LD, Sanecki RK, Gordon DE, et al: Juvenile renal disease in Miniature Schnauzer dogs, *Vet Pathol* 27:455–458, 1990.

Navasota Texas (NAV) Dogs

Cox ML, Lees GE, Kashtan CE, et al: Genetic cause of X-linked Alport syndrome in a family of domestic dogs, *Mamm Genome* 14:396–403, 2003.

Lees GE, Helman RG, Kashtan CE, et al: New form of X-linked dominant hereditary nephritis in dogs, *Am J Vet Res* 60:373–383, 1999.

Newfoundland

Koeman JP, Biewenga WJ, Gruys E: Proteinuria associated with glomerulosclerosis and glomerular collagen formation in three Newfoundland dog littermates, *Vet Pathol* 31:188–193, 1994.

Norwegian Elkhound

Finco DR: Familial renal disease in Norwegian Elkhound dogs: Physiologic and biochemical examinations, *Am J Vet Res* 37:87–91, 1976.

Finco DR, Duncan JR, Crowell WA, et al: Familial renal disease in Norwegian elkhound dogs: Morphologic examinations, *Am J Vet Res* 38:941–947, 1977.

Finco DR, Kurtz HJ, Low DG, et al: Familial renal disease in Norwegian elkhound dogs, *J Am Vet Med Assoc* 156:747–760, 1970.

Persian Cat

Barrs VR, Gunew M, Foster SF, et al: Prevalence of autosomal dominant polycystic kidney disease in Persian cats and related breeds in Sydney and Brisbane, *Aust Vet J* 79:257–259, 2001.

Barthez PY, Rivier P, Begon D: Prevalence of polycystic kidney disease in Persian and Persian related cats in France, *J Feline Med Surg* 5:345–347, 2003.

Beck C, Lavelle RB: Feline polycystic kidney disease in Persian and other cats: A prospective study using ultrasonography, *Aust Vet J* 79:181–184, 2001.

Biller DS, Chew DJ, DiBartola SP: Polycystic kidney disease in a family of Persian cats, *J Am Vet Med Assoc* 196:1288–1290, 1990.

Biller DS, DiBartola SP, Eaton KA, et al: Inheritance of polycystic kidney disease in Persian cats, *J Hered* 87:1–5, 1996.

Bosje JT, van den Ingh TS, van der Linde-Sipman JS: Polycystic kidney and liver disease in cats, *Vet Q* 20:136–139, 1998.

Cannon MJ, MacKay AD, Barr FJ, et al: Prevalence of polycystic kidney disease in Persian cats in the United Kingdom, *Vet Rec* 149:409–411, 2001.

Eaton KA, Biller DS, DiBartola SP, et al: Autosomal dominant polycystic kidney disease in Persian and Persian-cross cats, *Vet Pathol* 34:117–126, 1997.

Helps CR, Tasker S, Barr FJ, et al: Detection of the single nucleotide polymorphism causing feline autosomal-dominant polycystic kidney disease in Persians from the UK using a novel real-time PCR assay, *Mol Cell Probes* 21:31–34, 2007.

Lyons LA, Biller DS, Erdman CA, et al: Feline polycystic kidney disease mutation identified in PKD1, *J Am Soc Nephrol* 15:2548–2555, 2004.

Miller RH, Lehmkuhl LB, Smeak DD, et al: Effect of enalapril on blood pressure, renal function, and the renin-angiotensin-aldosterone system in cats with autosomal dominant polycystic kidney disease, *Am J Vet Res* 60:1516–1525, 1999.

Pedersen KM, Pedersen HD, Haggstrom J, et al: Increased mean arterial pressure and aldosterone-to-renin ratio in Persian cats with polycystic kidney disease, *J Vet Int Med* 17:21–27, 2003.

Stebbins KE: Polycystic disease of the kidney and liver in an adult Persian cat, *J Comp Pathol* 100:327–330, 1989.

Rottweiler

Cook SM, Dean DF, Golden DL, et al: Renal failure attributable to atrophic glomerulopathy in four related rottweilers, *J Am Vet Med Assoc* 202:107–109, 1993.

Wakamatsu N, Surdyk K, Carmichael KP, et al: Histologic and ultrastructural studies of juvenile onset renal disease in four Rottweiler dogs, *Vet Pathol* 44:96–100, 2007.

Samoyed

Bernard MA, Valli VE: Familial renal disease in Samoyed dogs, *Can Vet J* 18:181–189, 1977.

Bloedow AG: Familial renal disease in Samoyed dogs, *Vet Rec* 108:167–168, 1981.

Chen D, Jefferson B, Harvey SJ, et al: Cyclosporine A slows the progressive renal disease of Alport syndrome (X-linked hereditary nephritis): Results from a canine model, *J Am Soc Nephrol* 14:690–698, 2003.

Grodecki KM, Gains MJ, Baumal R, et al: Treatment of X-linked hereditary nephritis in Samoyed dogs with angiotensin converting enzyme (ACE) inhibitor, *J Comp Pathol* 117:209–225, 1997.

Jansen B, Thorner P, Baumal R, et al: Samoyed hereditary glomerulopathy. Evolution of splitting of glomerular capillary basement membrane, *Am J Pathol* 125:536–545, 1986.

Jansen B, Thorner PS, Singh A, et al: Animal model of human disease: Hereditary nephritis in Samoyed dogs, *Am J Pathol* 116:175–178, 1984.

Jansen B, Tryphonas L, Wong J, et al: Mode of inheritance of Samoyed hereditary glomerulopathy: An animal model for hereditary nephritis in humans, *J Lab Clin Med* 107:551–555, 1986.

Jansen B, Valli VE, Thorner P, et al: Samoyed hereditary glomerulopathy: Serial clinical and laboratory (urine, serum biochemistry and hematology) studies, *Can J Vet Res* 51:387–393, 1987.

Jansen BS, Valli VE, Thorner PS, et al: Scanning electron microscopy of cellular and acellular glomeruli of male dogs affected with Samoyed hereditary glomerulopathy and a carrier female, *Can J Vet Res* 51:475–478, 1987.

Thorner P, Baumal R, Binnington A, et al: The NC1 domain of collagen type IV in neonatal dog glomerular basement membranes: Significance in Samoyed hereditary nephropathy, *Am J Pathol* 134:1047–1054, 1989.

Thorner P, Baumal R, Valli VE, et al: Abnormalities in the NC1 domain of collage type IV in GBM in canine hereditary nephritis, *Kidney Int* 35:843–850, 1989.

Thorner PS, Baumal R, Valli VE, et al: Production of anti-NC1 antibody by affected male dogs with X-linked hereditary nephritis: A probe for assessing the NC1 domain of collagen type IV in dogs and humans with hereditary nephritis, *Virch Arch A Pathol Anat Histopathol* 421:467–475, 1992.

Thorner P, Jansen B, Baumal R, et al: Samoyed hereditary glomerulopathy. Immunohistochemical staining of basement membranes of kidney for laminin, collagen type IV, fibronectin, and Goodpasture antigen, and correlation with electron microscopy of glomerular capillary basement membranes, *Lab Invest* 56:435–443, 1987.

Thorner PS, Jansen B, Liang J, et al: Quantitation of anionic sites in glomerular capillary basement membranes of Samoyed dogs with hereditary glomerulopathy, *Virch Arch A Pathol Anat Histopathol* 411:79–85, 1987.

Thorner PS, Zheng K, Kalluri R, et al: Coordinate gene expression of the alpha3, alpha4, and alpha5 chains of collagen type IV. Evidence from a canine model of X-linked nephritis with a COL4A5 gene mutation, *J Biol Chem* 271:13821–13828, 1996.

Valli VE, Baumal R, Thorner P, et al: Dietary modification reduces splitting of glomerular basement membranes and delays death due to renal failure in canine X-linked hereditary nephritis, *Lab Invest* 65:67–73, 1991.

Zheng K, Thorner PS, Marrano P, et al: Canine X chromosome-linked hereditary nephritis: A genetic model for human X-linked hereditary nephritis resulting from a single base mutation in the gene encoding the alpha 5 chain of collagen type IV, *Proc Natl Acad Sci U S A* 91:3989–3993, 1994.

Shar Pei

DiBartola SP, Tarr MJ, Webb DM, et al: Familial renal amyloidosis in Chinese Shar pei dogs, *J Am Vet Med Assoc* 197:483–487, 1990.

Johnson KH, Sletten K, Hayden DW, et al: AA amyloidosis in Chinese Shar-pei dogs: immunohistochemical and amino acid sequence analysis, *Amyloid* 2:92–99, 1995.

Loeven KO: Spontaneous hepatic rupture secondary to amyloidosis in a Chinese Shar pei, *J Am Anim Hosp Assoc* 30:577–579, 1994.

May C, Hammill J, Bennett D: Chinese Shar pei fever syndrome: A preliminary report, *Vet Rec* 131:586–587, 1992.

Rivas AL, Tintle L, Kimball ES, et al: A canine febrile disorder associated with elevated interleukin-6, *Clin Immunol Immunopathol* 64:36–45, 1992.

Rivas AL, Tintle L, Meyers-Wallen V, et al: Inheritance of renal amyloidosis in Chinese Shar pei dogs, *J Hered* 84:438–442, 1993.

Soft-Coated Wheaten Terrier

Afrouzian M, Vaden SL, Harris T, et al: Immune complex mediated proliferative and sclerosing glomerulonephritis in soft coated wheaten terriers (SCWT): Is this an animal model of IgA nephropathy or IgM mesangial nephropathy? *J Am Soc Nephrol* 12:670A, 2001.

Eriksen K, Grondalen J: Familial renal disease in soft-coated Wheaten terriers, *J Small Anim Pract* 25:489–500, 1984.

Littman MP, Dambach DM, Vaden SL, et al: Familial protein-losing enteropathy and protein-losing nephropathy in Soft Coated Wheaten Terriers: 222 cases (1983-1997), *J Vet Int Med* 14:68–80, 2000.

Nash AS, Kelly DF, Gaskell CJ: Progressive renal disease in soft-coated Wheaten terriers: Possible familial nephropathy, *J Small Anim Pract* 25:479–487, 1984.

Vaden SL, Hammerberg B, Davenport DJ, et al: Food hypersensitivity reactions in Soft Coated Wheaten Terriers with protein-losing enteropathy or protein-losing nephropathy or both: Gastroscopic food sensitivity testing, dietary provocation, and fecal immunoglobulin E, *J Vet Int Med* 14:60–67, 2000.

Vaden SL, Sellon RK, Melgarejo LT, et al: Evaluation of intestinal permeability and gluten sensitivity in Soft-Coated Wheaten Terriers with familial protein-losing enteropathy, protein-losing nephropathy, or both, *Am J Vet Res* 61:518–524, 2000.

Standard Poodle

DiBartola SP, Chew DJ, Boyce JT: Juvenile renal disease in related Standard poodles, *J Am Vet Med Assoc* 183:693–696, 1983.

Welsh Corgi

Moore FM, Thornton GW: Telangiectasia of Pembroke Welsh Corgi dogs, *Vet Pathol* 20:203–208, 1983.

7 Diseases of the Glomerulus

INTRODUCTION

A. Glomerular diseases affect primarily the glomeruli. However, destruction of the glomerulus renders the remainder of the nephron nonfunctional and progressive destruction of glomeruli can lead to decreased glomerular filtration rate, azotemia, and renal failure.

B. Glomerular disease is an important cause of chronic renal failure in humans and has been increasingly recognized in veterinary medicine.

C. The two important glomerular diseases of domestic animals are glomerulonephritis (GN) and glomerular amyloidosis.

D. Marked, persistent proteinuria is the hallmark of glomerular disease.

E. The term nephrotic syndrome traditionally has been used to describe patients with proteinuria, hypoalbuminemia, hypercholesterolemia, and edema or ascites. Human patients excreting more than 3.5 grams of protein per 1.73 m^2 body surface area per day in their urine are said to have nephrotic range proteinuria. Patients with several different glomerular diseases can present as having nephrotic syndrome.

NORMAL GLOMERULAR ANATOMY AND FUNCTION

A. The glomerulus is a unique vascular structure consisting of a capillary bed between two arterioles (Figure 7-1).

B. An ultrafiltrate of plasma is forced through the glomeruli as blood is pumped through the kidney by the heart.

C. The filtration barrier of the glomerulus consists of three layers (from the vascular space to the urinary space) (Figure 7-2):

   1. Endothelium.

      a. The fenestrated capillary endothelium is 100 to 500 times more permeable to water and crystalloids than are systemic capillaries.

      b. Negatively-charged surface contributes to charge selectivity.

   2. Glomerular basement membrane.

      a. A trilaminar structure consisting of a central dense region (lamina densa) and outer less dense regions (lamina rara interna, lamina rara externa).

      b. Contains type IV collagen, proteoglycans, laminin, fibronectin, and water.

      c. Proteoglycans are large, highly negatively charged molecules consisting of a protein backbone with polysaccharide (glycosaminoglycans) side chains. The proteoglycans are responsible for the charge selectivity of the basement membrane.

      d. Type IV collagen in the basement membrane forms a mesh that contributes to the size selectivity of the glomerular capillary wall.

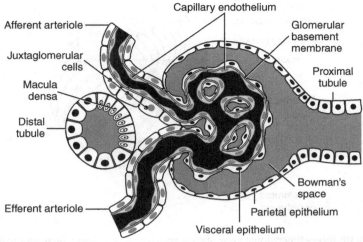

FIGURE 7-1 ■ Schematic representation of normal glomerular morphology at the light microscopic level. (Drawn by Tim Vojt.)

3. Visceral epithelial cells (podocytes).
   a. Cover the filtration barrier on the urinary side by means of primary and interdigitating secondary foot processes.
   b. Secondary foot processes are separated by slit or filtration diaphragms.
   c. Negative charge contributes to charge selectivity by virtue of negatively charged cell surface (sialoglycoproteins).
   d. Synthesize the glomerular basement membrane.
   e. Podocytes are phagocytic and may engulf macromolecules trapped in the filtration barrier.
D. The glomerular filter functions as a size and charge selective barrier.
   1. Size selectivity: The glomerular filter excludes particles of <35 Å in radius (serum albumin has a molecular weight of 70,000 daltons and molecular radius of 36 Å).
   2. Charge selectivity: For any given size, negatively charged macromolecules will experience greater restriction to filtration than neutral ones.
E. Other components of the glomerulus.
   1. Mesangial cells provide structural support for the glomerular capillary loops and also possess contractile and phagocytic properties (Figure 7-3).
      a. Reside in the glomerular interstitium in areas where the podocytes do not completely surround the capillary endothelium.
      b. Produce mesangial matrix, which is similar to the basement membrane in composition.
      c. Are phagocytic and may clear filtration residues from the mesangial space.
      d. Contain contractile elements that can alter the amount of glomerular surface area available for filtration.
      e. May play a role in the normal turnover of the glomerular basement membrane.
      f. May undergo fibrous metaplasia leading to glomerular sclerosis.
      g. The mesangium is an early site of deposition of immune complexes and amyloid fibrils.
   2. Parietal epithelial cells line the urinary side of the glomerular capsule (Bowman's capsule) and are continuous with the visceral epithelial cells at the vascular pole of the glomerulus and with the proximal tubule at the urinary pole.

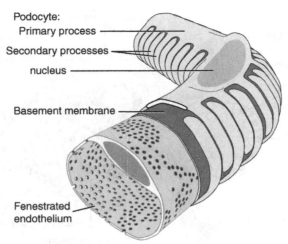

FIGURE 7-2 ■ Schematic three-dimensional view of glomerulus demonstrating the scanning electron microscopic appearance of the glomerulus. The three layers of the glomerular capillary barrier are indicated in the cutaway section. (Drawn by Tim Vojt.)

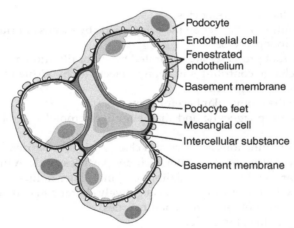

FIGURE 7-3 ■ Schematic transverse section of glomerulus showing the location of mesangial cells. (Drawn by Tim Vojt.)

3. The juxtaglomerular apparatus, at the vascular pole, consists of specialized smooth muscle cells of the afferent and efferent arterioles containing electron dense renin granules, and the macula densa, a specialized segment of the distal tubule. The juxtaglomerular apparatus mediates tubuloglomerular feedback.

PATHOGENESIS OF GLOMERULAR DISEASE

Glomerular Injury May Be Either Immune-Mediated or Nonimmune
1. Immune-mediated GN is associated with immune complex deposition in the glomeruli.
2. Nonimmune-mediated glomerular disease may be inflammatory (e.g., GN) or noninflammatory (e.g., amyloid fibril deposition, glomerular sclerosis secondary to hyperfiltration).

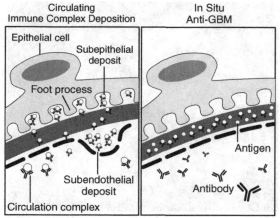

FIGURE 7-4 ■ Immune-complex GN: Deposition of subepithelial and subendothelial circulating immune complexes (left panel) and intramembranous complexes formed in situ (right panel). *GBM,* glomerular basement membrane. (Drawn by Tim Vojt.)

Immune-Mediated Glomerulonephritis

1. Immune-complex GN is a disease of glomeruli caused by deposition of immunoglobulin or complement in the glomerular capillary wall.
2. Immune complexes deposit in the glomerular filter in two ways (Figure 7-4):
   a. Soluble circulating immune complexes are trapped in the glomerulus in conditions of antigen-antibody equivalence or slight antigen excess (the classic example is serum sickness). In antibody excess, immune complexes tend to be large and insoluble and are rapidly removed from the circulation by phagocytic cells. In large antigen excess, immune complexes do not readily bind complement and are less likely to produce immune injury.
   b. Immune complexes may be formed in situ either in response to endogenous glomerular antigens, endogenous nonglomerular antigens, or exogenous antigens deposited or "planted" in the glomerular filter.
3. Immune complexes may be deposited in a subepithelial, subendothelial, or intramembranous position. Complexes also may deposit in the mesangium.
4. Factors affecting the location of deposition include size of the complexes (dependent on antigen-to-antibody ratio), charge of the complexes, removal of complexes by phagocytosis, and damage to the basement membrane itself.
   a. Subepithelial complexes are small and form at approximate antigen-antibody equivalence.
   b. Subendothelial complexes are large or highly negatively charged, and, therefore, do not easily pass through the basement membrane.
   c. Mesangial cells may remove large complexes and deposit them in the mesangium.
   d. Basement membrane damage may allow complexes to adhere or pass into intramembranous or subepithelial locations. Autoantibody directed against basement membrane components may lead to intramembranous deposition.
5. The location of deposition determines the histologic changes observed and the severity of glomerular dysfunction.
   a. Subepithelial complexes are associated with basement membrane thickening and minimal inflammatory cell infiltration. Proteinuria may be severe.

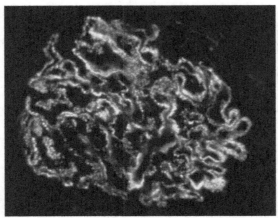

FIGURE 7-5 ■ *Lumpy bumpy* immunofluorescent appearance of the discontinuous deposition of immune complexes in GN. Note discrete areas of immune complexes positive for immunoglobulin G (IgG). (Fluorescein isothiocyanate-labeled rabbit anti-dog IgG, IgA, and IgM, ×400.)

  b. Subendothelial complexes are associated with recruitment of inflammatory cells and basement membrane thickening, but proteinuria may only be moderate in severity.
  c. Intramembranous deposition is most commonly associated with antiglomerular basement membrane disease.
  d. Mesangial complexes may be asymptomatic.
6. Immune complexes can be detected in the glomeruli by staining histologic sections with fluorescein-labeled antibody against immunoglobulins or complement of the species being studied. This technique requires renal biopsy specimens to be frozen in liquid nitrogen or stored for less than 7 days in special preservative solutions (e.g., Michel solution). More recently, immunohistochemistry using peroxidase-antiperoxidase methods can be applied to specimens preserved routinely in 10% buffered formalin.
  a. Glomerular deposition of preformed immune complexes usually results in a *lumpy bumpy* or granular discontinuous immunofluorescence pattern with mesangial and subendothelial location of the immune complexes (Figure 7-5).
  b. In situ formation of immune complexes can occur within glomeruli when circulating antibodies react with endogenous glomerular antigens or "planted" nonglomerular antigens in the glomerular capillary wall. In this instance, a smooth linear continuous pattern of immunofluorescence usually results.
  c. True autoimmune glomerulonephritis (anti-GBM GN) with antibodies against endogenous glomerular basement membrane antigens has not been conclusively identified in domestic animals.

Mechanisms of Immune Injury
  1. Deposition of immune complexes in the mesangium may or may not be associated with pathologic lesions or glomerular dysfunction.
  2. Immune complex deposition in glomeruli may reduce the amount of fixed negative charge and enhance filtration of negatively charged circulating macromolecules (e.g., albumin).
  3. Complement activation results in membrane damage and proteinuria. Soluble complement components also recruit inflammatory cells.

4. Platelet activation and aggregation may occur due to endothelial damage or antigen anti-body interaction and exacerbate glomerular damage by release of a variety of mediators. These mediators cause activation and proliferation of mesangial cells and endothelial cells, vasospasm and increased coagulation.
5. Mesangial cells contribute to glomerular inflammation by release of eicosanoids, cyto-kines, and growth factors and by increased matrix production.
6. Inflammatory cells also contribute to glomerular injury.
    a. Neutrophils and macrophages localize in the glomeruli in response to soluble media-tors including complement components, platelet activating factor, platelet-derived growth factor, and eicosanoids.
    b. Activated neutrophils release reactive oxygen species and proteinases, leading to fur-ther damage.
    c. Macrophages produce proteinases, oxidants, eicosanoids, growth factors, cytokines, complement fragments, and coagulation factors.
7. Many bioactive mediators may be involved in these interactions. Such mediators are produced by resident glomerular cells (mesangial cells, endothelial cells) or by recruited blood cells (neutrophils, platelets) in response to deposition of immune complexes in the glomerular basement membrane. Important mediators include:
    a. Eicosanoids (prostaglandins, thromboxanes, and leukotrienes) are products of arachi-donic acid metabolism. Thromboxanes, and leukotrienes cause vasoconstriction and mesangial cell contraction, both of which may result in decreased glomerular filtration rate (GFR). These mediators also attract and activate neutrophils.
    b. Cytokines and growth factors are produced by inflammatory cells and resident glo-merular cells. These include tumor necrosis factor, interleukin-1, interleukin-6, platelet-derived growth factor, transforming growth factor, and epidermal growth factor, and contribute to mesangial cell activation (cellular proliferation, matrix production) and incite inflammation.
    c. Other factors such as platelet activating factor, endothelin, and nitric oxide contribute to glomerular damage via activation of inflammatory and mesangial cells or by stimu-lating coagulation.
8. Several infectious and inflammatory diseases have been associated with glomerular depo-sition or in situ formation of immune complexes in dogs and cats (Box 7-1). In most cases, however, the antigen source or underlying disease process is not identified and the glo-merular disease is referred to as idiopathic.

Nonimmune Glomerular Injury
1. Most idiopathic GN in animals is thought to be immune-mediated, but glomerular dam-age also may occur by nonimmune mechanisms.
2. Whereas the primary target for immune-mediated glomerular disease is the filtration bar-rier, the primary target for nonimmune injury appears to be the endothelial cell.
3. Damaged endothelial cells release factors (e.g., endothelin) that have vasoactive, proliferative and proinflammatory effects. Additionally, endothelial damage stimulates coagulation.
4. Factors that may damage endothelial cells are:
    a. Hemodynamic factors: Intraglomerular hypertension secondary to hyperfiltration may physically damage endothelial cells.
    b. Coagulation followed by activation of the platelet release reaction may lead to endo-thelial damage.
    c. Hyperlipemia may cause endothelial damage directly.

■ BOX 7-1
■ **CAUSES OF IMMUNE-MEDIATED GLOMERULONEPHRITIS IN DOGS AND CATS**

Dogs
 I. Pyometra: Commonly associated with proliferative or membranoproliferative GN. Continuous high levels of bacterial antigens are thought to be responsible for immune complex formation and deposition, although these antigens have not been demonstrated in the kidney. The glomerular changes usually disappear once ovariohysterectomy is performed.
 II. *Dirofilaria immitis* infection: Also commonly associated with GN and proteinuria. One theory is that immune complexes form in response to shed microfilarial antigens. Another is that the mechanical presence or products of the microfilaria damage the glomerular vessels.
 III. Canine adenovirus-1 (infectious canine hepatitis): Associated with mild proliferative GN and interstitial nephritis. Dense deposits suggestive of immune complexes are seen in the glomerular basement membrane, and tubular epithelial antigens are shed in the urine. Intranuclear inclusion bodies may be present in endothelial cells.
 IV. Systemic lupus erythematosus (SLE): Antinuclear antibodies are responsible for the complexes.
 V. Other infectious diseases:
    A. Bacterial endocarditis
    B. Ehrlichiosis
    C. Brucellosis
    D. Borreliosis
       1. Membranoproliferative GN in Bernese Mountain dogs inherited as an autosomal recessive trait has a strong association with seropositivity for *Borrelia burgdorferi*
    E. Leishmaniasis
    F. Rocky Mountain spotted fever
    G. Trypanosomiasis
    H. Other chronic bacterial infections
 VI. Neoplasia
    A. Mastocytoma
    B. Lymphosarcoma
    C. Other
 VII. Other disease associations
    A. Immune-mediated polyarthritis
    B. Chronic skin disease
    C. Chronic prostatitis
    D. Proteinuria has been observed in dogs with hyperadrenocorticism, and normal dogs treated with glucocorticoids develop proteinuria and glomerular lesions (e.g., hypercellularity, thickened glomerular basement membranes, foot process fusion, glomerular adhesions) but no deposition of immune complexes.
    E. Pancreatitis
    F. Thickening of glomerular capillary wall but without proteinuria in dogs with congenital portosystemic shunts
 VIII. Most cases of GN in dogs are idiopathic
 IX. Familial glomerular disease
    A. Familial membranous or membranoproliferative GN in soft-coated Wheaten terriers
       1. Associated with protein-losing enteropathy in many affected dogs
       2. Progressive leading to glomerulosclerosis and end-stage renal disease
    B. Membranoproliferative GN associated with hereditary deficiency of complement component III in Brittany spaniels
    C. Autosomal recessive type IV collagen defect in English Cocker spaniels

---

■ BOX 7-1
■ **CAUSES OF IMMUNE-MEDIATED GLOMERULONEPHRITIS IN DOGS AND CATS—cont'd**

    D. X-linked dominant type IV collagen defect in Samoyeds
    E. Suspected basement membrane disorders in Doberman pinschers and Bull terriers
    F. Glomerulopathy with increased collagen deposition and glomerular sclerosis in young Newfoundland dogs

Cats

    I. Feline leukemia virus infection: Frequently associated with membranous GN with or without signs of renal dysfunction. These cats usually do not die from renal failure.
    II. Feline immunodeficiency virus
    III. Feline infectious peritonitis
    IV. Chronic progressive polyarthritis (*Mycoplasma gatae*)
    V. Most cases of GN in cats are idiopathic
    VI. Other:
        A. Pancreatic fat necrosis
        B. SLE
        C. Hemolymphatic neoplasia (e.g., lymphosarcoma)
        D. Familial: Sibling cats with GN

Progression of Glomerular Disease

1. Continued deposition of complexes and release of inflammatory mediators eventually lead to glomerulosclerosis.
2. Secondary antibodies directed against immune complexes may form in situ and exacerbate disease.
3. Glomerular disease may induce tubulointerstitial disease and progress to end-stage kidney disease and chronic renal failure.
   a. Obstruction of glomerular capillaries may result in ischemia of the tubules and tubulointerstitial disease.
   b. Proteinuria may lead to an interstitial immune response resulting in tubulointerstitial disease.
   c. Protein in the ultrafiltrate is taken up and degraded by proximal tubular cells. Overload of the lysosomal systems of these cells may lead to hypoxia and cell death. Increased protein uptake also may lead to increased transcription of inflammatory mediators.
   d. Inflammatory mediators from damaged glomeruli may lead to tubular and interstitial damage.

Resolution of Glomerular Disease

1. GN may resolve by:
   a. Solubilization of complexes via complement or excess antigen.
   b. Phagocytosis of immune complexes by macrophages.
   c. Degradation of immune complexes by extracellular proteases.
2. Removal of the causative antigen may result in resolution of GN (e.g., ovariohysterectomy in dogs with pyometra, treatment of heartworm disease).

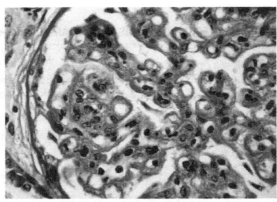

FIGURE 7-6 ■ Membranous GN. Note distinct thickening of the capillary loops. (Periodic acid schiff, ×400.)

LESIONS OF GLOMERULAR DISEASE

A. Histologic lesions of GN.
   1. Basement membrane thickening.
   2. Hypercellularity.
   3. Fibrosis.
B. GN is classified morphologically according the presence of basement membrane thickening, hypercellularity, or both.
   1. Disease characterized primarily by basement membrane thickening is called membranous GN (Figure 7-6).
   2. Disease characterized primarily by increased glomerular cellularity (due to inflammatory cell influx or mesangial cell proliferation) is called proliferative GN.
   3. Disease characterized by both basement membrane thickening and increased cellularity is called membranoproliferative GN.
   4. Disease characterized primarily by fibrosis of the glomeruli is called glomerulosclerosis.
C. Chronic changes include glomerular and periglomerular fibrosis with eventual glomerular sclerosis. Sclerotic glomeruli are nonfunctional.
D. Ultrastructural lesions of glomerular disease.
   1. The presence of immunoglobulin deposits in the basement membrane and podocyte foot process fusion may be detected by electron microscopy.
   2. Ultrastructural changes may include thickening or splitting of the basement membrane, podocytes foot process fusion, changes in the number and types of cells in the mesangium, presence of dense deposits, and other changes.
   3. The clinical relevance of these changes is not known in dogs and cats with GN, because ultrastructural examination is uncommonly performed.
   4. In human medicine, specific ultrastructural changes may be helpful in the diagnosis of specific disease syndromes.
E. Histologic lesions in other compartments.
   1. The presence of tubular protein casts, often accompanied by hyaline droplets in proximal tubular cells, is suggestive of glomerular disease.
   2. Chronic GN is accompanied by tubular dilatation and atrophy, interstitial lymphoplasmacytic inflammation, and interstitial fibrosis.

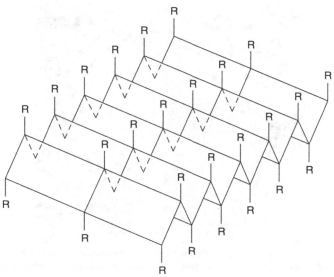

FIGURE 7-7 ■ β-Pleated sheet configuration of amyloid fibrils. *R*, side chain of amino acids comprising the amyloid protein P.

CAUSES OF GLOMERULONEPHRITIS IN DOGS AND CATS

A. In dogs and cats, most GN is idiopathic, and the cause is never determined.

B. Specific syndromes and infectious agents can cause GN (see Box 7-1). Important causes in dogs and cats include:

　1. Feline leukemia virus (FeLV) and feline infectious peritonitis in cats.

　2. Pyometra and heartworm disease in dogs.

　3. Chronic bacterial, parasitic, and neoplastic diseases.

　4. Autoimmune diseases.

Amyloidosis

CHARACTERISTICS

A. Amyloidosis refers to a diverse group of diseases characterized by extracellular deposition of fibrils formed by polymerization of protein subunits with a specific biophysical conformation called the β-pleated sheet (Figure 7-7). This specific biophysical conformation is responsible for the unique optical and tinctorial properties of amyloid deposits as well as their insolubility and resistance to proteolysis in vivo.

B. Amyloid deposits have a homogeneous, eosinophilic appearance when stained by hematoxylin and eosin and viewed by conventional light microscopy (Figure 7-8). They demonstrate green birefringence after Congo red staining when viewed under polarized light. The clinical diagnosis of amyloidosis is based on this finding.

C. Amyloid fibrils are variable in length, nonbranching, and 7 to 10 nm in width when viewed by transmission electron microscopy.

D. Congo–red-stained amyloid deposits from patients with reactive (secondary) amyloidosis lose their affinity for Congo red after permanganate oxidation. This feature is useful in the preliminary differentiation of reactive from other types of amyloidosis.

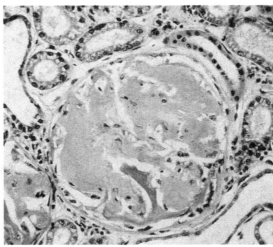

FIGURE 7-8 ■ Light microscopic appearance of advanced glomerular amyloidosis in a dog. Note the hypocellularity of the glomerulus due to deposition of an eosinophilic extracellular material (amyloid). (Hematoxyln and cosin, ×160.)

E. Amyloid syndromes may be classified by distribution of the deposits (i.e., systemic or localized) and by the nature of the responsible protein.
   1. Localized syndromes usually affect one organ and are uncommon in domestic animals. Examples of localized amyloidosis include pancreatic islet cell amyloid in domestic cats, solitary extramedullary plasmacytomas of the gastrointestinal tract or skin that produce immunoglobulin-associated amyloid, and amyloid deposits in the respiratory tract.
   2. Systemic syndromes affect more than one organ and include reactive, immunoglobulin-associated, and heredofamilial syndromes.
      a. Reactive (secondary) amyloidosis is a systemic syndrome characterized by tissue deposition of amyloid A protein (AA amyloid). Naturally occurring systemic amyloidosis in domestic animals is an example of reactive amyloidosis. Familial amyloid syndromes in the Abyssinian, Siamese and Oriental shorthair breeds of cat and in the Shar pei, beagle and English foxhound breeds of dog are additional examples of reactive systemic amyloidosis in veterinary medicine.
      b. Immunoglobulin-associated (primary) amyloidosis is characterized by tissue deposition of amino terminal fragments of immunoglobulin light chains (AL amyloid). In human patients, immunoglobulin-associated amyloidosis usually is systemic (e.g., amyloidosis complicating plasma cell dyscrasias such as multiple myeloma).
      c. In human beings, amyloidosis associated with genetic variants of transthyretin (prealbumin) may be systemic or localized. This type of amyloid has not been recognized in veterinary medicine.
   F. Tissue deposits from animals with reactive systemic amyloidosis contain amyloid A protein, which is an amino terminal fragment of an acute phase reactant called *serum amyloid A protein* (SAA).
   1. SAA is one of several acute phase reactants synthesized by the liver in response to tissue injury. Cytokines (e.g., interleukin-1, interleukin-6, tumor necrosis factor) released from macrophages after tissue injury stimulate hepatocytes to synthesize and release SAA.
   2. The normal serum concentration of SAA is approximately 1 mg/L but its concentration increases 100-fold to 500-fold after tissue injury (e.g., inflammation, neoplasia, trauma,

infarction). SAA concentration decreases to baseline by 36 to 48 hours if the inflammatory stimulus is removed. If inflammation persists, SAA concentration remains increased.

3. SAA presumably has a critical role in the body's response to tissue injury, but its actual biological function remains a mystery.

4. SAA serves as the precursor of amyloid A protein in tissues and the concentration of SAA is increased in plasma before amyloid deposits are observed in tissues.

5. Chronic inflammation and a prolonged increase in SAA concentration are necessary prerequisites for development of reactive amyloidosis. Despite this, only a small percentage (<5%) of individuals with chronic inflammatory disease develop reactive amyloidosis. Thus, other factors must also be important in development of amyloidosis.

6. Among the domestic animals, reactive amyloidosis is most common in the dog. It is relatively uncommon in other species.

7. Diseases that have been observed in association with reactive systemic amyloidosis in the dog include chronic infectious or noninfectious inflammatory diseases and neoplasms, but there is no discernible associated inflammatory or neoplastic disease in the majority of dogs and cats presented with reactive systemic amyloidosis.

8. The cause of the specific tissue tropisms of different amyloid proteins is poorly understood.
   a. AA amyloid has a predilection for kidney, spleen, and liver.
   b. AL amyloid has a predilection for the kidney, spleen, liver, tongue, heart, and musculoskeletal system.
   c. Transthyretin (prealbumin) has a predilection for the peripheral nervous system and heart.

9. The cause of species differences in the tissue tropisms of reactive amyloid deposits also is unknown.
   a. In the dog, amyloid AA deposits are most common in the kidney and clinical signs are due to renal failure and uremia. The spleen, liver, adrenal glands, and gastrointestinal tract also may be involved, but associated clinical signs are rare.
   b. In the cat, there is widespread deposition of amyloid deposits but clinical signs are due to renal failure and uremia.
   c. The Shar pei dog, Siamese cat, and Oriental shorthair cat are exceptions to these general rules. Severe liver deposition of amyloid can cause rupture of the liver and presentation as acute hemoabdomen in these breeds.

10. Within the kidney itself, the distribution of amyloid deposits varies among species. For example, amyloidosis is primarily a glomerular disease in the dog whereas amyloid deposits may have a predominant medullary distribution in the cat.

CLINICAL FINDINGS

Signalment

1. Most animals with glomerular disease are middle-aged or older at presentation.

2. There is no sex predilection in most species, but approximately 75% of cats with GN are males.

3. Any breed can be affected by glomerular disease but,
   a. Familial forms of membranoproliferative GN have been reported in soft-coated Wheaten terriers (thought to be associated with abnormal processing of dietary antigens), Brittany spaniels (associated with hereditary deficiency of the third component of complement), and Bernese Mountain dogs (often associated with positive serology for *Borrelia burgdorferi*).

    b. Hereditary defects of glomerular basement membrane type IV collagen occur as an autosomal recessive trait in English Cocker spaniels and as an X-linked dominant trait in male Samoyed dogs. Basement membrane defects are also suspected to occur in Doberman pinschers and Bull terriers.

    c. Familial renal amyloidosis occurs in young Abyssinian, Siamese, and Oriental short-hair cats and in Shar pei dogs. Familial amyloidosis has also been reported in beagles and English foxhounds. See Chapter 6 on Familial Renal Diseases of Dogs and Cats for more information about familial glomerular disease.

History: Six Possible Presentations of Glomerular Disease

1. Signs may be related to presence of chronic renal failure if more than 75% of the nephron population has become nonfunctional (e.g., anorexia, weight loss, lethargy, polyuria, polydipsia, vomiting). This is the most common presentation.
2. Signs may be related to an underlying infectious, inflammatory or neoplastic disease.
3. Proteinuria may be an incidental finding detected during diagnostic evaluation of another medical problem.
4. Signs may be related to classical nephrotic syndrome (e.g., ascites, subcutaneous edema).
5. Signs may be related to thromboembolism (e.g., sudden onset of dyspnea with pulmonary embolism, sudden onset of paraparesis with iliac or femoral artery embolism).
6. Sudden blindness may occur due to retinal detachment resulting from systemic hypertension.

PHYSICAL EXAMINATION FINDINGS

A. Usually related to the presence of chronic renal failure and uremia.
    1. Poor body condition.
    2. Poor hair coat.
    3. Dehydration.
    4. Oral ulceration.
    5. Small, firm, irregular but occasionally normal-sized kidneys.
B. Other physical findings may be related to the presence of underlying infectious, inflammatory, or neoplastic diseases. Affected Shar pei dogs may have a previous history of so-called *Shar pei fever* (episodic joint swelling usually involving the tibiotarsal joints and high fever that resolve within a few days, regardless of treatment).
C. Some physical findings may be related to severe protein loss (e.g., ascites, edema, poor body condition, poor hair coat).
D. Retinal hemorrhages, vascular tortuosity, and retinal detachment may occur due to systemic hypertension.

LABORATORY FINDINGS

Urinalysis

1. Marked persistent proteinuria with an inactive sediment is the hallmark of glomerular disease.
    a. Dipstick tests use a colorimetric method (tetrabromphenol blue indicator).
    b. Recognizes albumin more than globulins.
    c. Semiquantitative and detects as little as 10 mg/dL protein in urine.
2. Hyaline and granular casts.
3. Lipid droplets.

4. Isosthenuria if more than 67% of the nephron population has become nonfunctional. Early loss of concentrating ability may occur in animals with medullary deposition of amyloid (Abyssinian cats, Shar pei dogs).
5. Red cell casts and dysmorphic red cells (red cells with abnormal shape due to passage through the glomerular capillaries) may occur in human patients with GN but these findings have not been reported in domestic animals with GN.

Biochemistry
1. Either GN or amyloidosis can lead to chronic renal failure (CRF) with the expected biochemical abnormalities (e.g., azotemia, hyperphosphatemia, metabolic acidosis).
2. Hypoalbuminemia occurs in many dogs with glomerular disease (up to 75% of dogs with amyloidosis and 60% of dogs with GN).
3. Hypercholesterolemia occurs in most dogs with glomerular disease (up to 60% of dogs with GN and 90% of dogs with amyloidosis) but is a nonspecific finding in cats with renal disease. Hypercholesterolemia may be due in part to increased hepatic synthesis of cholesterol-rich lipoproteins secondary to chronic hypoalbuminemia.

Special Laboratory Tests
1. Urine protein-to-creatinine ratio.
   a. Avoids the confounding effect of total urine solute concentration (i.e., specific gravity) on qualitative assessment of proteinuria.
   b. Correlated with 24-hour urinary protein loss but easier to measure (i.e., does not require a 24-hour urine sample).
   c. Magnitude of increase in urine protein-to-creatinine ratio is roughly correlated with nature of glomerular disease.
   d. Values are highest in dogs with glomerular amyloidosis (often >10) and lowest in those with interstitial renal disease (usually <10). Animals with GN have very variable values (normal to >30).
   e. Presence of hematuria or pyuria can make the urine protein-to-creatinine ratio difficult to interpret (i.e., may cause a false-positive result).
   f. Normal urine protein-to-creatinine ratio is <0.3 in dogs and cats.
   g. As glomerular disease advances and GFR decreases, less protein is filtered and the urine protein-to-creatinine ratio can decrease. This decrease does not indicate improvement, and is a poor prognostic sign.
   h. Proteinuria is mild or absent in animals with renal medullary amyloidosis but without glomerular amyloidosis (e.g., some cats and Shar pei dogs with amyloidosis).
2. Normal 24-hour urinary protein loss is <20 to 30 mg/kg/day in dogs and cats, but collecting a 24-hour sample is cumbersome and this test has been replaced by the urine protein-to-creatinine ratio.
   a. 24-hour urinary protein loss usually is <500 mg/kg/day in GN.
   b. 24-hour urinary protein loss usually is >100 mg/kg/day in amyloidosis.
3. Renal biopsy is the only reliable way to differentiate GN from glomerular amyloidosis.
   a. A renal cortical biopsy will reliably differentiate GN from glomerular amyloidosis.
   b. Medullary tissue will be needed to diagnose renal medullary amyloidosis.
   c. Congo red stain is used to diagnose amyloidosis histologically.
   d. Light microscopic lesions may be minimal in GN. Immunopathologic methods using fluorescence microscopy or peroxidase-immunoperoxidase staining are helpful to diagnose and characterize immune complex GN.

    e. Transmission electron microscopy allows recognition of the ultrastructural pathology in GN but is not widely available to veterinarians.
4. Cytology of ascitic fluid reveals a pure transudate with low cell count and low total protein concentration.
5. Measurement of fibrinogen and antithrombin III concentrations may identify animals at risk for thromboembolism.

MANAGEMENT

General Principles

1. Identify and treat any underlying predisposing inflammatory or neoplastic disease process (i.e., remove the offending antigen if possible).
2. If CRF is present, it is treated according to the principles outlined in Chapter 5, Chronic Renal Failure.
3. Supportive treatment of hypertension.
   a. Low salt diet (<0.3% on a dry matter basis).
   b. Angiotensin converting enzyme (ACE) inhibitors (e.g., enalapril, benazepril) reduce glomerular capillary hydraulic pressure by decreasing postglomerular arteriolar resistance and, thus, reduce proteinuria. This beneficial effect must be balanced against their potential to worsen azotemia. In one study, enalapril (0.5 mg/kg PO every 12-24 hours) reduced proteinuria (as assessed by urine protein-to-creatinine ratio), reduced blood pressure, and slowed progression of renal disease in dogs with GN.
   c. Diuretics (e.g., furosemide) may be used in refractory cases but overzealous use may result in dehydration and prerenal azotemia.
   d. Other drugs that may be used in the management of hypertension include amlodipine, hydralazine, prazosin, and propranolol.
4. Prevention of thromboembolism.
   a. Heparin may be of limited usefulness when antithrombin III concentration is low (heparin requires AT III as a cofactor).
   b. Coumadin (warfarin) is a vitamin K antagonist anticoagulant but its use is not recommended because of the risk of hemorrhage and limited experience with it in domestic animals.
   c. Low dose aspirin therapy (0.5 mg/kg/day) has been used in dogs with GN to inhibit platelet aggregation.

Glomerulonephritis

1. No studies in veterinary medicine are available to demonstrate effectiveness of any specific therapy for GN. Likewise, in human medicine, little consensus exists on the treatment of many types of GN that cause nephrotic syndrome.
2. Immunosuppressive drugs (e.g., corticosteroids, azathioprine, cyclophosphamide, chlorambucil, cyclosporine).
   a. One controlled trial in dogs failed to show a benefit of cyclosporine treatment (15 mg/kg PO every 24 hours).
   b. Corticosteroid administration can cause proteinuria in dogs and one retrospective study suggested that corticosteroid therapy actually may be detrimental in dogs with idiopathic GN. Corticosteroids may be beneficial (or at least not detrimental) in cats with GN.
   c. Azathioprine (2.2 mg/kg PO every 24 hours) may be tried for immunosuppression in dogs (but not cats) with idiopathic GN. Azathioprine should not be used in cats

because they metabolize the drug very slowly and develop bone marrow suppression and severe leukopenia when given dosages similar to those used in dogs.

   d. Cyclophosphamide (2.2 mg/kg every 24 hours for 3 days then off for 4 days) also may be considered but it is more likely than azathioprine to be associated with side effects (e.g., myelosuppression).

   e. Demonstration of effectiveness is confounded by variable biological behavior of disease (e.g., some animals spontaneously resolve, some have stable proteinuria for long periods of time, and some progress to end-stage renal failure).

   f. The immunosuppressive drug mycophenolate mofetil also has been used (along with benazepril and aspirin) to treat GN in some dogs.

3. Thromboxane synthetase inhibitors (e.g., CGS 12970) can reduce proteinuria in experimental GN in dogs and may play a role in management of GN in the future.

4. Platelet inhibition (e.g., aspirin, dipyridamole) may reduce intraglomerular coagulation. In dogs, an aspirin dosage of 0.5 mg/kg PO once a day may selectively inhibit platelet cyclooxygenase without preventing the beneficial effects of prostacyclin formation (e.g., vasodilatation, inhibition of platelet aggregation).

5. Omega-3 polyunsaturated fatty acids (ω-3 PUFA) (e.g., fish oil) may suppress glomerular inflammation and coagulation by interfering with production of pro-inflammatory prostanoids.

6. Allopurinol (10 mg/kg PO every 12 hours) was useful in decreasing proteinuria and preventing progression of renal disease in dogs with visceral leishmaniasis and GN.

Amyloidosis

1. No specific therapy has been shown to be beneficial.
2. Dimethyl sulfoxide (DMSO).
   a. Experimentally, DMSO given during the rapid deposition phase will cause resolution of amyloid deposits and a persistent decrease in SAA concentration.
   b. May improve renal function by reduction of interstitial inflammation and fibrosis in the kidney.
   c. May reduce concentration of the acute phase reactant precursor of amyloid protein A (SAA).
   d. One case report in a dog with amyloidosis showed a beneficial effect (e.g., less proteinuria, improved GFR) of DMSO when used at a dosage of 80 mg/kg/wk administered SC.
   e. Another study of several affected dogs showed no effect of DMSO (i.e., dogs had similar amounts of amyloid in their kidneys at necropsy as in renal biopsies taken before instituting DMSO treatment).
3. Colchicine.
   a. Impairs the release of SAA from hepatocytes by binding to microtubules and preventing its secretion.
   b. Prevents development of amyloidosis in human patients with familial Mediterranean fever (FMF).
      (1) FMF is a genetic disorder of people of Middle Eastern ancestry that is characterized by recurrent self-limiting febrile episodes associated with serosal inflammation (e.g., pleuritis, peritonitis, synovitis).
      (2) FMF is caused by mutations in the pyrin (marenostrin) gene, which is expressed in neutrophils and normally inhibits inflammation provoked by minor insults.
      (3) If untreated, most people with FMF develop reactive amyloidosis, nephrotic syndrome, and renal failure in middle age.

(4) Colchicine prevents most febrile attacks and prevents development of amyloidosis.

  c. Colchicine (0.03 mg/kg/day) may be beneficial in Shar pei dogs with recurrent fever and joint swelling (so-called *Shar pei fever*) that may be at risk for development of systemic amyloidosis, but no prospective placebo-controlled study is available to support this treatment. Adverse effects of colchicine include gastrointestinal upset and rare development of neutropenia.

COMPLICATIONS OF GLOMERULAR DISEASE

Hypoalbuminemia

 1. The hypoalbuminemia of nephrotic syndrome is only partially explained by urinary loss of albumin.
 2. Hepatic albumin synthesis is increased in nephrotic syndrome but this increase is insufficient for the degree of hypoalbuminemia. In some other situations (e.g., chronic ambulatory peritoneal dialysis in humans), albumin loss can exceed that observed in nephrotic syndrome, but increased synthesis of albumin by the liver in these situations is sufficient to replenish the albumin loss.
 3. Low plasma oncotic pressure is thought to be the primary stimulus for increased hepatic synthesis of albumin in the nephrotic syndrome.
 4. Renal catabolism of albumin is increased in nephrotic syndrome due to increased reabsorption of filtered protein.
 5. Although an increase in dietary protein stimulates hepatic albumin synthesis it does not correct hypoalbuminemia in patients with nephrotic syndrome and only worsens the urinary losses of protein.

Sodium Retention

 1. The *underfill* hypothesis of edema and ascites formation in the nephrotic syndrome involves activation of the renin angiotensin-aldosterone system (RAAS):
    a. Progressive loss of albumin through the glomeruli and inadequate hepatic synthesis of albumin lead to hypoalbuminemia.
    b. Hypoalbuminemia leads to decreased oncotic pressure with loss of water and electrolytes from the vascular compartment.
    c. Decreased circulating volume leads to decreased renal blood flow and activation of the RAAS.
    d. Activation of the RAAS leads to aldosterone production and release with consequent renal conservation of sodium and water.
    e. Attempted restoration of circulating volume is unsuccessful because hypoalbuminemia and decreased oncotic pressure prevent retention of water in the vascular compartment.
    f. In addition to the RAAS, nonosmotic stimulation of antidiuretic hormone release and increased sympathetic nervous system activity could be invoked by decreased circulating volume and also would promote renal water and sodium retention.
 2. The *overfill* hypothesis is based on evidence for a primary intrarenal mechanism of sodium retention in nephrotic syndrome.
    a. Aldosterone concentrations frequently are normal or even low in human patients with nephrotic syndrome, and treatment with ACE inhibitors does not always prevent sodium retention.
    b. Primary intrarenal sodium retention in nephrotic syndrome occurs in the distal nephron (independent of aldosterone) and contributes to extracellular fluid volume expansion and edema formation.

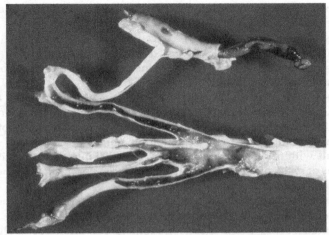

FIGURE 7-9 ■ Iliac thromboembolism with thrombi in the iliac arteries and one iliac vein. The pulmonary artery is another common location of thromboembolism in dogs with nephrotic syndrome.

     c. Patients with nephrotic syndrome also demonstrate a blunted response to atrial natriuretic peptide (ANP).

  3. Reconciling the *underfill* and *overfill* hypotheses of sodium retention and edema formation in the nephrotic syndrome:

     a. Intrarenal sodium retention in nephrotic patients with adequate serum albumin concentration and intravascular oncotic pressure could result in expansion of circulating volume and suppression of the RAAS (as described in the overfill hypothesis).

     b. In patients with severe hypoalbuminemia and low circulating volume due to reduced intravascular oncotic pressure, the RAAS would be activated (as described in the underfill hypothesis) despite the presence of an intrarenal mechanism for sodium retention.

Thromboembolism (Figure 7-9)

  1. The nephrotic syndrome is a hypercoagulable state. Occasionally, thromboembolic phenomena are responsible for the major presenting signs and overshadow the underlying renal disease, thus complicating the clinical course and delaying the primary diagnosis.

  2. Hypercoagulability and thromboembolism associated with the nephrotic syndrome occur secondary to several abnormalities in the coagulation system.

     a. Mild thrombocytosis and platelet hypersensitivity occur in association with hypoalbuminemia and result in increased platelet adhesion and aggregation. Plasma arachidonic acid normally is protein-bound, and more arachidonic acid is free to bind to platelets in the presence hypoalbuminemia. This may result in increased thromboxane production by platelets and platelet hyperaggregability. Hypercholesterolemia also may contribute to platelet hyperaggregability by altering platelet membrane composition or affecting platelet adenylate cyclase response to prostaglandins.

     b. Loss of antithrombin III (MW 65,000) in urine also results in hypercoagulability. Antithrombin III acts in concert with heparin to inhibit serine proteases (clotting factors II, IX, X, XI, and XII) and normally has a vital role in modulating thrombin and fibrin production.

    c. Decreased plasma concentrations of factors IX, XI, and XII occur due to urinary loss of these proteins.

    d. Increased fibrinogen (factor I) concentration and decreased fibrinolysis contribute to hypercoagulability. Decreased fibrinolysis occurs as a result of decreased concentration of plasminogen and increased concentration of α2 macroglobulin (a plasmin inhibitor).

    e. Increased concentration of large molecular weight coagulation factors (factors II, V, VII, VIII, and X) may lead to a relative increase in coagulation factors as compared with regulatory proteins. This increase may result from increased protein synthesis by the liver as it attempts to correct hypoalbuminemia.

    f. Animals with fibrinogen concentrations of >300 mg/dL and antithrombin III concentrations of <70% of normal are considered at risk for thromboembolism and anticoagulant therapy should be considered.

3. Thromboembolism occurs in 15% to 25% of dogs with nephrotic syndrome. It is rare (but has been reported) in cats with glomerular disease.

4. The pulmonary artery is the most common site for thromboembolism, but emboli also may lodge in mesenteric, renal, iliac, coronary, and brachial arteries as well as in the portal vein. Dogs with pulmonary thromboembolism usually are dyspneic and hypoxic with minimal pulmonary parenchymal radiographic abnormalities.

Hyperlipidemia

1. Hypercholesterolemia and hyperlipidemia are commonly associated with nephrotic syndrome. Decreased plasma oncotic pressure due to hypoalbuminemia and possibly increased loss of regulatory factors for lipid metabolism in urine cause increased hepatic synthesis of lipoproteins and decreased peripheral catabolism of ipoproteins.

2. Large molecular weight, cholesterol-rich lipoproteins that are not easily lost through the damaged glomerular capillary wall accumulate, whereas smaller molecular weight proteins such as albumin and antithrombin III are lost in the urine.

3. In nephrotic patients, plasma albumin concentrations are inversely correlated with plasma cholesterol and triglyceride concentrations, and cholesterol and lipid concentrations tend to increase as albumin concentration decreases.

4. Decreased hepatic catabolism of lipoproteins occurs due to abnormal lipoprotein lipase function. Normal lipoprotein lipase function requires heparin sulfate as a cofactor and concentrations of heparin sulfate frequently are decreased in nephrotic patients. The decrease in heparin sulfate has been linked to increased urinary loss of another glycoprotein, orosomucoid. Diversion of necessary sugar intermediates as the liver replaces the lost orosomucoid causes decreased production of heparin sulfate. Orosomucoid also has an important role in maintaining normal glomerular permselectivity. Consequently, urinary loss of orosomucoid not only contributes to the hyperlipidemia of the nephrotic syndrome but also exacerbates proteinuria.

Hypertension

1. Systemic hypertension may occur in dogs and cats with glomerular disease due to sodium retention, activation of the RAAS, and impaired release of normal renal vasodilator substances.

2. Systemic hypertension has been associated with immune-mediated GN, glomerulosclerosis, and glomerular amyloidosis and may occur in up to 50% or more of dogs with glomerular disease.

3. Retinal hemorrhage, retinal vascular tortuosity, and retinal detachment may result from systemic hypertension, and blindness may be the presenting complaint in hypertensive dogs and cats.

4. Blood pressure measurements (by Doppler technique) should be obtained in all dogs and cats with suspected glomerular disease because control of systemic hypertension may slow progression of the glomerular disease.

5. Enalapril (0.5 mg/kg PO every 12-24 hours) is recommended for treatment of hypertension in dogs and cats with glomerular disease because, in addition to reducing systemic hypertension, enalapril may reduce proteinuria. Patients treated with enalapril should be monitored to be sure their blood urea nitrogen (BUN) and serum creatinine concentrations remain stable.

PROGNOSIS

A. Amyloidosis is a progressive disease with a poor prognosis. Affected animals often are in renal failure at the time of presentation and generally live less than 1 year after diagnosis.

B. GN has a variable course, and a poor prognosis should not be given unless there is evidence of progression to CRF. The following may occur:
1. Spontaneous remission.
2. Stable course with ongoing proteinuria for several months to years.
3. Progression to CRF over months to years.

C. Lesions of GN can be observed at necropsy without there having been any clinical evidence of renal failure during life.

WHAT DO WE DO?

- Diagnose protein-losing diseases before the development of azotemia. Early diagnosis depends on monitoring patients for development of proteinuria before clinical signs become apparent.
- Distinguish between GN and amyloidosis by renal biopsy because the prognosis for these diseases is potentially very different (e.g., some patients with GN experience resolution of their disease whereas amyloidosis generally is a progressive disease).
- Measure systolic blood pressure using Doppler methodology in all patients with protein-losing glomerulonephropathy and treat hypertension as necessary.
- Provide a renal diet, low-dose aspirin, and ACE inhibitors to patients with GN.
- Follow the magnitude of proteinuria (as well as serum creatinine concentration) during treatment. A suggested goal of therapy is to reduce the magnitude of proteinuria by 50% without a substantial increase in serum creatinine concentration.
- Monitor plasma antithrombin activity in an effort to predict which patients are at greatest risk to develop thromboembolism.
- Obtain renal tissue for microscopic examination before development of azotemia to determine a morphologic diagnosis and identify the extent of interstitial inflammation and fibrosis.
- Screen for infectious diseases that potentially are associated with GN (e.g., dirofilariasis, ehrlichiosis, brucellosis, FeLV, feline immunodeficiency virus [FIV]).

THOUGHTS FOR THE FUTURE

- Supplementation with omega-3 polyunsaturated fatty acids may be beneficial specifically in animals with glomerular disease and in animals with chronic renal failure in general.
- Thromboxane synthetase inhibition could be a powerful tool should such drugs become commercially available in the future.

SUMMARY TIPS

- Monitor urinary protein concentration as measured by urine protein-to-creatinine ratio or identification of microalbuminuria.
- Increases in the urine protein-to-creatinine ratio or microalbuminuria indicate the possibility of progressive renal injury and justify additional diagnostic evaluation and more aggressive treatment interventions.
- Renal biopsy should be obtained before azotemia develops to determine the nature of the underlying glomerular disease.
- Evaluate the nutritional status of patients with protein-losing glomerulonephropathy that are fed protein-restricted renal diets using serial body weight, body condition score, and serum albumin concentration because these patients may be more likely to develop protein-calorie malnutrition than animals with other causes of chronic renal failure.

COMMON MISCONCEPTIONS

- Renal biopsy results are unlikely to change treatment. This statement sometimes is true, but it is important to distinguish GN and amyloidosis because treatment and prognosis are substantially different for these diseases. The severity of the glomerular lesion and associated tubulointerstitial disease also may warrant a more aggressive treatment approach. The benefit-to-risk ratio has been improved with the development of ultrasound-guided renal biopsy techniques.
- Nothing much can be done therapeutically when the glomerular lesion is advanced and proteinuria is severe. Actually, treatment with ACE inhibitors can lower intraglomerular pressure, decrease proteinuria, and slow progression of renal disease independent of their effects on systemic blood pressure.
- Any pathologist can adequately evaluate the renal lesions. Most pathologists should be able to provide a light microscopic diagnosis, but the light microscopic lesions of GN can be subtle and immunohistochemical and ultrastructural studies carried out by a pathologist with a special interest in nephropathology will provide more definitive and useful information.

FREQUENTLY ASKED QUESTIONS

Q: **A dog with weight loss has reasonably concentrated urine (urine specific gravity [USG] 1.026) and a urine protein-to-creatinine ratio of 12:1. The reference laboratory indicates that amyloidosis is the likely diagnosis. Is this a reliable method to make a diagnosis of glomerular amyloidosis?**

A: Although it is generally true that patients with glomerular amyloidosis tend to have the highest urine protein-to-creatinine ratios, glomerular amyloidosis cannot be reliably differentiated from GN by the magnitude of proteinuria alone. Some animals with amyloidosis have lower urine protein-to-creatinine ratios and patients with GN can have very high urine protein-to-creatinine ratios. Renal biopsy with use of appropriate stains (e.g., Congo red) and techniques (e.g., immunohistochemistry using peroxidase-antiperoxidase methodology) are necessary to accurately distinguish glomerular amyloidosis from glomerulonephritis.

Q: **An otherwise healthy 6-year-old spayed female mixed breed dog had normal hemogram and serum biochemistry results. The USG was 1.032 and the urine sediment was inactive, but 2+ proteinuria was identified by dipstrip analysis. The urine protein-to-creatinine ratio was 0.5 and microalbuminuria of 12 mg/dL was identified. Should this small amount of proteinuria be ignored until the dog's next annual wellness visit?**

A: The presence of microalbuminuria indicates some dysfunction of glomerular barrier function. The damage could have occurred in the past and be nonprogressive or the microalbuminuria could indicate an early stage of what may become progressive glomerular injury despite the absence of clinical signs. Thus, follow-up monitoring of microalbuminuria in this asymptomatic dog is warranted. If microalbuminuria and the urine protein-to-creatinine ratio increase over time, glomerular injury is ongoing and its cause should be investigated because the animals potentially is at risk for development of chronic renal disease and failure. Blood pressure also should be evaluated to see if systemic hypertension could be a factor contributing to the proteinuria.

Q: A dog with biopsy-confirmed glomerular amyloidosis has a serum creatinine concentration of 2.6 mg/dL, USG of 1.015, and proteinuria of 3+ dipstrip analysis. Hyaline and waxy casts are observed on urine sediment examination. Given the grave prognosis for amyloidosis, should euthanasia be recommended to the owner?

A: Renal amyloidosis generally is a relentlessly progressive disease, and the presence of moderate to severe azotemia warrants a grave prognosis. Most experience in veterinary medicine, however, has been with dogs with amyloidosis and advanced renal failure. Such patients have relatively short survival times (months). The prognosis may not be as grave when amyloidosis is discovered at an earlier stage (i.e., proteinuria with minimal azotemia). In one recent study in human patients with AA amyloidosis, median survival was correlated with serum amyloid A (SAA) protein concentration and patients with the lowest SAA concentrations had very long median survival times. Similar studies have not been performed in dogs. It is unknown whether or not treatment with ACE inhibitors is beneficial for dogs with glomerular amyloidosis, as is the case with GN.

Q: Over the past month, a dog with renal failure has had a stable serum creatinine concentration of 8.0 to 9.0 mg/dL. The urine sediment is inactive, the protein dipstrip reaction is 4+, and the urine protein-to-creatinine ratio is greater than 10. The kidneys are hyperechoic and small on ultrasound examination. Should a renal biopsy be performed?

A: A renal biopsy is unlikely to be helpful in this situation and may be harmful. Technical difficulties are more likely when performing a biopsy of a small kidney. Renal bleeding may be substantial. Furthermore, the small kidneys may have extensive interstitial fibrosis and it may not be possible to determine the underlying primary lesion (e.g., glomerular, interstitial, tubular) that led to chronic renal failure. The likelihood of obtaining useful diagnostic information is small compared with the risk of complications for the patient.

SUGGESTED READINGS

Center SA, Smith CA, Wilkinson E, et al: Clinicopathologic, renal immunofluorescent, and light microscopic features of glomerulonephritis in the dog: 41 cases (1975-1985), *J Am Vet Med Assoc* 190:81–90, 1987.

Center SA, Wilkinson E, Smith CA, et al: 24-hour urine protein/creatinine ratio in dogs with protein-losing nephropathies, *J Am Vet Med Assoc* 187:820–824, 1985.

Cook AK, Cowgill LD: Clinical and pathological features of protein-losing glomerular disease in the dog: A review of 137 cases, *J Am Anim Hosp Assoc* 32:313–322, 1996.

DiBartola SP, Benson MD: Review: The pathogenesis of reactive systemic amyloidosis, *J Vet Int Med* 3:31–41, 1989.

DiBartola SP, Tarr MJ, Parker AT, et al: Clinicopathologic findings in dogs with renal amyloidosis, *J Am Vet Med Assoc* 195:358–364, 1989.

Grauer GF: Canine glomerulonephritis: New thoughts on proteinuria and treatment, *J Small Anim Pract* 46:469–478, 2005.

Grauer GF, Greco DS, Getzy DM, et al: Effects of enalapril versus placebo as a treatment for canine idiopathic glomerulonephritis, *J Vet Int Med* 14:526–533, 2000.

Lachmann HJ, Goodman HJ, Gilbertson JA, et al: Natural history and outcome in systemic AA amyloidosis, *N Engl J Med* 356:2361–2371, 2007.

8 Cystitis and Urethritis: Urinary Tract Infection

INTRODUCTION

A. Urinary tract infection (UTI) is defined as bacterial colonization of portions of the urinary tract that normally are sterile (i.e., kidneys, ureters, bladder, proximal urethra).
   1. UTI can occur superficially on luminal surfaces, deeper within the parenchyma, or in both locations.
   2. Infection with fungal or chlamydial organisms is rare. Viral infections have not been conclusively identified as a cause of lower urinary tract clinical signs.
B. UTI most commonly is discovered when animals are presented with clinical signs of lower urinary tract distress (i.e., symptomatic bacteriuria) such as hematuria, pollakiuria, and increased frequency of urination.
   1. UTI may exist without clinical signs (i.e., asymptomatic bacteriuria). In these instances, infection is diagnosed fortuitously.

! UTI may be asymptomatic.

   2. As many as 10% of hospitalized dogs (with a variety of illnesses) have asymptomatic UTI.
C. UTI is common in dogs, but not in cats.
   1. UTI may be the most common infectious disease of dogs.
      a. An estimated 10% of dogs presented to veterinarians for any reason have UTI.
      b. Approximately 14% of dogs will have at least one UTI during their lifetime.

! UTI may be the most common infectious disease in dogs.

      c. Female dogs have a higher risk of developing UTI than do male dogs.
      d. UTI occurs as a single episode in 75% of affected dogs.
      e. Multiple episodes of UTI occur in some dogs, with predisposing factors favoring recurrence. Of all dogs presented to a referral hospital, 0.3% were estimated to have recurrent UTI.
   2. UTI occurs in only 0.1% to 1% of all cats.

! UTI is uncommon in cats.

      a. Geriatric cats are more commonly affected.
      b. Siamese cats may have a higher risk for developing UTI than other breeds.

    c. Increased incidence of UTI in male cats is related to the increased use of urinary catheters to relieve urinary obstructions in males. When it does occur, UTI is a single episode in 85% of affected cats.

    d. In cats older than 10 years of age presenting with signs of lower urinary tract irritation, more than 50% are expected to have UTI. Most of these cats have underlying chronic renal disease with submaximal ability to concentrate urine.

D. The term cystitis often is used to refer to bacterial UTI. The urinary bladder primarily is involved in these disorders, but the urethra may also be part of the process. Cystourethritis may be a better term.

    1. It is difficult to assess the involvement of the urethra in UTI because of limitations of the commonly used diagnostic tests.

    2. Urethroscopy provides a method to determine the extent of urethral involvement.

PATHOGENESIS AND PATHOPHYSIOLOGY

Bacteria Associated with Urinary Tract Infection

    1. Bacteria commonly associated with urinary tract infection in dogs and cats are shown in Figures 8-1 and 8-2.

    2. Most UTIs are caused by a single organism (monomicrobic). A single organism is isolated in 75% of cases, two organisms are isolated in 20%, and three organisms are isolated in 5% of UTI.

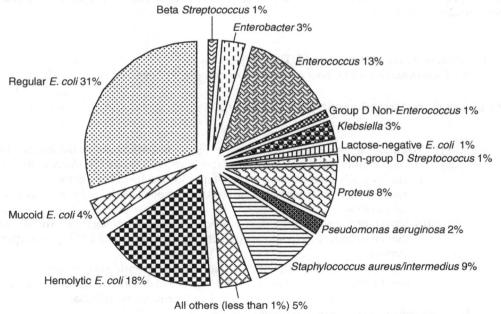

FIGURE 8-1 ■ Bacteria associated with urinary tract infection in dogs. Organisms isolated in significant quantitative growth from cystocentesis samples in dogs. 5,060 urine samples were cultured yielding growth in 28% and no growth in 72%. Organisms listed as less than 1% each (<5% total) included *Acinetobacter, Citrobacter, Clostridium,* coagulase-negative *Staphylococcus, Corynebacterium* sp, *Klebsiella oxytoca, Lactobacillus, Malassezia, Mycoplasma, Pasteurella multocida, Pasteurella* sp, *Pseudomonas* sp, *Serratia,* and yeast. (Courtesy of The Ohio State University Microbiology Laboratory, January 2000-April 2007.)

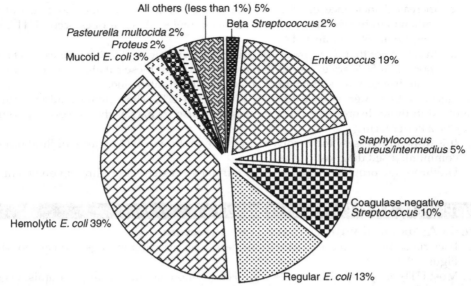

FIGURE 8-2 ■ Bacteria associated with urinary tract infection in cats. Organisms isolated in significant quantitative growth from cystocentesis samples in cats. 1429 urine samples were cultured yielding growth in 15% and no growth in 85%. Organisms listed as less than 1% each (<5% total) included *Corynebacterium, Enterobacter, Klebsiella*, lactose-negative *E. coli, Pasteurella* sp, *Moganella, Serratia*, and yeast. (Courtesy of The Ohio State University Microbiology Laboratory, January 2000-April 2007.)

3. Gram-negative bacteria cause UTI in 75% of cases.
   a. *Escherichia coli* is the most common uropathogen in dogs and cats.

> ❗ *Escherichia coli* is the most common uropathogen in dogs and cats.

        (1) Coagulase-negative *Staphylococcus* species can be pathogenic in the urinary tract of cats, accounting for about 20% of isolates in recent reports (*Staphylococcus felis*).
          (a) Traditionally, coagulase-negative staphylococci have been considered contaminants. *S. felis* is a normal commensal organism of the skin, conjunctiva, and saliva of cats.
          (b) Most laboratories report staphylococci as "coagulase-negative" and do not further characterize as to species (which requires ribosomal RNA gene sequencing technology).
          (c) *S. felis* UTI is associated with a higher urinary specific gravity than that encountered with other causes of UTI. All *S. felis* isolates are urease-positive, which is associated with alkaline urinary pH and struvite crystalluria.
    b. *Pasteurella* is an occasional pathogen in cats.
4. Sex differences.
    a. Multiple organism (i.e., polymicrobic) infections are more common in female dogs.
    b. Male dogs have a higher incidence of *Klebsiella* infections than females.
    c. Female dogs have a higher incidence of *Proteus* and *Enterococcus* infections than males.

5. Breed differences.
   a. German shepherd dogs, miniature and toy poodles, Labrador retrievers, dachshunds, Doberman pinschers, and miniature Schnauzers may have increased incidence of UTI.
   b. In Labrador retrievers and Dalmatians, more males are affected than females.
   c. In dachshunds and English Springer spaniels, more females are affected than males.
   d. In dachshunds, males are unlikely to have UTI caused by *Staphylococcus*.
   e. Origin of bacteria (route of entry).
6. Ascent of bacteria.
   a. Ascension of fecal flora is the most common pathogenesis of UTI.
      (1) Fecal flora contaminate the perineum, ascend the urethra, and enter the bladder.

> **!** Ascent of fecal bacteria is the most common route of infection.

      (2) Organisms that successfully gain entry into the bladder then have the potential to ascend the ureters, cross the renal pelvic epithelium, and enter renal parenchymal tissue.
      (3) Fecal flora is the most common source of organisms for UTI though they can also arise from the skin.
   b. Ascending organisms can originate from the environment (e.g., hospital flora).
   c. Ascending organisms can arise from the vagina, prepuce, and distal urethra.
7. Hematogenous and lymphogenous.
   a. These routes of infection occasionally are encountered, especially during septicemia.
   b. Organisms can localize in the kidney initially, with the potential to inoculate the lower urinary tract.
8. Direct extension from an infected site near the urinary tract.
   a. Uterine stump abscess.
   b. Laparotomy sponge infection.
   c. Osteomyelitis.
   d. Perirenal abscess.
9. Urinary catheterization.
   a. Introduction of normal flora during catheterization; contamination with fecal or hospital flora is also possible.
   b. Indwelling catheter (i.e., migration of bacteria between the catheter and urethral mucosa or through the lumen of the catheter).

Normal Host Defenses Against Establishment of Urinary Tract Infection

1. Abrogation of some aspect of the normal host defense system may allow UTI to be established.
2. Normal flora of the distal urethra, vagina, and prepuce may be protective. Normal flora may occupy uroepithelial receptors and consume micronutrients, preventing pathogenic bacteria from establishing an infection.
3. Urine from healthy animals inhibits the growth of bacteria.
   a. Urea in urine has antibacterial properties.
   b. High urine osmolality inhibits bacterial growth. This mechanism may be particularly important in cats.

      c. Highly acidic urine can be bacteriostatic or bactericidal.

      d. Ammonia in urine may contribute antibacterial effects.

  4. Host defense mechanisms exist for the perineum, vagina, prepuce, urethra, bladder, ureters, renal pelvis, and renal parenchyma.

      a. Very little is known about perineal host defense mechanisms.

      b. Urethral host defense mechanisms.

        (1) Epithelial cells lining the urethra (i.e., urothelium) can physically trap bacteria and bar their ascent.

        (2) The mid-urethra has a functionally important high-pressure zone that helps prevent bacterial ascension.

        (3) Urethral length, width, and distance from anus.

          (a) The female urethra is wider and shorter than the male urethra, conceivably making it easier for bacteria to ascend into the bladder. Since the anus is closer to the urethral orifice of female dogs than males, there is a greater chance of fecal contamination and inoculation of organisms for female dogs. Male dogs may have additional protective mechanisms due to antibacterial prostatic secretions.

        (4) Timely, forceful, and complete emptying of bladder urine mechanically flushes out low numbers of bacteria that may have ascended the urethra (so-called hydrokinetic washout).

      c. Urinary bladder.

> **❗ Host defense mechanisms must be decreased for UTI to occur.**

        (1) Hydrokinetic washout of small numbers of bacteria from the bladder may be important.

        (2) Normal glycosaminoglycans (GAG) on the uroepithelium inhibit attachment of bacteria (antiadherence properties).

        (3) Bladder urothelium has some inherent bactericidal properties, but bacteria must be in close apposition for this effect to be valuable.

        (4) Some poorly characterized secretions of the normal bladder are antibacterial.

        (5) Local secretion of immunoglobulin can occur, but is not of major importance. A systemic immunoglobulin response also can occur, but is not protective.

      d. Ureters.

        (1) The distal movement of urine (i.e., from kidney to bladder) inhibits ascent of bacteria. However bacteria in the ureters can ascend by Brownian motion against the flow of urine.

        (2) The normal oblique intramural passage of the ureters into the bladder provides functional closure of the ureters as the bladder fills.

      e. Kidneys.

        (1) Renal pelvic epithelium.

        (2) Renal medulla.

          (a) The renal medulla is much more susceptible to bacterial colonization after ascending or hematogenous infection than is the renal cortex.

          (b) Low medullary blood flow and high interstitial osmolality impair the inflammatory response.

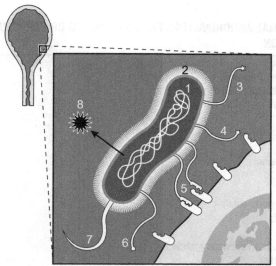

FIGURE 8-3 ■ Uropathogenic Escherichia coli and uorepithelial cell. Structure with pili, adhesions, and virulence factors. In order for a UTI to become established it is necessary for adhesins on the end of fimbria to interact with specific receptors on the uroepithelial cells. 1, Supercoiled bacterial DNA; 2, Lipopolysaccharide (LPS) of bacterial wall; 3, 4, and 6, show fimbria without adhesins that fit into uroepithelial receptors; 5, Shows fimbria with adhesins that specifically fit into the uroepithelial receptors—binding with these receptors is pivotal in allowing the establishment of UTI; 7, Flagellum; 8, Various virulence factors produced by the organisms that favor pathogenicity. (Drawn by Tim Vojt.)

Requirements for Development of Urinary Tract Infection
1. Exposure to sufficient numbers of uropathogenic bacteria (Figure 8-3).
2. Presence of epithelial receptors for uropathogens.
3. Failure of normal urinary defenses.
   a. Reduced anti-adherence properties of the uroepithelium.
   b. Decreased antibacterial properties of urine.
   c. Abnormal patterns of voiding.
   d. Reduced integrity of intrinsic mucosal defenses.
   e. Presence of anatomic abnormalities.

Increased Risk for Development of Urinary Tract Infection
1. Anatomic abnormalities of the genitourinary system (Boxes 8-1 and 8-2).
   a. Urachal remnants may provide a reservoir of stagnant urine, have decreased GAG, and be associated with microabscesses.
   b. Ectopic ureters.
      (1) Most common in female dogs.
      (2) Higher incidence in Siberian huskies, toy and miniature poodles, golden retrievers, Labrador retrievers, fox terriers, West Highland white terriers, collies, soft coated Wheaten terriers, and Welsh corgis.
      (3) Low incidence in cats, but males are more commonly affected.
      (4) Most ectopic ureters terminate in the urethra of females and may allow vaginal bacteria to ascend the ureter into the kidney.

■ BOX 8-1
■ **ANATOMIC AND FUNCTIONAL ABNORMALITIES PREDISPOSING TO OR PERPETUATING URINARY TRACT INFECTION**

Bladder atony (high residual urine volume)
Deep-seated cystitis (chronic bladder wall changes)
Ectopic ureters (developmental)
Emphysematous cystitis
Encrusting cystitis
Metritis or pyometra
Neoplasia of the bladder or urethra
Peri-urachal microabscesses
Polypoid cystitis
Poor vulvar conformation (developmental)
Prostatitis (sexually intact male dogs)
Pyelonephritis
Small urinary calculi that have been previously missed
Urachal remnant (developmental)
Ureterocoele
Urethral fistula
Urethral sphincter incompetence with urinary incontinence
Urethral stricture
Vestibulovaginal stenosis (developmental)

■ BOX 8-2
■ **METABOLIC CONDITIONS PREDISPOSING TO URINARY TRACT INFECTION**

Chemotherapy
Diabetes mellitus
Exogenous corticosteroid administration
Hyperadrenocorticism
Hyperthyroidism (cats)
Immunosuppression
Renal failure (especially cats)

    (5) Incontinence is the most common sign.
    (6) UTI may be present without clinical signs.

> **!** Animals receiving long-term exogenous corticosteroids and those with hyperadrenocorticism or diabetes mellitus are at increased risk for developing UTI, with or without clinical signs. Cats with CRF are also at high risk for developing UTI.

    2. Exogenous corticosteroid use in dogs.
       a. About 40% of dogs receiving long-term corticosteroid therapy (6 months or longer) for chronic skin disease have UTI.
       b. Greater risk in females, and castrated male dogs.

    c. Many do not have clinical signs of UTI, and urinalysis can be normal. Pyuria often is absent.

    d. Urine culture is necessary for diagnosis.

3. Endogenous corticosteroids in dogs (i.e., hyperadrenocorticism).

    a. UTI occurs in 46% of dogs with hyperadrenocorticism.

    b. Many do not have clinical signs of UTI, and urinalysis can be normal.

    c. Urine culture is necessary to identify UTI in dogs with hyperadrenocorticism.

4. Diabetes mellitus.

    a. UTI occurs in 37% of dogs and 12% of cats with diabetes mellitus.

    b. Many do not have clinical signs of UTI, and urinalysis can be normal.

    c. Urine culture is necessary to identify UTI in dogs and cats with diabetes mellitus.

5. Decreased systemic immunity.

6. Abnormal mucosal defenses.

7. Abnormal micturition.

8. Clitoral hyperplasia, especially in greyhounds.

9. Urolithiasis.

    a. Urine culture obtained by cystocentesis may be negative in animals with urolithiasis.

    b. Bacteria may adhere to bladder mucosa or uroliths, and the bladder biopsy specimen and uroliths should be cultured at surgery.

10. Perineal urethrostomy in dogs and cats.

11. Indwelling urinary catheter in dogs and cats.

> **!** **Urinary catheterization increases the risk of UTI.**

    a. Persistent UTI often develops even when using a closed system of urine drainage.

    b. In dogs and cats with indwelling catheters, 50% develop UTI within days, even if receiving antimicrobials.

    c. Bacterial organisms migrate along the outside of the catheter in the periurethral space.

    d. Normal bacterial flora are carried into the urinary bladder during catheterization.

12. Single episode of urinary catheterization in female dogs.

    a. UTI develops in 20% of female dogs within 3 days after passage of a urinary catheter.

13. Cats with chronic renal failure (CRF).

    a. UTI occurs in approximately 30% of cats with CRF, often within 1 year of diagnosis.

    b. Females with CRF are more likely to have UTI.

    c. *E. coli* typically is isolated.

    d. UTI may be a factor in the progression of CRF in cats.

14. Cats with hyperthyroidism.

    a. UTI occurs in approximately 12% of cats with hyperthyroidism.

    b. Urine culture is recommended, because many cats have no clinical signs of UTI.

15. Incontinence.

    a. Urine scalding may change the resident perineal bacterial population.

    b. Wicking action of urine may allow ascent of organisms.

    c. Excessive perivulvar skin folds and pyoderma (especially in recurrent UTI).

       (1) Episioplasty or vulvoplasty increases exposure of external genitalia to air and eliminates excessive skin folds.

        (2) The bacterial population in the perivulvar region is reduced, thus decreasing the likelihood of bacterial ascent.
    f. Vestibulovaginal stenosis.
        (1) So-called vestibulovaginal stenosis is unlikely to be a major predisposing factor in development of UTI.
        (2) What has been called *stenosis* most likely is a normal variant of the junction of the vestibule with the vagina in the area of the cingulum.

HISTORY

Dogs
1. Age at presentation with first UTI ranges from 0.3 to 16 years, with a median of 7 years.

Cats
1. Affected males have a mean age of 6.3 years at presentation, and females have a mean age of 10.6 years.
2. Cats older than 10 years of age that present for irritative voiding and signs of lower urinary tract disease (LUTD) commonly have bacterial UTI, unlike young cats presented with similar signs.

> **!** Older cats with lower urinary tract disease (LUTD) signs commonly have bacterial UTI whereas young cats with LUTD signs typically do not have bacterial UTI.

3. Many affected cats have a history of dilute urine, perineal urethrostomy, or previous urinary catheterization.

CLINICAL SIGNS

A. Most animals with UTI present with clinical signs of lower urinary tract distress (i.e., symptomatic bacteriuria).
1. Hematuria.
2. Pollakiuria.
3. Stranguria or dysuria.
4. Urination in inappropriate locations.
5. Incontinence.
6. Decreased volume of urine voided also may occur in animals with partial obstruction of the urethra (e.g., granulomatous urethritis).
B. Animals with UTI may have no clinical signs (i.e., asymptomatic bacteriuria).
1. Eighty percent of all dogs with UTI have no clinical signs.
2. As many as 10% of hospitalized dogs with a variety of illnesses have UTI without clinical signs.

PHYSICAL EXAMINATION

A. A thickened or painful urinary bladder may be palpated.
B. Thickening or induration of the urethra sometimes is detected during rectal examination when the urethra is involved.
C. The prostate gland may be palpably abnormal in sexually intact male dogs.

DIAGNOSIS

Hematology and Serum Biochemistry

1. Complete blood count (CBC) and routine serum biochemistry are normal if UTI is limited to the lower urinary tract.

> ❗ Complete blood count (CBC) and serum biochemistry are normal if UTI is limited to the lower urinary tract.

Urinalysis

Urine Specific Gravity (USG)

a. Urine usually is concentrated if UTI is limited to the lower urinary tract.

b. Dilute urine may occur in the presence of pyelonephritis or when lower UTI is associated with systemic absorption of bacterial endotoxin, which impairs the responsiveness of the collecting ducts to antidiuretic hormone.

c. UTI caused by *E. coli* tends to be associated with USG of <1.025.

d. UTI caused by staphylococci or streptococci tends to be associated with USG of more than 1.025.

e. Varying combinations of hematuria, pyuria, proteinuria, and bacteriuria usually are identified on urinalysis.

f. UTI caused by *E. coli* is associated with pyuria but not hematuria.

g. UTI caused by streptococci is associated with hematuria.

Pyuria

a. The combination of pyuria in association with bacteriuria increases the likelihood that bacteria actually are present in the urine sample. Clumps of white blood cells (WBCs) also add credence to the presence of bacteria.

(1) Dipsticks designed to detect neutrophils in urine do not work well in the urine of dogs or cats (false negatives are common in dogs and false positives are common in cats). The urine sediment must be evaluated microscopically to determine if pyuria is present.

> ❗ Dipsticks to detect WBCs in the urine are not accurate in dogs and cats. Urinary sediment examination must be performed microscopically.

(2) The WBC response (i.e., severity of pyuria) may vary among individuals and over time.

(3) Decreased WBC numbers are seen in animals with UTI that also have diabetes mellitus, hyperadrenocorticism, *Pseudomonas* UTI, or very dilute urine and in those that have received exogenous corticosteroids or antineoplastic drugs.

Urine pH

a. Consistently alkaline urine pH (>7.0) can be supportive of UTI associated with urease-producing organisms such as *Staphylococcus aureus* and *Proteus* spp.

b. Many UTI occur in acidic urine, however.

Urine Sediment

a. Failure to observe bacteria in wet mounts of urine sediment does not exclude their presence (i.e., false negative).

> ❗ Failure to visualize bacteria in urine sediment does *not* rule out UTI, and presence of bacteria does not necessarily mean UTI is present.

   b. Bacteria also can be reported in wet mounts of urine sediment when they are not pres-
      ent (i.e., false-positive). False-positive results are especially common in the urine of
      cats, which may contain artifacts that resemble bacteria (pseudobacteria).

Direct Examination of Urine
   a. Place one drop of well-mixed, fresh urine on a slide. Do not smear. Allow to air dry
   b. Gram stain and examine under oil immersion (1000×).
   c. Visualization of 2 bacteria or more per oil immersion field is indicative of bacterial UTI.
      This method is very specific and sensitive for diagnosis of UTI.

Modified Wright Stain of Urine Sediment
   a. One drop of urine sediment applied to a slide. Air dry and stain with modified Wright's
      stain.
   b. Evaluate 20 fields at 1000× (oil immersion).
   c. Enumerate as none, occasional (1-4), few (5-9), moderate (10-20), many (>20).
   d. Good correlation with quantitative culture results—superior to that estimated by
      routine wetmount of urine sediment. Less false-positive and false-negative results.

Urine Culture
   a. Collect urine for culture by cystocentesis (highly preferred) or urinary catheterization.
      (1) Do not culture voided urine due to the high likelihood of growth of bacterial
          contaminants.

> ❗ Do *not* culture voided urine.

      (2) Culture of urine obtained by urinary catheterization is not recommended for
          routine purposes.
   b. Plate collected urine on blood agar and MacConkey media within 15 minutes of
      collection.
      (1) Most bacteria will grow within 18 to 24 hours at 37° C. Most veterinary isolates
          of *Mycoplasma* grow within 3 days on routine blood agar plates (unusual strains
          can require 7 days or longer) and special media. *Corynebacterium* can require up to
          4 days to grow following inoculation.
      (2) If growth appears, the plate can be submitted to a microbiology laboratory for
          identification and susceptibility testing.
   c. Bacterial growth.

> ❗ Quantitative urine culture is necessary to positively identify causative bacteria and to choose the most
> appropriate antibacterial treatment.

      (1) Large quantitative bacterial growth occurs in approximately 75% of dogs with UTI
          caused by one organism (Figure 8-4).
      (2) 10^5 colony-forming units (cfu)/mL is seen in 74% of males and 79% of affected
          females.
      (3) Less quantitative growth occurs in approximately 25% of affected dogs.
      (4) 10^4 cfu/mL but <10^5 cfu/mL in 6% of males and females.
      (5) 10^3 cfu/mL but <10^4 cfu/mL in 8% of males and 7% of females.
      (6) <10^3 cfu/mL in 11% of males and 7% of females (growth of this magnitude can
          indicate UTI, but also can arise from skin contamination during cystocentesis).
      (7) If obtaining urine for culture through an indwelling urinary catheter, fewer num-
          bers of bacteria isolated on quantitative culture are supportive of a diagnosis of
          true bacterial UTI.

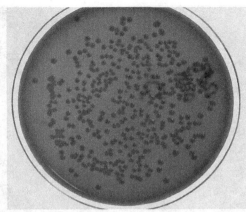

FIGURE 8-4 ■ Substantial quantitative growth of a urinary pathogen on blood agar in a Petri dish after 24 hours of incubation. The number of colonies that grow are counted and then multiplied by the dilution factor (usually 100 or 1000) to report growth in colony-forming units (cfu)/mL.

    d. Bacterial characteristics.
       (1) Gram staining.
          (a) Gram-negative bacteria.
             (i) *E. coli.*
             (ii) *Proteus* spp.
             (iii) *Klebsiella* spp.
             (iv) *Enterobacter* spp.
             (v) *Pseudomonas aeruginosa.*
          (b) Gram-positive bacteria.
             (i) Staphylococci.
             (ii) Enterococci.
             (iii) *Pasteurella* spp.
             (iv) *Streptococcus* Group D non-enterococcus.
          (c) *Mycoplasma* are too small to identify by Gram staining.
    e. Presumptive in-house identification of urinary bacterial isolates.
       (1) Rods in acidic urine: *E. coli* (*Klebsiella* spp, *Pseudomonas* sp, *Enterobacter* spp less often).
       (2) Rods in alkaline urine: *Proteus* spp.
       (3) Cocci in acidic urine: Streptococci or enterococci.
       (4) Cocci in alkaline urine: Staphylococci.

DIAGNOSTIC IMAGING

    A. Diagnostic imaging usually is not necessary for evaluation of dogs and cats with first occurrence of UTI.
    B. Diagnostic imaging is helpful in recurrent UTI to evaluate for the presence of functional and structural abnormalities.
    C. Plain abdominal radiographs.
       1. Useful to exclude or detect the presence of radiopaque urinary calculi.
       2. Useful for evaluation of bladder positioning if bladder is sufficiently full (i.e., exclude so-called pelvic bladder).

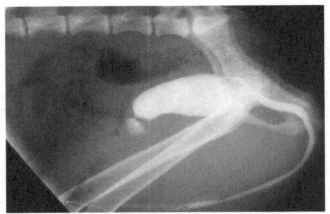

FIGURE 8-5 ■ Positive contrast urethrocystogram—urachal diverticulum. Note residual positive contrast. This anomaly can make it impossible to permanently eradicate UTI.

    3. Useful to evaluate before and after voiding (i.e., may help detect abnormal volume of residual urine).
    4. Useful for evaluation of kidneys to rule out upper UTI.
D. Contrast radiography.
    1. Positive contrast urethrogram.
      a. Useful to exclude urethral stricture.
      b. May be useful in dogs with prostatic disease.
    2. Double contrast cystogram.
      a. Superior to ultrasound for detection of small lesions.
      b. Useful in detection of small uroliths, polyps, masses, urachal diverticulum (Figure 8-5) and for evaluation of bladder wall thickness.
    3. Excretory urography (intravenous pyelography or IVP).
      a. Useful to evaluate kidneys for evidence of pyelonephritis (e.g., pyelectasia, dilated diverticula, dilated proximal ureter).
      b. Useful to evaluate ureteral termination (i.e., exclude ectopic ureter).
    4. Contrast vaginography.
      a. Useful for diagnosis of ectopic ureter.
      b. Useful to rule out so-called vestibulovaginal stenosis. Be careful not to over-interpret the normal narrowing of the junction of the vestibule with the vagina (i.e., cingulum).
E. Ultrasonography.
    1. Useful to evaluate the kidneys (e.g., exclude nephroliths or pyelectasia, evaluate renal contour and echotexture) (Figure 8-6).
    2. Useful to evaluate the bladder (i.e., exclude uroliths and bladder masses).
      a. Not useful to evaluate for presence of urachal diverticulum, unless it is very large.
      b. Can be used to evaluate bladder wall thickness if bladder is adequately filled.
      c. Useful to evaluate for polyps and masses (Figure 8-7).
      d. Useful to evaluate for presence of uroliths, especially those that are radiolucent.
    3. Occasionally useful to evaluate the urethra.
      a. Some ability to evaluate the proximal urethra.
      b. Cannot evaluate the remainder of the urethra.

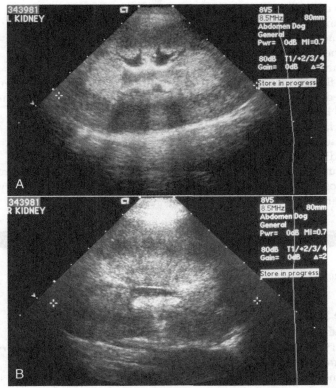

FIGURE 8-6 ■ Renal sonogram—pyelonephritis. The diverticula **(A)** and renal pelvis **(B)** are dilated, findings suggestive for pyelonephritis.

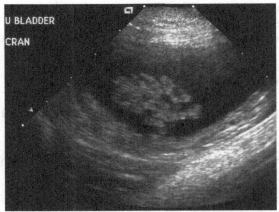

FIGURE 8-7 ■ Urinary bladder sonogram—polypoid cystitis. Notice thin-based masses projecting into the bladder lumen. Polyps can harbor bacteria, making it difficult to eradicate UTI.

4. Useful to evaluate the prostate gland.
   a. Size and echotexture.
   b. Presence of cyst, abscess, or paraprostatic cyst.
   c. Fine needle aspiration for cytology and culture.
F. Special referral techniques.
   1. IVP plus fluoroscopy for more definitive evaluation for ectopic ureter.
   2. Computed tomography (CT) plus IVP for further evaluation of urinary anatomy.
      a. Small lesions.
      b. Especially useful for exclusion of ectopic ureter.
   3. Uroendoscopy.
      a. May disclose small lesions missed by other imaging modalities.
      b. Very useful to definitively exclude ectopic ureter, evaluate vaginitis, determine presence of urachal diverticulum, determine presence of polypoid cystitis or transitional cell carcinoma.

TREATMENT

! Decide first if UTI is complicated or uncomplicated.

Urinary Tract Infection
Uncomplicated
a. History of only one or two episodes of UTI per year, or first occurrence.
b. Not immunosuppressed.
c. No underlying anatomic, metabolic, or functional abnormalities that would predispose to continuing infection.
d. Has not been on antibiotics for UTI or other problem within the past 1 to 2 months.
Complicated
a. Has defects in host defense mechanisms, including anatomic defects.
b. Has mucosal damage due to urolithiasis or neoplasia.
c. Has an alteration in urine volume or composition.
d. Has a concurrent systemic disorder (e.g., diabetes mellitus, hyperadrenocorticism, neoplasia).
e. Has received long-term treatment with corticosteroids.
f. Has a functional defect—cannot fully empty the bladder.

Potential Consequences of Untreated Urinary Tract Infection
1. Upper urinary tract infection (UUTI).
2. Renal failure from UUTI.
3. Urolithiasis, especially struvite urolithiasis secondary to urease-positive bacteria.
4. Bladder or urethral thickening.
5. Sepsis, especially after immunosuppressive treatment.
6. Infertility (both sexes).
7. Prostatitis.
8. Orchitis.
9. Discospondylitis.
10. Recurrent uveitis (dogs)—immune mediated.
11. Polyarthritis—immune mediated.

■ TABLE 8-1
■ ■ **Antimicrobial Agents, Dosages, and Urine Concentration Achieved in Normal Dogs**

Drug	Dosage	Mean Urine Concentration (μg/mL)
Amikacin	5 mg/kg SQ TID	342 ± 143
	(10 mg/kg SQ or IM BID)	
	15 mg/kg SID to reduce nephrotoxicity	
Amoxicillin	12 mg/kg PO TID	202 ± 93
Ampicillin	25 mg/kg PO TID	309 ± 55
Cephalexin	35 mg/kg PO TID	500
Chloramphenicol	35 mg/kg PO TID	124 ± 40
Doxycycline	5 mg/kg PO BID	53 ± 24
Enrofloxacin	2.5 mg/kg PO BID	≥40
Gentamicin	2.2 mg/kg SQ TID	107 ± 33
Hetacillin	25 mg/kg PO TID	300 ± 156
Kanamycin	5 mg/kg SQ TID	530 ± 151
Nitrofurantoin	4.4 mg/kg PO TID	100
Penicillin G	35,000 U/kg PO TID	295 ± 211 (U/mL)
Penicillin V	25 mg/kg PO TID	148 ± 99
Sulfisoxazole	22 mg/kg PO TID	1466 ± 832
Tetracycline	20 mg/kg PO TID	138 ± 65
Tobramycin	2.2 mg/kg SQ TID	145 ± 86
Trimethoprim-sulfonamide	12.5 mg/kg PO TID	246 ± 150
	2.5 mg/kg PO TID	55 ± 19

Data from Dr. G.V. Ling, School of Veterinary Medicine, University of California, Davis, except doxycycline and nitrofurantoin.

Drug Therapy

1. Antimicrobial drugs remain the cornerstone of treatment of UTI (Table 8-1) but correction of predisposing factors also is important.
   a. The concentration of antimicrobial that is achieved in the urine (μg/mL) is the most important factor in eradication of UTI.

! The concentration of antimicrobial achieved in urine is the single most important factor in eradication of UTI.

   b. Animals that produce large quantities of dilute urine may have decreased concentration of urinary antimicrobials.
   c. Tissue concentrations of the antimicrobial are important in animals with renal and prostatic infections as well as in animals with markedly thickened bladder walls from chronic infection.
2. Duration of antibacterial treatment.
   a. Uncomplicated UTI: 14 to 21 days.
   b. Upper UTI: 30 to 60 days.
   c. Sexually intact males with lower urinary tract infection (LUTI): 30 days.
3. Antimicrobial agents ideally should be selected after confirmation of UTI by quantitative culture. UTI can be treated on the basis of susceptibility testing (or on the basis of predicted biological behavior of the organism in animals with uncomplicated UTI).

! Choose an appropriate antimicrobial based on the results of quantitative urine culture.

   a. Most laboratories do not provide susceptibility testing for *Mycoplasma*. Typically, *Mycoplasma* are sensitive to tetracyclines. Chloramphenicol or tylosin may be considered as alternative treatments.

4. Most UTI can be successfully treated by the oral route using penicillins (especially those with clavulanate), trimethoprim-potentiated sulfonamides (Tribrissen), ormetoprim-potentiated sulfonamides (Primor), or first-generation cephalosporins such as cephalexin or cefadroxil.
   a. Adverse effects associated with trimethoprim-potentiated sulfonamides include keratoconjunctivitis sicca, cytopenias, hepatopathy, and immune-mediated polyarthritis.
   b. Ormetoprim-potentiated sulfonamides are not effective in prostate-associated UTI. Trimethoprim-potentiated sulfonamides should be used in dogs with UTI and prostatic disease.

5. Sulfonamides of any kind should not be prescribed for animals in which medical calculolytic protocols are in place. Sulfonamides can precipitate on the surface of the stone and decrease the rate of stone dissolution.

Do not use sulfonamides in patients undergoing urolith dissolution therapy.

6. Fluoroquinolones such as norfloxacin (Noroxin), ciprofloxacin (Cipro), enrofloxacin (Baytril), orbifloxacin (Orbax), marbofloxacin (Zeniquin), and difloxacin (Dicural) can be used orally to treat resistant bacteria.
   a. The quinolones have a wide spectrum of antibacterial activity (except against enterococci and anaerobes), achieve high tissue concentrations, and are not nephrotoxic.
     (1) There is little difference in activity of the various fluoroquinolones against urinary pathogens.
     (2) The minimum inhibitory concentration (MIC) of orbifloxacin often is somewhat higher than that of other fluoroquinolones, but adequate concentrations still are readily achievable in urine.
     (3) Marbofloxacin may have a lower MIC against *Pseudomonas* spp.
     (4) Ciprofloxacin usually has the most activity against *Pseudomonas* spp.
     (5) Difloxacin is excreted in bile, and consequently less is excreted in the urine.
   b. Quinolones should not be given to young, growing dogs (less than 6 to 18 months of age depending on breed) because of potential damaging effects on articular cartilage.
   c. Quinolones should be reserved for treatment when other therapeutic agents have failed.
   d. An association has been found between use of enrofloxacin and blindness in some cats. Enrofloxacin was used for many years before this adverse effect was observed. Mydriasis may be an early finding.
     (1) Blindness has not been noted in cats receiving other fluoroquinolones, but caution should be exercised.
     (2) Reports of blindness have dramatically decreased since a maximal dose of 5mg/kg once daily have been implemented. Fluoroquinolones exhibit retinal toxicity in experimental studies in cats when given at high doses.

Do not use fluoroquinolones in young, growing animals.

     (3) Increased risk to increase the concentration of drug and metabolites exist in those with hepatic or renal dysfunction. Drug dosage should be reduced to match decreases in liver or renal function.

7. Aminoglycosides.
   a. Reserved for highly resistant bacteria or for animals that have failed to respond to aggressive treatment with other antibacterial agents.
   b. Aminoglycosides can be nephrotoxic and are available for use only by injection.
8. Cephalosporins
   a. Ceftiofur sodium (Naxcel, Excenel).
      (1) A third-generation cephalosporin labeled for use in dogs with UTI.
      (2) Effective in eradication of UTI when given by once daily injection.
      (3) Good activity against *E. coli* and *Proteus,* but possesses little activity against *Pseudomonas* or *Enterococcus.*
   b. Cefpodoxime (Simplicef).
      (1) Third-generation oral cephalosporin.
      (2) Once daily.
      (3) Not generally effective against *Pseudomonas.*
   c. Cefovecin (Convenia).
      (1) Third-generation injectable cephalosporin.
      (2) Given subcutaneously once every 14 days.
9. In vitro susceptibility patterns of common uropathogens to antibiotics (Tables 8-2 and 8-3).
   a. Kirby-Bauer susceptibility testing can yield misleading results.
   b. Discs placed on the culture plate approximate concentrations of the antibacterial agent achievable in blood, whereas many antimicrobials achieve 10 to 100 times these concentrations in urine.
   c. An organism showing antimicrobial resistance by the Kirby-Bauer method may in fact be susceptible to the antimicrobial in question. Those antimicrobials reported as susceptible should be effective.
10. The likely response of uncomplicated UTI after appropriate antibacterial treatment is well known for the common uropathogens. Treatment in these instances is based solely on identification of the organism.
    a. Nearly 100% success is expected in eradication of UTI caused by *Staphylococcus aureus/intermedius* or *Streptococcus* after penicillin or ampicillin if the dog has not received antibiotics in the previous 2 to 3 months.
    b. Approximately 80% cure of UTI is expected after an appropriate course of potentiated sulfonamides for *E. coli,* ampicillin for *Proteus,* cephalexin for *Klebsiella,* and tetracycline for *Pseudomonas.* Doxycycline is not a good substitute for tetracycline as a urinary antimicrobial because doxycycline is excreted primarily in the bile though it still may be useful in special situations such as with encrusting cystitis.

Dietary Therapy
1. No diet has been shown to prevent development of UTI.
2. No diet has been shown to prevent recurrence of UTI.
   a. Consider a change in diet if the urine pH consistently is more than 6.5 at a time when the patient has sterile urine. Changing the diet to one that results in acidic urine (e.g., meat-based diet) may provide benefit from the inhibitory effects of acidic urine on bacterial growth.
3. Canned foods increase water turnover and urine production. Increased hydrokinetic washout can be protective, and encouraging increased water intake is a reasonable recommendation, as long as increased opportunities to void urine are provided concurrently.

■ TABLE 8-2
■ ■ Percentage Antimicrobial Susceptibility and Intermediate Susceptibility of Common Canine Uropathogens 2002-2006
(large quantitative bacterial growth)

Antibiotic	Regular *Escherichia coli*			Hemolytic *E. coli*			Mucoid *E. coli*			*Staphylococcus aureus/intermedius*			*Enterococcus*		
	Total No.	Inter (% of isolates)	Sus (% of isolates)	Total No.	Inter (%)	Sus (%)	Total No.	Inter (%)	Sus (%)	Total No.	Inter (%)	Sus (%)	Total No.	Inter (%)	Sus (%)
Amikacin	403	<1	97.7	221	<1	99.5	54	5.6	87	102	<1	99	185	<1	0
Ampicillin	413	8.9	45.3	226	9.7	69.9	54	9.3	16.7	108	<1	31.5	185	74.6	1.1
Cephalosporin	414	33.6	31.2	229	38.9	47.6	54	18.5	24.1	108	0	94.4	185	9.2	11.9
Amoxicillin/Clavamox	415	12.5	60.7	229	6.1	86.5	54	11.1	38.9	108	0	93.5	185	1.1	81.1
Enrofloxacin	414	<1	80	229	0	100	54	1.9	38.9	108	1.9	91.7	185	40.5	37.8
Furadantin	397	2.8	98.7	223	<1	99.6	51	7.8	80.4	59	0	100	168	1.8	95.2
Sulfamethoxazole/Trimethoprim	415	<1	75.4	229	0	96.9	54	0	37	108	16.7	75	172	0	90.7

Antibiotic	*Klebsiella*			*Enterobacter*			*Proteus*			*Pseudomonas aeruginosa*		
	Total No.	Inter (% of isolates)	Sus (% of isolates)	Total No.	Inter (%)	Sus (%)	Total No.	Inter (%)	Sus (%)	Total No.	Inter (%)	Sus (%)
Amikacin	46	0	100	48	0	97.9	99	0	100	36	0	97.2
Ampicillin	46	0	0	51	1.9	1.9	101	<1	95	37	0	0
Cephalosporin	47	2.1	70.2	52	3.8	9.6	100	3	94	37	0	0
Amoxicillin/Clavamox	47	0	72.3	52	0	15.4	101	0	97	37	0	0
Enrofloxacin	47	6.4	89.4	52	5.8	86.5	101	<1	98	37	21.6	54.1
Furadantin	46	39.1	45.7	51	33.3	54.9	96	0	1	31	0	3.2
Sulfamethoxazole/Trimethoprim	47	0	87.2	52	1.9	80.8	101	<1	93.1	37	0	0

Inter, intermediate susceptibility; *No.*, number; *Sus*, susceptible

Courtesy of Dr. Joseph P. Kowalski and The Ohio State University Microbiology Laboratory.

■ TABLE 8-3

■ ■ **Percentage Antimicrobial Susceptibility and Intermediate Susceptibility of Common Feline Uropathogens 2002-2006 (large quantitative bacterial growth)**

Antibiotic	Regular Escherichia coli			Hemolytic E. coli			Mucoid E. coli			Staphylococcus aureus/intermedius			Proteus		
	Total No.	Inter (%)	Sus (%)	Total No.	Inter (%)	Sus (%)	Total No.	Inter (%)	Sus (%)	Total No.	Inter (%)	Sus (%)	Total No.	Inter (%)	Sus (%)
Amikacin	15	6.7	93.3	61	1.6	96.7	4	0	100	5	0	100	4	0	100
Ampicillin	16	12.5	37.5	63	4.7	74.6	4	0	25	5	0	60	4	0	75
Cephalosporin	16	50	31.3	63	44.4	53.9	4	25	75	5	0	80	4	0	100
Amoxicillin/ Clavamox	16	31.3	62.5	63	9.5	88.9	4	0	100	5	0	80	4	0	100
Enrofloxacin	16	0	81.3	63	0	100	4	0	50	5	0	100	4	0	100
Furadantin	16	6.3	87.5	60	0	100	4	0	100	1	0	100	4	0	0
Sulfamethoxazole/ Trimethoprim	16	0	93.8	63	0	98.4	4	0	100	4	25	75	4	0	75

Antibiotic	Enterococcus			Pseudomonas aeruginosa			Coag. Neg. Staphylococcus		
	Total No.	Inter (%)	Sus (%)	Total No.	Inter (%)	Sus (%)	Total No.	Inter (%)	Sus (%)
Amikacin	26	0	0	3	0	100	18	11.1	88.9
Ampicillin	28	82.1	7.1	3	0	0	18	0	50
Cephalosporin	29	3.4	20.7	3	0	0	18	0	72.2
Amoxicillin/Clavamox	29	0	93.1	3	0	0	18	0	72.2
Enrofloxacin	29	31	55.1	3	33.3	66.7	18	0	94.4
Furadantin	27	0	96.3	2	0	0	5	0	100
Sulfamethoxazole/ Trimethoprim	29	0	89.7	3	0	0	18	0	66.7

Inter, intermediate susceptibility; *No.,* number; *Sus,* susceptible
Courtesy of Dr. Joseph P. Kowalski and The Ohio State University Microbiology Laboratory.

Supportive Therapy

1. Increase water intake sufficiently to result in polyuria.
2. The animal should be provided with increased opportunities to urinate.
3. Correct predisposing factors (anatomic and metabolic) if possible.

❗ Increase water intake with drinking water or canned foods to increase urine production.

a. Remove all uroliths if possible by surgery or voiding urohydropulsion.
b. Treat hyperadrenocorticism if present.
c. Maximize glycemic control in animals with diabetes mellitus.
d. Discontinue exogenous corticosteroids if possible. Consider alternative methods to control inflammatory diseases or decrease the dosage of corticosteroid.
e. Partial cystectomy can be performed in animals with urachal diverticula and in animals with severe cranial bladder wall thickening due to chronic cystitis.
f. Resect polyps in animals with polypoid cystitis.
   (1) Full-thickness resection of polyps traditionally has been employed using partial cystectomy.
   (2) Submucosal saline injection facilitates removal of lesions. More than 50% of the mucosa can be removed if necessary. This approach may be superior to removal of individual lesions.
g. Episioplasty (vulvoplasty) for recurrent UTI.
   (1) Some female dogs have increased risk for UTI associated with excessive perivulvar skin folds.
   (2) Many normal dogs however have similar excess perivulvar skin folds and do not seem to develop recurrent UTI.
   (3) Perivulvar dermatitis is common, but not necessarily present in dogs with excessive perivulvar skin folds.
   (4) Removal of the excessive skin folds may decrease recurrent UTI in affected dogs.

Alternative and Supplemental Treatments
Cranberry Extract
a. No protection from bacterial adherence was observed in a canine model of UTI.
b. No clinical data are available by which to judge this treatment.
Cranberry Juice
a. No clinical studies in dogs.
b. Prevents UTI in women, but does not facilitate resolution of existing UTI.
Glycosaminoglycans
a. GAGs have anti-adherence properties in the urothelium of healthy animals.
b. No clinical studies are available of the prevention or resolution of UTI or on the prevention of reinfection.
c. No difference was found in resolution of UTI using GAG treatment versus placebo in dogs with an induced UTI model but 7% of administered GAG was excreted in urine.

❗ Urinary acidifiers typically are not used because most commercial diets result in acidic urine.

Urinary Acidifiers
a. Highly acid urine can be antibacterial for some uropathogens.
b. This approach was more useful when the veterinary diets fed were not highly acidifying.

   c. Urinary acidifiers can be dangerous if given concurrently with acidifying diets (i.e., risk of metabolic acidosis).

Alpha Agonists (e.g., Phenylpropanolamine, Ephedrine, Pseudoephedrine)

   a. Dogs with urinary incontinence have been noted to be at increased risk for UTI due to a wicking effect of the urine-soiled perineum that facilitates ascent of bacteria.

   b. Dogs with a history of urinary incontinence may have fewer UTI after control of incontinence.

   c. Some dogs with recurrent UTI but without obvious incontinence also seem to benefit from drugs that increase urethral tone. This beneficial effect may be due to increased pressure in the mid-portion of the urethra which may inhibit ascent of bacteria to the bladder.

Estrogens (Diethylstilbestrol [DES], Conjugated Estrogens [Premarin])

   a. May be helpful for reasons similar to those noted above for phenylpropanolamine.

   b. Low concentrations of estrogens may be associated with decreased uroepithelial GAG. If so, replacement of estrogens could enhance the host defenses of the urothelium.

   c. Estrogen replacement increases vaginal blood flow and alters the vaginal epithelium, which may be helpful in preventing ascent of bacteria.

Prophylactic Therapy

1. Useful to prevent new infections after previous infection has been eliminated in patients that have had multiple UTI.
2. Low-dose intermittent antimicrobial therapy may be of value to prevent the occurrence of new infections.

> **!** Long-term prophylactic use of antibacterials may help prevent recurrence of UTI in some patients.

   a. Subtherapeutic doses of antimicrobials are given, but may prevent development of new UTI.

     (1) Bacterial numbers may be decreased.

     (2) Host defense systems may be able to handle the reduced number of bacteria.

     (3) Bacteria that are not directly killed by the antimicrobial may not express fimbria necessary to attach to urothelium, and consequently may be eliminated during voiding.

3. An appropriate antimicrobial is administered in the standard manner and then is followed by chronic administration of one third to one half of the total daily dose given once daily.

   a. The owner is instructed to give the medication at bedtime. This protocol favors a high concentration of the excreted antimicrobial in urine when it is being stored the most, thus facilitating maximal prophylactic effect.

   b. A trimethoprim-potentiated sulfonamide, cephalexin, or nitrofurantoin is recommended if UTI is caused by a gram-negative organism.

     (1) The risk of folate deficiency during long-term therapy with trimethoprim-potentiated sulfonamides has not been fully evaluated in clinical patients. Periodic assessment of the CBC is recommended to detect anemia.

     (2) Thrombocytopenia and hepatopathy rarely have been observed in patients receiving nitrofurantoin. CBC and liver function tests should be evaluated periodically.

     (3) A myasthenia gravis-type syndrome has also been reported in some dogs receiving nitrofurantoin.

   c. Use of ampicillin/clavulanate or trimethoprim-potentiated sulfonamide is effective if UTI is caused by gram-positive bacteria.

    d. The antibiotic previously used to eradicate the most recent UTI should be considered when designing a prophylactic program.

    e. A fluoroquinolone is prescribed to prevent ascent of highly resistant organisms.

4. Prophylaxis may be necessary for at least 6 consecutive months to prevent reinfection.

    a. Ideally, urine should be cultured monthly to ensure that it remains sterile.

    b. If the urine remains sterile for 6 months, the animal's urinary defense mechanisms may have improved, and further medication may no longer be needed. Most dogs that respond with negative urine cultures for 6 months will maintain sterile urine when prophylaxis is discontinued.

    c. Some animals require life-long prophylactic antibacterial therapy.

    d. If the urine remains sterile, administration of the drug every other day or twice weekly may be possible.

    e. High dose pulse (once weekly) antibacterial therapy also has been recommended for chronic prophylaxis. No comparisons between daily and pulse dose prophylaxis have been reported.

Treatment of Highly Resistant or Unique Organisms
Resistance

    a. Increased resistance of urinary tract strains of *E. coli* has been recently noted. Drugs that may overcome resistance include:

      (1) Fluoroquinolones.

      (2) Third-generation cephalosporins.

      (3) Methenamine.

      (4) Imipenem.

      (5) Meropenem is especially good for quinolone-resistant *E. coli*. It is administered at 8 to 10 mg SC twice daily, and is stable for 25 days in the refrigerator.

      (6) Aminoglycosides.

      (7) Ticarcillin.

      (8) Piperacillin.

Recurrent *Proteus* spp Infections

    a. Fluoroquinolones may provide increased tissue penetration.

Pseudomonas

    a. Fluoroquinolones.

    b. Tetracyclines other than doxycycline.

Enterococci

    a. Amoxicillin-clavulanate.

    b. Chloramphenicol.

    c. Nitrofurantoin.

Mycoplasma, *Ureaplasma*, or *Chlamydia*

    a. Tetracycline or doxycycline.

    b. Chloramphenicol.

Corynebacterium (Urealyticum, Jeikeium)

    a. Vancomycin—can be toxic.

    b. Teicoplanin (vancomycin-related glycopeptide).

    c. Tetracyclines (doxycycline controversial).

    d. Chloramphenicol.

    e. Fluoroquinolones—variable susceptibility.

Fungal Organisms

    a. Fluconazole (eliminated primarily in urine).

      b. Flucytosine (renal elimination).
         (1) Bone marrow toxicity possible.
         (2) Resistance may develop rapidly.
      c. Clotrimazole (intermittent bladder infusion).

Special Types of Urinary Tract Infections

1. *Corynebacterium urealyticum* is associated with a unique form of relapsing UTI in both dogs and cats in which encrustations of urinary tissue with struvite and calcium phosphate can prevent eradication of the organism with medical treatment alone.

    a. Gram-positive, non-hemolytic, urease-positive, catalase-positive, non-spore forming, aerobic bacillus. Resistant to multiple common antibiotics including amoxicillin, cephalosporins, and potentiated-sulfa. Susceptibility testing can be impossible, because some organisms are so slow growing.

    b. Normal skin flora of humans (suspected to be the same in dogs and cats).

    c. Often reported as "diphtheroids" and considered as contaminants since many saprophytes exist.

    d. Sometimes referred to as "encrusting cystitis" since the urease-producing activity of this infection is associated with struvite and calcium phosphate precipitations that can adhere to the mucosal surface. Calculi can be free moving, or small stones may adhere to the mucosal surface. Other UTI associated with urease-producing activity (*S. aureus*, *Proteus* spp.) are not associated with adherent plaque formation.

    e. Almost always discovered after several previous UTI with more common organisms and following multiple courses of antibacterial treatment.

    f. Nearly all have micturition abnormalities that predispose to this infection (e.g., chronic urinary incontinence, neurogenic bladder, atonic bladder, cystostomy tube placement, indwelling urinary catheterization, chronic recumbency from musculoskeletal or neurological disorders) or immunosuppression with glucocorticosteroids.

    g. Can be overlooked as a cause for UTI since the organism is slow-growing, growth of other organisms may overwhelm its growth in vitro, and "diphtheroids" are often considered to be contaminants.

    h. Hematuria, pyuria, and alkaline urine with struvite crystalluria are typical. Organisms may or may not be seen. Gram-positive reaction for rods.
       (1) Polymerase chain reaction (PCR) test for use in human medicine has not been evaluated in dogs or cats.

    i. Radiography may reveal stones or irregular mineralization along the mucosal surface. Contrast radiography usually shows a thickened bladder with an irregular mucosa, sometimes with filling defects from the encrustations and small stones.

    j. Ultrasonography reveals thickening of the bladder with irregular-shaped mucosal projections that are of varying echogenicity.
       (1) Heavy sediment may be observed within the bladder.
       (2) The mucosal surface may be highly hyperechogenic with or without shadowing. This is distinguished from the shadowing of stones that are homogenous in echotexture and shape.
       (3) Hydroureter and hydronephrosis may be seen in those with obstruction from severe cystitis. Dilatation of the renal pelvis is possible secondary to pyelitis or pyelonephritis.

    k. Cystoscopy reveals erythema and increased vascularity to the mucosa of the bladder and urethra. Distinctive yellow or white plaques that are firmly attached to the mucosa may be seen, as well as bands of encrusting debris.

l. Bladder histopathology is expected to reveal suppurative, necrotizing, ulcerating cystitis. Mineralization along the mucosa may be pronounced.

m. Ensure that the urine culture plate and broth are evaluated up to 5 days for bacterial growth in those in which typical urinary sediment and imaging findings described above are found.

n. Correction of the underlying predisposition to the UTI is necessary to achieve long-term urinary sterility.

o. Tetracycline and chloramphenicol are often the first choice antibacterial treatment. Fluoroquinolones are sometimes effective. Vancomycin is a tertiary choice due to toxicity and need to be given parenterally.

(1) Antibacterial therapy by itself is often ineffective, because the drug cannot eradicate the organisms in the encrustations and stones.

p. Surgery to remove any encrustations (plaque debridement, submucosal resection, or partial cystectomy) improves the chances that medical therapy can be effective.

q. Local installation of acidifying solutions into the bladder can be considered as an ancillary treatment.

r. Prognosis for long-term cure is guarded to poor for most cases.

s. *Corynebacterium jeikeium* UTI was recently diagnosed in a cat using gene sequencing for definitive identification. Clinical features were similar to those described earlier.

2. Emphysematous cystitis is a very rare complication of a bacterial UTI, particularly in diabetic patients or others with glucosuria. It has also been associated with other immunosuppressive diseases such as hyperadrenocorticism. Some of these animals may not demonstrate clinical signs but may have evidence of UTI on urinalysis.

a. Occurs when bacterial cystitis is caused by a gas-producing bacterium such as *Clostridium* spp. These bacteria create pockets of gas within the wall of the bladder that are apparent on radiographs and ultrasound. It has also been associated with *Corynebacterium* infection.

b. Can be diagnosed via abdominal ultrasound or survey radiographs (may see gas in the bladder wall).

c. Care should be taken in performing cystocentesis in these patients because the integrity of the bladder wall may be affected by the presence of gas within the bladder wall.

d. Aerobic cultures may be negative if an anaerobic organism is responsible.

e. Treatment with appropriate antibiotic therapy usually results in resolution of these lesions.

f. Surgical stripping of the bladder mucosa is rarely indicated.

Outcomes

1. Clinical signs resolve, and urine culture is negative. This occurs in most cases.
2. Clinical signs resolve, then return, and urine culture is positive.
   a. Reinfection.
      (1) New bacterial organism (reinfection due to poor host defenses).
   b. Relapse or persistent infection.
      (1) Same organism with same susceptibility pattern (antibiotic is ineffective).
         (a) Resistant organism may be protected in biofilms and survive therapy.
         (b) Antibiotic not reaching the organism.
      (2) Same organism with new susceptibility pattern (acquired resistance).
   c. Super-infection (uncommon)—previous organism is gone but a new one is present.
3. Clinical signs continue (with or without positive culture).

     a. Wrong diagnosis (sterile inflammation).
     b. UTI superimposed on neoplasia.
     c. Superinfection.

SUCCESS OF THERAPY

A. Success depends on maintaining sterile urine during treatment and after medication has been discontinued.
B. Resolution of clinical and laboratory signs (e.g., hematuria, proteinuria, microscopic bacteriuria) can be misleading because these can resolve due to reduced activity of the UTI but not necessarily its eradication.
C. Quantitative urine cultures are recommended 5 to 7 days, 1 month, and 3 months after medication has been discontinued to ensure that infection has been eradicated and urine sterility maintained.
D. It is difficult or impossible to resolve UTI in an animal with a predisposing anatomic factor.

! Anatomic abnormalities must be corrected for treatment of UTI to be successful.

E. Urine should be cultured after the animal with a recurrent UTI has received antibiotics for 3 to 5 days, especially when it is unclear whether or not the urine has ever been sterilized.
    1. This is an in vivo susceptibility test.
    2. Any growth of organisms of this time indicates that the infection is not likely to be sterilized with this treatment.

ADDITIONAL THERAPEUTIC CONSIDERATIONS

Therapeutic Failures (Box 8-3)

    1. Incorrect diagnosis (UTI is not present).
    2. UTI is present but secondary to another urinary tract disorder (e.g., neoplasia, ectopic ureter, uroliths).
    3. Medication was not given or was not absorbed (e.g., pills regurgitated, interfering substances in the gastrointestinal tract).
    4. The wrong antibacterial was selected (based on the suspected biological behavior of a specific pathogen).

! In cats, the most common reason for failure of antibiotics to eliminate clinical signs is that the disease is not bacterial.

    5. The wrong dose, interval, or duration of the antibacterial was prescribed.
    6. Lower concentration was achieved in urine than expected (e.g., decreased glomerular filtration rate, impaired urinary concentrating ability).
    7. The infecting organism is highly resistant.
    8. The organism has developed resistance during treatment.
    9. A second pathogen has emerged.
    10. The organism is not accessible to the antibacterial (e.g., sequestered due to polyps or fibrosis).
    11. Predisposing host factors have not been identified.
      a. Anatomic.
      b. Metabolic.
      c. Functional.

■ BOX 8-3
■ QUESTIONS TO CONSIDER WHEN URINARY TRACT INFECTION RECURS

Are you certain that the disease really is bacterial?
Have you made sure that there are no important predisposing anatomic abnormalities?
   Urolithiasis—lower and upper urinary tract
   Ectopic ureters
   Neoplasia of bladder, urethra, or prostate
   Urachal diverticulum
   Polypoid cystitis
   Recessed vulva
   Chronic bladder thickening with extensive tissue changes
   Pyelonephritis
   Prostatitis
Have you made sure that there are no important functional abnormalities?
   Can the animal completely empty its bladder? Is the residual volume normal?
   Is primary sphincter mechanism incompetence present (i.e., low urethral tone with urinary incontinence and
   wicking of bacteria)?
Have you made sure that there are no important metabolic conditions present?
   Diabetes mellitus?
   Hyperadrenocorticism?

! In dogs, the most common reason for failure of antibiotics to eliminate clinical signs is that underlying
anatomic, functional, or metabolic disorders have not been identified.

12. A new UTI has developed after urethral catheterization.
13. Systemic immunosuppression is present.
14. Failure of host urinary defense mechanisms has allowed a new UTI to develop.

Recurrent Urinary Tract Infection

1. Recurrent infections are repeated episodes of bacterial UTI (often associated with clinical
   signs) usually after therapy. Recurrent infections either are reinfections or relapsing infections. Serial quantitative culture results allow the distinction between relapse or reinfection (Table 8-4).
   a. Reinfection is another clinical episode of infection caused by a different organism than
      previously. The offending organism may be an entirely different genus and species or
      may be the same genus and species, but a different serotype (54% of recurrent UTI).

! Recurrent UTI occurs in approximately 0.3% of all dogs in a referral population; 5% of all positive urine
cultures are from recurrent cases.

      (1) This situation represents a new infection that typically occurs weeks to months
          after discontinuation of drug therapy for a previous UTI.
      (2) Long-term treatment usually is not indicated, because routine therapy will eradi-
          cate the current infection.
      (3) Multiple new infections suggest that the animal's host defense mechanisms are
          not operating properly. A search for predisposing factors including anatomic

■ TABLE 8-4
■ ■ **Schedule of Urine Cultures for Difficult or Recurrent Cases**

Initial Presentation	Identify Organism and Determine Susceptibility
After 3-5 days on treatment	Document effective eradication in urine
	Rule out persistent infection
	Change in MIC if persistent?
	Rapid emergence of resistance?
3 days before treatment ends	Rule out super-infection (rare)
	New organism identified?
7-10 days after treatment ends	Rule out relapse
1, 2, 3, 6, and 12 months after treatment	Identify reinfection

      defects, urolithiasis, urinary retention (e.g., neurologic dysfunction), neoplasia, and metabolic disorders (e.g., hyperadrenocorticism, diabetes mellitus, immunosuppression) should be undertaken. Often no predisposing factors are found, indicating primary failure of host defense mechanisms.

   b. Relapsing infection is another clinical episode caused by the same organism (i.e., same serotype) and implies persistence of an organism that was never eradicated (44% of recurrent UTI).

     (1) This situation suggests that the infection is deep-seated within the tissues. Clinical signs tend to occur soon after discontinuation of medications, usually within days to a week.

> ! It is important to distinguish between reinfection and relapsing infection because the causes and treatment are different.

     (2) Long-term therapy for 30 to 60 days or longer is indicated.
     (3) A search for predisposing factors should be undertaken to exclude:
       (a) Pyelonephritis.
       (b) Obstructive nephropathy.
       (c) Urolithiasis.
       (d) Chronic bladder wall changes allowing sequestration of bacteria.
       (e) Anatomic defects.
       (f) Urinary retention.
       (g) Re-inoculation of the bladder from prostatic or uterine infection.
   c. Persistent infection is a variant of relapsing infection in that the same organism is present, but it has never been eradicated, even transiently.
     (1) Persistent infection occurs in approximately 2% of all recurrent UTI.
     (2) It implies severe abrogation of local host defenses or an organism highly resistant to the antimicrobial agent presently being used to treat the infection.
 2. Female dogs typically have recurrent infections with *Staphylococcus*, *Enterococcus* sp, or *P. aeruginosa*.
 3. Male dogs with recurrent UTI are more likely to have *Klebsiella*, *Providentia*, *Salmonella* sp, *Corynebacterium* sp, *Acinetobacter* sp, or *Actinomyces* sp infections.
 4. In recurrent infections, 20% of affected dogs have two bacterial organisms isolated and 4% have three isolated.

Diagnostic Imaging Studies

1. Diagnostic imaging studies (e.g., plain radiography, contrast urography, ultrasonography, cystoscopy) also are important in the evaluation of recurrent UTI.

WHAT DO WE DO?

- We quantitatively culture the urine of all dogs and cats with clinical signs related to the lower urinary tract. This procedure allows us to know if a bacterial UTI is present or not. Definitive identification of the organism and the numbers present (cfu/mL) make a difference in our degree of certainty that UTI is real and may provide a clue as to how difficult it will be to eradicate the organism.
- We culture urine from cats with CRF at initial presentation and periodically thereafter regardless of whether or not they have clinical signs, because many CRF cats have a UTI at some point in their clinical course.
- We institute surveillance of dogs with hyperadrenocorticism and those that have received long-term treatment with corticosteroids regardless of whether or not they have pyuria on urine sediment examination.
- We pursue diagnostic imaging if more than one infection has occurred within a 6-month period.
- We culture urine during the administration of antibacterial agents in difficult cases to ensure that the urine is sterilized while the animal is on medication.
- We culture the urine 5 to 7 days after stopping antibacterial agents and then again 1 and 3 months later in animals with recurrent UTI.
- We institute chronic prophylactic antibacterial treatment at subtherapeutic doses in animals with recurrent UTI in which no predisposing factors can be found after a full course of antibacterial treatment has sterilized the urine. We culture the urine periodically to ensure that breakthrough infection has not occurred.
- We select antimicrobial agents on the basis of susceptibility test results in animals with recurrent UTI.

SUMMARY TIPS

DO's	DON'Ts
Culture urine in all dogs and cats with signs of lower urinary tract disease.	Don't blindly pick an antibacterial agent, unless financial constraints of the owner dictate otherwise.
Collect urine by cystocentesis for culture.	Don't culture voided urine.
Periodically culture urine from cats with CRF, from dogs and cats receiving corticosteroids, and from those with diabetes mellitus or hyperadrenocorticism.	Don't ignore the likelihood of UTI in patients with CRF, diabetes mellitus, and hyperadrenocorticims. UTI in such patients often is asymptomatic.
Perform a direct examination of fresh urine, and culture the urine.	Don't assume urine is sterile if bacteria are not seen in urine sediment. Don't assume that "bacteria" in sediment are real, especially in the absence of pyuria.
Use urine sediment examination to visualize WBCs.	Don't depend on dipsticks to detect WBCs in urine. They are unreliable in dogs and cats.
Perform urinary catheterization when medically or surgically necessary, but be aware of the risk of introducing UTI.	Don't ignore the risk of UTI after urinary catheterization. Don't carelessly administer antibiotics to animals with indwelling urinary catheters. Infection may be delayed but not prevented, and resistant organisms are likely.
Culture urine after treatment to ensure sterility of urine.	Don't rely on resolution of clinical signs to indicate that urine is sterile.
Follow a full course of antibacterial therapy.	Don't discontinue treatment early just because the patient looks or feels better.
Treat all cases of UTI, even those that are asymptomatic.	Don't ignore the potential consequences of untreated UTI.

COMMON MISCONCEPTIONS

- Bacterial urine cultures are of limited value. Actually, quantitative culture of urine is the gold standard that indicates whether UTI actually exist or not. Many things look like bacteria in the urine; hence, culture is necessary to confirm whether bacteria are actually present in abundance or not.
- It is reasonable to culture voided urine. Definitely not true in most instances, because of the high degree of contamination of the urine sample from bacteria that reside in the distal urethra, vestibule, or prepuce.
- Young cats frequently have bacterial UTI. Not true. Young cats have exquisite defense mechanisms that protect them against bacteria that could otherwise cause UTI. It may be that the cat's extremely high urine-concentrating capacity is especially protective compared with that in dogs.
- Urine culture is of no value while an animal is receiving antimicrobial agents. It is true that urine culture taken while an animal is receiving antibacterial medication often results in no growth of bacteria even when they are present, because their growth is inhibited in the laboratory by the presence of the antimicrobial agent. However, during assessment of difficult cases with recurrent UTI, culture of urine while on medication can be valuable. If an organism grows, it means that the organism is either very resistant to the medication chosen or the agent is not getting to where the organism is hiding.
- Dipstick WBC measurements are useful in the documentation of pyuria. Dipstick pads for WBC are designed to detect WBC esterase. This test is frequently negative in dogs despite the presence of WBC and positive in cats despite the absence of WBC.

FREQUENTLY ASKED QUESTIONS

Q: Do I really need to culture urine on an animal's first episode of presumed bacterial UTI?

A: Ideally, yes, but it may not be essential the first time. Most animals with their first UTI will respond to a routine course of antimicrobial treatment. If antimicrobial agents have been given for another reason within the past few months, it is a good idea to culture the urine rather than assuming the UTI will respond to treatment.

Q: Why do most of my urine cultures from cats with signs of LUTD come back negative?

A: Cats younger than 10 years of age with signs of irritative voiding rarely (<1% of the time) have bacterial UTI. Cats have excellent urinary host defenses (such as high urine osmolality) that make it very difficult for UTI to become established. Bacterial UTI in cats is more common in cats that have had perineal urethrostomies or in those that have had urethral catheterization within the past 6 months. Cats older than 10 years of age with signs of irritative voiding have a greater likelihood of having a bacterial UTI, often in association with CRF. Diagnosis of bacterial UTI in cats often is erroneously based on the observation of so-called bacteria in urine sediment. Unfortunately, many things in the urine sediment of cats can look like bacteria, but actually are not bacteria. Dipstrip tests for WBC in urine based on leukocyte esterase reactions frequently are falsely positive in cats that do not have pyuria.

Q: Why is it important to distinguish between reinfection and relapsing infection? How do I approach these differently?

A: Relapsing infection is diagnosed when the same organism is isolated a few days to one week after discontinuing antibacterial medication. Presence of a relapsing infection means the original organism was never completely eradicated, and that it is still present. A relapsing UTI implies a deeply seated infection (e.g., one in the kidneys, prostate gland, or thickened bladder wall or one complicated by other factors such as uroliths, polypoid cystitis, or a urachal remnant). Usually, the solution to a relapsing infection is to prescribe antimicrobial treatment for a much longer period of time or to enhance tissue penetration by switching to an antibiotic with better distribution to the affected tissue. Also, the organism may have become resistant to the antibiotic that has been chosen. Reinfections are detected weeks to months after antibiotic therapy. An initial follow-up urine culture taken 5 to 7 days after medication has been discontinued is sterile. The implication is that the organism was easy to eliminate, and that colonization by a new organism has occurred. A routine course of antibiotic is indicated again, and longer courses do not increase the likelihood that another infection will be prevented. Newer, more expensive antibiotics also are not the answer because the initial infection usually is easily treated using conventional antibiotics.

Q: How often does UTI occur in the absence of pyuria? In the absence of visible bacteriuria in urinary sediment?

A: Most UTI are accompanied by pyuria. The odds of a UTI being present are higher if the WBCs are seen with bacteria. Cats with CRF and dogs with hyperadrenocorticism, diabetes mellitus, or exogenous corticosteroid administration can have a true bacterial UTI without pyuria or bacteriuria and with or without lower urinary tract clinical signs. Such patients should have quantitative urine cultures performed periodically. Bacteria may not be visible during evaluation of wet mounts of urine sediment despite the presence of a true UTI. A critical number of bacteria must be present before the human eye can detect them in the urinary sediment. Remember also that not everything reported to be bacteria in the urinary sediment really is bacteria. Many particulate artifacts occur in urine sediment and can be confused with bacteria.

Q: How often are bacteria really in urine, but fail to grow in the microbiology laboratory?

A: Most common uropathogens grow readily on blood agar within 12 to 24 hours in an incubator. Similar results are achieved even if urine has been refrigerated for up to 6 hours. Refrigeration for 24 hours or more reduces bacterial growth, but usually the infecting organism can be isolated and a diagnosis made. Typically, if the organism is there, it will grow using conventional methods. If you are concerned that you are getting false-negative results due to storage of urine samples or that growth has been inhibited during transport to the laboratory, consider plating out the urine sample immediately after collection, and send the plate to the laboratory after initial incubation if overnight growth is detected.

Q: What are treatable predisposing factors that either initiate or potentiate UTI in dogs? In cats?

A: Inadequate opportunities for dogs to void, infection-related uroliths, urachal diverticulum, ectopic ureter, polypoid cystitis, recessed vulva (dogs), diabetes mellitus, hyperadrenocorticism, exogenous corticosteroid exposure, urinary incontinence, CRF (cats), and proliferative urethritis (dogs) are some recognized predisposing problems.

Q: How frequently is UTI associated with highly resistant bacterial organisms?

A: Fortunately, most UTI are associated with organisms that are highly susceptible to routinely used antibacterial agents. More resistant organisms are encountered in animals with recurrent UTI, in which susceptibility testing is clearly indicated. Recent reports of bacterial susceptibility in dogs with UTI indicate the emergence of increased bacterial resistance to enrofloxacin, possibly due to widespread use of this drug.

Q: In general, how long do you administer antimicrobials to an animal with UTI?

A: In uncomplicated cases, antibiotics usually are given for 2 to 3 weeks.

Q: How would you change the length of antimicrobial treatment in an upper UTI compared with a lower UTI?

A: Upper UTI poses a special challenge to eradicate the bacterial organisms. It takes at least 4 to 6 weeks and possibly 2 to 3 months to sterilize renal tissue. In some instances, it is not possible to sterilize the kidneys.

Q: When do you re-culture urine during or after treatment for UTI?

A: In difficult cases, urine can be cultured during antibiotic treatment as a form of in vivo susceptibility testing. If bacteria are present in urine during antibiotic treatment (i.e., persistent infection), then the urine is not being sterilized by the selected therapy and a different antibiotic or dosing regimen should be chosen. Urine culture should be performed after treatment in all cases, if possible and financially feasible for the owner. Clinical signs are not reliable to document successful eradication of UTI.

Q: How can it be that an organism is reported by the laboratory as resistant to a specific antimicrobial agent, when actually it is susceptible in the animal's urinary tract?

A: Kirby-Bauer testing uses discs that contain concentrations of the antibacterial agents comparable to what can be achieved in serum. The concentration of the antimicrobial is likely to be much higher in urine than in serum. Consequently, the organism may be reported as resistant to the antimicrobial agent in question when in reality it is susceptible at concentrations of the drug that can be achieved in urine.

SUGGESTED READINGS

Bailiff NL, Westropp JL, Jang SS, Ling GV: *Corynebacterium urealyticum* urinary tract infection in dogs and cats: 7 cases (1996-2003), *J Am Vet Med Assoc* 226:1676–1680, 2005.

Bartges J: Lower urinary tract diseases in geriatric cats, *Proceedings of the ACVIM*, Lake Buena Vista, Fla., 1997, 322–324.

Cooke CL, Singer RS, Jang SS, Hirsh DC: Enrofloxacin resistance in *Escherichia coli* isolated from dogs with urinary tract infections, *J Am Vet Med Assoc* 220:190–192, 2002.

Davidson AP, Ling GV, Stevens F, et al: Urinary tract infections in cats: A retrospective study 1977-1989, *California Veterinarian* 5:32–34, 1992.

Forrester SD, Troy GC, Dalton MN, et al: Retrospective evaluation of urinary tract infection in 42 dogs with hyperadrenocorticism or diabetes mellitus or both, *J Vet Intern Med* 13:557–560, 1999.

Gelatt KN, van der Woerdt A, Ketring KL, et al: Enrofloxacin-associated retinal degeneration in cats, *Vet Ophthalmol* 4:99–106, 2001.

Lightner BA, McLoughlin MA, Chew DJ, et al: Episioplasty for the treatment of perivulvar dermatitis or recurrent urinary tract infections in dogs with excessive perivulvar skin folds: 31 cases (1983-2000), *J Am Vet Med Assoc* 219:1577–1581, 2001.

Ling GV, Norris CR, Franti CE, et al: Interrelations of organism prevalence, specimen collection method, and host age, sex, and breed among 8,354 canine urinary tract infections (1969-1995), *J Vet Intern Med* 15:341–347, 2001.

Litster A, Moss SM, Honnery M, et al: Prevalence of bacterial species in cats with clinical signs of lower urinary tract disease: Recognition of *Staphylococcus felis* as a possible feline urinary tract pathogen, *Vet Microbiol* 121:182–188, 2007.

Mayer-Roenne B, Goldstein RE, Erb HN: Urinary tract infections in cats with hyperthyroidism, diabetes mellitus and chronic kidney disease, *J Feline Med Surg* 9:124–132, 2007.

Norris CR, Williams BJ, Ling GV, et al: Recurrent and persistent urinary tract infections in dogs: 383 cases (1969-1995), *J Am Anim Hosp Assoc* 36:484–492, 2000.

Seguin MA, Vaden SL, Altier C, et al: Persistent urinary tract infections and reinfections in 100 dogs (1989-1999), *J Vet Intern Med* 17:622–631, 2003.

Swenson CL, Boisvert AM, Kruger JM, Gibbons-Burgener SN: Evaluation of modified Wright-staining of urine sediment as a method for accurate detection of bacteriuria in dogs, *J Am Vet Med Assoc* 224:1282–1289, 2004.

Wilson BJ, Norris JM, Malik R, et al: Susceptibility of bacteria from feline and canine urinary tract infections to doxycycline and tetracycline concentrations attained in urine four hours after oral dosage, *Aust Vet J* 84:8–11, 2006.

9 Urolithiasis

INTRODUCTION, TERMINOLOGY, AND GENERAL PATHOPHYSIOLOGY

Urine Is a Complex Solution Containing Many Organic and Inorganic Solutes

1. More of a given solute can remain in solution in urine than in water because of the complex interactions that occur among the various organic and inorganic constituents in urine.
2. For several possible reasons (e.g., diet, decreased water intake, altered urine pH, relative lack of inhibitors, or presence of promoters of crystallization), the solubility product of a particular solute may be exceeded, crystals may form, and these crystals may aggregate and grow. (Figure 9-1.)
   a. If the crystals precipitate spontaneously, the process is called homogenous nucleation. Homogenous nucleation probably does not occur in urine.
   b. If another substance (e.g., desquamated epithelial cells, inflammatory cells and debris, bacteria, foreign body) acts as a nidus for crystal precipitation, the process is called heterogenous nucleation.
   c. Crystals must reside in the urinary tract for a sufficient time for a urolith to form, so factors that predispose to urinary stasis play an important role in urolithiasis. Conversely, factors that increase voiding such as increased water intake may be protective.
3. A crystalloid is a component of a crystal (e.g., an ion).
4. A urolith is an organized concretion found in the urinary tract and containing primarily organic or inorganic crystalloid and a much smaller amount of organic matrix.

❗ Most uroliths are identified in the lower urinary tract.

   a. When 70% or more of the urolith is composed of one type of crystalloid it is named for that crystal. Secondary crystalloids can comprise up to 30% of the total weight. Most stones in dogs and cats have one major crystal component (Figures 9-2 and 9-3). More than 90% of stones submitted for quantitative analysis are collected from the lower urinary tract.
   b. When <70% of the urolith is composed of one mineral but without identifiable nidus, shell, or surface crystals, it is called a mixed urolith.
   c. A matrix urolith contains organic matrix without appreciable crystalloid.
   d. A urolith with an identifiable nidus composed of one mineral with one or more surrounding layers of different mineral composition is called a compound urolith.
5. Calculus is a general term referring to a solid concretion formed in ducts of hollow organs.
6. Matrix is the noncrystalline organic components of a urolith.

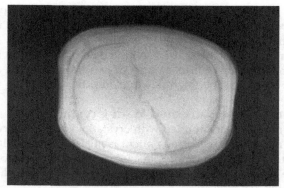

FIGURE 9-1 ■ Note lamellar pattern of large urolith shown on radiograph after stone had been removed surgically.

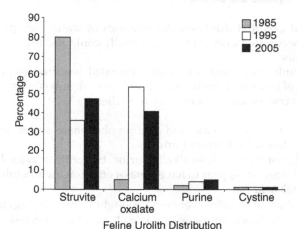

FIGURE 9-2 ■ Percentage of urolith type from cats submitted to the Minnesota Urolith Center, Courtesy of Minnesota Urolith Center, University of Minnesota College of Veterinary Medicine, St. Paul, Minn.

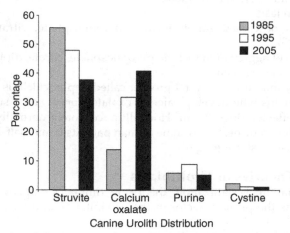

FIGURE 9-3 ■ Percentage of urolith type from dogs submitted to the Minnesota Urolith Center, Courtesy of Minnesota Urolith Center, University of Minnesota College of Veterinary Medicine, St. Paul, Minn.

    a. Albumin, globulins, Tamm-Horsfall mucoprotein (uromucoid), hexose, hexosamine, and matrix substance A have been identified in uroliths, but normally make up a very small portion of the total weight of the urolith.

    b. Calculi composed solely of dried solidified blood have been removed from all regions of the upper and lower urinary tract of cats. Most affected cats also have hematuria (> 100 red blood cells per high-power field [RBCs/hpf]).

Urine Is Commonly Supersaturated With Crystalloids

1. Urine is commonly supersaturated with crystalloids, and observation of individual crystals does not necessarily mean the patient is at risk for urolithiasis. Cooling of the urine specimen during storage promotes in vitro crystal precipitation, and observed crystals may not have been present at the time the sample was collected. Supersaturation of urine with crystalloids depends on:

Amount of solute ingested and excreted
Urine Volume

    a. Dogs and cats that drink smaller volumes of water may produce small volumes of more concentrated urine, which potentially could predispose them to development of urolithiasis.

    b. In one study, miniature Schnauzers urinated less frequently and produced smaller volumes of urine with higher pH and higher calcium concentration than did Labrador retrievers consuming the same dry food diet.

Urine pH

    a. Struvite, calcium carbonate, and calcium phosphate are less soluble in alkaline urine.

    b. Cystine is less soluble in acid urine.

    c. Uric acid is more soluble in alkaline urine, but urate is less soluble in alkaline urine.

    d. Urine pH does not appear to have a major effect on the solubility of silicate and oxalate.

Promoters of Urolithiasis

    a. Abnormal urine proteins were once thought to promote aggregation and growth. No conclusive evidence for (or against) this theory has emerged.

    b. Precipitation of one crystal on the surface of another, a process called epitaxy, can promote growth of crystals with similar lattice configurations, such as uric acid, calcium oxalate, and calcium phosphate.

Inhibitors of Urolithiasis

    a. Inhibitors of crystallization include pyrophosphate, citrate, and various cations (e.g., Mg^{+2}).

    b. Inhibitors of aggregation include pyrophosphate, citrate, diphosphonates, and glycosaminoglycans (GAGs).

    c. A urinary inhibitor of crystal growth called nephrocalcin is biochemically altered in some humans who develop calcium oxalate stones, and a similar change may occur in some affected dogs. Tamm-Horsfall mucoprotein normally protects against crystal aggregation in urine, but in some human patients it may self-aggregate and fail to protect against crystal aggregation.

Three General Theories of Urolithiasis

1. The precipitation-crystallization theory incriminates supersaturation of urine with crystalloids as the primary factor in the precipitation and subsequent growth of calculi (Figure 9-4).

❗ Calculi collected from the lower urinary tract are assumed to have formed there.

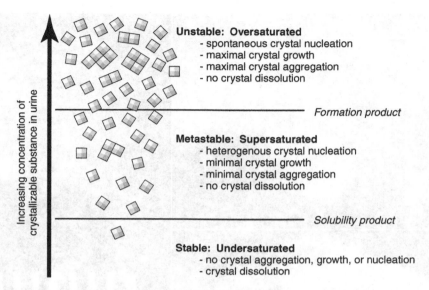

FIGURE 9-4 ■ Crystal dissolution, formation, and growth as a function of the concentration of crystalloids.

2. The matrix-nucleation theory implies that some abnormal substance in the urine is responsible for the initial development of calculi.
3. The crystallization-inhibition theory suggests that the absence of some critical inhibitor (or presence of a promoter) of crystal formation is the primary factor in the development of calculi.
4. It possible that elements of all three theories contribute to the development of urolithiasis.
5. It has been assumed that calculi initially identified in the lower urinary tract actually formed in that location, but this has not been proven. Based on recent data about urolith formation in human patients, it is thought that uroliths may originate from abnormal processes in the kidneys themselves.

PATHOPHYSIOLOGY OF INDIVIDUAL STONE TYPES

Struvite Urolithiasis
1. For many years, struvite was the most common type of urolith found in dogs and cats comprising 60% to 70% of uroliths in dogs and up to 95% of uroliths found in cats. Between 1981 and 2001, the frequency of calcium oxalate urolithiasis increased and that of struvite decreased. Today, struvite comprises 40% to 50% of uroliths in dogs and cats. The increase in calcium oxalate urolithiasis began to level off between 1998 and 2001. (see Figures 9-2 and 9-3.)
2. The major crystalloid in these uroliths is $MgNH_4PO_4\cdot6H_2O$ (struvite). Calcium phosphate as carbonate apatite often is present in small amounts (2%-10%). The presence of three cations (i.e., Ca^{+2}, Mg^{+2}, and NH_4^+) detected by early qualitative analytical methods was responsible for the name "triple phosphate" previously used for these stones. They also have been called magnesium ammonium phosphate stones.
3. Struvite uroliths are spherical, ellipsoidal, or tetrahedral in shape and may be present singly or in large numbers of varying sizes. (Figure 9-5.)

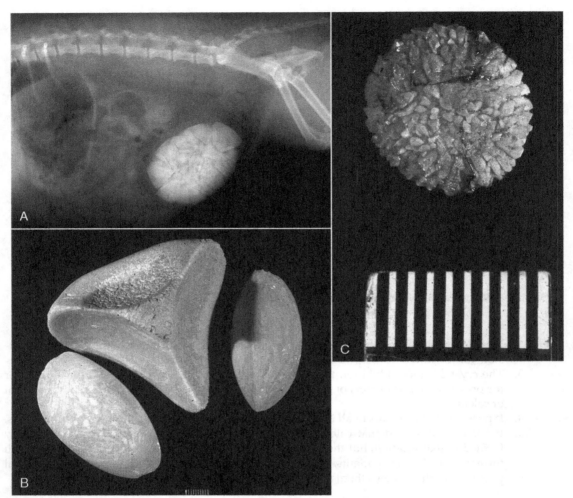

FIGURE 9-5 ■ **A,** Note multiple large cystic calculi composed of struvite from a dog with a urinary tract infection. **B,** Large struvite stones from a dog. Notice how the surfaces of stones growing near each other mold to fit. **C,** Single flat cystic calculus from a cat with sterile urine removed during surgery. They can appear *wafer* like.

4. In dogs and cats, the bladder is the most common site of struvite uroliths, although they may occur at any site in the urinary tract.
5. In dogs, struvite calculi tend to recur after surgical removal, and the recurrence rate in one study was 21%.

> ❗ Most dogs with struvite urolithiasis have underlying UTI that promotes urolith growth. Most cats with struvite urolithiasis have sterile urine when their calculi are first recognized.

6. Infection of the urinary tract by urease-positive bacteria (especially staphylococci and *Proteus* sp) plays the most important role in the pathogenesis of struvite urolithiasis in dogs. More than 95% of dogs with struvite urolithiasis have infection as an underlying cause for the urolith growth. In almost all cats with struvite urolithiasis, infection is not present and

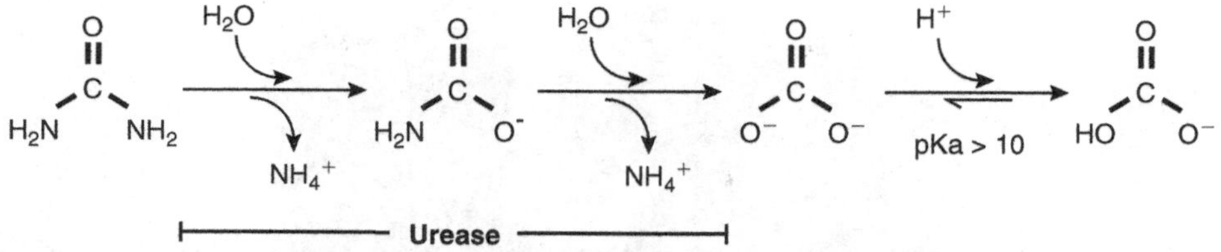

FIGURE 9-6 ■ How urease-positive UTI changes urinary chemistry to favor struvite crystal formation.

the calculi are thought to be metabolic in origin. However, a family of Cocker spaniels with recurrent sterile struvite urolithiasis has been reported.

   a. The solubility of struvite is markedly reduced in alkaline urine. Struvite becomes progressively less soluble as the pH increases above 6.7.
   b. Hydrolysis of urea by urease-positive bacteria liberates ammonia and carbon dioxide, which alkalinizes the urine and increases availability of ammonium and phosphate ions for struvite crystal formation (Figure 9-6).
   c. Experimentally, induction of urease-positive staphylococcal urinary tract infection (UTI) in dogs is followed in 2 to 8 weeks by the development of struvite calculi.
7. Struvite solubility is decreased in animals with persistently alkaline urine even in the absence of UTI. In dogs that form struvite stones in the absence of UTI, predisposing factors that may be associated with alkaline urine (e.g., family history of struvite stones, diet based on vegetable proteins, distal renal tubular acidosis) should be considered.
8. UTI usually is not present in cats with struvite stones. More than 95% of cats with struvite urolithiasis have sterile urine.
9. Diets formulated with high magnesium, phosphorus, calcium, chloride, or fiber, and moderate protein content are associated with increased risk of struvite urolithiasis in cats. Diets with high fat content, low in sodium or potassium, and those formulated to maximize urine acidity are associated with decreased risk of struvite urolithiasis in cats.

Oxalate Urolithiasis

1. Calcium oxalate stones are the most common type of urolith in humans, and their frequency has increased in dogs and cats and during the past 25 years.
2. Risk factors for development of oxalate urolithiasis in dogs.
   a. Age older than 4 years. Affected dogs are older than 1 year of age and the highest risk occurs between 8 and 12 years of age. The average age of occurrence is between 8 and 9 years.
   b. Neutered males are at highest risk.
   c. Breeds at highest risk are miniature and standard Schnauzer, Lhasa apso, Yorkshire terrier, Bichon frise, Shih tzu, miniature and toy poodle. Golden retriever, German shepherd, and Cocker spaniel are at lowest risk for oxalate urolithiasis.
   d. Overweight dogs have higher risk.
   e. Pet dogs have higher risk than working dogs.
   f. Hypercalcemia (usually as a consequence of primary hyperparathyroidism) is a contributing factor in approximately 4% of dogs with calcium oxalate urolithiasis.
3. Risk factors for development of oxalate urolithiasis in cats.
   a. The increase in frequency of oxalate urolithiasis in cats over the past 25 years does not seem to be related to changes in the age, breed, sex, or reproductive status of the cat population during this time.

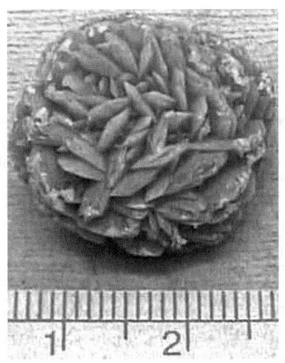

FIGURE 9-7 ■ Calcium oxalate stone from the urinary bladder of a dog removed at surgery. Note the jagged edges which are commonly seen in oxalates.

  b. Exclusive feeding of an acidifying diet without provision of different brands of food or table scraps is a strong risk factor for development of calcium oxalate urolithiasis in cats.
  c. Middle-aged to older cats usually are affected.
  d. Males (usually neutered) are affected more commonly than females.
  e. Persian, Himalayan, Ragdoll, Havana Brown, and Scottish Fold breeds are at increased risk for development of oxalate urolithiasis whereas Siamese and Abyssinian cats are at decreased risk.
  f. Cats kept indoors exclusively are at increased risk.
 4. Calcium oxalate stones are composed of calcium oxalate monohydrate (whewellite) or calcium oxalate dihydrate (weddellite). Oxalate often is not detected by qualitative analysis, and quantitative analysis of stones is necessary for reliable identification.
 5. Calcium oxalate calculi usually are white in color and very hard. They often have sharp, jagged edges and may be single or multiple in number. (see Figure 9-7.)
 6. Oxalate stones often are found in the bladder and urethra, but they also are the most common type of urolith found in the kidney and ureter of both dogs and cats. A 10-fold increase in urolithiasis in the upper urinary tract of cats has been reported over the past 25 years.
 7. The recurrence rate for oxalate urolithiasis is high (between 25 and 48%).
 8. Oxalate is derived both from the diet and endogenously from the metabolism of ascorbic acid (vitamin C) and the amino acid glycine. In human beings, increased dietary oxalate, increased gastrointestinal absorption of oxalate, vitamin B_6 deficiency, and inherited

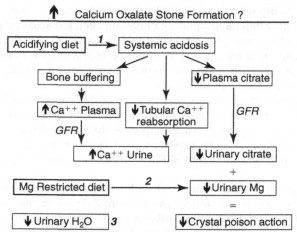

FIGURE 9-8 ■ Interaction of systemic acidosis, urinary calcium excretion, reduction in oxalate crystal poisons, and reduced urinary water—a working hypothesis to explain an increased frequency of calcium oxalate urolithiasis. *GFR*, glomerular filtration rate

defects of oxalate metabolism can predispose to development of calcium oxalate stones. The role of such factors in development of calcium oxalate stones in animals is not known.

9. Altered calcium metabolism may play a role in development of oxalate urolithiasis (Figure 9-8).

a. Increased urinary excretion of calcium (hypercalciuria) can result from increased absorption of calcium from the intestinal tract (*absorptive* hypercalciuria), from increased urinary loss of calcium (*renal leak* hypercalciuria), or from increased release of calcium from bone (*resorptive* hypercalciuria). In absorptive as compared to renal leak hypercalciuria, urinary calcium excretion is higher after feeding than during fasting.

b. In one study, miniature Schnauzers had higher urinary calcium excretion during fasting than did beagles and urinary calcium excretion increased 3-fold after feeding (i.e., hypercalciuria seemed to be absorptive).

c. Dogs or cats with hypercalcemia due to primary hyperparathyroidism may develop calcium oxalate or calcium phosphate uroliths due to parathyroid hormone-mediated mobilization of calcium from bone (resorptive hypercalciuria).

d. Chronic acidosis may be associated with increased urinary excretion of calcium due to increased calcium release from bone as a buffering mechanism. Long-term feeding of an acidifying diet may contribute to this resorptive hypercalciuria and may partially explain the increase in calcium oxalate urolithiasis in cats during the past 25 years (i.e., increased feeding of acidifying diets to prevent struvite urolithiasis). Decreased magnesium concentration in the urine also may contribute, because magnesium is a crystal inhibitor for calcium oxalate.

e. Dogs with hyperadrenocorticism are predisposed to development of calcium oxalate and calcium phosphate uroliths possibly as a result of decreased renal reabsorption of calcium (i.e., renal leak hypercalciuria) and effects that increase bone resorption of calcium (i.e., resorptive hypercalciuria).

f. Hypercalcemia occurs in approximately one third of cats with calcium oxalate stones, and idiopathic hypercalcemia in cats has become increasingly common in the past

15 years. Many cats with idiopathic hypercalcemia also have calcium oxalate stones. Affected cats often have a history of having been fed acidifying diets, and chronic subclinical acidosis may play a role in development of hypercalcemia, hypercalciuria, and calcium oxalate urolithiasis. High fiber diets and prednisone therapy have been used to manage cats with idiopathic hypercalcemia, but it is not yet clear if this approach decreases occurrence of urolithiasis.

10. Citrate forms a soluble complex with calcium and normally may be an inhibitor of calcium oxalate formation. Acidosis may be associated with decreased urinary citrate excretion and, thus, may predispose to calcium oxalate stone formation.

11. The role of diet in oxalate urolithiasis in dogs and cats is unclear. The following conclusions are based on recent studies of diet composition and risk of calcium oxalate urolithiasis:

   a. One predictor of stone mineral crystallization and growth is the degree of urine supersaturation with the crystalloid in question. Relative supersaturation (RSS) is the ratio of the activity product to the solubility product for stone-forming salts such as calcium oxalate and magnesium ammonium phosphate. RSS values of >1 indicate supersaturation and values of <1 indicate undersaturation. Computer programs have been developed to determine RSS using urine pH and the concentrations of various inorganic and organic urinary electrolytes (Robertson WG, et al. 2002).

   b. Higher RSS of urine with calcium oxalate has been observed in dogs with a history of forming calcium oxalate stones as compared with non–stone-forming dogs of similar age, breed, and sex (Stevenson AE, et al. 2003).

   c. In dogs, canned food diets with the highest amounts of protein, fat, calcium, phosphorus, magnesium, sodium, potassium, chloride, or moisture were associated with decreased risk of calcium oxalate urolithiasis. Canned food diets with the highest amount of carbohydrate were associated with increased risk of calcium oxalate urolithiasis (Lekcharoensuk C, et al. 2002).

   d. In cats, diets low in sodium or potassium or formulated to maximize urine acidity and those with moderate fat or carbohydrate content were associated with increased risk of calcium oxalate urolithiasis. Diets with high moisture or protein content and with moderate magnesium, phosphorus, or calcium contents were associated with decreased risk of calcium oxalate urolithiasis (Lekcharoensuk C, et al. 2001). Widespread use of acidifying diets in cats may play a role in development of urolithiasis in this species.

   e. RSS of urine with calcium oxalate was compared in normal miniature Schnauzers and Labrador retrievers fed a 7% moisture diet with 0.06 g sodium/100 kcal as compared to the same diet supplemented with water (73% moisture) or sodium (0.2 to 0.3 g sodium/100 kcal). Increased moisture decreased calcium oxalate RSS in the miniature Schnauzers but not in the Labrador retrievers. Increased sodium content decreased calcium oxalate RSS in both breeds (Stevenson AE, et al. 2003). This study contradicts previous concerns that diets with large amounts of sodium may facilitate calciuresis and predispose to calcium oxalate urolithiasis.

   f. In dogs, dry food diets with the lowest concentrations of sodium, phosphorus, calcium, chloride, protein, magnesium, or potassium were associated with increased risk of calcium oxalate urolithiasis. Diets with high urinary acidifying potential and low moisture content also were associated with increased risk of calcium oxalate urolithiasis (Lekcharoensuk C, et al. 2002).

   g. In a comparison of nutrient intake and urine composition in calcium oxalate stone-forming dogs as compared with healthy control dogs, stone-forming dogs had lower

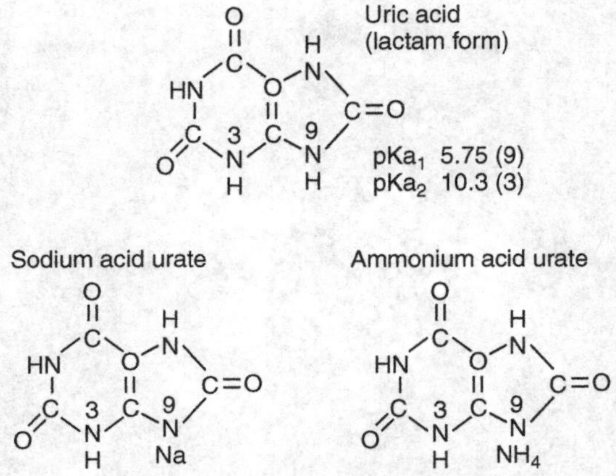

FIGURE 9-9 ■ Different forms of urate in urine.

intakes of sodium, calcium, potassium, and phosphorus and higher urinary calcium and oxalate concentrations, calcium excretion, and calcium oxalate RSS. Feeding Royal Canin's Urinary SO Diet for 1 month resulted in increased intake of moisture, sodium, and fat and decreased intake of potassium and calcium and decreased urinary concentrations of calcium and oxalate, calcium excretion, and calcium oxalate RSS (Stevenson AE, et al. 2004).

h. Although it may seem paradoxical that a low calcium diet would be associated with a higher risk of calcium oxalate urolithiasis, this increased risk presumably occurs because diets restricted in calcium but not oxalate can result in decreased formation of insoluble, poorly absorbed calcium oxalate complexes in the gastrointestinal tract. As a consequence, more oxalate is absorbed, leading to hyperoxaluria, which is a bigger risk factor for calcium oxalate urolithiasis than hypercalciuria alone.

i. Healthy beagle dogs were fed a canned diet designed to decrease calcium oxalate urolith recurrence (Hill's Prescription Diet u/d) with and without NaCl supplementation (1.2% versus 0.24% sodium on a dry matter basis). On the sodium-supplemented diet, 24-hour urine volume and calcium excretion increased, but there was no change in urine calcium concentration. Urine oxalate concentration and calcium oxalate RSS were lower on the NaCl supplemented diet. Hence, propensity to calcium oxalate crystallization was decreased on the NaCl-supplemented diet despite an increase in 24-hour urinary excretion of calcium (Lulich JP, et al. 2005).

j. The urine activity product for calcium oxalate was decreased in oxalate stone-forming cats after feeding a diet designed to prevent recurrence of calcium oxalate stones (Hill's Prescription Diet x/d).

12. UTI, when it occurs, is thought to be a complication rather than a predisposing factor to oxalate urolithiasis.

Urate Urolithiasis

1. Urate stones in dogs usually are composed of the monobasic ammonium salt of uric acid (ammonium acid urate) (Figure 9-9). In human beings, they usually are composed of uric acid. Urate stones found in dogs with portosystemic shunts often contain struvite in addition to urate.

2. Urate stones are found most often in the Dalmatian and English bulldog. Other breeds also may be affected (e.g., miniature Schnauzer, Yorkshire terrier, Shih tzu). Urate stones may be

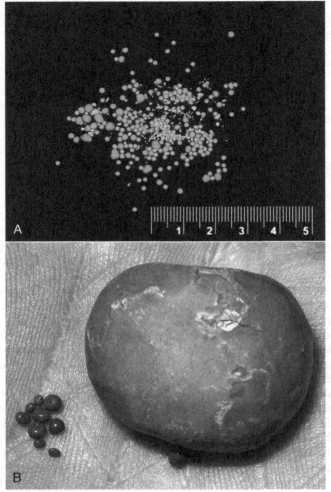

FIGURE 9-10 ■ **A,** Multiple small ammonium urate calculi removed from the bladder of a Dalmatian dog by voiding urophydropulsion. **B,** Several small and a few large urate calculi were removed from the bladder of a dog with a portosystemic shunt (PSS); the stones are shown in the palm of a hand.

found in dogs with portosystemic shunts, possibly due to reduced conversion of ammonia to urea and uric acid to allantoin. Urate stones generally occur uncommonly in cats.

3. Males are clinically affected much more commonly than females (especially in Dalmatians) possibly because the small stones become lodged in the urethra of males, leading to signs of urinary tract obstruction. Dalmatian dogs may be asymptomatic for their urate stones until an episode of obstruction occurs or the stones become quite large.

4. Urate calculi are small, brittle, spherical stones with concentric lamination. They usually are multiple in number and light yellow, brown, or green in color. (Figure 9-10.)

5. They are found most often in the bladder and urethra.

6. The recurrence rate for urate urolithiasis in the dog may be as high as 30% to 50%.

7. When it occurs, UTI is a complication of urate urolithiasis rather than a predisposing cause.

FIGURE 9-11 ■ Generation of xanthine, uric acid, and allantoin during purine metabolism. Allopurinol acts as a competitive inhibitor of the enzyme xanthine oxidase by virtue of its structural similarity to hypoxanthine.

8. A defect in uric acid metabolism in the Dalmatian dog is a predisposing factor for urate urolithiasis. This defect is a predisposing factor and not a primary cause of urolithiasis because Dalmatian dogs that do not develop stones also excrete large amounts of urate in their urine and other breeds (e.g., English bulldog) also may develop urate urolithiasis.
    a. Uric acid is derived from the metabolic degradation of purines (Figure 9-11).
    b. In dogs other than Dalmatians, uric acid is converted to allantoin in the liver by the enzyme uricase.
    c. Dalmatian dogs have higher plasma uric acid concentrations and excrete much more uric acid in their urine than do other dogs.
    d. The defect in uric acid metabolism in the Dalmatian is not caused by absence of hepatic uricase. The enzyme is present in the liver of Dalmatians in amounts comparable with those found in other breeds. Impaired transport of uric acid into hepatocytes may reduce the rate of hepatic oxidation in Dalmatians.
    e. The proximal tubules of Dalmatians appear to reabsorb less and secrete more urate than do the kidneys of other dogs, leading to increased urinary urate excretion.

Cystine Urolithiasis
1. Cystine stones are uncommon in dogs and rare in cats.
2. Cystine stones have been reported in many breeds of dog including English bulldogs, Newfoundlands, dachshunds, Irish terriers, Basset hounds, and bullmastiffs.
3. In most studies, cystine stones are found almost exclusively in male dogs. However, both male and female Newfoundlands are affected.
4. Affected dogs usually are middle-aged (4 to 6 years at presentation).
5. Canine cystinuria is an inherited disorder of renal tubular transport involving cystine or cystine plus other amino acids (often ornithine, lysine, and arginine). Not all dogs with cystinuria develop urolithiasis. Therefore, cystinuria is considered to be a predisposing rather than a primary causative factor.

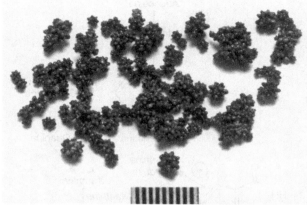

FIGURE 9-12 ■ Multiple silicate uroliths removed from the bladder of a dog. They characteristically have a *jack* like appearance.

6. Cystinuria is inherited as an autosomal recessive trait in the Newfoundland and is associated with a mutation in the *SLC3A1* amino acid transporter gene. Where tested in other breeds of dog with cystinuria, the *SLC3A1* gene was not involved, supporting the suspicion that cystinuria is genetically heterogenous in dogs as it is in humans.
7. Cystinuria decreases in severity with age (especially >5 years of age) in some affected dogs.
8. Cystine stones are composed entirely of cystine. Qualitative kits for stone analysis may give false positive reactions for cystine, which may have falsely increased the frequency of cystine stones in early surveys. Hence, quantitative analysis of stones is necessary.
9. They are small, spherical, and light yellow, brown, or green in color.
10. They occur most commonly in the bladder and urethra and usually are multiple.
11. The recurrence rate for cystine urolithiasis may be as high as 47% to 75%.
12. When it occurs, UTI usually is a complication of cystine urolithiasis rather than a predisposing cause.
13. Cystine crystals have a characteristic hexagonal shape, and when observed in urine should be considered abnormal.

Silicate Urolithiasis

1. Silicate urolithiasis is uncommon in dogs and extremely rare in cats.
2. These stones are composed primarily of silica (as silicon dioxide) but small amounts of other minerals such as struvite also may be present. Qualitative stone analysis kits do not detect silica, and quantitative analysis is necessary.
3. In dogs, silicate stones are gray-white or brownish and usually multiple in number. They frequently have a jack-like appearance. (Figure 9-12.) Not all silica stones have this jack-like appearance, however, and not all jack-stones are silicates. Urate and struvite stones also may have a jack-like appearance.
4. Silica stones usually are found in the bladder and urethra of affected dogs.
5. Silicate calculi occasionally recur following surgical removal.
6. The role of diet in spontaneously occurring silicate urolithiasis of dogs has not been determined, but diets high in corn gluten or soybean hulls are suspected to be contributory. An experimental atherogenic diet containing 12% silicic acid and 3% magnesium silicate resulted in silicate urolithiasis involving the kidneys, bladder, and urethra of dogs after as short a time as 4 months on the diet.

7. UTI, when it occurs, appears to be a complication of rather than a predisposing factor to silicate urolithiasis.
8. There is no clear relation between silica urolithiasis and urine pH.

SIGNALMENT

Struvite Calculi
1. Any breed of dog or cat, but increased risk in miniature Schnauzer, Bichon frise, Shih tzu, Lhasa apso, Yorkshire terrier.
2. Female dogs more commonly than males; no sex predilection in cats.
3. No age predilection (middle-aged but generally younger than those with oxalate calculi).
4. Calculi that occur in dogs younger than 1 year of age frequently are composed of struvite.

Oxalate Calculi
1. Any breed, but increased risk in miniature Schnauzer, Bichon frise, Shih tzu, Lhasa apso, Yorkshire terrier.
2. Persian and Himalayan cats.
3. Male dogs and cats more commonly than females.
4. No age predilection (generally older than those with struvite calculi).

Urate Calculi
1. Most common in Dalmatians and English bulldogs.
2. Male dogs more commonly than females; no sex predilection in cats.
3. No age predilection.
4. Young dogs with portosystemic shunts are predisposed to formation of urate stones and there is no sex predilection in this clinical setting.

Cystine Calculi
1. English bulldog, Newfoundland, dachshund, Irish terrier, Basset hound, bullmastiff, Rottweiler, and many other breeds; very rare in cats.
2. Male dogs much more commonly than females (except in Newfoundlands).
3. Young to middle-aged dogs.

Silicate Calculi
1. German Shepherds, Old English sheepdog, and many other breeds.
2. Male dogs much more commonly than females.
3. Middle-aged dogs.

HISTORY

A. The history in animals with urolithiasis depends on the anatomic location of the calculi, the duration of their presence, their physical features, the presence or absence of urinary tract obstruction and if present whether it is partial or complete, and the presence or absence of UTI. Risk of nephrolithiasis and ureterolithiasis is higher in cats than in dogs, where stones more often occur in the bladder.

Cystic (bladder) Calculi
1. No clinical signs.
2. Signs of bladder inflammation or infection (e.g., dysuria, increased frequency of urination, hematuria).

Urethral Calculi
1. Urethral obstruction in the male (urethral obstruction is rare in females).
   a. Frequent unsuccessful attempts to urinate.
   b. Passage of very small amounts of urine (paradoxical overflow of urine).
   c. Dribbling of urine.
   d. Nonspecific signs of postrenal azotemia (e.g., lethargy, anorexia, vomiting).
2. Signs of urethral inflammation.
   a. Dysuria.
   b. Increased frequency of urination.
   c. Hematuria.

Renal Calculi
1. No clinical signs.
2. Painless hematuria.
3. Signs of pyelonephritis or pyonephrosis.
   a. Anorexia.
   b. Lethargy.
   c. Fever.
   d. Polyuria/polydipsia.
   e. Flank pain.
4. Nonspecific signs of primary renal azotemia if there has been sufficient destruction of renal parenchyma (e.g., bilateral renal calculi).

Ureteral Calculi
1. Ureteral calculi are uncommon in dogs but have become much more commonly diagnosed in cats in the past 10 years.
2. May have no clinical signs.
3. Flank pain associated with acute ureteral obstruction and hydronephrosis is most likely to be observed in dogs.
4. In most cats with ureteral calculi, signs are nonspecific and include anorexia, vomiting, lethargy, and weight loss.
5. Ureteral calculi are identified by radiographs or ultrasound in 90% of affected cats.
6. Ureteral obstruction is identified in 92% of cats with ureteral calculi.
7. Most cats with ureteral calculi are azotemic even when calculi are unilateral, indicating presence of renal disease in the contralateral kidney. This suspicion is confirmed by ultrasound examination.
8. On quantitative analysis, 98% of ureteral calculi removed from affected cats were calcium oxalate stones.
9. Only 8% of affected cats had positive urine cultures.
10. Ureteroliths in dogs may be struvite, calcium oxalate, or calcium phosphate, and UTI is common with struvite calculi.

PHYSICAL EXAMINATION FINDINGS DEPEND ON THE LOCATION OF THE CALCULI

Urinary Bladder
1. Palpable stones.
   a. May be difficult to palpate if the bladder is distended with urine. Palpation should be repeated when the bladder is empty.
   b. Many small stones palpated in the bladder will create a "crepitant" sensation.
   c. Thickened bladder wall.

Urethra

1. Large, distended bladder suggestive of urethral obstruction.
2. Detection of a stone on rectal palpation of the urethra, external palpation of the perineal urethra, and evaluation of the penile urethra (especially just proximal to the os penis).
3. If the bladder has ruptured before presentation, the diagnosis may be confused by inability to palpate the bladder. In this instance, pain and tenderness may be noted on abdominal palpation in small animals.

Kidney

1. Renomegaly if there is obstruction at the renal pelvis causing hydronephrosis or pyonephrosis.
2. Physical examination findings compatible with uremia if there has been sufficient destruction of renal parenchyma.
3. No abnormal physical findings.

Ureter

1. Renomegaly due to hydronephrosis or pyonephrosis.
2. Pain and tenderness on abdominal palpation due to uroabdomen if the ureter has ruptured.
3. No abnormal physical findings.

DIAGNOSIS

Urinalysis

Urine Sediment Findings Often Indicate Inflammation or Infection

a. Pyuria.
b. Hematuria.
c. Proteinuria.
d. Bacteriuria.

Urine pH Is Variable

a. In dogs with struvite calculi and UTI due to a urease-positive organism, the urine pH often is alkaline.
b. The urine pH may be acidic in dogs with cystine stones.
c. The urine pH is variable in dogs with oxalate, silicate, and urate stones.
d. The urine pH of dogs with metabolic stones (e.g., urate, cystine, oxalate) may be alkaline if a urease-positive UTI is present.

Crystals

a. Cystine crystals are not found in normal urine samples, but the presence of struvite, oxalate, or urate crystals is not necessarily pathologic.

> **!** Crystalluria may be found in animals without urolithiasis and may be absent in animals with urolithiasis.
> The crystals present in the urine sediment may differ from the composition of the uroliths.

b. Struvite crystals have a "coffin-lid" appearance.
c. Calcium oxalate monohydrate crystals have a "picket fence" appearance whereas calcium oxalate dehydrate crystals have a "Maltese cross" or "square envelope" appearance.
d. Urate crystals have a "thornapple" appearance.
e. Cystine crystals are flat and hexagonal in shape but can be confused with struvite, which have more of a three-dimensional appearance.

Microbiology

1. Urine culture and sensitivity should be performed in animals with urolithiasis to detect presence of UTI and formulate appropriate antibiotic therapy.
2. In dogs, UTI by a urease-positive organism (usually staphylococci or *Proteus* sp) typically accompanies struvite urolithiasis.
3. In cats with struvite urolithiasis, urine cultures usually are negative.
4. In animals with urate, cystine, oxalate, and silicate stones, UTI is a complication of urolithiasis rather than a predisposing cause.
5. If bacteriologic culture is negative on a urine sample obtained by cystocentesis, culture of the bladder wall and the center of the calculus may provide more accurate assessment of the bacteriologic status of the urinary tract.

Blood Count

1. Complete blood count (CBC) usually is normal in uncomplicated cases of urolithiasis. If pyelonephritis or pyonephrosis is present, leukocytosis with a left shift may be observed.

Serum Biochemistry

1. Increased blood urea nitrogen (BUN), creatinine, and phosphorus concentrations will be present if there is postrenal azotemia secondary to urinary tract obstruction. Primary renal azotemia may occur if there has been sufficient renal parenchymal destruction due to bilateral hydronephrosis, pyonephrosis, or pyelonephritis.

Stone Analysis

1. An educated guess ("guesstimate") about a urolith's composition can be made based on signalment, diet, urine culture results, urine pH, and radiographic density of the urolith, but such "guesstimates" can be inaccurate (especially considering the two most common urolith types are both radiodense). Consequently, it is recommended to submit all removed uroliths for laboratory analysis. In animals with recurrent urolithiasis, the current urolith may differ from the type previously identified (e.g., xanthine urolith in a dog with previous urate urolithiasis treated with allopurinol; struvite urolith in a dog with previous oxalate urolithiasis). Although not optimal, "guesstimates" of urolith composition may be necessary in patients that are treated without surgical intervention.
2. Uroliths should never be placed in 10% formalin, because doing so prevents accurate quantitative analysis.
3. In the past, qualitative analysis of stones using commercial kits was commonly performed. Unfortunately, such kits often yield inaccurate results.
   a. Xanthine and silicate are not detected.
   b. Oxalate frequently is not detected.
   c. False-positive results may occur for cystine and urate.
   d. Detection of secondary mineral components and failure to identify the primary crystalloid will cause confusion and may lead to inappropriate therapy.
   e. With qualitative analysis there is no way to tell which minerals constitute the primary component and which are secondary.
4. For these reasons, quantitative analysis by optical crystallography is recommended for routine analysis.
5. The nucleus of the stone as well as its outer shell should be analyzed. Primary metabolic stones may have an outer covering of struvite, which could lead to confusion if only the outer portion of the stone were analyzed.

IMAGING OF THE URINARY TRACT: RADIOGRAPHY AND ULTRASONOGRAPHY

A. Radiodensity
  1. Calcium phosphate, calcium oxalate, struvite, and silicate calculi are the most radiodense.
  2. Cystine and urate calculi are the least radiodense.
  3. In many instances, calculi will be dense enough to be observed on plain radiographs after proper patient preparation (e.g., enemas to remove fecal material). Calculi as small as 3 to 4 mm can be observed radiographically if they are sufficiently radiodense.
  4. If there is a clinical suspicion of urolithiasis but calculi cannot be observed on plain radiographs, positive or double-contrast radiographic studies should be performed. Calculi usually will appear lucent when surrounded by the denser contrast agent.
B. Although calculi occur more commonly in the bladder and urethra of the dog and cat, a radiographic evaluation of the entire urinary tract is recommended to rule out renal or ureteral calculi.
C. Care should be taken not to confuse blood clots and bubbles of air for lucent calculi on contrast studies of the bladder and urethra.
D. Objects that may cause confusion during radiographic interpretation:
  1. Teats in female dogs.
  2. Radiodense material in the gastrointestinal tract.
  3. Calcified mesenteric lymph nodes or adrenal glands.
E. Ultrasound examination of the urinary tract may identify uroliths that are not radiodense. Ultrasonography provides evaluation of only the most proximal portion of the urethra, and thus should not be used in place of plain and contrast radiography of the urethra. In general, ultrasound examination is more sensitive and less specific than radiography for identification of uroliths.
F. Ultrasonography of the ureter and kidneys is useful to determine the presence or absence of urinary tract obstruction in patients with uroliths. Obstruction can be identified when hydroureter, hydronephrosis, or pyelectasia is observed. In cats, administration of furosemide (1-3 mg/kg IV) will increase urine flow and can facilitate visualization of a dilated renal pelvis or ureters.

GENERAL PRINCIPLES OF MANAGEMENT

A. Relief of lower urinary tract obstruction and re-establishment of urine flow.
  1. Decompressive cystocentesis can be used to decrease bladder pressure opposing the passage of a urinary catheter.
  2. Pass a well-lubricated, small diameter catheter alongside and beyond the obstructing urethral calculus and into the bladder.
  3. A technique of retrograde urohydropulsion has been described for dislodgement of urethral calculi in both male and female dogs. This technique involves fluid distension of the urethra around the obstructing calculus using a combination of sterile saline and lubricating gel (Figure 9-13).
  4. If these techniques fail, repeated decompressive cystocentesis may be needed, or emergency urethrotomy may be performed after medical stabilization.
B. Correction of fluid, electrolyte, and acid-base imbalances associated with obstruction and postrenal azotemia (see Chapter 11, Obstructive Uropathy and Nephropathy). Medical treatment of cats with ureteral calculi (fluid administration to promote diuresis) usually is of limited effectiveness.

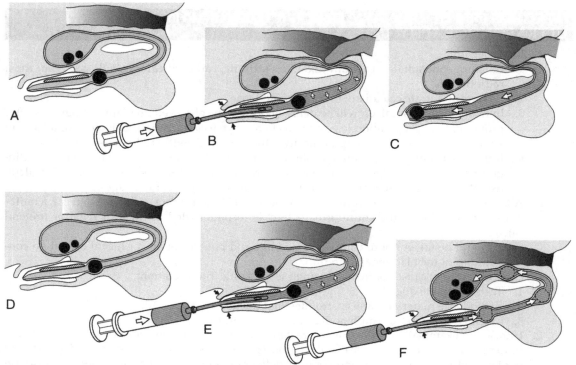

FIGURE 9-13 ■ Retrograde urohydropropulsion to move urethral stones into the bladder. Retropulsion of urethral calculus into urinary bladder of male dog. **A,** Calculus lodged in urethra. **B,** Passage of a standard urinary catheter into the distal urethra accompanied by digital occlusion of the urethra around the catheter by a gloved finger per rectum. **C,** Dilatation of urethra and explusion of urethral calculus after injection of sterile irrigating solution under pressure followed by removal of catheter. **D,** Calculus lodged in urethra. **E,** Passage of a standard urinary catheter into the dista urethra accompained by digital occlusion of the urethra around the catheter by a gloved finger per rectum. **F,** Urethrolith has been successfully retropulsed into the urinary bladder. (Drawn by Tim Vojt.)

C. Nonsurgical retrieval of calculi for analysis or treatment.
   1. Voiding urohydropulsion of bladder stones (Figure 9-14).
      a. Stones should be small: <7 mm in female dogs, <5 mm in male dogs, <5 mm in female cats, and <1 mm in male cats.
      b. Procedure should be performed under general anesthesia.
      c. The bladder is distended with sterile saline administered via a cystourethroscope (preferable) or transurethral catheter (largest diameter possible).
      d. The catheter or cystourethroscope then is removed. The following procedure requires two operators: Hold the animal vertically relative to the table. Shake bladder. Apply steady digital pressure transabdominally to induce micturition. Maintain pressure on abdomen to facilitate flow and keep urethra dilated. Repeat as necessary until no more uroliths are expelled.
      e. Take abdominal radiographs to verify removal of stones.
      f. Submit stones for analysis.
      g. Complications.
         (1) Hematuria (common).
         (2) Stones lodged in urethra.
         (3) Bladder rupture (rare, but increased risk if previous bladder surgery).

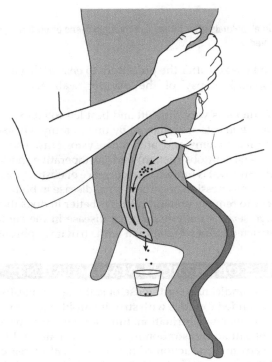

FIGURE 9-14 ■ Technique for voiding urohydropropulsion of small urinary stones. This technique is especially effective in female dogs and cats. The patient is held vertically by an assistant and then the bladder (which has been filled with sterile saline by catheter) is expressed with digital pressure to expell small stones that fall by gravity from the bladder, into the urethra, and out into the container. Based on technique developed by Dr. Jody Lulich. (Drawn by Tim Vojt.)

2. Small stones in the bladder of male dogs also can be collected for analysis using catheter-assisted retrieval even if larger cystic calculi cannot be removed. Quantitative analysis of removed stones allows the clinician to determine whether or not medical dissolution is likely to be successful and to design stone-specific prevention protocols.

3. Lithotripsy can be used to break up stones in dogs and facilitate their removal from the urinary tract. This technique requires specialized equipment and expertise not available to most veterinarians. During intracorporeal laser lithotripsy, the photoacoustic effects of the laser create cavitation bubbles in the urolith that in turn generate shock waves when they collapse and cause the stone to fragment. This procedure is used for urethral and bladder calculi. In extracorporeal shock wave lithotripsy the shock waves are generated outside of the body and directed at the uroliths through water while the patient is partially submerged in a water bath. This procedure usually is used for nephroliths and ureteroliths. Some transient renal injury (e.g., hemorrhage) occurs during this procedure. Stone fragments that enter the ureters usually pass into the bladder without complications. Cystine nephroliths are resistant to fragmentation.

SURGICAL REMOVAL OF CALCULI

A. At the time of surgery, a search for any predisposing anatomic abnormalities (e.g., urachal diverticulum) or foreign bodies (e.g., suture material, catheter fragments) should be made and such abnormalities corrected.

> **!** Radiographs should be taken in all animals after removal of multiple cystic or urethral calculi to confirm that all stones have been removed.

B. Radiographs should be taken after the procedure to ensure that all stones were removed.

C. Culture, sensitivity, and biopsy of the bladder wall also may be performed at this time.

D. Surgery of the feline ureter is very difficult and best left to an experienced soft tissue surgeon. Proximal ureteral calculi in cats are removed by ureterotomy whereas distal ureteral calculi are removed by partial ureterectomy and ureteroneocystostomy. The complication rate was 31% (e.g., urine leakage, persistent obstruction) and postoperative mortality was 18% in one large study of affected cats. Survival is limited by recurrence of obstruction postoperatively and by the common presence and progression of chronic renal disease in both kidneys.

E. Survival after surgery to remove ureteral calculi is better in dogs than in cats and affected dogs do not typically have serious underlying renal disease in the contralateral kidney. However infection of the obstructed kidney is common with struvite nephroliths or ureteroliths.

GENERAL PRINCIPLES OF MEDICAL MANAGEMENT

A. Unless there is a contraindication for the use of salt (e.g., congestive heart failure), induction of polyuria is recommended for dogs with struvite urolithiasis to reduce urine specific gravity (USG) and increase frequency of urination, thus reducing the concentration of crystalloids in the urine. The role of salt administration in calcium oxalate urolithiasis is unclear. Although there has been concern that induction of natriuresis will increase calciuresis, some studies have shown that high sodium intake is associated with decreased risk of calcium oxalate urolithiasis. There also has been concern that natriuresis may increase urinary excretion of cystine.

1. Sodium chloride is added to the diet at an empirical dosage of 0.5 to 10 g/day depending upon the size of the dog (one teaspoon of table salt is approximately equivalent to 6 g NaCl).

2. The aim is to reduce the USG to <1.025 or to double urine output.

3. The animal should be allowed frequent opportunities to void to prevent bladder distension and urine stasis.

4. Controlled studies designed specifically to assess the effectiveness of salt therapy in the prevention of urolithiasis in dogs or cats are not available but some experimental studies of urine in normal cats and dogs suggest increased salt intake may be useful as a prevention strategy.

B. All dogs with urolithiasis should have their urine cultured. If UTI is present, appropriate antibiotic therapy and careful follow-up should be instituted to ensure elimination of infection.

MEDICAL MANAGEMENT OF INDIVIDUAL STONE TYPES

Struvite Stones

1. Because of the primary role of UTI by urease-positive organisms in struvite urolithiasis of dogs, careful elimination of infection by appropriate antibiotic therapy and repeated patient follow-up to demonstrate eradication of infection are the most important aspects of medical management to prevent recurrence.

2. The use of urinary acidifiers to maintain urine pH in the range of 6.0 to 6.5 has been suggested in dogs because struvite and hydroxyapatite are most soluble in acidic urine. In most dogs with struvite urolithiasis, eradication of UTI will return urine pH to

the acidic range. Use of urinary acidifiers in the face of infection by a urease-positive organism is not useful. If urine pH remains alkaline after elimination of UTI, other potential causes (e.g., dietary, familial, metabolic) of alkaline urine should be investigated. In cats with struvite urolithiasis without UTI, urinary acidifiers may play a more important role. Many commercial cat foods have been reformulated to reduce urine pH. Urine acidifiers should only be given to cats with urine pH of >6.5 measured under ad libitum feeding conditions. Addition of acidifying compounds to cat foods may have contributed to the increased incidence of calcium oxalate stones in this species over the past 25 years.

3. One calculolytic diet (Prescription Diet Canine s/d, Hill's Pet Products, Topeka, Kans.) has been used successfully to induce dissolution of struvite calculi in dogs.
   a. S/d for dogs is low in phosphorus and magnesium, and high in sodium chloride.
   b. It is low in protein to reduce urea availability to urease-positive organisms capable of converting urea to ammonia and carbon dioxide.
   c. The diet promotes undersaturation of the urine with ions necessary for formation of struvite uroliths and, thus, promotes dissolution of existing struvite calculi.
   d. The added NaCl induces diuresis and dilution of urine. Additional salt should not be added to the diet of the dog unless diuresis does not occur on s/d.
   e. Concurrent antibiotic therapy is recommended to eradicate UTI.
   f. In dogs with struvite uroliths and UTI, dissolution is expected to take 2 to 3 months. The diet is used for 1 month beyond radiographic evidence of urolith dissolution.
   g. The following clinical and laboratory findings are expected in dogs on s/d diet:
      (1) Polyuria/polydipsia and dilute urine (urine specific gravities as low as 1.010 can be expected in animals being fed s/d diet).
      (2) Decreased BUN is expected soon after starting to feed s/d diet.
      (3) Increased alkaline phosphatase (hepatic isoenzyme) may occur after several weeks of feeding s/d diet.
      (4) Decreased serum phosphorus concentration.
      (5) Decreased serum albumin may occur after weeks to months of feeding s/d diet.
   h. The clinician can make an educated guess (i.e., "guesstimate") as to the likelihood that a given stone is composed of struvite based on finding a urease-positive UTI (usually staphylococci), alkaline urine, struvite crystalluria, and radiodense calculus.
   i. Certain precautions should be observed when considering use of canine s/d diet. Canine s/d should not be fed to cats because of its extremely low protein content, nor should it be fed to growing puppies or to pregnant or lactating bitches. Occasionally, nephroliths that have decreased in size after institution of s/d diet may pass into the ureter causing ureteral obstruction and hydronephrosis.
   j. Feline s/d diet (an acidifying diet with a higher protein content than Canine s/d diet but restricted magnesium content and supplemental sodium) has been used successfully to dissolve stones in cats with struvite urolithiasis.
      (1) The average time for dissolution of sterile struvite stones in affected cats fed Feline s/d was about 30 days.
      (2) Treatment was successful in 93% of cases in one study.
      (3) Dissolution in cats with UTI and struvite stones (an uncommon occurrence) took longer (60-90 days).

         (4) Urinary acidifiers should not be given to cats fed c/d, s/d, or soft-moist diets because these foods already are acidified.

    k. Similar results (i.e., dissolution of struvite cystic calculi within 30 days in 31/39 cats) recently were obtained using canned and dry formulations of an acidifying, magnesium-restricted diet manufactured by Veterinary Medical Diets (Guelph, Ontario, Canada).

Oxalate Stones (Figure 9-15)

  1. Attempts to dissolve calcium oxalate stones in dogs and cats so far have been unsuccessful and surgery or voiding urohydropulsion typically is used to remove these stones.

  2. Several dietary recommendations have been considered in attempts to prevent recurrence of calcium oxalate urolithiasis.

    a. *Water*: Diets with high water content are associated with decreased risk of calcium oxalate urolithiasis. Thus, high moisture diets are preferred over dry formulations. High moisture diets promote production of an increased volume of urine with decreased concentration of calculogenic crystalloids.

    b. *Calcium*: Based on theoretical considerations, a diet low in calcium and oxalate may be helpful. Diets restricted in calcium but not oxalate, however, may be associated with hyperoxaluria and increased risk of calcium oxalate urolithiasis. Nondietary calcium supplements (given between meals) have minimal effect on gastrointestinal absorption of oxalate and may increase the risk of calcium oxalate urolithiasis by contributing to hypercalciuria. Some studies have shown a decreased risk of calcium oxalate urolithiasis in dogs consuming diets high in calcium and an increased risk in dogs consuming diets low in calcium. Also, in one study, stone-forming dogs had lower calcium intake than non-stone-forming dogs. The higher calcium diet may allow insoluble calcium oxalate to form in the gastrointestinal tract and avoid absorption. Thus, the role of dietary calcium in calcium oxalate urolithiasis is uncertain.

    c. *Oxalates*: Dietary ingredients (e.g., spinach, soy beans, sardines, sweet potatoes, asparagus, tofu) rich in oxalate should be avoided.

    d. *Phosphorus*: Dietary phosphorus should not be restricted because reduced phosphorus could result in increased activation of vitamin D_3 to calcitriol by 1-α-hydroxylase in the kidney and cause increased intestinal absorption of calcium. Also, urinary pyrophosphate may function as an inhibitor of calcium oxalate formation.

    e. *Magnesium*: Dietary magnesium should not be restricted because it may serve as an inhibitor of calcium oxalate formation.

    f. *Sodium*: Increased dietary sodium may be associated with increased urinary excretion of calcium. The additional dietary sodium, however, increases urine volume, and limits any increase in urinary calcium concentration that would otherwise occur.

    g. *Potassium*: Diets with higher potassium content may be associated with decreased risk of calcium oxalate urolithiasis due to decreased urinary excretion of calcium and formation of potassium oxalate salts in the urine, which are more soluble than calcium oxalate.

    h. *Protein*: A diet with less animal protein may be beneficial because a diet high in animal protein may be acidifying and could promote bone loss of calcium.

    i. *Citrate*: Supplementation of the diet with citrate may be helpful because urinary citrate may complex with calcium to form calcium citrate, which is much more soluble than calcium oxalate. It is unclear if urinary citrate excretion can be increased in dogs and cats using conventional dosages of citrate. The alkalinizing effect of citrate, however,

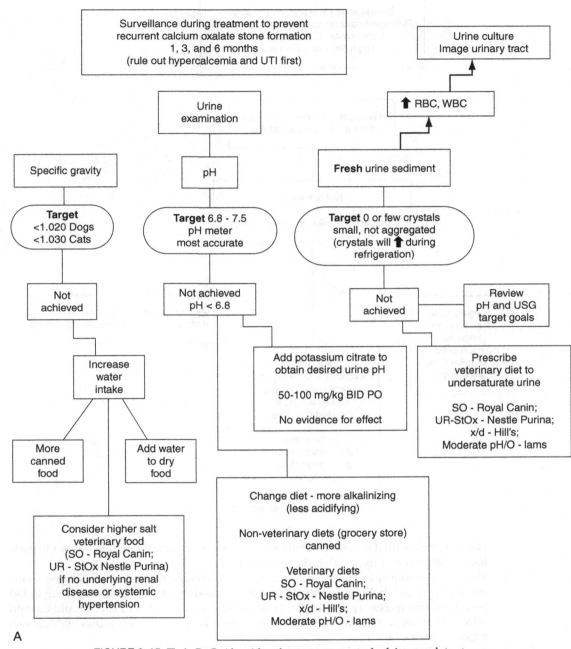

FIGURE 9-15 ■ **A, B, C,** Algorithm for management of calcium oxalate stones.

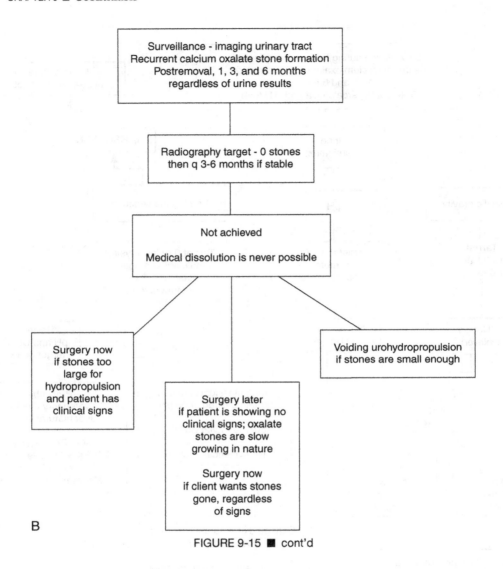

FIGURE 9-15 ■ cont'd

also may be useful if chronic acidosis associated with an acidifying diet has led to bone loss of calcium and hypercalciuria (see later).

j. *Vitamins*: Avoidance of excessive amounts of vitamin C is recommended because ascorbic acid is a metabolic precursor of oxalate. Excessive vitamin D should be avoided because it will increase gastrointestinal absorption of calcium. The diet should contain adequate amounts of vitamin B_6 because vitamin B_6 deficiency promotes endogenous production of oxalate.

3. Commercial diets that have been used in attempts to prevent recurrence of oxalate stones include Hill's Prescription Diets u/d, k/d, w/d and x/d. Prescription Diet u/d often is recommended for dogs with a history of oxalate urolithiasis. U/d reduced both calcium and oxalate excretion in dogs in one study. It is important to reduce both calcium and oxalate in the diet because reduction of calcium alone may result in increased gastrointestinal

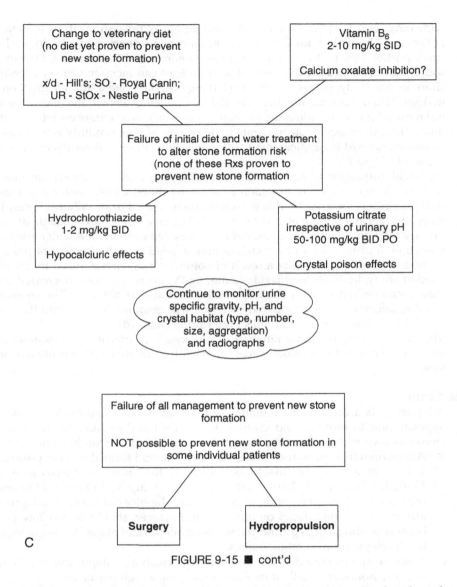

C

FIGURE 9-15 ■ cont'd

absorption of oxalate due to insufficient calcium in the diet to bind with oxalate and form non-absorbable calcium oxalate complexes. Urinary SO Diet (Royal Canin, St. Charles, Mo.) has been designed to undersaturate the urine with struvite and promote dissolution of struvite uroliths while at the same time decreasing RSS for calcium oxalate and helping to prevent recurrence of calcium oxalate urolithiasis. Purina also makes veterinary diets designed to manage struvite (Purina UR, Nestlé Purina Pet Care, St. Louis, Mo.) and struvite or oxalate (Purina UR St/Ox) urolithiasis in cats.

4. Administration of citrate as potassium citrate has been recommended because urinary citrate may act as an inhibitor of calcium oxalate aggregation and its alkalinizing effect may reduce bone release of calcium. Beyond this effect, therapeutic manipulation of urine pH is not known to be beneficial because oxalate solubility is relatively unaffected by a

wide range of urine pH. The recommended dosage of potassium citrate is 50 to 75 mg/kg PO every 12 hours but this dosage may not increase urinary citrate in dogs where a very small portion (1% to 3%) of filtered citrate is eliminated in the urine. Do not substitute sodium citrate because the increased sodium load can increase urinary excretion of calcium. In one study, potassium citrate (150 mg/kg/day) had a limited effect on urine pH in dogs. This dosage did not affect the RSS of calcium oxalate in the urine of normal dogs but reduced it in three miniature Schnauzers and increased citrate excretion in these three dogs. Thus, the specific role of citrate in dogs with oxalate urolithiasis is unclear but Prescription Diet u/d is supplemented with potassium citrate and results in slightly alkaline urine (pH 7.0 to 7.5).

5. Hydrochlorothiazide (2 mg/kg PO every 12 hours) reduced urinary calcium excretion with no change in oxalate excretion in dogs. Its diuretic effect also caused increases in sodium, potassium, and chloride excretion and increased urine volume. It may be used in dogs and cats at a dosage of 2 to 4 mg/kg PO twice a day. Chlorothiazide did not reduce urinary calcium excretion in dogs, but dogs were fed canned food with added water. The reduction in urine calcium by thiazides may depend on enhancement of proximal tubular reabsorption of calcium as a result of volume contraction induced by the diuretic. In another study, hydrochlorothiazide (2 mg/kg PO every 12 hours) decreased urinary calcium excretion in dogs with a history of calcium oxalate urolithiasis. The greatest decrease in urine calcium concentration and excretion was obtained in dogs simultaneously fed a low calcium, low protein diet (Hill's Prescription Diet u/d).

6. Vitamin B_6 promotes transamination of glyoxylate (a precursor of oxalate) to glycine, but it is unknown if it is valuable to administer it to an animal that is not deficient in this vitamin.

Urate Stones

1. Allopurinol is a competitive inhibitor of the enzyme xanthine oxidase which converts hypoxanthine to xanthine and xanthine to uric acid in the course of purine metabolism. One of its own metabolites, oxypurinol, also is an inhibitor of xanthine oxidase.
   a. Allopurinol therapy reduces the amount of uric acid formed from hypoxanthine.
   b. It is recommended in dissolution protocols for urate urolithiasis at a dosage of 15 mg/kg PO every 12 hours. A dosage of 5 to 10 mg/kg PO every 12 hours has been recommended for prevention of recurrence. The bioavailability of allopurinol is not affected by feeding. Dogs on allopurinol, however, should be fed low purine diets because feeding a high purine diet while on allopurinol places the dog at increased risk for development of xanthine stones.
   c. Xanthine stones may develop in some dogs receiving allopurinol at >15 mg/kg PO every 12 hours, especially if they are consuming a high purine diet.
   d. Xanthine stones also have been reported to occur spontaneously as a familial trait (suspected autosomal recessive) in Cavalier King Charles spaniels, possibly due to a defect in xanthine oxidase. Rare sporadic case reports also exist in other dog breeds (dachshund) and in a cat.
   e. Adverse effects of allopurinol administration in dogs are extremely rare (e.g., immune-mediated reactions).
   f. The dosage of allopurinol should be reduced in the presence of renal failure, because it is excreted by the kidneys.
2. The usefulness of $NaHCO_3$ therapy in urate urolithiasis is uncertain.
   a. Most urate calculi in dogs are composed of ammonium acid urate and rarely of uric acid. In humans, most urate stones are uric acid. Uric acid becomes more soluble in alkaline urine, but urate becomes less soluble.

    b. Hydrogen and ammonium ions contribute to growth of ammonium urate crystals in urine. Administration of $NaHCO_3$ or potassium citrate increases urine pH and decreases urinary ammonium ion concentration.

    c. If additional urine alkalinization is required, potassium citrate (100-150 mg/kg PO every 12 hours) may be preferable to sodium bicarbonate because of concern that natriuresis will enhance calciuresis.

3. A diet low in organ-derived meats reduces the ingested purine load because organ-derived products are rich in nucleic acids, which are the metabolic precursors of purines. Feeding a low protein, low purine diet has been shown to reduce urinary excretion of urate in normal dogs.

4. A 10% to 11% casein-based low protein, low purine diet containing potassium citrate as an alkalinizing agent without supplemental sodium (Hill's Prescription Diet u/d) has been studied extensively in normal dogs and is recommended for dissolution of urate stones and prevention of recurrence.

    a. U/d Diet (compared to p/d Diet) decreases urinary excretion of uric acid, ammonia, and titratable acid and increases urinary excretion of bicarbonate resulting in an alkaline urine pH of 7.0 to 7.5 (vs. 6.0 to 6.5 in dogs fed Hill's p/d).

    b. Successful use of this diet should eliminate urate crystals from the urine sediment. Owner compliance can be identified by finding BUN of <10 mg/dL, USG of <1.020, and urine pH >7.0 in the treated dog.

    c. The protein content of u/d is very low and it should not be used in pregnant or lactating bitches, and it should be avoided in immature growing dogs. In young growing dogs, surgery is recommended for removal of urate uroliths.

    d. U/d diet is very low in protein, and serum albumin concentration, body weight and body condition score should be monitored in patients fed this diet to evaluate for development of protein depletion.

    e. Also, low purine diets should not be used in English bulldogs, because of the risk of developing dilated cardiomyopathy (this rarely may occur in Dalmatians as well). It is hypothesized that English bulldogs with urate stones may also have defective renal reabsorption of cystine and carnitine and that carnitine deficiency may contribute to the development of dilated cardiomyopathy.

    f. Treatment of dogs with urate stones using Prescription Diet u/d and allopurinol results in complete dissolution in 33% of affected dogs, partial dissolution in 33%, and no dissolution in 33%.

    g. Time to dissolution ranges from 1 to 10 months with an average of between 3 and 4 months.

    h. Success of the dissolution protocol in dogs with urate stones and portosystemic shunts is less clear.

    i. During attempted dissolution, the size of the urate stones should be monitored by double contrast cystourethrography, and male dogs should be monitored for development of urethral obstruction that could occur as stones become smaller.

5. The preventive protocol for dogs with a history of urate urolithiasis involves feeding the low purine, low protein alkalinizing diet (Prescription Diet u/d) and monitoring patient response (i.e., urate crystals in the urine sediment, urine pH, USG). If crystals still are seen in the urine sediment, allopurinol can be added at a dosage of 5 to 10 mg/kg PO every 12 hours. It is important to continue the low purine diet while the dog is on allopurinol so as to avoid development of xanthine stones.

6. UTI is a common complication of urate urolithiasis and may occur in up to 33% of affected dogs. UTI should be treated by appropriate antibiotic therapy and eradication of UTI should be documented by follow-up urine cultures.

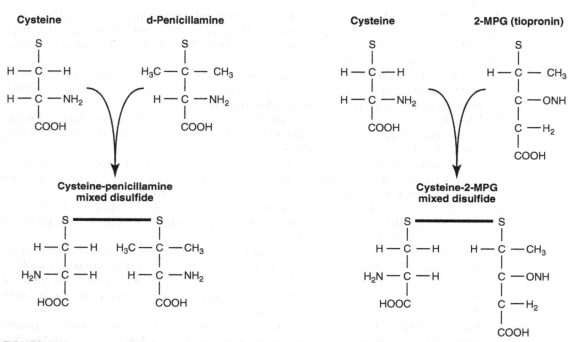

FIGURE 9-16 ■ D-penicillamine and 2-MPG interactions with cysteine that increase its solubility in urine. (Drawn by Tim Vojt.)

7. The low protein, low purine diet (Prescription Diet u/d) results in increased urine output and decreased USG presumably due to decreased concentrating ability resulting from reduced renal medullary urea content. Thus, additional sodium usually is not necessary to increase urine output. Increased sodium can increase urinary excretion of calcium, which is not desirable (increased risk of calcium oxalate, sodium calcium urate, or ammonium calcium urate stones).

8. In one study, male dogs with urate urolithiasis that were treated by cystotomy for stone removal followed by scrotal urethrostomy and dietary modification had the best outcome in terms of recurrent clinical signs.

Cystine Stones (Figure 9-16)
Thiol Disulfide Exchange Drugs (D-Penicillamine, 2-MPG)
a. D-penicillamine forms a disulfide with cysteine and, thus, reduces the cystine content of urine.

(1) Cysteine-penicillamine mixed disulfide is 50 times more soluble than cystine in the urine. D-penicillamine is administered at a dosage of 15 mg/kg PO twice a day and is most effective at neutral to alkaline urine pH.

(2) The major side effect in dogs is vomiting. Giving the drug with food, using anti-emetics, or reducing the dosage slightly (10 to 20 mg/kg/day) may prevent this adverse effect.

(3) Many toxic side effects have been observed in humans including fever, rash, proteinuria, and blood dyscrasias, but these have not been reported in the dog.

(4) D-penicillamine has an antipyridoxine (vitamin B_6) effect and has been reported to adversely affect wound healing by interfering with collagen cross-linking.

b. 2-mercaptopropionylglycine (2-MPG, tiopronin).

(1) 2-MPG acts by a thiol disulfide exchange reaction similar to that of D-penicillamine.

(2) 2-MPG also has adverse effects in dogs (about 13% of treated dogs). The most disturbing include aggressiveness, myopathy, and proteinuria, thrombocytopenia, and anemia (immune-mediated type reaction). Other adverse effects include skin lesions (pustules, dry crusty nose), increases in liver function tests (enzymes, bile acids), lethargy, and a sulfur smell to the urine. Adverse effects disappear when the drug is discontinued.

(3) 2-MPG can be used at a dosage of 15 to 20 mg/kg PO every 12 hours to dissolve cystine stones. Dissolution occurs in 60% of treated dogs and takes between 1 and 3 months. Consider surgery if dissolution has not occurred by 3 months.

(4) The protocol for prevention of cystine stones in dogs with a history of cystine urolithiasis includes tiopronin (2-MPG) at 15 mg/kg PO every 12 hours along with addition of water (not sodium) to food and alkalinization of urine using potassium citrate (100 to 150 mg/kg/day). In one study, recurrence was prevented in 86% of treated dogs. If recurrence occurs, the dissolution protocol should be started again.

Alkalinization of Urine

a. Cystine has limited solubility in urine with a pH range of 5.5 to 7.0 and is twice as soluble in urine of pH 7.8 as it is in urine of pH 6.5.

b. $NaHCO_3$ can be administered at a dosage of 0.5 to 1g per 5 kg body weight PO every 12 hours for urine alkalinization. One-half teaspoon of baking soda is equivalent to approximately 2g $NaHCO_3$. Bicarbonate therapy may not be very effective based on one study, and the increased sodium load may increase cystinuria.

c. Potassium citrate may be a preferable alkalinizing agent because the sodium in $NaHCO_3$ may increase urinary sodium excretion, which in human beings has been shown to increase urinary cystine excretion.

d. The risk of struvite urolithiasis also may be increased if urine is maintained in an alkaline range.

Diet

a. A low protein diet may result in lower urine specific gravity (less urea available to contribute to medullary interstitial hypertonicity) and increased urine pH. Hill's Prescription Diet u/d has been recommended for this purpose.

Silicate Stones

1. The effects of urine pH on silicate solubility are not established, and no recommendations can be made concerning therapeutic alterations of urine pH.

2.. Diets high in plant proteins (e.g., soybean, corn gluten) may predispose to silicate urolithiasis and should be avoided.

PROGNOSIS

A. The prognosis for survival in dogs and cats with lower urinary tract urolithiasis is good.
B. Complications are the major factors affecting prognosis in individual cases.

COMPLICATIONS

A. Recurrence is highest for the metabolic stones (i.e., oxalates, urates, cystine) and may be somewhat lower for struvite stones.
B. Postrenal azotemia.
C. Urethral obstruction.
 1. Ruptured bladder.
 2. Ruptured urethra.
D Adverse drug effects.
E. Urinary tract infection.

WHAT DO WE DO?

• Make every attempt to retrieve a urolith and submit it for quantitative analysis.
• Make educated guesses ("guesstimates") about urolith composition only when none is available for laboratory analysis.
• Take abdominal radiographs (and be sure to include the urethra) after surgery or urohydropulsion to remove cystic and urethral calculi to ensure that all calculi were removed.
• Design a regular regimen of reevaluation visits (*stone surveillance*) for all dogs and cats with a history of urolithiasis. USG, urine pH, and urine bacteriologic culture should be assessed during follow-up visits, and dietary and treatment strategies should be modified as necessary to maintain moderately dilute urine, appropriate urine pH (depending upon stone type), and sterile urine.
• Remember that UTI almost always precedes development of struvite stones in dog. Consequently, obtain urine samples on a regular basis (regardless of the absence or presence of clinical signs) in dogs with a history of struvite urolithiasis to be sure that their urine remains sterile.
• Remember that adequate water intake may be the single most important factor in determining whether or not recurrent urolithiasis develops.

COMMON MISCONCEPTIONS

• Stone analysis is optional. False, since the basis for medical dissolution or prevention of recurrence of stones depends on knowing their chemical composition. Though "guesstimates" can frequently line up with the chemical analysis quantitative analysis remains the gold standard.
• Qualitative stone analysis provides all of the necessary information for proper patient management. False, as there are both false positives and negatives as to the presence of certain chemicals in the stone and no idea of their relative presence is provided.
• All different types of uroliths can be dissolved medically using the appropriate regimen. Struvite is the most amenable to dissolution. Some urates and cystine stones can be dissolved using medical protocols. A protocol has not been designed that effectively dissolves calcium oxalates.
• Medical and dietary protocols can be designed to prevent the recurrent of urolithiasis in all affected animals. Protocols have been designed to prevent the recurrence of metabolic stones though shockingly little has actually been proven to be effective in doing so.
• The presence of crystalluria indicates that uroliths already are present or they are inevitable. Absolutely not true. Many normal animals have crystalluria and will never develop a stone. Crystalluria

can be a normal physiological phenomenon especially when the urine sample is stored under refrigeration (the crystals may not have been there at the time the sample was collected).

- The absence of crystalluria insures that no uroliths are present in the urinary tract. Not true. Many animals with confirmed urinary stones have no crystals at the time the sample was collected (they may be all in the stone).
- When a urolith is present in the urinary tract, its chemical composition is always reflected in the type of crystals observed in the urine sediment. Not true – a surprising number of animals with confirmed stone type have a different type of crystal or none at all reported in their urinalysis.
- Radiography after surgery or urohydropulsion to remove cystic or urethral calculi is not routinely necessary. Not true. A surprising number of cystic calculi are left behind after cystotomy for their removal. It is in your best interest and that of the patient to guarantee that all stones were removed at the time of surgery by taking radiographs immediately post-operatively. If only one or two large stones were initially present, radiographs are not necessary.

FREQUENTLY ASKED QUESTIONS

Q: Is it essential to submit uroliths for quantitative analysis?

A: Making an educated guess (a "guesstimate") is necessary if uroliths are not available for analysis and the clinician intends to attempt medical dissolution. In this situation, information about species, breed, urine pH, presence or absence of UTI, crystalluria, radiodensity of the urolith, and dietary history can be used to speculate about the chemical composition of a urolith. However, quantitative analysis remains the gold standard and should always be used to make treatment decisions when uroliths are available for laboratory submission.

Q: A dog with a radiodense cystic calculus, urine culture positive for *Staphylococcus aureus*, and urine pH of 6.8 has been treated using a diet advocated for dissolution of struvite uroliths. The urolith has not changed in size after 8 weeks of feeding the diet and treating with amoxicillin on the assumption that the urolith is composed of struvite. What is the explanation for treatment failure?

A: First, determine whether or not the owner is feeding only the dissolution diet to the dog. Don't forget to consider treats the owner may be feeding the animal. For a dissolution diet to be successful, it must be fed exclusively. If the owner has been feeding the prescribed diet exclusively, the patient's BUN is expected to be low and the USG should be in the range of 1.007 to 1.018. If the diet has been fed exclusively, it is possible that the urolith is composed of something other than struvite (e.g., oxalate). If so, consider surgical removal (and quantitative analysis) of the urolith.

Q: Many uroliths were removed from a cat's urinary bladder two weeks earlier. The uroliths were 100% calcium oxalate based on quantitative analysis. At the time of suture removal 14 days after surgery, the cat was noted to be straining to urinate and additional abdominal radiographs were taken. Three small uroliths were identified in the bladder. During surgery, a conscientious attempt was made to lavage the bladder thoroughly and all calculi were thought to have been removed. Do these calculi represent new uroliths that have formed in the time between surgery and suture removal?

A: It is likely these calculi were left behind during surgery 2 weeks ago. A surprising number of stones (especially small calcium oxalate uroliths) can be left behind after routine cystotomy. It takes several months for new calcium oxalate stones to become large enough to be visible on radiographs, and rapid growth of new calculi likely does not account for the appearance of these uroliths 2 weeks after surgery. Failure to evacuate all calculi may be more likely to occur when the bladder is lavaged antegrade (i.e., from bladder to urethra) rather than retrograde (i.e., urethra to bladder). Calculi also sometimes can be moved into the urethra during removal of indwelling urinary catheters. Performance of postoperative radiography (being sure to include the urethra on the film) provides reasonable assurance that all calculi were removed during surgery, especially when many small cystic calculi are present preoperatively and cannot be definitively counted on the preoperative radiographs. If calculi are not observed in the bladder or urethra on follow-up radiographs, acquired UTI or a suture reaction should be considered as alternative explanations for the straining.

Q: A 9-year-old neutered male domestic shorthair cat has had three episodes of urolithiasis. Several years ago a cystotomy was performed to remove struvite stones, and within the past year calcium oxalate stones were removed from the bladder. Since that time, the cat has been fed a diet designed to prevent recurrence of calcium oxalate stones. The owner is reluctant to have a third surgery performed and asks about medical treatment options. The urine specific gravity is 1.042, pH is 7.0, and urine culture is negative.

A: Older cats are more likely to form calcium oxalate stones than struvite stones. Based on the cat's age, the likelihood of recurrent oxalate urolithiasis is high. Effective medical dissolution protocols for calcium oxalate stones are not available. Surgery is likely still the best option for this cat because voiding urohydropulsion is less successful in males than in females. Alternatively, a 4- to 8-week trial of a diet designed to dissolve struvite calculi could be fed in the event that the current stone is composed of struvite. If this approach is not successful, another surgery remains the best option.

SELECTED READINGS

Abdullahi SU, Osborne CA, Leininger JR, et al: Evaluation of a calculolytic diet in female dogs with induced struvite urolithiasis, *Am J Vet Res* 45:1508–1519, 1984.

Albasan H, Lulich JP, Osborne CA, et al: Evaluation of the association between sex and risk of forming urate uroliths in Dalmatians, *J Am Vet Med Assoc* 227:565–569, 2005.

Aldrich J, Ling GV, Ruby AL, et al: Silica-containing urinary calculi in dogs (1981-1993), *J Vet Int Med* 11:288–295, 1997.

Bartges JW, Osborne CA, Lulich JP, et al: Canine urate urolithiasis: Etiopathogenesis, diagnosis, and management, *Vet Clin N Amer* 29:161–191, 1999.

Bartges JW, Kirk C, Lane IF: Update: Management of calcium oxalate uroliths in dogs and cats, *Vet Clin North Am Small Anim Pract* 34:969–987, 2004.

Case LC, Ling GV, Franti CE, et al: Cystine-containing urinary calculi in dogs: 102 cases (1981-1989), *J Am Vet Med Assoc* 201:129–133, 1992.

Case LC, Ling GV, Ruby AL, et al: Urolithiasis in Dalmatians: 275 cases (1981-1990), *J Am Vet Med Assoc* 203:96–100, 1993.

Collins RL, Birchard SJ, Chew DJ, et al: Surgical treatment of urate calculi in Dalmatians: 38 cases (1980-1995), *J Am Vet Med Assoc* 213:833–838, 1998.

Dalby AM, Adams LG, Salisbury SK, et al: Spontaneous retrograde movement of ureteroliths in 2 dogs and 5 cats, *J Am Vet Med Assoc* 229:1118–1121, 2006.

Davidson EB, Ritchey JW, Higbee RD, et al: Laser lithotripsy for treatment of canine uroliths, *Vet Surg* 33:56–61, 2004.

Hoppe A, Denneberg T: Cystinuria in the dog: Clinical studies during 14 years of medical treatment, *J Vet Int Med* 15: 361–367, 2001.

Houston DM, Rinkardt NE, Hilton J: Evaluation of the efficacy of a commercial diet in the dissolution of feline struvite bladder uroliths, *Vet Ther* 5:187–201, 2004.

Kyles AE, Hardie EM, Wooden BG, et al: Clinical, clinicopathologic, radiographic, and ultrasonographic abnormalities in cats with ureteral calculi: 163 cases (1984-2002), *J Am Vet Med Assoc* 226:932–936, 2005.

Kyles AE, Hardie EM, Wooden BG, et al: Management and outcome of cats with ureteral calculi: 153 cases (1984-2002), *J Am Vet Med Assoc* 226:937–944, 2005.

Lekcharoensuk C, Lulich JP, Osborne CA, et al: Association between patient-related factors and risk of calcium oxalate and magnesium ammonium phosphate urolithiasis in cats, *J Am Vet Med Assoc* 217:520–525, 2000.

Lekcharoensuk C, Lulich JP, Osborne CA, et al: Patient and environmental factors associated with calcium oxalate urolithiasis in dogs, *J Am Vet Med Assoc* 217:515–519, 2000.

Lekcharoensuk C, Osborne CA, Lulich JP, et al: Association between dietary factors and calcium oxalate and magnesium ammonium phosphate urolithiasis in cats, *J Am Vet Med Assoc* 219:1228–1237, 2001.

Lekcharoensuk C, Osborne CA, Lulich JP, et al: Associations between dietary factors in canned food and formation of calcium oxalate uroliths in dogs, *Am J Vet Res* 63:163–169, 2002.

Lekcharoensuk C, Osborne CA, Lulich JP, et al: Associations between dry dietary factors and canine calcium oxalate uroliths, *Am J Vet Res* 63:330–337, 2002.

Lekcharoensuk C, Osborne CA, Lulich JP, et al: Trends in the frequency of calcium oxalate uroliths in the upper urinary tract of cats, *J Am Anim Hosp Assoc* 41:39–46, 2005.

Ling GV, Thurmond MC, Choi YK, et al: Changes in proportion of canine urinary calculi composed of calcium oxalate or struvite in specimens analyzed from 1981 through 2001, *J Vet Intern Med* 17:817–823, 2003.

Lulich JP, Osborne CA: Catheter-assisted retrieval of urocystoliths from dogs and cats, *J Am Vet Med Assoc* 210:111–113, 1992.

Lulich JP, Osborne CA, Carlson M, et al: Nonsurgical removal of uroliths in dogs and cats by voiding urohydropropulsion, *J Am Vet Med Assoc* 203:660–663, 1993.

Lulich JP, Osborne CA, Lekcharoensuk C, et al: Effects of diet on urine composition of cats with calcium oxalate urolithiasis, *J Am Anim Hosp Assoc* 40:185–191, 2004.

Lulich JP, Osborne CA, Lekcharoensuk C, et al: Effects of hydrochlorothiazide and diet in dogs with calcium oxalate urolithiasis, *J Am Vet Med Assoc* 218:1583–1586, 2001.

Lulich JP, Osborne CA, Sanderson SL, et al: Effects of dietary supplementation with sodium chloride on urinary relative supersaturation with calcium oxalate in healthy dogs, *Am J Vet Res* 66:319–324, 2005.

Midkiff AM, Chew DJ, Randolph JF, et al: Idiopathic hypercalcemia in cats, *J Vet Intern Med* 14:619–626, 2000.

Osborne CA, Lulich JP, Kruger JM, et al: Medical dissolution of feline struvite uroliths, *J Am Vet Med Assoc* 196:1053–1063, 1990.

Robertson WG, Jones JS, Heaton MA, et al: Predicting the crystallization potential of urine from cats and dogs with respect to calcium oxalate and magnesium ammonium phosphate (struvite), *J Nutr* 132:1637S–1641S, 2002.

Snyder DM, Steffey MA, Mehler SJ, et al: Diagnosis and surgical management of ureteral calculi in dogs: 16 cases (1990-2003), *N Z Vet J* 53:19–25, 2005.

Sorenson JL, Ling GV: Diagnosis, prevention, and treatment of urate urolithiasis in Dalmatians, *J Am Vet Med Assoc* 203:863–869, 1993.

Sorenson JL, Ling GV: Metabolic and genetic aspects of urate urolithiasis in Dalmatians, *J Am Vet Med Assoc* 203:857–862, 1993.

Stevenson AE, Blackburn JM, Markwell PJ, et al: Nutrient intake and urine composition in calcium oxalate stone-forming dogs: Comparison with healthy dogs and impact of dietary modification, *Vet Ther* 5:218–231, 2004.

Stevenson AE, Hynds WK, Markwell PJ: Effect of dietary moisture and sodium content on urine composition and calcium oxalate relative supersaturation in healthy miniature schnauzers and labrador retrievers, *Res Vet Sci* 74:145–151, 2003.

Stevenson AE, Markwell PJ: Comparison of urine composition of healthy Labrador retrievers and miniature schnauzers, *Am J Vet Res* 62:1782–1786, 2001.

Stevenson AE, Robertson WG, Marwell PJ: Risk factor analysis and relative supersaturation as tools for identifying calcium oxalate stone-forming dogs, *J Small Anim Pract* 44:491–496, 2003.

Westropp JL, Ruby AL, Bailiff NL, et al: Dried solidified blood calculi in the urinary tract of cats, *J Vet Int Med* 20:828–834, 2006.

10 Nonobstructive Idiopathic or Interstitial Cystitis in Cats

TERMINOLOGY

Feline Urological Syndrome (FUS) and Feline Lower Urinary Tract Disease (FLUTD)

1. Previously used terminology is confusing and reflects a lack of understanding of the etiopathogenesis of this syndrome.
2. These terms originally were used to describe a syndrome in cats characterized by pollakiuria, stranguria, hematuria, and inappropriate urination.
3. They are nonspecific terms and do not indicate if clinical signs arise from the bladder, urethra, or both.
4. In private practice, cats with idiopathic cystitis account for 1.5% to 6.0 % of all feline visits.

Feline Idiopathic Cystitis (FIC)

1. Describes signs of abnormal or irritative voiding behavior associated with absent or minimal cellular inflammation in the lower urinary tract. This type of inflammation is called neurogenic and is characterized by vasodilatation, edema, vascular leakage, diapedesis of red blood cells, but minimal inflammatory cellular infiltration.
2. FIC is a diagnosis of exclusion made after ruling out urolithiasis, bacterial urinary infection, anatomic abnormalities, behavioral disturbances, and neoplasia.
3. The disease process is multifactorial and involves interactions among the bladder, other organs (e.g., adrenal glands), the central nervous system (CNS), husbandry practices, and the environment.
4. It can be an acute or chronic condition.
5. In severe cases, affected cats may have a variety of comorbid disorders, and lower urinary tract signs are a manifestation of some underlying disorder.
6. Most male cats with urethral obstruction have lower urinary tract signs related to FIC after relief of the obstruction.

Interstitial Cystitis

1. Originally used to describe a bladder pain syndrome in humans that is very similar to FIC.
2. Original guidelines for diagnosis required visualization of glomerulations (submucosal petechial hemorrhages) by cystoscopy, but these findings are no longer required for diagnosis.
3. Interstitial cystitis refers to a chronic condition that waxes and wanes in severity and often is exacerbated by stress. Flares are acute episodes of clinical signs superimposed on the underlying chronic condition.
4. The term feline interstitial cystitis was coined to include cats with FIC that had undergone cystoscopic evaluation for the presence of glomerulations (submucosal petechial hemorrhages).

PATHOPHYSIOLOGY

A. The pathophysiology of chronic FIC is not completely understood, but appears to involve abnormalities in many body systems including the bladder, nervous system, hypothalamic-pituitary-adrenal (HPA) axis, and possibly other body systems. Bladder lesions observed in cats with FIC may be a result of abnormalities in other body systems and not the actual cause of the disease.

B. Little is known about the acute pathophysiology of FIC because clinical signs often spontaneously resolve in <5 to 7 days even without treatment. Most studies have focused on cats with recurrent FIC.

C. Subclinical systemic abnormalities persist in cats with recurrent FIC even when clinical signs are not present.
   1. Urothelial integrity, bladder permeability, glycosaminoglycan (GAG) excretion, adrenal function during stress, and CNS function are all abnormal in cats with FIC even when detectable clinical signs are not present.
   2. No correlation exists among clinical signs, cystoscopic appearance of the bladder, and histologic findings. Cystoscopy often reveals severe changes in the bladder mucosa of cats currently in remission.

D. Histopathologic lesions in the bladder of affected cats are nonspecific (Figure 10-1).
   1. Urothelium may be damaged or intact.
   2. Submucosal edema.
   3. Dilatation of submucosal blood vessels with marginated neutrophils.
   4. Submucosal hemorrhage.
   5. Increased mast cell infiltration.
   6. Minor increases in numbers of lymphocytes and plasma cells in the submucosa.
   7. Neutrophilic infiltration is not common.
   8. Fibrosis.
   9. Increased sensory nerve fiber density (identified by special stains).

E. Urothelial integrity is compromised in chronic FIC, and this change may be an initiating or perpetuating factor in the disease process (Figure 10-2).
   1. In a normal bladder, GAG (specifically GP-51) contributes to the mucous layer that coats the intact urothelium and provides a barrier that inhibits bacterial attachment and repels noxious substances in urine, thus preventing urothelial damage.

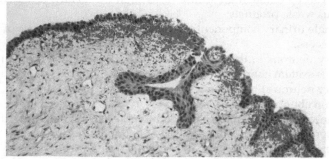

FIGURE 10-1 ■ Histopathologic lesions in the bladder of cat with FIC. Note predominantly hemorrhagic inflammation in the submucosa just below the uroepithelium. The submucosa is also edematous. Substantially lacking is any identifiable infiltration with neutrophils.

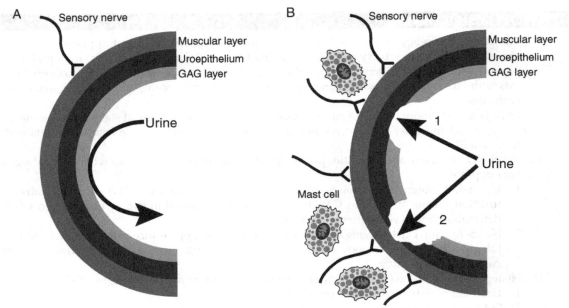

FIGURE 10-2 ■ **A,** Normal bladder. Urine is repelled by the normal uroepithelium of the bladder and the glycosaminoglycan (GAG) layer. **B,** Chronic FIC showing increased bladder permeability. The GAG layer (1) or the GAG layer and the uroepithelium (2) have been damaged, allowing urine to permeate the bladder wall. Increased permeability in chronic FIC cats has been demonstrated even when cats were not showing signs of active inflammation. Infiltration with mast cells and increased numbers of sensory nerve fibers are a result. (Drawn by Tim Vojt.)

2. Chronic FIC is characterized by a decrease in urinary GAG excretion. In some but not all studies, this is seen to occur as a result of decreased GAG synthesis or increased GAG adherence to damaged uroepithelial cells. The underlying reason for these changes in GAG and the uroepithelium is unknown. Whether the change is a primary abnormality or secondary to other changes in the bladder remains to be determined.
3. Decreases in the urothelial GAG layer may lead to an increase in bladder permeability allowing noxious substances in urine to permeate the bladder wall, causing tissue irritation and activation of the nervous system.
    a. Urine can be damaging because of its high osmolality, low pH, and the presence of noxious waste products.
    b. No single urinary component has been identified as the cause of irritation to the bladder mucosa.
    c. Sensory neurons in the bladder wall are stimulated by urine and may contribute to nervous system abnormalities.
    d. Sensory neuron stimulation also initiates pelvic pain.
F. Sensory neuron abnormalities.
    1. C-fiber sensory neurons in the bladder are more sensitive in cats with FIC than in normal cats and contribute to altered activation of neural pathways.
        a. Sensory neurons innervate the bladder via the pelvic and hypogastric nerves, which originate from the dorsal horn of the sacral and lumbar spinal cord, respectively.
        b. These nerves include unmyelinated, nociceptive fibers referred to as C-fibers.

  c. These fibers are more sensitive to bladder distension in cats with FIC than in normal cats.

  d. There are increased numbers of these sensory fibers in addition to increased sensitivity to pain stimulation in cats with FIC.

2. Changes in sensory neuron excitability are not limited to the bladder and appear to represent a general neurologic malfunction, which, in turn, may explain why clinical signs of FIC are not necessarily limited to the bladder.

G. CNS alterations in FIC are associated with increased sympathetic nervous system activity.

> **!** Increased sympathetic nervous system outflow from the brain stem is a pivotal event in the neurogenic model of inflammation in FIC.

1. Altered activity in the locus coeruleus (LC), Barrington's nucleus, and the paraventricular nucleus of the hypothalamus increase sympathetic outflow.

2. The LC is the most important source of norepinephrine in the feline CNS.

  a. Perception of threat or bladder distension stimulates activity in the LC.

  b. The LC increases sympathetic nervous system output to the periphery, including the bladder.

  c. Chronic activation of this pathway increases levels of tyrosine hydroxylase (TH), the rate-limiting enzyme for the synthesis of catecholamines, in the LC.

  d. Increases in TH contribute to increases in norepinephrine in cerebrospinal fluid and nervous tissue, bladder and colon, plasma, and urine in cats with FIC.

  e. Cats with FIC have increased tyrosine hydroxylase immunoreactivity (THIR) in the LC.

H. Stress, inflammation, and bladder pain are key components of FIC that are integrated at the level of the sympathetic nervous system.

1. Stress, inflammation, and pain all activate the sympathetic nervous system.

2. Environmental stressors combined with increased sympathetic activity play a key role in the disease process.

  a. Even in healthy animals, stress activates the sympathetic nervous system, which may initiate and perpetuate inflammation.

  b. Norepinephrine contributes to vigilance, arousal, analgesia, and visceral responses to stress in cats.

  c. In FIC, increased THIR and the corresponding increase in plasma norepinephrine concentration indicate an exaggerated sympathetic response even in the absence of stress.

  d. This finding may explain why cats with FIC often exhibit a disease course that waxes and wanes and why environmental stressors intensify clinical signs.

  e. Development of clinical signs of FIC seems to result from a *sensitive cat in a provocative environment* as depicted in Figure 10-3.

I. Increased sympathetic nervous system activity potentiates clinical signs in several ways.

1. Increased sympathetic nervous system activity promotes release of inflammatory mediators throughout the body, and these mediators are linked with pain that is not limited to the bladder. Norepinephrine also initiates the release of prostaglandins.

> **!** Increased sympathetic nervous system activity enhances the inflammatory potential of the bladder and urethra.

2. Increased sympathetic outflow to the bladder alters urothelial permeability and initiates neurogenic inflammation via C-fibers (Figure 10-4).

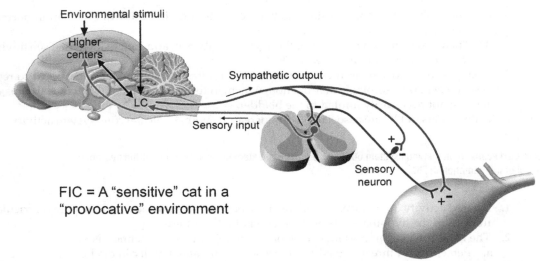

FIGURE 10-3 ■ Interactions among environmental stimuli, the central nervous system, and the bladder can produce clinical signs of FIC when a sensitive cat is exposed to a provocative environment. Over activation of the brain stem from sensory nerve stimulation from the bladder activates adrenergic outflow from the locus coeruleus (LC) to the spinal chord, dorsal root ganglia, and the bladder wall, which upregulates the inflammatory response. The LC also can be activated directly from external stressors or through input from the cerebral cortex. (Drawn by Tim Vojt.)

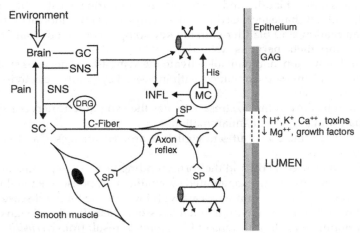

FIGURE 10-4 ■ Neurogenic inflammation in FIC. Sensory neurons (C-fibers) transmit action potentials via the dorsal root ganglia (DRG) to the spinal cord (SC) and brain. These signals may be interpreted as pain by the brain. Sensory fibers also can propagate a local axon reflex without central transmission. The local axon reflex results in release of peptide neurotransmitters such as substance P (SP) by the nerve endings. Interaction of SP with receptors on vessel walls results in vascular leakage, which can be augmented by SP-induced release of histamine by mast cells. These actions may result in the submucosal petechial hemorrhages (i.e., glomerulations) observed at cystoscopy. Receptors for SP also are present on smooth muscle. Also shown are the uroepithelium and glycosaminoglycan (GAG) layer overlying the mucosa. Damage to either or both of these layers permits hyperosmolar (>2000 mOsm/L) urine and its constituents (e.g., protons, potassium ions) to activate the sensory fibers. Stress may result in descending efferent sympathetic (SNS) signals stimulating the DRG and inducing peripheral release of neuropeptides. Local release of neurotransmitters by bladder sympathetic fibers also may stimulate sensory fibers. (Drawn by Tim Vojt.)

a. Increased urothelial permeability allows noxious components of urine to gain access to the bladder wall and activate C-fibers.

b. Increased C-fiber activity initiates local inflammatory pathways that lead to vasodilatation and mast cell infiltration.

c. Chronic C-fiber activation may overload the brain with sensory information, which over time causes an increase in the density of C-fibers in the bladder.

3. Alpha 2-adrenoceptors also appear to function abnormally in cats with FIC in ways that may enhance inflammation.

a. Alpha 2-adrenoceptors are found throughout the CNS, including in the LC and spinal cord. Receptors in the brain function to prevent catecholamine release and those in the spinal cord dampen nociceptive input to the brain.

b. Peripheral alpha 2-adrenoceptors can be found in the bladder and urethral mucosa, where they regulate blood flow.

c. Alpha 2-adrenoceptors in the bladder and in the spinal cord of cats with FIC appear to be relatively desensitized.

(1) In the bladder, there is an increase in the inflammatory response, because of changes in blood flow.

(2) Nociceptive input to the brain increases, because the receptors in the spinal cord no longer dampen sensory input.

J. Abnormalities in the HPA axis help explain increased sympathetic activity.

1. Activity of the HPA axis in the healthy cat.

a. Corticotropin releasing factor is released by the hypothalamus and communicates with the pituitary to initiate the release of adrenocorticotrophic hormone (ACTH) and also activates the sympathetic nervous system in the brain stem.

> ❗ Feline stressors often are unappreciated by the owner and attending veterinarian. Stress is a powerful stimulus for increased sympathetic nervous system activity and subsequent neurogenic inflammation.

b. ACTH stimulates the release of cortisol and other corticosteroids from the adrenal cortex.

c. Cortisol participates in a negative feedback loop to decrease production of ACTH and limit activation of the sympathetic nervous system.

2. Increased concentrations of corticotropic-releasing factor and ACTH and an impaired cortisol response have been identified during periods of stress in cats with FIC (Figure 10-5).

3. Decreased adrenal corticosteroid production may be involved in the pathogenesis of FIC.

a. During stressful situations in FIC cats, a disproportionate activation of sympathetic outflow may occur because of the deficient adrenocortical response.

b. Epithelial permeability may be adversely affected because, normally, cortisol enhances tight junction integrity.

4. Glucocorticoid therapy does not provide any long-term benefit to cats with FIC, indicating that inadequate production of other adrenal steroids may play a role in the pathophysiology. Only cortisol has been studied thus far.

5. Decreased adrenal gland volume per kilogram of body weight was found in cats with FIC compared with healthy cats.

a. No histologic abnormalities were identified in the adrenal glands of FIC cats.

b. The zona fasciculata and zona reticularis of the adrenal cortex (areas responsible for corticosteroid production) were significantly smaller in FIC cats compared with healthy cats.

c. The adrenal medulla (the area responsible for catecholamine production) was slightly larger in FIC cats compared with healthy cats.

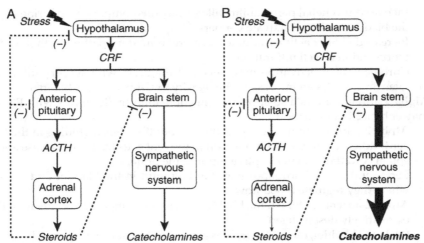

FIGURE 10-5 ■ Imbalances in the neuroendocrine system in FIC. . **A,** Normal stress response. **B,** Abnormal stress response. Excitatory sympathetic nervous system (SNS) outflow is inadequately restrained by cortisol and other adrenal corticosteroids. This enhanced sympathetic activity can increase tissue permeability, resulting in increased sensory afferent activity. Feedback inhibition at the level of the anterior pituitary and hypothalamus also is decreased, which perpetuates release of corticotrophin releasing factor (CRF). Neurosteroid production by the adrenal cortex, which normally enhances central nervous system (CNS) inhibitory tone during chronic stress, also may be reduced. The *bold solid arrows* indicate stimulation, and the *dotted arrows* indicate inhibition. Line thickness indicates signal intensity.

SIGNALMENT

Age
1. Range: 1 to 10 years of age.
2. Peak occurrence: 2 to 7 years of age.
3. Decreased risk in cats younger than 1 year of age.

Sex
1. No difference in occurrence between males and females.

Breed
1. Persian cats may be at increased risk.
2. Siamese cats may be at decreased risk.

Behavioral Characteristics of Affected Cats
1. Over-reactive to their environment.
2. Nervous, fearful, defensive, or aggressive.
3. May have a neurotic attachment to their owners.

Factors That Have Been Associated With Increased Risk
1. Neutered (versus intact).
2. Indoor housing.
3. Use of a litter box for urination and defecation.
4. Diet consisting of 75% to 100% dry food.

5. Obesity.
6. Sedentary lifestyle.
7. Multi-cat household.
8. Decreased water intake.
9. Stressful interactions with owners or environment.
10. Recent moves or changes in routine.
11. Genetics and epigenetic modulation.

CLINICAL SIGNS

A. We use the acronym "FISH" to describe the principal lower urinary tract signs associated with idiopathic cystitis:
   1. Increased *frequency.*
   2. *Inappropriate* urinations. Also called periuria (i.e., urinating outside the litter box). This is the most common clinical sign reported by owners, and in some cases may be the only reported sign.
   3. *Stranguria.*
   4. *Hematuria and howling* (vocalization) during urination.
B. Clinical signs may be acute or chronic.
   1. An attempt should be made to determine if the problem has been chronic.
   2. Chronic recurrent signs mandate a more extensive diagnostic evaluation and treatment plan.
   3. Urethral obstruction may be a sequela to FIC in male cats.
C. The development of clinical signs appears to require the presence of predisposing internal abnormalities (i.e., brain, bladder, adrenal glands) as well as external factors (i.e., stressors) that bring the cat to a threshold at which clinical signs will be exhibited.
D. Recent studies have shown that 50% or more of cats with FIC will develop episodic or persistent signs within 1 year of the first episode.

DIFFERENTIAL DIAGNOSES

Cats Younger Than 10 Years of Age
   1. FIC accounts for 60% to 70% of cats presented for clinical signs of irritative voiding (Figure 10-6).

> **!** FIC is the most common diagnosis in cats younger than 10 years of age with signs of irritative voiding.

   2. Urolithiasis accounts for 10% to 20%.
   3. An anatomic abnormality (e.g., urachal diverticulum, urethral stricture) accounts for 10%.
   4. A behavioral disorder accounts for 10%.
   5. Bacterial urinary infection accounts for < 2%.
   6. Neoplasia accounts for <1%.

Cats Older Than 10 Years of Age
   1. FIC accounts for only 5% of cats presented for clinical signs of irritative voiding.
   2. Bacterial urinary tract infection (UTI) accounts for more than 50%. Bacterial UTI in older cats often occurs in association with urolithiasis or chronic kidney disease (with production of submaximally concentrated urine).

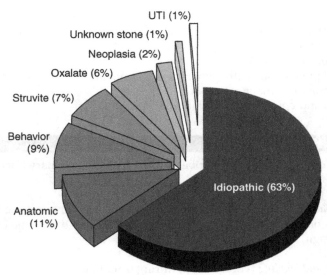

FIGURE 10-6 ■ Distribution of diagnoses in young cats presented for signs of lower urinary tract distress. (From Buffington CA, Chew DJ, Kendall MS, et al: Clinical evaluation of cats with nonobstructive urinary tract diseases. *J Am Vet Med Assoc* 210:46-50, 1997.)

HISTORY

A. See Figure 10-7 for lower urinary tract (LUT) Environmental and Resource Questionnaire.
B. Effective client communication will facilitate accurate diagnosis and increase the likelihood of successful treatment.
C. Establish a bond with the client, ask open-ended questions, practice reflective listening, and provide empathic statements to obtain a thorough history and build client confidence.
D. Ask questions about early adverse events the cat may have experienced and that may serve as vulnerability factors (e.g., maternal stress, orphaned, bottle-fed, early neutering).
E. Attempt to identify comorbid conditions that may be present:
   1. Gastrointestinal disturbances.
      a. Regurgitation.
      b. Vomiting (hair or food).
      c. Soft stool.
      d. Diarrhea.
   2. Skin lesions (e.g., a diagnosis of flea allergy dermatitis with no fleas present).
   3. Behavior problems (e.g., frightened, withdrawn, hiding, aggressive, overly attached).
   4. Cardiac conditions.
      a. Heart murmur.
      b. Gallop rhythm.
      c. Cardiomyopathy.
F. Gather information about litter box use and maintenance.
   1. Number and location.
      a. Cat owners should have one litter box for each cat (or cat group) in the household plus one additional box.
      b. Boxes should be easily accessible and kept away from noisy household appliances that may frighten the cat and keep it from using the litter box.

Clinical Signs History Form

Owner Name: _____

Pet Name: _____ Date: _____

Directions: For items below, please use the following choices to describe how many times you have seen your pet experience the symptom:

Score =

0 = I have **NEVER** seen   3 = I've seen at least **ONCE per MONTH**
1 = I have seen **ONCE**   4 = I've seen at least **ONCE per WEEK**
2 = I've seen at least **ONCE per YEAR**   5 = I see it **DAILY**

Sign – please circle applicable signs and symptoms. Comments/explanation – as appropriate.

Score	How often does your cat:	Comments/explanation
	Cough (± productive, sound)	
	Sneeze	
	Have difficulty breathing	
	Vomit (character/contents)	
	Have hairballs	
	Have diarrhea (color, consistency, urgency)	
	Have constipation	
	Defecate outside the litter box	
	Strain to urinate	
	Have frequent attempts to urinate	
	Urinate outside the litter box	
	Have blood in the urine	
	Sprays urine on vertical surfaces	
	Grooms abdomen/perineum excessively	
	Have excessive hair loss	
	Scratch excessively (please note locations)	
	Have discharge from eyes (color, consistency)	
	Appear nervous (anxious)	
	Appear fearful	
	Appear aggressive	

A

FIGURE 10-7 ■ Detailed Environmental History and Assessment Forms for use in cats with FIC. Results from these forms are designed to assist the attending veterinarian in a comprehensive assessment of the cat's living environment. **A,** Clinical Signs History Form.

2. Size and depth.
   a. Boxes may be too small for large cats or too deep for arthritic cats to easily enter.
   b. As a rule of thumb the litter box should be as long as the cat.
3. Hooded or uncovered.
4. Automatic cleaning. Although these devices keep litter boxes clean, some cats are frightened by the noise created by the machine.
5. Type of litter used and how often the owner changes the litter.
   a. Clumping versus nonclumping.
   b. Scented versus nonscented.
   c. Cats sometimes demonstrate definite substrate preferences.
      (1) Substrate preference can be determined by testing different substrates in separate boxes and allowing the cat to choose.
      (2) The type of substrate should not be changed frequently, because doing so may induce stress, unless the new substrate is provided in a separate litter box.

"9-Lives" Checklist

The "9-Lives" checklist is intended to get an idea of the level of stress in the household that might be affecting the cat. Positive responses to any of the top three suggest that empathic, emotion-focused responses (may not be able to change the situation) may be indicated; whereas the rest suggest that more action-focused responses may be useful.

Owner Name: _____

Cat's Name: _____ Date: _____

Just like people, some cats may be more sensitive to changes in their environment than others. Please review the attached checklist of common "life events" that can happen in the homes of indoor-housed cats, and place a check mark next to any event your cat has experienced during the past 12 months. Please also indicate the approximate date of the event. If you noticed that any of the events affected the cat's disease symptoms, please put a ✓ in the appropriate box in the last columns next to any events that affected your cat's disease.

Scoring:

↓↓ = Much worse, ↓ = worse, ↔ = no change, ↑ = better, ↑↑ = much better

Check, if appropriate	Event During the past 12 months, my cat has experienced	Approximate Date	Change in Disease				
			↓↓	↓	↔	↑	↑↑
	Death or departure of a pet family member						
	Death or departure of a human family member						
	Serious hassle in the household (injury, illness, other)						
	New human in the household (spouse, baby, friend, child, other relative)						
	New pet(s) in the household						
	Change in schedule (work, school, travel, vacation, retirement)						
	Visitors (friends, relatives, etc.)						
	Construction around the house (inside or outside)						
	Changes of season						
	Weather changes/severe storm/earthquake						
	New house/apartment						
	Frequent loud noises (house/car alarms, neighbors, etc.)						
	Boarding						
	Remodeling						
	Moving/rearranging furniture						
	Neighborhood cats outdoors						
	Exam time (for students)						
	Holidays						
	Change in diet						
	Change in litter						
	Travel (car, train, plane)						
	Other (please describe below)						

B

FIGURE 10-7, cont'd ■ B, "9-Lives" Checklist.

The **Resource Checklist and Client Action Plan** is designed to be completed by clients (except for the action column) and reviewed with them by the technician (veterinarian). I primarily use the "No" and "DK" columns. Checks in the NO column are candidates for intervention, whereas those in the DK column are opportunities for investigation (or a warning that the wrong person filled out the form). I suggest that turning items checked as NO or DK into YES may help, and ask clients which of the item(s) checked they think may be most important to change or which they want to change first. I do this to try to obtain "buy-in" and to (hopefully) enhance compliance. Clients are then given detailed help in changing **this factor only** to avoid information overload. They are told that when this is under control we can work on other issues as needed.

Resource Checklist and Client Action Plan

The following questions ask about the indoor environment of your cat(s). There are no right or wrong answers; we just want to learn more about your cat's environment. Please check Yes or No after each question. If a question does not apply to your home, please check NA; if you don't know, please check DK. If you want to comment on any of the questions, please write the number of the question and your comments in the space below the questionnaire

Diet – Wet food (check one)	□ None □ 25% □ 50% □ 75% □ 100%
Diet – Dry food (check one)	□ None □ 25% □ 50% □ 75% □ 100%
How many hours each day, on average, does your cat spend indoors? (check one)	□ 0–6 hours □ 18–24 hours □ 6–12 hours □ Indoor only □ 12–18 hours
How many total cats live in your house?	

If you have more than one cat, what is their relationship?(check one)
  □ Not related   □ Parent-offspring
  □ Littermate   □ Single cat household
  □ Sibling □ Other	

Where did you obtain your cat (source)? (check one) □ Shelter □ Offspring from a pet I already own(ed) □ Obtained from a friend □ Gift □ Purchased from a pet shop □ Purchased from a breeder □ Stray/orphan □ Other	

Food and Water	Yes	No	NA	DK	Action Client Target Date/Priority
Does each cat have its own food bowl?					
Does each cat have its own water bowl?					
Are the bowls located in a convenient location that provides some privacy while it eats or drinks					
Are bowls located such that another animal cannot sneak up on this cat while the cat eats or drinks?					
Are bowls washed regularly (at least weekly) with a mild detergent?					
Are bowls located away from appliances and air ducts that could make noise unexpectedly?					

C

FIGURE 10-7, cont'd ■ **C,** Resource Checklist and Client Action Plan. (Developed by the Indoor Cat Initiative, The Ohio State University [www.vet.ohio-state.edu/indoorcat.htm] and used by permission.)

Space	Yes	No	NA	DK	Action Client Target Date/Priority
Does each cat have its own resting area in a convenient location that provides some privacy?					
Does each cat have a safe hiding area?					
Are perches provided so each cat can look down on their surroundings?					
Can each cat move about freely, explore, climb, stretch, and play if it chooses to?					
Is a radio or TV left playing when the cat is home alone?					

Social Contact	Yes	No	NA	DK	Action Client Target Date/Priority
How many hours a day are you in sight of your cat?	_____ (hours/day)				
How many minutes a day do you spend petting your cat?	_____ (min/day)				
How many minutes a day do you spend playing with your cat?	_____ (min/day)				
Does each cat have a variety of toys to play with?					
Does each cat have many toys to choose from?					
Do your cats like to play with toys?					
Can each cat play with other animals or the owner if it chooses to?					

Body Care	Yes	No	NA	DK	Action Client Target Date/Priority
Are horizontal scratching posts provided?					
Are vertical scratching posts provided?					
How many litter boxes are in your house?					
Does each cat have its own litter box?					
Are litter boxes located in a convenient, well-ventilated location that still gives the cat some privacy while using them?					
Are litter boxes located on more than one level in multi-level homes?					
Are litter boxes located so that the cat has easy access to and from the box?					
Are litter boxes located away from appliances and air ducts that could make noise unexpectedly?					
Are litter boxes washed regularly?					
Is unscented litter used?					
Is clumping litter used?					
Is the type of litter used kept consistent?					
Is the litter scooped as soon after use as possible (just as we flush after each use); at least daily?					

FIGURE 10-7, C, cont'd

6. Cleaning schedule.
   a. How often is the box scooped for urine and feces (i.e., once daily, twice daily, every other day, weekly)?
   b. How often is the litter completely removed and the box refilled?
7. Does the cat fully cover its urine and feces in the box? Failure to do so suggests an unsatisfactory litter box environment.

G. Ask detailed questions about inappropriate eliminations to identify periuria.
   1. The location, number, and size of urine spots may help determine if FIC or a behavioral problem is more likely.
      a. Large spots may indicate polyuria with overflow.
      b. Small spots in numerous locations may indicate increased urgency and pain from cystitis.
   2. Distinguish litter box problems from inappropriate eliminations associated with FIC. Toileting (defined as the deposition of normal urine and feces outside the litter box without signs of irritative voiding) suggests litter box management problems.

> **!** Determine if inappropriate urinations are normal toileting events or related to irritation of the lower urinary tract.

   a. Characterized by the presence of a moderate amount of urine in one spot.
   b. Paw markings on the carpet around the urine spot suggest an attempt to cover the area (a normal behavior associated with urination).
   c. The cat may prefer the substrate in the area in which it is toileting (e.g., carpet texture).
   d. Toileting problems indicate the litter box must be cleaned more frequently.
   e. Toileting problems may indicate the cat has developed an aversion to the current litter. Aversion to a particular litter type can develop during acute episodes of FIC, after which the cat may associate a particular litter type with painful attempts at urination. Toileting in only one location suggests litter box avoidance.
   f. Urinations on vertical locations (e.g., walls) indicate spraying or marking behavior.
   g. Litter box problems should be considered likely if the owner reports deposition of both feces and urine outside of the litter box.
   3. Irritative voiding results in deposition of small volumes of urine in multiple places.

H. Stress in the cat's or owner's life should be identified if possible during the history because stress can play an important role in initiating and perpetuating clinical signs. Determination of the degree of stress in an individual cat's life can be difficult.
   1. Moving to a new living space or a change in the owner's schedule are very stressful experiences for a cat.
   2. Many other stressors are possible and may arise from other animals, humans, the living space itself, and husbandry (e.g., diet, water, litter box).
   3. Earthquakes and dramatic changes in weather conditions (as seasons change) also have also been reported to increase risk for episodes of FIC.
   4. The amount of activity in the cat's environment can affect the stress response.

PHYSICAL EXAMINATION

A. Perform a complete physical examination of all other body systems before focusing on the urinary tract to ensure identification of all comorbid conditions that may be present.
B. Evaluate the cat for pain on abdominal palpation of the bladder or elsewhere.

C. A thickened bladder wall may be identified in some cats with chronic disease. During flares of FIC, the bladder will be small due to irritative voiding.

D. The remainder of the physical examination usually is normal.

E. Excessive grooming or biting of the hair on the caudal abdomen may be a sign of referred pain in some cats (so-called *barbering*). Some cats also will pull hair out in clumps from the flanks and tail base.

F. Gallops, murmurs, hypertrophic cardiomyopathy, obesity, odontoclastic resorptive dental lesions, gastrointestinal disease, and nervousness potentially are comorbid conditions that occur with increased frequency in cats with FIC.

DIAGNOSIS

Evaluation

1. An exhaustive diagnostic evaluation is not necessary in a young cat experiencing its first episode of FIC. A diagnosis of FIC however cannot be made until urolithiasis, bacterial UTI and neoplasia have been excluded as possible causes of clinical signs. Most cats with an acute episode of FIC experience spontaneous remission of clinical signs within 1 week of onset.

   a. Survey abdominal radiographs will allow exclusion of radiopaque cystic calculi.

   b. A urinalysis will establish baseline results for urine specific gravity (USG), protein concentration, hematuria, and pyuria.

   c. Although bacterial UTI is uncommon in cats younger than 10 years of age with lower urinary tract signs, a urine culture will eliminate UTI as a diagnostic consideration.

Routine Laboratory Tests

Urinalysis

   a. Urinalysis findings are neither sensitive nor specific for FIC.

   b. USG.

   (1) Healthy cats eating canned foods typically have USG of >1.025.

   (2) Healthy cats eating dry foods typically have USG of >1.035.

   (3) Cats with lower urinary tract signs and USG of <1.025 should be evaluated for systemic disease. Renal disease or renal failure, hyperthyroidism, and diabetes mellitus all impair the ability of the kidneys to produce concentrated urine.

   (4) An extremely high USG (i.e., 1.060-1.080) may increase the risk for perpetuation of FIC if therapy to lower the USG is not initiated.

   c. Urine pH.

   (1) Urine pH is of no diagnostic importance in FIC.

   (2) There is no scientific evidence to support the idea that urine pH contributes to development of FIC or that manipulation of pH is useful in the treatment of FIC.

   (3) Urine pH depends on the interaction of many factors including diet, postprandial alkaline tide, stress-induced respiratory alkalosis, urease-producing bacteria in UTI, and the presence of plasma in the urine associated with bleeding.

   (4) Most cats in North America eat commercial cat foods that acidify their urine.

   (5) Stress induced by transport to the veterinarian's office has been shown to cause acute respiratory alkalosis that results in alkaline urine in some cats.

   d. Hematuria and proteinuria are common in cats with FIC but often wax and wane over time and even between urinations on the same day.

❗ Hematuria is the predominant abnormal finding on urinalysis of cats with flares of FIC.

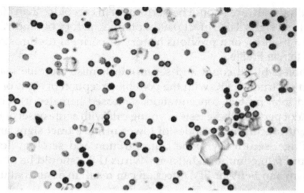

FIGURE 10-8 ■ Many red blood cells in the urine sediment of a cat with acute FIC. This is sometimes called *hemorrhagic inflammation* because of the predominance of red blood cells and the absence of neutrophils. A few struvite crystals are also in this figure, but they have no pathological significance in FIC.

    e. So-called hemorrhagic inflammation (i.e., many red blood cells with few white blood cells) is common in the urine sediment of cats with FIC (Figure 10-8). Red cells and protein can enter urine during cystocentesis. Therefore, it is difficult to assess the importance of hematuria in samples collected from cats using this method.

    f. Crystals often are not present or are present in low numbers in fresh urine from cats with FIC.

       (1) Refrigeration can cause ex vivo formation of crystals that were not present in vivo.

       (2) The presence of crystals has no known diagnostic relevance in cats with nonobstructive FIC.

       (3) Crystal formation does not lead to lower urinary tract damage and lower urinary tract signs. Struvite and calcium oxalate crystals do not appear to damage healthy urothelium.

       (4) Sterile inflammation initially damages the urothelium and allows plasma protein exudation into urine, increasing urine pH and allowing struvite crystals to precipitate as a secondary event. Urine stasis due to incomplete voiding also may play a role.

Microbiology

    a. Bacterial culture reveals growth in 1% to 2% of cats younger than 10 years of age with lower urinary tract signs.

    b. Cultures for ureaplasma and mycoplasma are also negative in most cats with lower urinary tract signs.

! Urine culture is negative in cats with FIC. The urine sediment may contain elements that look like bacteria, but these elements usually are artifacts.

    c. It generally is not necessary to submit urine cultures in cats younger than 10 years of age that have a USG of >1.040 and <5 white blood cells per high power field in their urine sediment. The likelihood for a bacterial UTI in this setting is low. However negative results of a urine culture will eliminate bacterial UTI as a diagnostic possibility.

d.   Urine cultures always should be performed in cats older than 10 years of age with lower urinary tract signs, USG of <1.040, azotemia, history of urethral catheterization within the past 6 months, or a previous history of perineal urethrostomy.

Blood Count and Serum Profile

a.   The complete blood count and serum biochemistry profile usually are normal in cats with non-obstructive FIC with the possible exception of signs of hemoconcentration (i.e., increased total protein concentration, increased hematocrit). Consequently, many clinicians do not perform these tests in young cats with acute onset of lower urinary tract signs.

b.   In cats with recurrent episodes of lower urinary tract signs and in cats older than 10 years of age, serum thyroxine concentration and serology for feline leukemia virus (FeLV) and feline immunodeficiency virus (FIV) should be performed because hyperthyroidism and FeLV or FIV infection can result in abnormal urinary behavior.

IMAGING

Radiography

1.   Survey radiographs will identify radiopaque cystic calculi (e.g., calcium oxalate, struvite) 2 to 3 mm or more in diameter. Cats that experience recurrent episodes or persistent clinical signs require more extensive imaging.

> **!** Advanced imaging techniques such as contrast cystourethrography and ultrasonography are useful in cats that fail to respond to initial treatment or in those with recurrent clinical signs.

2.   Double contrast cystourethrography.
   a.   Results are normal in approximately 85% of cats with recurrent FIC.
   b.   Focal or diffuse thickening of the bladder is noted in cats with longstanding FIC.
   c.   Contrast material may be seen permeating the bladder wall or through the bladder wall and into the peritoneal space in some cats with FIC.
   d.   Filling defects in the contrast pool may represent blood clots or cellular debris.
   e.   Focal urethral stricture sometimes is diagnosed in male cats with positive contrast urethrography making this form of imaging extremely valuable in male cats. Stricture is more likely in cats with signs of FIC that have recently been catheterized. Stricture also can develop in male cats that have not been catheterized, and may occur as a consequence of chronic urethral inflammation.
   f.   Double contrast cystourethrography also facilitates identification of small or radiolucent calculi, neoplasia, and urachal diverticula.

Ultrasonography

1.   Ultrasound examination is a useful and less invasive form of imaging than contrast cystourethrography but it does not replace radiographic studies.
2.   Bladder wall thickness, which is increased in some cats with FIC, should be measured when the bladder is adequately distended with urine. Inadequate distension of the bladder can result in overestimation of wall thickness (Figure 10-9).
3.   Both radiolucent and radiopaque calculi can be identified during an ultrasound examination if they are >2 mm in diameter. Small stones may not shadow well and are difficult to distinguish from hyperechoic urinary debris that sometimes does shadow.
4.   Ultrasonography allows for evaluation of the proximal urethra, but most of the distal urethra is obscured by the pelvis on ultrasound examination.
5.   Polyps and neoplasia can be identified on ultrasonography.

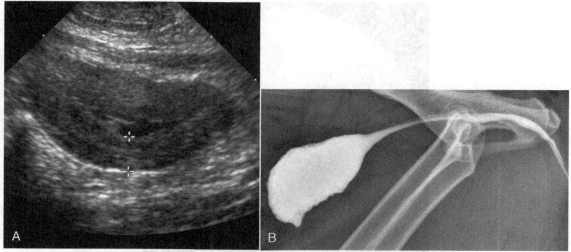

FIGURE 10-9 ■ Disparity in perceived thickness of the bladder wall between ultrasonography (left) and contrast cystography (right). Note the bladder is relatively empty in the image on the left, potentially resulting in the impression that the bladder wall is markedly thickened. The bladder is more distended in the image on the right, taken during positive contrast cystography. The bladder wall in the radiographic image on the right is thickened but not as much as suggested by the ultrasound image on the left. Also note the urachal diverticulum at the cranioventral location of the bladder in the positive contrast cystogram.

Cystoscopy

1. Cystoscopy allows direct visualization of the bladder mucosa. It is rarely necessary but can ensure that an underlying problem has not been missed. Cystoscopy can be used instead of contrast cystography in female cats.
2. The most commonly identified bladder lesions in cats with FIC are increased vessel density and tortuosity, edema and submucosal hemorrhage, and glomerulations (submucosal petechial hemorrhages) (Figure 10-10).
3. An increase in the number and size of glomerulations often occurs in cats with FIC when higher bladder filling pressures (≥ 80 cm water) are used during cystoscopy. This finding does not occur in normal bladders and allows for a specific diagnosis of interstitial cystitis.
4. A rigid pediatric cystoscope is the instrument of choice to obtain images of the bladder and urethra in female cats 3 kg or more. Small lesions are readily identified due to the degree of magnification achieved. Biopsies obtained through the operating port often are not very informative due to their small size.

Urethroscopy

1. The urethra of male cats can be evaluated for erosions, hemorrhages, and urethral strictures using a small fiberoptic endoscope.
2. Urethral lesions are identified in approximately 40% of male cats with FIC.
3. Female cats with FIC rarely have lesions in the urethra.

HISTOPATHOLOGY

A. Biopsy is not necessary in most cats with lower urinary tract signs suspected to have FIC.
B. Biopsy of the bladder should be performed in cats in which neoplasia cannot be excluded (e.g., highly irregular bladder mucosa or mass observed on cystography or ultrasonography).

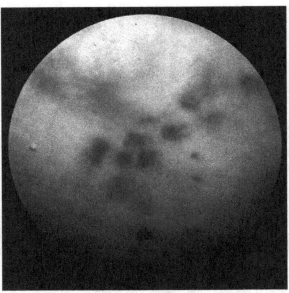

FIGURE 10-10 ■ Cystoscopic findings in a cat with FIC. Note the circular submucosal petechial hemorrhages (also called glomerulations). Also note the edema that obscures normal background vessels.

C. Histopathologic findings in cats with FIC are not specific (see later section, "Pathophysiology" for additional information).
D. When biopsy is performed, a toluidine blue stain should be requested in addition to routine hematoxylin and eosin staining to identify mast cells that sometimes are present in the bladder wall of affected cats.

TREATMENT
A. Step-wise approach is taken in the management of FIC (Figure 10-11).

General Aims of Treatment for Cats With Feline Idiopathic Cystitis

> **!** Cats with FIC are extremely sensitive to changes in their environment and their response to stress includes exaggerated sympathetic nervous system activity.

1. Intra-episode: Decrease the severity and duration of clinical signs during acute episodes.
2. Inter-episode: Increase the interval between episodes of active disease (flares) in cats with recurrent FIC.

Aims of Treatment of Interstitial Cystitis in Humans
1. Decrease irritants in urine.
2. Improve barrier function of the bladder so that it becomes less permeable.
3. Decrease mast cell activation in the bladder wall.
4. Decrease the stress response.
5. Decrease bladder and urethral spasms.
6. Provide analgesia.

Lower Urinary Tract Signs

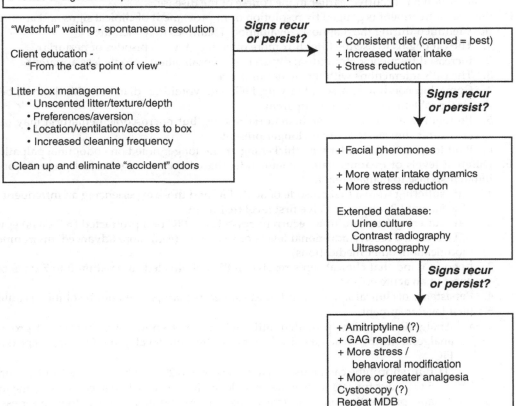

Minimum database: Urinalysis + Abdominal radiograph if signs >7 days
Urinary history (vertical vs. horizontal periuria? Irritative voidings?)
Detailed environmental history

Provide analgesia/antispasmodics for "flare": Acepromazine + Buprenorphine

"Watchful" waiting - spontaneous resolution

Client education -
    "From the cat's point of view"

Litter box management
    • Unscented litter/texture/depth
    • Preferences/aversion
    • Location/ventilation/access to box
    • Increased cleaning frequency

Clean up and eliminate "accident" odors

*Signs recur
or persist?*

+ Consistent diet (canned = best)
+ Increased water intake
+ Stress reduction

*Signs recur
or persist?*

+ Facial pheromones

+ More water intake dynamics
+ More stress reduction

Extended database:
    Urine culture
    Contrast radiography
    Ultrasonography

*Signs recur
or persist?*

+ Amitriptyline (?)
+ GAG replacers
+ More stress /
    behavioral modification
+ More or greater analgesia
Cystoscopy (?)
Repeat MDB

FIGURE 10-11 ■ Step-wise approach to the management of FIC using the multimodal environmental modification (MEMO) approach. *MDB,* minimum database.

PATHOPHYSIOLOGY

A. Based on the pathophysiology of the disease, decreasing sympathetic nervous system activity is crucial in cats with FIC.
B. Modify husbandry practices to decrease stress.
C. Provide analgesia.
   1. Like stress, chronic pain activates sympathetic nervous system activity.
   2. Systemic analgesia is more important than local analgesia in the bladder.

TREATMENT

A. Insofar as possible, treatment should address modification of external and internal risk factors.
   1. It may not be possible to modify internal risk factors (i.e., vulnerability of the brain, bladder, and adrenal glands) so as to increase the threshold at which clinical signs occur in an individual cat with FIC.

2. Consequently, modification of husbandry practices and attempts to decrease environment stressors become crucial components of effective therapy for FIC.

B. In a given cat with FIC, successful treatment depends on the willingness of the owner and veterinarian to work together to identify contributing husbandry practices and environmental stressors and to implement effective control strategies.

C. Cats with severe, longstanding clinical signs are more difficult to manage than those in which intervention has occurred earlier in the course of the disease.

D. Success of treatment is gauged by resolution or improvement of clinical signs and abnormalities identified during the diagnostic evaluation. Examples may include:

1. The cat begins to use the litter box more often (i.e., fewer episodes of periuria).
2. Increased frequency, stranguria, dysuria, and vocalization become less apparent.
3. The cat's interactions with the owner improve.
4. Comorbid conditions associated with FIC (e.g., vomiting, diarrhea, skin lesions, behavioral problems) become less apparent.
5. Proteinuria and macroscopic hematuria resolve, but microscopic hematuria may persist even after clinical signs are no longer present.
6. Bladder pain and bladder wall thickening are no longer noted on abdominal palpation.

E. Different levels of treatment are recommended based on the cat's clinical presentation and initial response to management.

1. Cats suffering from a first episode of acute FIC and those experiencing an infrequent flare of recurrent FIC should receive first level treatment.
2. Cats suffering from multiple recurrent episodes of FIC or a protracted (> 7 days) episode of FIC should receive additional levels of treatment (e.g., more advanced environmental modification, other medications).
3. Keep in mind that clinical signs resolve in 85% of affected cats within 5 to 7 days of the onset of an acute episode.
4. Persistence of clinical signs beyond 7 days suggests that spontaneous resolution is unlikely.
5. First level treatment.
   a. Analgesia should be provided, although it is not known whether or not providing analgesia during an acute episode has any effect on development of future episodes of FIC.
      (1) Buprenorphine can be used at a dosage of 5 to 20 μg/kg PO every 6 to 12 hours for 5 to 7 days for cats with acute episode of FIC. We have had success using the injectable preparation orally in many cats. This preparation appears to be odorless and tasteless to cats.
      (2) Butorphanol also has been used, but its effects are not as potent and do not last as long as those of buprenorphine.
      (3) Nonsteroidal anti-inflammatory drugs (NSAIDs).

> **!** Administration of buprenorphine and acepromazine for 5 to 7 days is a useful treatment for cats with an acute episode of FIC.

      (a) No studies of the safety or effectiveness of NSAIDs for treatment of FIC have been reported.
      (b) Some anecdotal evidence supports their use.
      (c) Chronic use of NSAIDs could predispose cats to the development of acute intrinsic renal failure.
      (d) NSAIDs have been ineffective in pain management of interstitial cystitis in humans.

b. Sedation is helpful for cats that are extremely anxious during an acute episode or flare of FIC.
   (1) Acepromazine.
       (a) 0.05 mg/kg SC every 8 to 12 hours. Or,
       (b) 1.25 to 2.5 mg per cat given PO every 8 to 12 hours to effect (i.e., mild sedation, prolapse of the nictitans membrane).
       (c) Acepromazine also acts as an alpha-2 antagonist and has an antispasmodic effect on the urethra.
c. Cleaning of urine-soiled areas in the cat's environment.
   (1) Ineffective cleaning can cause other cats in the household to begin urinating in the same areas and may cause the affected cat to continue using these areas for urination.
   (2) Kits are available to inject enzymes that can break down urine that has soaked into carpet padding. Chemical deodorizers may render these enzyme treatments ineffective.
   (3) Products with strong odors are not recommended because they decrease the effectiveness of feline facial pheromone preparations that can be used in the treatment of FIC (see later).

> **!** MEMO is the most important treatment for cats with FIC.

   (4) It may not be possible to clean large, heavily soiled areas with injector kits. Replacement of carpeting may be necessary.
   (5) Properly cleaned areas should be treated with aversive stimuli such as aluminum foil, adhesive tape, or citrus deodorants to keep the cat from returning to these locations.
6. Second level treatment: Introduction to multimodal environmental modification (MEMO; see Figure 10-11).
   a. Behavioral studies suggest that captivity and a monotonous indoor lifestyle elicit a stress response in cats because these features drastically differ from the lifestyle of cats in the wild. However a chaotic unpredictable environment also can be stressful for some cats.
   b. Cats did not evolve as pack animals as did dogs and humans. They are considered solitary but not antisocial, and they have relatively large home ranges.
   c. In the wild, cats eat 10 to 20 small meals a day consisting of insects, birds, and rodents.
   d. Large carnivores including dogs are the cat's natural predators.
   e. Cats do not display any circadian rhythm in their daily activities in the wild.
   f. House cats have limited space for hunting and roaming, are not provided with prey, must adapt their activities to their owner's schedule and often must live in close proximity to humans, dogs and other cats.
   g. Living in close confinement with other cats may be stressful and can be a source of conflict that goes unnoticed by cat owners and veterinarians.

> **!** Cats are solitary and not pack animals like dogs and humans.

   h. Indoor housing and monotonous environments do not cause FIC, but the associated stress may play a role in its development and maintenance.

   i. As a result of neuroendocrine abnormalities, cats with FIC are sensitized to stress and may have more need for environmental enrichment than do healthy cats.
   j. MEMO can take time to implement successfully. Many cats require 3 to 6 weeks and owners should be advised of this time course so as to expect gradual changes.
   k. The goal of MEMO is to alter litter box management, diet, water intake and the indoor environment to decrease anxiety, conflict, and stress in the cat's life.
   l. The goal of modifying these external factors is to increase the cat's threshold for development of clinical signs (i.e., decrease the likelihood of episodes of FIC).
   m. Good client communication and education are essential to make MEMO successful.
      (1) Any changes in the environment should be tailored to the individual limitations of the cat, owner, and household.
      (2) Specific stressors should be identified and quantified by talking with the owner to properly initiate MEMO.
      (3) The veterinarian also must help keep the owner calm as a maneuver to decrease stress in the cat's life.
         (a) Treating FIC is difficult and time-consuming, and many owners become frustrated.

! MEMO often decreases clinical signs of FIC and should be considered before drug treatments other than analgesia and sedation for acute episodes.

         (b) To make clients feel more secure, it is important to listen carefully, explain the problem and treatment steps thoroughly, and show empathy and concern for the owner's fear and frustration.
   n. Successful MEMO may eliminate the need for drugs. Approximately 80% of cats with recurrent FIC experience significant reduction in clinical signs during the year after implementation of MEMO.
   o. A website called "The Indoor Cat Initiative" by Dr. Tony Buffington (www.indoorcat.org) provides resources for clients and veterinarians wishing to implement MEMO.
7. MEMO Level 1.
   a. Manage litter box practices effectively.
      (1) The litter box should be an inviting place for the cat to use frequently. Anything that discourages use of the litter box will favor urine retention and increase the likelihood that noxious components of urine will permeate the bladder wall and stimulate nociceptors (see earlier).
      (2) Owners should follow the "1 plus 1" rule: One litter box for each cat (or cat group) in the house plus one additional litter box.
      (3) Litter boxes should be placed in quiet, easily accessible locations with an available escape route. Providing an escape route will minimize the possibility of dominant cats preventing access to less dominant cats.
      (4) Place litter boxes in different locations and (if possible) on different levels of the house to maximize use.
      (5) Increase the frequency of scooping and cleaning of the litter boxes.
         (a) Litter should be scooped twice daily.
         (b) Litter should be discarded and replaced with new litter weekly.
         (c) Do not use detergents with strong odors that may discourage use.

(6) The litter box must be large and deep enough to accommodate the cat. Experimenting with different sizes and types may allow the owner to determine the kind of litter box the cat prefers. For example, some cats may prefer the privacy of hooded litter boxes. However owners may not clean them frequently enough because they minimize odors and prevent owners from recognizing when the litter box needs to be cleaned.

(7) Unscented clumping litters are recommended.

    (a) Scented litters deter some cats from using the litter box.

    (b) Whether cats actually prefer clumping litter or if its use merely encourages owners to clean the litter box more frequently and thoroughly is unknown.

(8) Trials with different litter substrates may allow the owner to determine the cat's preferences.

    (a) Place two boxes next to each other, each containing a different substrate.

    (b) Failure to adequately cover urine and feces with litter may indicate the cat's dislike for that particular substrate.

    (c) It may take trials using several different types of litter to identify one the cat prefers.

(9) One study reported that the use of an odor eliminator spray (Zero Odor) in the litter box appeared to increase the attractiveness of the litter box to cats.

b. Increase water intake.

(1) Cats with FIC often have very concentrated urine (USG ranging from 1.060-1.080) especially if they consume only commercial dry foods.

(2) Highly concentrated urine may be more irritating to the more permeable bladder wall of cats with chronic FIC.

(3) Cats with lower USG produce more urine and urinate more frequently, which decreases the amount of time potentially noxious urinary constituents spend in contact with the bladder wall. Dilute urine also has lower concentrations of these noxious substances.

(4) Feeding canned food (as compared with the same nutrients in a dry form) significantly decreased signs of recurrent FIC over a 12-month follow-up period.

(5) Adding water to the food will increase water intake and lower USG.

    (a) The highest possible percentage of the cat's daily food intake should come from canned food (ideally 100%) and water should be added to the remaining semimoist and dry foods that the cat is consuming.

    (b) Adding water to semimoist food in pouches generates gravy that often is very palatable.

(6) Water intake potentially can be increased by altering the flavor, depth, freshness, and movement of the water, as well as the water bowl shape, according to the cat's preferences.

    (a) Water fountains or dripping faucets can be used.

    (b) Clam, tuna, or chicken juice from canned products designed for human consumption can be added for flavor.

    (c) Bottled water may be more appealing to cats in areas where tap water is chlorinated or heavily mineralized.

    (d) Some cats seem to prefer having their water bowls in unusual places.

    (e) Some cats prefer large, wide water bowls.

    (f) "Topping off" the water bowl several times a day seems to increase water intake in some cats.

   c. Salt food to increase water intake and lower USG.
- (1) Whether long-term increased dietary salt intake in cats is associated with increased risk of hypercalciuria, hypertension, and renal injury is unclear.
  - (a) There is no evidence that feeding high salt diets to normal cats causes chronic renal injury. There is some evidence that high dietary salt intake can exacerbate underlying chronic renal disease and contribute to renal disease progression.
  - (b) Feeding high salt diets may increase urinary calcium excretion but not its concentration in urine, because more water also is excreted. Thus, the risk for formation of calcium-containing calculi should not be increased.
- (2) Salt intake should be increased gradually until a target USG of 1.030 or less is reached, but any decrease in USG potentially is helpful.

❗ Increased water intake and increased production of more dilute urine are cornerstones of FIC management.

- (3) Cats have been shown to tolerate foods containing up to 4% sodium chloride and this level of salt supplementation was associated with a 70% increase in water consumption.

   d. Manage feeding practices.
- (1) Feeding practices should not be drastically altered. In two studies, MEMO in the absence of dietary modification resolved clinical signs of FIC.
- (2) Dietary changes ultimately are the cat's choice.
- (3) Diet changes should focus primarily on increasing water intake by transitioning the cat to canned food.
  - (a) In the transition to canned food, both dry and canned should be offered.
  - (b) If the cat shows interest in the canned food, the dry food can slowly be withdrawn as a choice.
- (4) Some cats may have an aversion to canned food, especially those cats that have eaten dry food exclusively all of their lives.
- (5) Some cats seem to prefer both dry and canned foods to be fed.
- (6) Some cats do not seem to like canned and dry foods mixed in the same bowl.
- (7) Canned or semi-moist foods may provide a more positive feeding experience due to how the food feels in the cat's mouth (so-called *hedonics* or *mouth feel*). This may have a beneficial effect on the cat's nervous system.
- (8) Feeding moist food allows for potentially beneficial feeding-related interactions between the cat and owner due to the associated ritual of food preparation and presentation.
- (9) Provide opportunities for simulated predatory behavior by hiding small amounts of food around the house or by placing it in containers from which the cat will need to extract the food.
- (10) Once a change is made, maintain the constancy (type of food), consistency (water content), and composition (nutrient content) of the diet.
- (11) Some cats develop an aversion to the foods they were eating at the time they developed FIC and in these instances a dietary change is indicated.
- (12) There is no need to further acidify the urine to prevent struvite crystalluria because struvite crystals have not been shown to damage the urothelium or aggravate nonobstructive FIC.
- (13) The optimal diet for cats with FIC has not been identified, and currently there are no veterinary prescription diets specifically for this condition.

e. Decrease conflict among cats in multiple cat households.
  (1) Conflict develops among cats as a result of perceived threats to their status or territory from other cats in the environment.
  (2) Open conflict is easily identified, but silent conflict is much harder to recognize. Threatened cats avoid other cats, decrease their activity, and spend time away from the family in less-used areas of the house.
  (3) Threatened cats are more likely to develop elimination problems.
  (4) Competition for resources (e.g., food, space, water, litter boxes, perching spots) is the most common cause of conflict among cats even when limitations of these resources are not apparent to the owner.
  (5) Provide separate resources for each cat in an area where the resources can be accessed without being seen by the other cats. Cardboard boxes work well to provide hiding places during periods of stress.
  (6) Neuter all cats in the household.
  (7) Regularly trim the nails of all cats in the household.
  (8) When supervision is not possible, the threatened cat should be provided its own separate space for refuge.
  (9) Outside cats also can be a source of conflict. Cats do not see windows as a barrier or form of protection from the outside world. The owner may consider making the yard or garden less appealing to stray animals.
f. Offer toys that promote behaviors practiced in the wild.
  (1) Small moving objects may mimic prey and provide opportunities for stalking and pouncing behavior (e.g., laser pointers, bright objects on strings).
  (2) Containers or toys that periodically release food stimulate hunting behavior.
  (3) The owner may be able to identify the cat's prey preference (e.g., bird, small mammal, insect) by paying close attention to the cat's responses to different items.
  (4) Expandable tunnels provide opportunities for play and also for hiding.
  (5) Provide a variety of toys and bring them out at playtime to keep the cat interested.
    (a) Toys should be available on different levels of the house.
    (b) Toys on the ground or hanging from door knobs for the cat to swat can be useful.
    (c) As long as the owner is not a source of stress for the cat, he or she can be involved in playtime.
  (6) Catnip, honeysuckle, and valerian root produce relaxing behaviors in many cats. Catnip also is available in a spray that can be used on scratching posts, sleeping areas, and other preferred areas.
  (7) DVDs that provide visual stimulation and images of prey seem to appeal to some cats.
  (8) Certain types of music appear to be soothing for some cats.
g. Increase available space.
  (1) Provide horizontal and vertical scratching posts.
  (2) Areas should be available for hiding, climbing (e.g., boxes), playing, and resting.
    (a) Wooden ladders can be effective for climbing and scratching, and can be used for hanging toys.
    (b) Cats prefer to monitor their surroundings from an elevated vantage points, making climbing frames, hammocks, window seats, and kitty condos ideal toys.

    h. Consider pheromone therapy.
- (1) Cats normally rub their faces on objects in their environment to mark them with naturally occurring pheromones that communicate familiarity and identify objects as nonthreatening.
- (2) Synthetic feline facial pheromones are available (Feliway, Abbott Laboratories, Abbott Park, Ill.), and the room diffuser product will continually disperse the pheromone for approximately 30 days.
- (3) Place diffusers in areas of the home the cat seems to find most stressful (e.g., windows, soiled furniture, litter box).
- (4) Pheromones may decrease vigilance and have a calming effect on the cat. A decrease in vigilance may reflect decreased sympathetic nervous system activity.
- (5) Although no statistically significant effect of pheromones as compared with placebo could be demonstrated in a study of facial pheromones, a positive trend was noted and they may be useful in some cats with FIC.

    i. Minimize stress from administration of medications as much as possible.
- (1) Orally administered liquid or injectable medications should be considered over tablets or capsules.
- (2) Medications delivered in so-called *pill pockets* are well tolerated by many cats.
- (3) Providing medications before meals may provide additional positive reinforcement.

8. MEMO Level 2 can be implemented if MEMO Level 1 strategies have not sufficiently decreased clinical signs of FIC. At this point, it is important to review with the client what modifications already have been made, how they were implemented, which worked, and which did not. Alternative approaches to Level 1 MEMO can be discussed, and the client may wish to make additional attempts. Alternatively, MEMO Level 2 can be implemented.

❗ Exposure to the outdoors sometimes effectively decreases clinical signs of FIC.

---

    a. Exposure to the outdoors for several hours each day results in dramatic improvement in some cats. Enclosed patios, yards, or other contained areas can provide safe access to the outdoors.

    b. Provide a safe haven for very sensitive cats with FIC. The approach presumably allows the cat to feel more secure, and many cats will only use the safe haven when they feel threatened by changes in their environment.
- (1) The safe haven can be a room, a dog crate, the basement, or some other private area designed by the owner.
- (2) Add the cat's favorite items to this area (e.g., bed, toys, food, perches).
- (3) Add a Feliway diffuser nearby.
- (4) Consider adding quiet music or video material.
- (5) If a crate is used, and depending on its size, the litter box can either be placed in the crate or nearby outside of it.
- (6) The safe haven should be kept dark and quiet.
- (7) The cat should not be disturbed for any reason (e.g., medication administration) while in its safe haven.
- (8) Other pets and children should be excluded from the safe haven.

(9) Allow the cat to remain in its safe haven if it is experiencing an active flare of FIC so as to avoid overstimulation. Resolution of this current episode of FIC often will occur within a few days.

(10) Free access crate training (FACT) is available on the website www.mmilani.com for owners who wish to establish a safe haven using a crate.

c. Beyond analgesia and sedation, we do not recommend additional drug therapy until conscientious attempts have been made to implement all of the environmental modifications described above (MEMO Level 1 and Level 2). Drugs used in the treatments of FIC are listed in Table 10-1.

■ TABLE 10-1
■ ■ **Drugs Used in the Management of Feline Idiopathic Cystitis**

Acute Therapy

Drug	Class	Indications	Dosage	Potential Adverse Effects
Acepromazine (PromAce)	Phenothiazine derivative	Sedation, anti-spasmodic	0.05 mg/kg TID SC	Sedation, hypotension
Butorphanol (Torbugesic)	Synthetic partial opioid agonist	Analgesia, acute episode	0.2-0.4 mg/kg TID PO or SC	Sedation
Buprenorphine (Buprenex)	Synthetic partial opioid agonist	Analgesia, acute episode	0.01-0.02 mg/kg BID to q8h PO or SC	Sedation
Fentanyl (Duragesic)	Opioid agonist	Analgesia, acute episode	25 µg/hr	Respiratory depression, bradycardia
Phenoxybenzamine (Dibenzyline)	Alpha 1-adrenoceptor antagonist	Anti-spasmodic	2.5 mg per cat BID PO	Sedation, hypotension
Prazosin (Minipress)	Alpha 1-adrenoceptor antagonist	Anti-spasmodic	0.5 mg per cat BID PO	Sedation, hypotension

Chronic therapy

Drug	Class	Indications	Dosage	Potential Adverse Effects
Amitriptyline (Elavil)	Tricyclic antidepressant	Feline idiopathic cystitis (FIC)	0.5 to 2.0 mg/kg per cat SID PO	Sedation, anti-cholinergic effects, weight gain, urine retention, urolith formation
Buspirone (BuSpar)	Non-benzodiazpine anxiolytic	FIC, urine spraying, anxiety	2.5 to 5.0 mg per cat BID PO	Rare: Sedation, other neurologic effects
Clomipramine (Clomicalm, Anafranil)	Tricyclic antidepressant	FIC, urine spraying	0.5 mg/kg SID PO	Sedation, anti-cholinergic effects
F3 fraction of feline facial pheromones (Feliway)	Synthetic pheromone	Anxiety, FIC	1 spray in affected area SID or room diffuser	None reported
Fluoxetine (Prozac)	Selective serotonin reuptake inhibitor	FIC, urine spraying	1 mg/kg SID PO	Rare: Decreased food intake, vomiting, lethargy
Pentosan polysulfate sodium (Elmiron)	Glycosaminoglycan (GAG) supplement	FIC	8 to 16 mg/kg per cat BID PO	Rare: Vomiting, diarrhea

(1) Tricyclic antidepressants (TCA).
    (a) TCAs are classified as serotonin and norepinephrine reuptake inhibitors.
    (b) TCAs can decrease clinical signs in cats with the severe, recurrent FIC.
    (c) Amitriptyline is the TCA that has been most studied in cats with FIC.
        (i) Stabilizes mast cells that may infiltrate the bladder in cats with FIC.
        (ii) Decreases detrusor contractions by anticholinergic actions.
        (iii) Decreases sensory nerve fiber activity in the bladder.
        (iv) Downregulates norepinephrine release from the brain.
    (d) In a study of cats with recurrent FIC, amitriptyline resolved clinical signs for one year in 60% of cases. A dose of 10 mg amitriptyline PO daily given in the evening was used.
    (e) Alternatively, 5 mg PO every 24 hours can be used and the dose gradually increased in increments of 2.5 mg up to a maximal dose of 12.5 mg.
    (f) Amitriptyline (or other TCA) should not be discontinued abruptly because so-called *abrupt withdrawal syndrome* can result in exacerbation of clinical signs.
    (g) No improvement in the cystoscopic appearance of the bladder was observed in this study despite resolution of clinical signs.
    (h) Other studies have shown no benefit of TCA when administered to cats with acute FIC.
    (i) Adverse effects.
        (i) Somnolence may occur after the start of treatment, but dissipates with time and usually is not problematic if the medication is given in the evening.
        (ii) Behavioral changes such as decreased grooming may occur.
        (iii) Weight gain.
        (iv) Alterations in liver enzyme activity may occur and serum biochemistry should be monitored while the cat is receiving amitriptyline.
        (v) Chronic use rarely can cause neutropenia or thrombocytopenia and hemograms should be evaluated periodically.
        (vi) TCA may cause arrhythmias and should be used cautiously if at all in cats with known heart disease.
    (j) Clomipramine (Clomicalm) is another TCA that may be considered in cats with refractory FIC at a dosage of 0.25 to 0.5 mg/kg PO every 24 hours.
(2) Fluoxetine (Prozac) is a selective serotonin reuptake inhibitor that may be considered at a dosage of 0.5 to 1.0 mg/kg PO every 24 hours for cats with refractory FIC.
(3) GAG supplementation has not been shown to be of benefit in cats with FIC.
    (a) No beneficial effect of glucosamine or pentosan polysulfate (PPS) supplementation over placebo administration was observed in cats with FIC despite the fact that GAG excretion has been shown to be decreased in cats with FIC.
    (b) Adverse effects of GAG supplementation occasionally include diarrhea (at low dosages) and potentially coagulopathies (at high dosages). We have observed diarrhea but not coagulopathies with GAG supplementation in cats with FIC.

(c) In a multicenter study of FIC cats treated with PPS or placebo, no significant difference between treatments was observed. Interestingly, all treated cats (PPS and placebo) showed considerable improvement in their clinical signs. This observation emphasizes the importance of the cat's environment in FIC. The beneficial effects may have resulted from a positive change in interaction between the cats and their owners that led to decreased stress.

d. Bacteria do not play a primary role in the pathogenesis of FIC and antibiotics are of no value in cats with FIC unless it is complicated by other factors (e.g., predisposition to bacterial UTI by catheterization or previous perineal urethrostomy).

e. Referral to an animal behaviorist should not be considered a last resort.
 (1) Primary care veterinarians can provide information that can help clients better understand feline husbandry (as described earlier for MEMO), but it can sometimes be difficult to differentiate an inflammatory condition such as FIC from a behavioral problem.
 (2) Also, FIC and behavioral problems may coexist in the same cat.
 (3) Reasonable diagnostic efforts to exclude bacterial UTI, urinary calculi, anatomic abnormalities, and neoplasia should be performed before referral.
 (4) Behaviorists have expertise in dealing with difficult clients. This expertise includes issues of noncompliance by the owners, the human-animal relationship, and instability in the household.

! Some cats with severe refractory FIC cannot be helped despite MEMO and drug therapy. These cats often are euthanized because of the cat's distress and the owner's frustration.

WHAT DO WE DO?

• Rule out other causes of lower urinary tract signs (e.g., bacterial UTI, calculi, neoplasia) in cats suspected of having FIC.
• Provide analgesia (e.g., buprenorphine) and mild tranquilization (e.g., acepromazine) during the first few days of an acute episode of FIC.
• Avoid using nonsteroidal anti-inflammatory drugs and corticosteroids in cats with FIC.
• Do not prescribe antibiotics to cats with FIC.
• Promote increased water intake by dietary change (i.e., canned food) and other strategies to increase water consumption.
• Emphasize multimodal environmental modification (MEMO) in an attempt to decrease stress in the lives of cats with FIC.
• Request advanced diagnostic imaging procedures for cats that do not respond to initial treatment.
• Consider alternative diagnoses in cats with low USG (e.g., hyperthyroidism, chronic renal failure).
• Consider use of feline facial pheromones (Feliway) as part of stress-reduction treatment.
• Prescribe amitriptyline for cats with severe recurrent FIC when MEMO alone is not successful.
• Consider potential beneficial clinical effects of GAG replacers despite little scientific evidence of efficacy.

THOUGHTS FOR THE FUTURE

• Additional work may elucidate the salutary effects of the placebo arm of controlled clinical trials in cats (i.e., possible beneficial effect of increased interaction of the owner with the cat).
• Adrenal steroids other than glucocorticoids will be shown to be important in the pathophysiology of FIC and its treatment.

- Additional work will resolve the question of whether or not infectious agents play a role in the pathogenesis of FIC.
- The effect of maternal stress on the development of adrenal glands in the fetus and the role of small adrenal glands in the pathogenesis of FIC will be better understood.
- The neurobiology of stress and its role in development of FIC will be better understood and lead to improved treatment.
- It will become clear that FIC is just one of several chronic disease conditions in cats characterized by excessive activity of the sympathetic nervous system.
- Diets specifically for FIC will become available and will be designed to increase water excretion in the urine without excessive urinary acidification.

COMMON MISCONCEPTIONS

- Struvite crystalluria plays an important role in the pathogenesis of FIC. Actually crystals play no role in the nonobstructive forms of FIC. Crystals do contribute to urethral plug formation, but form secondary to the underlying FIC. Neither struvite nor calcium oxalate crystals are known to "harpoon" the mucosa.
- Antibiotic treatment is responsible for the resolution of acute signs of FIC. The acute signs of FIC often abate within one week, many times within a few days, regardless of treatment. This disease has a natural waxing and waning course.
- High urine pH plays an important role in the pathogenesis of FIC. Alkaline urine in and of itself is not damaging to the bladder or urethral mucosa. It can contribute to the precipitation of struvite crystals, but they have no important role in nonobstructive FIC.
- High magnesium content of the diet plays an important role in the pathogenesis of FIC. High magnesium content can contribute to struvite crystalluria, but this has no role in the development or maintenance of FIC.
- Bacterial UTI is common in cats presenting for an initial acute episode of FIC. Bacterial UTIs are exceedingly uncommon in cats younger than 10 years of age presenting for signs of urinary urgency. Some confusion about the diagnosis of UTI exists when urine that is collected by voiding or by urinary catheterization is cultured (contaminants are isolated).
- Fastidious bacterial organisms that cannot be routinely cultured are important in the pathogenesis of FIC. As far as we can tell, this is not true, because special techniques to isolate fastidious or unusual organisms have failed to do so.

SUMMARY TIPS

- FIC can be thought of as a disease of a sensitive cat in a provocative environment.
- Ideally MEMO should be the standard of care for all cats housed indoors.
- Most cats with FIC recover from their first episode in <5 to 7 days regardless of treatment. This fact can be used to positively motivate clients to adopt MEMO and other treatments.
- More than 50% of cats with FIC will have a recurrent episode (or flare) within 1 year, especially when MEMO is not implemented.
- Inappropriate urination (i.e., periuria) sometimes is the only clinical sign noted by the owner of cats with FIC that later is documented by cystoscopy. Thus, a history of only inappropriate urinations does not necessarily mean the cat has a behavioral disorder.
- Crystals often are an artifact of sample storage (i.e., refrigeration) and have no known role in the pathophysiology of nonobstructive FIC. They do play a role in urethral plug and calculus formation.
- Although hematuria and proteinuria often are detected during a flare of FIC, their presence waxes and wanes. Microscopic hematuria and proteinuria can persist despite resolution of clinical signs.

- Although FIC is characterized by neurogenic inflammation, it rarely responds well to corticosteroids or NSAIDs.
- Remember that the placebo effect (increased interaction between owner and cat during medication) can have unexpected salutary effects; thus, empowering the owner can be an effective tool in management.

FREQUENTLY ASKED QUESTIONS

Q: Almost every time I prescribe amoxicillin for a cat with FIC, it gets better and my clients are happy. I have followed this practice for years with success. Now you are telling me that antibiotics have no place in the treatment of FIC. How can you say that?

A: FIC is not a bacterial disease, and it is not rational to use antibiotics to treat it. In most cats with an acute episode of FIC, clinical signs resolve in <5 to 7 days regardless of treatment. FIC is a waxing and waning disease that often is self-limiting, at least initially. After an initial episode of FIC, the client should be advised to institute dietary changes that will increase the cat's water intake and to institute MEMO Level 1.

Q: Our practice has used meloxicam or piroxicam (off-label use) as a treatment for FIC. We give it every other day for a few weeks after the initial episode. What is the role of NSAIDs in treatment of FIC?

A: There is no evidence that NSAIDs have a beneficial effect in cats with FIC. A double-blind placebo-controlled clinical trial would be necessary to evaluate the use of NSAIDs in FIC. NSAIDs don't work very well for pain control in humans with interstitial cystitis and the potential for renal injury (especially in cats with decreased water intake and possible dehydration) has made us reluctant to use NSAIDs in FIC.

Q: I've heard that cranberry juice is beneficial for cats with recurrent FIC. Is this true?

A: Cranberry juice is unlikely to have a specific benefit for cats with FIC beyond the increase in fluid intake. Cranberry extract seems to be helpful in humans to prevent bacterial UTI, but FIC is not caused by bacterial infection. The additional acid load may decrease urine pH, but this effect is unlikely to be helpful because high urine pH is not a primary causative factor in FIC.

Q: I have observed a few cats with chronic FIC that underwent remission of clinical signs after contrast cystography. Is this just coincidental or is there an explanation for this effect?

A: We have also observed this effect in some cats. One possibility is that distension of the bladder during cystography has had a beneficial effect. Hydrodistension (to approximately 60 cm water pressure) may deplete sensory neuropeptides from the chronically inflamed bladder and provide some relief from pain. Is so, this effect is likely to be transient.

Q: Because GAG excretion is decreased in FIC, it makes sense that supplementation with GAGs would be beneficial in these cats.

A: Decreased GAG excretion also may occur in some humans with interstitial cystitis, and pentosan polysulfate (Elmiron) is licensed for use in these patients. It seems to provide a modest benefit over placebo for a small percentage of people with interstitial cystitis. In a multi-center study of cats with FIC, pentosan polysulfate had an effect no different from that of placebo. Interestingly, both groups of cats (pentosan polysulfate-treated and placebo-treated) showed some improvement, suggesting possibly that increased interaction of the owner with the cat may have had a positive effect.

Q: Is surgery useful in the management of FIC?

A: Surgery doesn't play a role in the management of nonobstructive FIC. Rarely, a full-thickness bladder biopsy is obtained by surgery when the bladder thickening is so severe or irregular that the clinician is concerned about neoplasia. In young cats with such bladder thickening, FIC usually still is the cause. Full thickness bladder biopsy can definitively exclude neoplasia and be supportive of (but not pathognomonic for) FIC. A toluidine blue stain for mast cells should be requested because mast cells cannot be identified with routine hematoxylin and eosin staining. Mast cells often infiltrate the bladder in cats with FIC, but their pathophysiological significance is unknown. Surgical stripping of the bladder mucosa using a blade or gauze sponge in an effort to "convert a chronic to an acute process" has not been effective and is not recommended. If a urachal diverticulum is present, its removal occasionally alleviates clinical signs of FIC. However it is difficult to determine if improvement is a consequence of surgery or merely reflects spontaneous remission.

Q: Are high salt diets useful in cats with FIC?

A: High salt diets are given to FIC cats because they have the potential to increase water intake, increase urine volume, and decrease USG. More dilute urine is thought to protect against future episodes of FIC. Whether or not high salt diets contribute to hypertension, hypokalemia, and progression of underlying chronic renal disease in cats is not clear. In general, high salt diets do not seem to be dangerous in cats without underlying renal disease.

Q: I see cats with lower urinary tract signs in which the urine dipstick reaction is positive for white cells but urine culture is negative. Should these cats be treated with antibiotics?

A: No. The dipstrip reaction for white cells was designed to detect the presence of leukocyte esterase in human white cells. This color pad reaction often is positive in cats despite the absence of white cells. Pyuria in cats (and dogs) needs to be identified based on microscopic evaluation of fresh urinary sediment.

Q: I sometimes see bacteria in the urine sediment of cats with lower urinary tract signs but get no growth on urine culture. I believe these cats have urinary tract infection caused by a fastidious organism and treat them with antibiotics. They frequently recover with a week. Is this reasonable?

A: Remember that most cats with an acute episode of FIC will recover in <5 to 7 days regardless of treatment. Also, remember that particulate debris in the urine sediment can resemble bacteria and also that urinary stains (e.g., Sedi-Stain, BD, Franklin Lakes, N.J.) can be contaminated by bacteria that then can be observed in the stained urine sediment. FIC is not a bacterial disease and consequently antibiotics are not indicated in its treatment.

Q: How much effort should be put into differentiating periuria associated with a purely behavioral condition from periuria associated with FIC? It sounds like the treatment approaches can be quite similar. Is uncertainty about the underlying cause of periuria an acceptable clinical approach?

A: Yes. In one study, cystoscopic abnormalities consistent with FIC were observed in more than 50% of cats with periuria even when no diagnostic abnormalities were identified on urinalysis and diagnostic imaging. We recommend implementation of MEMO in all cats with periuria. The few cats that do not respond to this approach may respond to various pharmacological approaches.

Q: A middle-aged female cat with a history of FIC that I manage had been doing well for some time after implementation of MEMO. On the Fourth of July, the cat was stressed by the loud fireworks. I thought its clinical signs would abate, but unfortunately they have not. The owner has implemented all elements of MEMO. What else can we do?

A: You have identified a specific stressor (holiday fireworks) that precipitated an acute flare of FIC in this cat. Once a cat has an episode of FIC, it may be predisposed to future episodes for the remainder of its life as a consequence of some individualized environmental sensitivity. Repeated exposure to specific stressors can result in acute flares of FIC in such predisposed cats. Usually, treating such an episode using orally administered acepromazine and buprenorphine for 3 to 5 days often will break the cycle of pain and inflammation. If not, additional reduction in stimulation can be achieved by providing the cat with a *safe haven* for a few days in a dark quiet room that contains all the cat's resources. The cat then may be gradually reintroduced into its wider environment and praised by the owner. When all of these approaches fail, you may want to consider a tricyclic antidepressant such as amitriptyline for the cat.

SUGGESTED READINGS

Barsanti JA, Brown J, Marks A, et al: Relationship of lower urinary tract signs to seropositivity for feline immunodeficiency virus in cats, *J Vet Intern Med* 10:34–38, 1996.

Birder LA, Barrick SR, Roppolo JR, et al: Feline interstitial cystitis results in mechanical hypersensitivity and altered ATP release from bladder urothelium, *Am J Physiol Renal Physiol* 285:F423–429, 2003.

Buffington CA: Comorbidity of interstitial cystitis with other unexplained clinical conditions, *J Urol* 172:1242–1248, 2004.

Buffington CA, Blaisdell JL, Binns SP Jr, Woodworth BE: Decreased urine glycosaminoglycan excretion in cats with interstitial cystitis, *J Urol* 155:1801–1804, 1996.

Buffington CA, Chew DJ, Kendall MS, et al: Clinical evaluation of cats with nonobstructive urinary tract diseases, *J Am Vet Med Assoc* 210:46–50, 1997.

Buffington CA, Chew DJ, Woodworth BE: Feline interstitial cystitis, *J Am Vet Med Assoc* 215:682–687, 1999.

Buffington CA, Chew DJ, Woodworth BE: Interstitial cystitis in humans, and cats? *Urology* 53:239, 1999.

Buffington CA, Pacak K: Increased plasma norepinephrine concentration in cats with interstitial cystitis, *J Urol* 165:2051–2054, 2001.

Buffington CA, Teng B, Somogyi GT: Norepinephrine content and adrenoceptor function in the bladder of cats with feline interstitial cystitis, *J Urol* 167:1876–1880, 2002.

Buffington CA, Westropp JL, Chew DJ, Bolus RR: Clinical evaluation of multimodal environmental modification (MEMO) in the management of cats with idiopathic cystitis, *J Feline Med Surg* 8:261–268, 2006.

Chew DJ, Buffington CA, Kendall MS, et al: Amitriptyline treatment for severe recurrent idiopathic cystitis in cats, *J Am Vet Med Assoc* 213:1282–1286, 1998.

Chew DJ, Buffington T, Kendall MS, et al: Urethroscopy, cystoscopy, and biopsy of the feline lower urinary tract, *Vet Clin North Am Small Anim Pract* 26:441–462, 1996.

Cottam N, Dodman NH: Effect of an odor eliminator on feline litter box behavior, *J Feline Med Surg* 9:44–50, 2007.

Filippich LJ: Feline lower urinary tract disease: Dietary considerations, *Aust Vet J* 71:326–327, 1994.

Gerber B, Boretti FS, Kley S, et al: Evaluation of clinical signs and causes of lower urinary tract disease in European cats, *J Small Anim Pract* 46:571–577, 2005.

Griffith CA, Steigerwald ES, Buffington CA: Effects of a synthetic facial pheromone on behavior of cats, *J Am Vet Med Assoc* 217:1154–1156, 2000.

Gunn-Moore DA, Cameron ME: A pilot study using synthetic feline facial pheromone for the management of feline idiopathic cystitis, *J Feline Med Surg* 6:133–138, 2004.

Gunn-Moore DA, Shenoy CM: Oral glucosamine and the management of feline idiopathic cystitis, *J Feline Med Surg* 6:219–225, 2004.

Hostutler RA, Chew DJ, DiBartola SP: Recent concepts in feline lower urinary tract disease, *Vet Clin North Am Small Anim Pract* 35:147–170, 2005.

Kruger JM, Conway TS, Kaneene JB, et al: Randomized controlled trial of the efficacy of short-term amitriptyline administration for treatment of acute, nonobstructive, idiopathic lower urinary tract disease in cats, *J Am Vet Med Assoc* 222:749–758, 2003.

Kruger JM, Osborne CA, Goyal SM, et al: Clinical evaluation of cats with lower urinary tract disease, *J Am Vet Med Assoc* 199:211–216, 1991.

Lavelle JP, Meyers SA, Ruiz WG, et al: Urothelial pathophysiological changes in feline interstitial cystitis: A human model, *Am J Physiol Renal Physiol* 278:F540–F553, 2000.

Lekcharoensuk C, Osborne CA, Lulich JP: Epidemiologic study of risk factors for lower urinary tract diseases in cats, *J Am Vet Med Assoc* 218:1429–1435, 2001.

Markwell PJ, Buffington CA, Chew DJ, et al: Clinical evaluation of commercially available urinary acidification diets in the management of idiopathic cystitis in cats, *J Am Vet Med Assoc* 214:361–365, 1999.

Osborne CA, Kruger JM, Lulich JP, Polzin DJ: Feline urologic syndrome, feline lower urinary tract disease, feline interstitial cystitis: What's in a name? *J Am Vet Med Assoc* 214:1470–1480, 1999.

Pereira DA, Aguiar JA, Hagiwara MK, Michelacci YM: Changes in cat urinary glycosaminoglycans with age and in feline urologic syndrome, *Biochim Biophys Acta* 1672:1–11, 2004.

Reche Junior A, Buffington CA: Increased tyrosine hydroxylase immunoreactivity in the locus coeruleus of cats with interstitial cystitis, *J Urol* 159:1045–1048, 1998.

Scrivani PV, Chew DJ, Buffington CA, Kendall M: Results of double-contrast cystography in cats with idiopathic cystitis: 45 cases (1993-1995), *J Am Vet Med Assoc* 212:1907–1909, 1998.

Westropp JL, Buffington CA: In vivo models of interstitial cystitis, *J Urol* 167:694–702, 2002.

Westropp JL, Kass PH, Buffington CA: Evaluation of the effects of stress in cats with idiopathic cystitis, *Am J Vet Res* 67:731–736, 2006.

Westropp JL, Kass PH, Buffington CA: In vivo evaluation of alpha(2)-adrenoceptors in cats with idiopathic cystitis, *Am J Vet Res* 68:203–207, 2007.

Westropp JL, Welk KA, Buffington CA: Small adrenal glands in cats with feline interstitial cystitis, *J Urol* 170:2494–2497, 2003.

11 Obstructive Uropathy and Nephropathy

INTRODUCTION

A. Obstructive nephropathy refers to the functional and anatomical effects of obstruction on the kidney.

B. Obstructive uropathy refers to local effects on the urinary tract at the site of obstruction as well as to effects on sites proximal to the obstruction, including the kidneys.
1. Urothelial damage.
2. Hemorrhage.
3. Inflammation.
4. Necrosis.
5. Erosion.
6. Perforation.
7. Rupture under pressure proximal to the obstruction.

C. Total obstruction of one kidney eventually results in the total destruction of the renal parenchyma.

D. Partial obstruction, or complete short-term obstruction, results in decreased renal function that may be reversible if adequate urine flow can be re-established promptly.

E. Total obstruction of both kidneys is not compatible with life, and death occurs in experimental animals with complete obstruction after 3 to 5 days.

F. A predictable sequential loss of renal function occurs during progressive obstruction.
1. Decreased concentrating ability.
2. Decreased acidifying ability.
3. Decreased glomerular filtration rate (GFR).
4. Decreased renal blood flow (RBF).

G. Types of obstructions.
1. Unilateral (affecting one kidney).
2. Bilateral (affecting both kidneys).
3. Partial.
4. Complete.
5. Acute.
6. Chronic.
7. Combinations of the above.

H. Location of obstruction.
1. Renal pelvis.
2. Ureters.
3. Urinary bladder.
4. Urethra (most common site of obstruction).

ETIOLOGY OF OBSTRUCTION

A. Urolithiasis (most common in dogs).
B. Urethral plugs (common in cats).
C. Idiopathic urethral (most common in cats).
D. Functional (increased urethral tone).
   1. Neurologic.
   2. Idiopathic.
E. Neoplasia (intraluminal or extraluminal).
F. Strictures.
   1. Posttraumatic (including after indwelling urinary catheterization).
   2. Postsurgical.
   3. Idiopathic.
   4. Congenital.
G. Accidental placement of ligature around a ureter during ovariohysterectomy.
H. Suture granuloma.
I. Severe ureteritis or cystitis.
J. Proliferative (granulomatous) urethritis.
K. Prostatic enlargement (severe).
L. Perineal hernia entrapment.
M. Congenital anomaly (e.g., ectopic ureter, urethral abnormalities).
N. *Dioctophyma renale* (renal pelvic worm).

LOWER URINARY TRACT OBSTRUCTION

A. Obstruction within the urethra is the most common cause (Figure 11-1).
   1. Urethral calculi in dogs.
      a. Males more commonly are obstructed due to their long narrow urethra as compared with females.
      b. Obstructing calculi often are trapped behind the os penis of male dogs.
   2. Idiopathic urethritis or urethral plugs in cats.
   3. Urethral or trigonal neoplasia in older animals.
B. Obstruction of urine outflow also can occur from masses in the trigone region of the bladder.
C. Clinical and laboratory abnormalities depend on the extent and duration of obstruction.
   1. Signs of lower urinary tract distress (e.g., stranguria, pollakiuria).
   2. Paradoxical (overflow) incontinence.
   3. Oliguria or anuria.

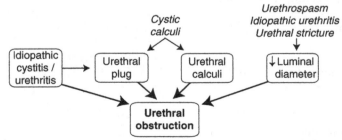

FIGURE 11-1 ■ Underlying causes and mechanisms of urethral obstruction.

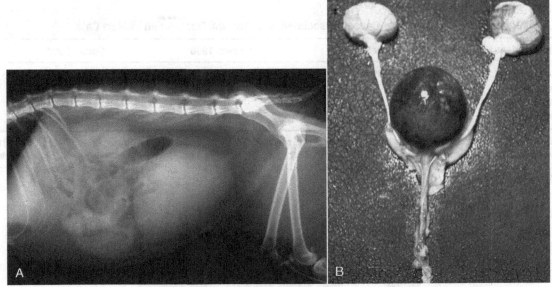

FIGURE 11-2 ■ Overdistended bladder–urethral obstruction. **A,** Lateral radiograph. **B,** Necropsy specimen.

    4. Azotemia (acute postrenal failure and uremic syndrome).
    5. Postobstructive diuresis.
    6. Bladder atony.
    7. Azotemia (chronic postrenal failure and uremic syndrome).
    8. Polyuria without azotemia as a result of impaired urinary concentrating ability.
  D. Bladder overdistension decreases blood supply to the bladder wall (Figure 11-2).
    1. Ischemia contributes to bladder injury when the bladder is distended and subject to increased hydrostatic pressure.
    2. Referred to as detrusor atony (bladder atony) or hyporeflexia.
    3. Bladder overdistension disrupts the continuity of detrusor smooth muscle fibers.
      a. Tight junctions between cells are separated.
      b. Loss of detrusor reflex usually is temporary.
    4. Urine retention results because the patient cannot urinate, despite relief of obstruction.

URETHRAL OBSTRUCTION (UO) IN MALE CATS

Causes and Associations

    1. Idiopathic urethritis/cystitis, urethral plugs, and uroliths are the most common causes of UO in male cats. Urethral plugs and idiopathic urethritis/cystitis are responsible for obstruction in more than half of affected cats (Table 11-1).

Urethral Plugs (Figure 11-3)
      a. According to conventional wisdom, UO in cats usually is associated with urethral plugs.
      b. Recent studies, however, show that only 18% of UO episodes were associated with urethral plugs. This is consistent with findings from an unpublished pilot study at The Ohio State University using urethroscopy at the time of initial evaluation.

■ TABLE 11-1
■ ■ **Frequency of Occurrence for Causes Associated With Urethral Obstruction in Male Cats**

Characteristic	Kruger 1991	Barsanti 1996	Gerber 2008
Urethral plugs	59%	42%	18%
Idiopathic	29%	42%	53%
Uroliths	12%	5%	29%
Strictures	0%	11%	0%

Kruger JM, Osborne CA, Goyal SM, et al: Clinical evaluation of cats with lower urinary tract disease. *J Am Vet Med Assoc* 199:211-216, 1991; Barsanti JA, Brown J, Marks A, et al: Relationship of lower urinary tract signs to seropositivity for feline immunodeficiency virus in cats. *J Vet Intern Med* 10:34-38, 1996; Gerber B, Eichenberger S, Reusch CE: Guarded long-term prognosis in male cats with urethral obstruction. *J Feline Med Surg* 10:16-23, 2008.

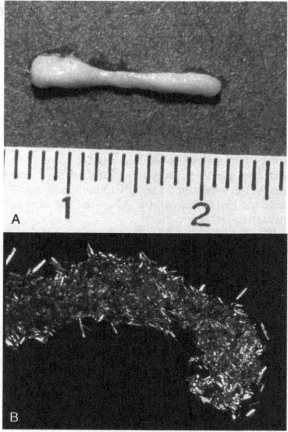

FIGURE 11-3 ■ Urethral plug. **A,** Salubrious mucoid plug cm marker. **B,** Plug with mostly mineral component. (No stain, ×400) Dissecting scope.

> ❗ Urethral plugs are less commonly associated with urethral obstruction in cats than has previously been assumed.

   c. Urethral plugs have minimal intrinsic cohesive structure but often are cylinder-shaped after extrusion from the urethra.

   d. Urethral plugs are fundamentally different from calculi that lodge within the urethra (i.e., urethroliths).

     (1) Uroliths have an organized internal structure with much less matrix and are not easily compressed or distorted.

     (2) Urethral plugs consist largely of matrix mucoprotein with embedded minerals.

     (3) The predominant mineral composition in most plugs is magnesium ammonium phosphate hexahydrate (i.e., struvite). This is true despite the fact that cats form calcium oxalate and struvite uroliths with nearly equal frequency.

     (4) Secondary components can contribute to plug formation, including inflammatory exudate (i.e., white cells, proteins), red cells, cellular debris, sloughed tissue (i.e., epithelial cells), struvite crystals, and combinations of these (Figure 11-4).

     (5) Virus-like particles resembling calicivirus and bacteria also have been observed in urethral plugs examined by transmission electron microscopy.

       (a) Finding virus-like particles within urethral plugs does not prove that viruses create the plug or are contributory to the obstructive process.

       (b) Virus particles can be shed into urine during periods of stress and after recent vaccination.

   e. Most plugs are assumed to lodge within the penile urethra, but obstructions also can occur at more proximal sites (Figure 11-5).

   f. Definitive diagnosis of a urethral plug requires retrieval of the plug. Supportive evidence for the presence of a urethral plug can be seen on radiographs in some cats with UO (Figure 11-6).

     (1) Many veterinarians assume that a urethral plug has been dislodged during hydropulsion and attempts to pass a urethral catheter when the catheter suddenly advances.

     (2) This could indicate movement of a plug into the bladder or it could indicate that resistance caused by urethral spasm has been overcome.

     (3) Retrieval of a plug or retropulsion of the plug into the bladder does not always result in restoration of normal urine flow (several other factors initiate or maintain the obstructing process).

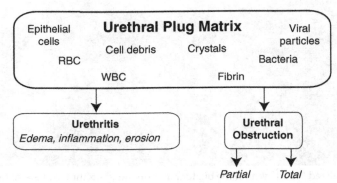

FIGURE 11-4 ■ Possible urethral plug composition. *RBC*, red blood cells; *WBC*, white blood cells.

g. Previously, the crystalline-matrix hypothesis proposed that plugs that then became embedded in a matrix formed secondary to precipitation of struvite crystals in the urine. According to this hypothesis, plugs created UO and urethritis.

h. It is now hypothesized that plugs form as a consequence of underlying idiopathic urethritis and cystitis (i.e., inflammation occurs first, followed by plug formation).

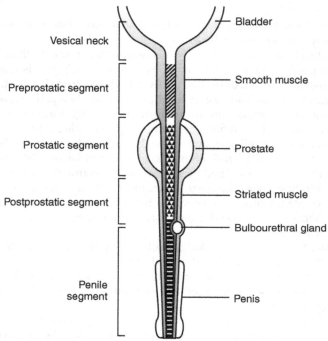

FIGURE 11-5 ■ Possible locations for obstruction in male cats. (Drawn by Tim Vojt.)

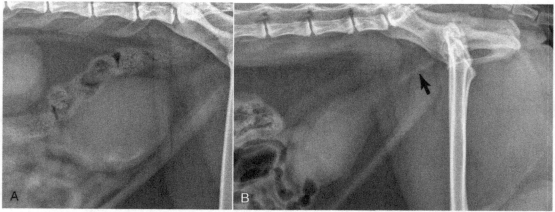

FIGURE 11-6 ■ Mineralized "sand" within the bladder and proximal urethra. **A,** Lateral radiograph mineralized material in a dependent location within the bladder. **B,** Mineralized debris within the urethra (arrow). (Courtesy of Dr. Edward Cooper, Columbus, Ohio.)

(1) Urine pH increases as plasma exudes into urine and the alkaline pH favors struvite precipitation.

(2) Urethral spasm and edema favor urine retention and struvite precipitation.

(3) Primary inflammatory changes (i.e., exudate, blood, edema) or changes within the urethral wall secondary to the presence of lodged intraluminal urethral plugs may contribute to the obstructive process.

> ❗ Urethral plugs develop secondary to underlying idiopathic urethritis and cystitis rather than as a primary event arising from crystalluria.

Urethral Calculi (Figure 11-7)
Idiopathic

a. Most common association in cats with UO.

b. This process is an extension of idiopathic/interstitial cystitis (see Chapter 10, Nonobstructive Idiopathic or Interstitial Cystitis in Cats).

> ❗ Most male cats with urethral obstruction have no identifiable cause (i.e., idiopathic).

(1) Some cats have signs of nonobstructive idiopathic/interstitial cystitis before UO.

(2) Many cats have signs of idiopathic/interstitial cystitis after relief of UO.

c. Obstruction is secondary to functional urethral spasm in addition to swelling of the urethra due to edema and hemorrhage.

(1) Refers to pathologic or neurogenic processes that cause contraction of the circular smooth or skeletal muscle of the urethra or both.

(2) Part of urethral tone maintained by the skeletal muscle (so-called *rhabdosphincter*) is influenced by sympathetic innervation.

(3) Stimulation of adrenoreceptors (particularly α-1) within the urethra increases urethral tone in normal cats. Pain and stress after UO increase sympathetic outflow from the central nervous system, leading to additional urethral spasm.

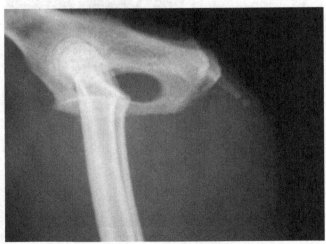

FIGURE 11-7 ■ Radiopaque urethral stones in a male cat with urethral obstruction.

    d. Bacterial urinary tract infection (UTI) is very uncommon before urethral catheterization. UTI deserves more consideration in cats with recurrent UO that have undergone urinary instrumentation.

    e. Urethral stricture may occur (Figure 11-8).

      (1) Especially in cats that have had previous indwelling urinary catheters.

      (2) Severe recurrent episodes of nonobstructive idiopathic/interstitial cystitis.

    f. Neoplasia of the urethra or bladder neck is rare.

    g. Phimosis is rare.

    h. Catheter fragment foreign body in urethra or bladder is rare.

SIGNALMENT AND HISTORY

A. The majority of cats with UO are relatively stable; approximately 10% are critically ill. Increased client awareness that male cats can have a life-threatening emergency associated with "urinary blockage" likely is responsible for these percentages.

B. Approximately 75% of cats presented with UO are experiencing their first episode.

C. The median age is 4 to 5 years old, but any age can be affected (0.5 to 16 years).

D. Most affected cats in the United States are neutered males. Intact males comprise 10% of cats with UO.

E. In the United States, more than 80% of affected cats are housed exclusively indoors.

F. Median duration of clinical signs before initial presentation was 3 days in a study of 223 cats. Signs include those of cystitis and partial obstruction before development of complete obstruction.

! Most cats presented with UO are experiencing their first episode.

G. Clinical signs depend on the completeness of the obstruction and its duration. Cats with long-standing obstruction display signs of uremia (e.g., vomiting, lethargy, dehydration) in addition to signs referable to the lower urinary tract (e.g., stranguria, pollakiuria, hematuria, pain, overflow incontinence).

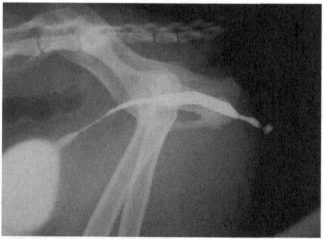

FIGURE 11-8 ■ Urethral stricture demonstrated on positive contrast urethrogram. (Courtesy of Dr. Jordan Jaeger, Carolina Veterinary Specialists Medical Center, Charlotte, N.C.)

H. The time required to develop clinical signs of uremia after UO varies widely.

> **!** Some cats with UO continue to urinate small volumes. Urine overflow from a large bladder with total or partial obstruction may occur.

1. Cats with experimental UO do not demonstrate signs of uremia until after 24 to 48 hours of complete obstruction (Figure 11-9).
2. By 48 hours, lethargy and vomiting are noted.
3. After 48 hours, clinical signs become severe.
4. By 72 hours, many cats are moribund and some die. Some cats can survive periods of UO up to 98 hours, however.

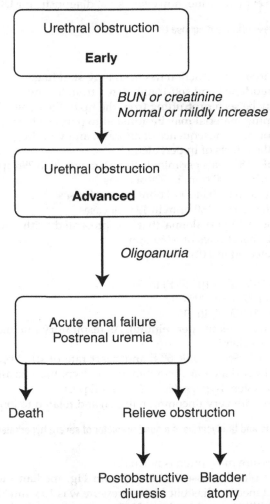

FIGURE 11-9 ■ Potential syndromes associated with urethral obstruction. *BUN,* blood urea nitrogen. (Drawn by Tim Vojt.)

5. Azotemia develops at a variable rate among individuals with the same degree of obstruction based on:
    a. Rate of urine formation at the time of obstruction.
    b. Distensibility of urinary tract proximal to the obstruction.
    c. Integrity of the urothelium at the time of obstruction. Cats with damaged urothelium develop azotemia more quickly as waste products traverse the bladder wall. This may explain why cats that immediately re-obstruct become sick and azotemic very quickly.

PHYSICAL EXAMINATION

A. A readily palpable bladder at a time when the cat is straining to urinate defines UO.
B. Urine is not readily expressible from an enlarged bladder (only gentle pressure should be applied). Failure to express urine, however, is not diagnostic for UO.

> **!** Do not rely on inability to express urine to diagnose UO.

C. A large, turgid bladder if obstruction has been long-standing.
D. The penis may be reddened and self-traumatized from licking.
E. A urethral plug may be seen protruding from the tip of the penis.
F. Already extruded plug material may be adhered to perineal hair.
G. Signs of dehydration as a consequence of anorexia and vomiting.
H. Bradycardia from the effects of hyperkalemia.
    1. Median heart rate, 187 beats per minute (bpm); range, 40 to 296 bpm (Lee and Drobatz, 2003).
    2. Severe bradycardia: <100 bpm in 5% of cases.
    3. Moderate bradycardia: 100 to 140 bpm in 6% of cases.
    4. Mild bradycardia: 140 to 160 bpm in 12% of cases.
    5. Most cats without hyperkalemia that are presented with severe illness and stress are expected to have heart rates of >160 bpm.
I. Arrhythmia was detected in 11%.
J. Hypothermia.
    1. Normothermia (100° F to 102.5° F) in 50%.
    2. Hypothermia (<100° F) in 39%.
    3. Hyperthermia (>102.5° F) in 11%.
K. Tachypnea (median, 36 breaths per minute). As respiratory rate increases, there is less likelihood of severe hyperkalemia.
L. Rectal temperature of <95° F to 96.6° F and heart rate of <120 bpm was the most accurate predictor of severe hyperkalemia. A combination of hypothermia and bradycardia was 98% to 100% predictive for severe hyperkalemia (> 8.0 mEq/L).
M. Twitching or seizures are very uncommon (0.5%) and related to ionized hypocalcemia.

> **!** The combination of hypothermia and bradycardia is a good predictor of severe hyperkalemia.

N. Systemic blood pressure most often is normal.
    1. Median systolic blood pressure was 135 mm Hg, median mean arterial pressure was 120 mm Hg, and median diastolic blood pressure was 108 mm Hg in a study of 28 affected cats (Malouin, Milligan, and Drobatz, 2007).
    2. No cat was hypotensive, 71% were normotensive, and 29% were hypertensive.

3. Less seriously affected cats tended to be hypertensive.
4. Pain, stress, and anxiety likely increased blood pressure.
5. Normal blood pressure at initial presentation may be misleading because of combinations of major stress, hypovolemia, and bradycardia.
6. Mean arterial pressure correlated inversely with serum potassium and directly with total serum calcium concentrations.
7. Major abnormalities on physical examination and serum biochemistry were encountered despite normal blood pressure.

> ❗ Normal systemic blood pressure does not preclude abnormal physical examination or biochemical findings.

DIAGNOSTICS

Serum Biochemistry

1. Severity of abnormalities varies depending on duration and extent (partial or complete) of obstruction.
2. Blood urea nitrogen (BUN): Median, 25 mg/dL; range, 8 to 257 mg/dL; 33% were above the reference range (Lee, Drobatz, 2003). We have observed BUN concentrations of >300 mg/dL.
3. Serum creatinine concentration: Median, 1.5 mg/dL; range, 0.8 to 7.7 mg/dL; 29% were above the reference range. We have observed serum creatinine concentrations of >20 mg/dL.

> ❗ Initial magnitude of BUN, serum creatinine, and serum phosphorus concentrations do not predict survival or failure to regain normal renal function. They may predict the severity of postobstructive diuresis.

4. Serum phosphorus concentration: Median, 5.0 mg/dL; range, 2.8 to 20 mg/dL; 25% were above the reference range and 6% were below the reference range. We have observed serum phosphorus concentrations between 20 and 30 mg/dL.
5. Serum potassium concentrations ranged from 3.4 to 10.5 mEq/L in 199 cats.
   a. Six percent were below the reference range, 41% were above the reference range, and 53% were in the reference range.
   b. Serum potassium concentration was:
      (1) <6.0 mEq/L in 66% of cases.
      (2) >6.0 but <8.0 mEq/L in 12% of cases.
      (3) >8.0 but <10.0 mEq/L in 12% of cases.
      (4) >10.0 mEq/L in <1% of cases.

> ❗ It is important to measure serum potassium concentration because some cats with severe hyperkalemia do not have classic ECG or physical examination findings.

   c. Hyperkalemia most often was encountered with acidosis (pH <7.2 in 74% of cases) and low serum ionized calcium concentration (<1.0 mmol/L in 75% of cases).

> ❗ Hyperkalemia does not occur in isolation and often is accompanied by acidosis and low serum ionized calcium concentration.

6. Blood gases.
    a. Median venous pH was 7.29 in 198 cats (range, 7.02 to 7.45); 40% were below the reference range and 4.5% were above the reference range.
        (1) pH of >7.35 in 25% of cases.
        (2) pH >7.2 but <7.35 in 60% of cases.
        (3) pH >7.1 but <7.2 in 9% of cases.
        (4) pH <7.10 in 6% of cases.
    b. Median venous pCO_2 was 40.2 mm Hg (range, 26.6 to 74.2 mm Hg); 13% were below the reference range and 30% were above the reference range.
    c. Median venous bicarbonate concentration was 19.2 mEq/L (range, 7 to 27.8 mEq/L); 30% were below the reference range and 7% were above the reference range.
7. Serum ionized calcium concentration.
    a. Median serum ionized calcium concentration was 1.10 mmol/L (range, 0.57 to 1.60 mmol/L) in 199 cats (median, 4.40 mg/dL; range, 2.28 to 6.44 mg/dL).
    b. Normal serum ionized calcium concentration for cats is 1.10 to 1.22 mmol/L or 4.40 to 4.88 mg/dL.
    c. Serum ionized calcium concentration was below the reference range in 34%, above the reference range in 19%, and in the reference range in 47% of cases.

❗ Approximately 33% of cats with UO are expected to have clinically relevant hypocalcemia based on serum ionized calcium concentration.

---

    d. Serum ionized calcium concentration was:
        (1) >1.2 mmol/L (> 4.8 mg/dL) in 23%.
        (2) >1.0 but <1.2 mmol/L (>4.0 but <4.7 mg/dL) in 57%.
        (3) >0.8 but <1.0 mmol/L (>3.2 but <4.0 mg/dL) in 14%.
        (4) ≤0.8 mmol/L (≤3.2 mg/dL) in 6%.
    e. Serum total calcium concentration in 51 cats was below the reference range in 39%, above the reference range in 0%, and within the reference range in 61%.
    f. Serum ionized calcium concentration was negatively correlated with BUN, serum creatinine, serum phosphorus, and serum potassium concentrations.
    g. Serum ionized calcium concentration was positively correlated with venous pH in contrast to the expected decrease in ionized calcium concentration associated with increasing pH under normal circumstances.
    h. Cats with low serum total calcium concentrations had moderate to severely decreased serum ionized calcium concentrations (Drobatz, Hughes, 1997.). In one study, more cats were found to have hypocalcemia when defined by measurement of serum ionized calcium concentration (75%) than when defined by serum total calcium concentration (27%).
    i. Serum parathyroid hormone (PTH) concentration was increased in 63% of cats with UO in one study, including 8 cats with low and 4 cats with normal serum ionized calcium concentrations (Drobatz, Ward, Graham, et al., 2005). Serum PTH concentration was much higher in cats with hypocalcemia as compared with those with normocalcemia. Serum 25-hydroxycholecalciferol status was not correlated to serum ionized calcium concentration.
    j. Low serum ionized calcium concentration is not a consequence of deficient secretion of PTH, nor does it appear related to serum concentrations of 25-hydroxycholecalciferol.

Rather, it likely is a consequence of increased serum phosphorus concentration. The potential role of decreased serum calcitriol concentration has not been studied.

Urinalysis

1. Urine specific gravity (USG) is unpredictable. USG can be >1.040 when evaluated early during UO. In more advanced cases, submaximal urine concentration can occur due to the effects of obstruction on renal tubular function.
2. Red blood cells (RBCs): Hematuria is almost always observed because of the presence of underlying idiopathic urethritis/cystitis and the effects of overdistension of the bladder wall with resultant hemorrhage.
3. White blood cells (WBCs): A mild increase can be observed, but numbers of WBCs in the sediment may be normal.
4. Epithelial cells: A mild increase can be seen; occasionally rafts of epithelial cells are observed in the urine sediment.
5. Bacteria usually are not present, but often are described as present because particulate matter in the urine sediment may resemble bacteria and be erroneously interpreted as such.
6. Crystals: Struvite crystals may be observed, especially if urine pH is alkaline. Crystals are more likely to be secondary to urine stasis or alkaline urine pH than a primary cause of obstruction.
7. Proteinuria usually is present due to hemorrhage.
8. pH often is neutral to alkaline due to anorexia and plasma protein exudation into urine from bleeding.
9. Glucosuria: Positive glucose oxidase dipstrip reactions are sometimes observed.
    a. Detected in 74% of cats with severe UO in one study (Burrows, Bovee, 1978). Detected in 40% of cats with less severe UO (Loeb, 1971).
    b. Thought to be a consequence of stress hyperglycemia. Moderate hyperglycemia occurs in many cats with UO, but frequently not above the renal threshold for glucose.
    c. Transient renal glucosuria may occur.
    d. 40% of cats with glucosuria actually had pseudo-glucosuria due to presence of a non-glucose, oxidizing substance that acts directly with the chromogen in the dipstrip pad; 60% had true glucosuria (Loeb, 1971).

Urine Culture

1. Nearly all cats with UO have sterile urine on original presentation for obstruction.
2. Bacterial culture at the time of urinary catheter removal is more likely to identify pathogenic bacteria.
3. Isolation of bacteria from cats with a previous history of UO is more likely than isolation from cats suffering an initial episode of obstruction.

❗ Expect no growth from urine culture in cats presented during their first episode of urethral obstruction.

Abdominal and Urinary Tract Imaging
Radiography

❗ All cats with UO should have radiography to determine if urolithiasis is contributing to obstruction.

a. Abdominal radiographs should be obtained in all cats with UO to rule out the presence of radiopaque calculi in the bladder or urethra. It is very important to include the perineal region in the radiographs to identify urethral calculi.

b. Evaluation of the kidneys and ureters to be sure nephroliths or ureteroliths are not part of the overall process is important because upper urinary tract involvement can markedly affect the overall prognosis.

c. Free fluid resulting in a loss of abdominal detail can be seen in some cats with severely distended urinary bladders.

d. Free fluid has been observed at surgery and necropsy in some UO cats in which no tear in the bladder or urethral wall could be demonstrated. This fluid likely arises from transmural movement across an inflamed and highly permeable bladder wall (i.e., underlying idiopathic cystitis) subjected to increased hydrostatic pressure from UO.

Contrast Radiographic Studies

a. Useful for cats with recurrent UO, especially after recent instrumentation of the urethra.

b. Positive contrast urethrography is helpful to rule out urethral stricture. It also is useful to document the presence of urethral rupture after urethral catheterization.

c. Double contrast cystography is useful to demonstrate small urinary calculi and blood clots.

Abdominal Ultrasonography

a. A small amount of free abdominal fluid sometimes is observed (more often on ultrasonography than on radiography).

b. Evaluation of bladder for blood clots and evaluation of bladder wall thickness are best accomplished by ultrasonography.

c. Small cystic calculi can be identified.

d. Urethral calculi are not reliably identified; only those in the proximal urethra can be seen.

! A small amount of free abdominal fluid may be identified at initial presentation and may be more easily detected on ultrasonography when a large bladder has been emptied.

Urethroscopy

1. A small number of cats have what appears on endoscopy to be plugs.
2. Many cats have urethral erosions and submucosal hemorrhage.
3. Some cats have increased urethral vascularity.
4. Some cats have crystalline material adherent to denuded areas of the urethra.
5. Cystoscopy at the time of obstruction usually is not rewarding due to the presence of hemorrhage and the need to use very small diameter flexible endoscopes.

TREATMENT OF URETHRAL OBSTRUCTION

A. Diagnostic testing and treatment of UO are performed simultaneously (Figure 11-10).

B. The severity of clinical signs from uremia, electrocardiographic (ECG) findings, and magnitude of bladder distension dictate how quickly and in what order treatments must be performed.

C. Cats in uremic crisis and those with very large turgid bladders are in need of prompt attention (Figure 11-11).

D. The causes of collapse and hypotension are multifactorial.

1. Hyperkalemia leads to venous dilatation and pooling of blood.
2. Bradycardia leads to decreased cardiac output.
3. Acidosis decreases vascular sensitivity to catecholamines.

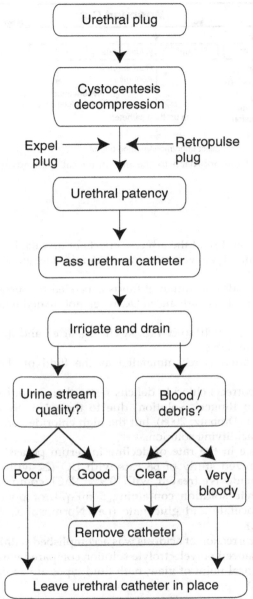

FIGURE 11-10 ■ A decision-making algorithm for management of urethral obstruction due to a urethral plugs in male cats.

4. Ionized hypocalcemia decreases myocardial contractility and causes peripheral vasodilatation.
5. Acute uremia contributes to myocardial depression and decreased cardiac output.
6. Hypothermia contributes to decreased mean arterial pressure, cardiac contractility, and cardiac output.

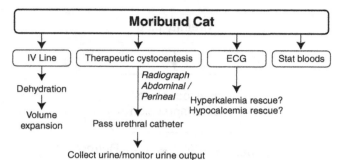

FIGURE 11-11 ■ Overview of the approach to the moribund cat with advanced urethral obstruction. *ECG*, electrocardiogram.

E. Stabilize the patient and treat the adverse effects of uremia, if present, before administering any anesthetic agents. Hypovolemia, hyperkalemia, metabolic acidosis, and hypocalcemia must be treated first.
1. Intravenous (IV) administration of fluids is needed for seriously ill cats with UO. Ten of 13 cats died after relief of advanced UO when not treated with IV fluids (Finco, Cornelius, 1977).
   a. IV fluid therapy at 10 to 20 mL/kg/hr is started and the rate adjusted as the animal becomes more stable.
   b. 0.9% NaCl often is recommended as the fluid of choice because it contains no potassium.
   c. 0.9% NaCl corrects chloride deficits faster than more balanced electrolyte solutions (e.g., lactated Ringer's solution) due to the relatively high chloride concentration (154 mEq/L) (Drobatz, 2008), but the high chloride concentration of 0.9% NaCl also makes it an acidifying solution.
   d. No difference in the rate of decline in serum potassium concentration was seen in a randomized study of 68 cats with UO (22 with hyperkalemia and 31 with metabolic acidosis) treated with 0.9% NaCl compared with a more balanced polyelectrolyte solution containing 5 mEq/L of potassium as well as the base precursors acetate and gluconate (i.e., Normosol-R, Abbott Laboratories, North Chicago, Ill.).
   e. More rapid correction of acidosis was accomplished within 12 hours of treatment with the more balanced polyelectrolyte solution compared with 0.9% NaCl.
   f. From a practical point of view, both fluid types are acceptable for treatment of most cats with UO.
   g. Severely affected cats with metabolic acidosis may benefit more from an alkalinizing polyelectrolyte solution (e.g., lactated Ringer's solution, Normosol-R).
2. Management of hyperkalemia will be needed in the approximately 12% of cats that have severe hyperkalemia and may be warranted in another 12% that have moderate hyperkalemia. No specific treatment is needed for cats with mild hyperkalemia.
   a. Restoration of normal renal function after relief of obstruction results in kaliuresis and a rapid decrease in serum potassium concentration.
   b. Calcium gluconate is the treatment of choice for cats with severe hyperkalemia (>8.0 mEq/L), heart rate of >140 bpm, and especially in cats with ECG abnormalities.

> ❗ Serum potassium concentration decreases soon after relief of urethral obstruction and often is normal by the time substantial decreases in BUN and serum creatinine concentrations are observed.

        (1) Conversion to a more normal ECG tracing is very rapid (minutes).

        (2) This treatment stabilizes the heart, but does nothing to change the severity of the hyperkalemia.

        (3) 50 to 100 mg/kg of calcium gluconate (0.5 to 1.0 mL/kg of 10% calcium gluconate) is given over 2 to 3 minutes with continuous ECG monitoring.

        (4) The beneficial effects are short-lived (about 20-30 minutes), and other methods to lower serum potassium concentration are needed.

    c. IV dextrose is helpful for longer term control of hyperkalemia, especially if serum potassium concentration initially is >8.0 mEq/L.

        (1) 0.5 g/kg dextrose bolus (1 mL/kg of a 50% dextrose solution).

        (2) Dextrose should be diluted to a final concentration of 10% to 20% before IV injection.

        (3) The goal is to create hyperglycemia that stimulates endogenous insulin release with subsequent translocation of potassium into cells.

    d. Some clinicians also give one unit regular insulin IV to further stimulate the transcellular shift of potassium. Insulin should always be given with a bolus injection of dextrose with or without a constant rate infusion of dextrose to prevent hypoglycemia.

    e. Sodium bicarbonate may be administered IV in cats with serum potassium concentration >10.0 mEq/L.

        (1) 1 mEq/kg (1 mL/kg of an 8.4% sodium bicarbonate solution) is the standard dosage of sodium bicarbonate.

        (2) 4 mEq/kg (4 mL/kg of an 8.4% sodium bicarbonate solution) is the maximal dosage of sodium bicarbonate.

        (3) A potentially serious disadvantage to this treatment is development of ionized hypocalcemia due to increased binding of calcium to albumin and intracellular translocation.

3. Management of acidosis will be needed in approximately 6% of cats with severe acidosis and may be warranted in another 9% with moderate acidosis. No specific treatment is needed for cats with mild acidosis.

    a. Restoration of normal renal function after relief of obstruction allows for rapid correction of metabolic acidosis, especially when an alkalinizing polyelectrolyte crystalloid solution (e.g., lactated Ringer's solution, Normosol-R) is used for IV fluid therapy.

    b. In cats with severe metabolic acidosis, 1 mEq/kg of sodium bicarbonate is given by IV infusion and then acid-base status is checked after 15 to 30 minutes to see if more sodium bicarbonate should be given. A partial increase in blood pH back toward normal is the goal rather than full restoration of normal blood pH.

4. Management of hypocalcemia.

    a. Specific treatment rarely is needed.

    b. Relief of obstruction usually results in rapid correction of serum calcium concentration as serum phosphorus concentration decreases toward normal.

    c. An IV infusion of calcium gluconate is administered until the desired effect is achieved in cats that have muscular twitching or seizures.

    d. Stop any infusion of $NaHCO_3$ because alkalinization will exacerbate ionized hypocalcemia.

F. Sedation and analgesia for relief of obstruction due to urethral plugs, idiopathic urethritis/cystitis, or urethral stones (Table 11-2).

1. An IV catheter is placed before sedation, analgesia, and anesthesia in unstable cats.
2. An IV catheter can be placed after sedation and analgesia in stable cats.
3. Nearly all cats benefit from preanesthetic analgesics to decrease pain and anxiety; these usually are given before decompressive cystocentesis and before anesthesia to pass a urinary catheter.
4. Urethral relaxation while the cat is sedated or under anesthesia may increase the likelihood of urethral plug dislodgment or facilitate urethral relaxation.
5. Little or no sedation is indicated for cats with severe uremia.
6. Many different sedation protocols are available, depending on the cat's condition and the clinician's comfort and familiarity with their use (Figure 11-12).
   a. Buprenorphine.
   b. Acepromazine.
   c. Hydromorphone or oxymorphone.
   d. Fentanyl.
   e. Diazepam or midazolam.

Decompressive (Therapeutic) Cystocentesis

1. Cystocentesis to empty the bladder should be performed as soon as possible in cats with very enlarged bladders to prevent rupture of the bladder and to allow renal excretory function to resume.
2. Cystocentesis allows for rapid reduction of urinary tract pressure and resumption of GFR compared with catheterization, which can take considerable time. Decompressive cystocentesis may stabilize the cat before anesthesia for urinary catheter placement.
3. Relief of bladder pressure before urethral catheterization also may facilitate efforts to dislodge urethral plugs, and allows collection of a superior urine sample for analysis before manipulation of the urinary tract and contamination by irrigation solutions.
4. Decompressive cystocentesis is considered controversial by some clinicians who fear that bladder rupture will occur or that urine will continue to leak from the bladder.
5. We have performed decompressive cystocentesis before passage of a urinary catheter in cats with UO for more than 15 years and have found the procedure to be safe.

❗ The benefits of decompressive cystocentesis outweigh potential adverse effects.

6. Some leakage of urine immediately after decompressive cystocentesis may occur, especially if the bladder is not adequately emptied.
7. The use of a 22-gauge needle on an extension set or use of a butterfly needle can minimize trauma and urine leakage during the procedure.
8. The needle should be directed toward the pelvic inlet so that that needle trauma to the bladder mucosa will not occur as bladder volume decreases. Continuous gentle pressure on the bladder during drainage will allow a maximal volume of urine to be removed.

G. The volume of urine removed by cystocentesis or obtained after the initial passage of a urinary catheter should be recorded.

1. We have removed up to 260 mL of urine by cystocentesis during treatment of cats with UO.
2. In one study, the median volume of urine removed by urinary catheter at the time initial obstruction was relieved in 28 cats was 85 mL (range, 35 to 280 mL) (Malouin, Milligan, Drobatz, 2007).
3. Cats normally void urine at bladder fill volumes of approximately 20 to 50 mL.

■ TABLE 11-2
■ ■ **Drugs Useful During the Management of Cats With Urethral Obstruction**

Drug	Dose	Indication/Mechanism of Action	Side Effects
Acepromazine	0.02 to 0.05 mg/kg Orally 0.25 to 0.50 mg/kg as needed	Target smooth muscle alpha -2 receptor (blocker) Decrease urethral tone Provide tranquilization	Hypotension
Phenoxy-benzamine	0.5 mg/kg SID or divided BID	Alpha blocker smooth muscle Slow onset of action orally Increase dose after 4 days	Hypotension
Prazosin	IV 0.1 mg/cat or 0.03 mg/kg Orally 0.25 to 0.50 mg per cat BID to TID	Alpha-1 smooth muscle blocker	Hypotension
Dantrolene	IV 1 mg/kg Oral dose is unknown Cats 0.5 mg/kg to 2.0 mg/kg BID to TID	Direct skeletal muscle relaxant—mid to distal urethra	
Diazepam	Orally 1.25 to 2.5 mg/cat BID to TID Short duration of action; Give pills 15 to 30 min prior to bladder expression IV 0.1 to 0.2 mg/kg	Acts on CNS—relaxes skeletal muscle of mid to distal urethra	Sedation; Transient hunger Oral toxicity at 1.25 to 2.0 mg SID or BID: Lethargy, anorexia, ataxia, jaundice, increased ALT, increased glucose, increased cholesterol Oral may be fatal due to acute hepatocellular damage Anecdotes of the same type of toxic reaction exist for the use of IV diazepam Whether midazolam is a safer alternative has not been studied
Propantheline	Orally 7.5 mg/cat every 72 hours 5.0 to 7.5 mg/cat BID to TID PO	Anticholinergic—decrease bladder hypercontractility	
Oxybutynin	Orally 0.50 to 1.25 mg/cat BID to TID	Anticholinergic (weak) and antispasmodic. Also has some direct analgesic effect in bladder; may be useful for detrusor hyperreflexia	

ALT, alanine aminotranferase.

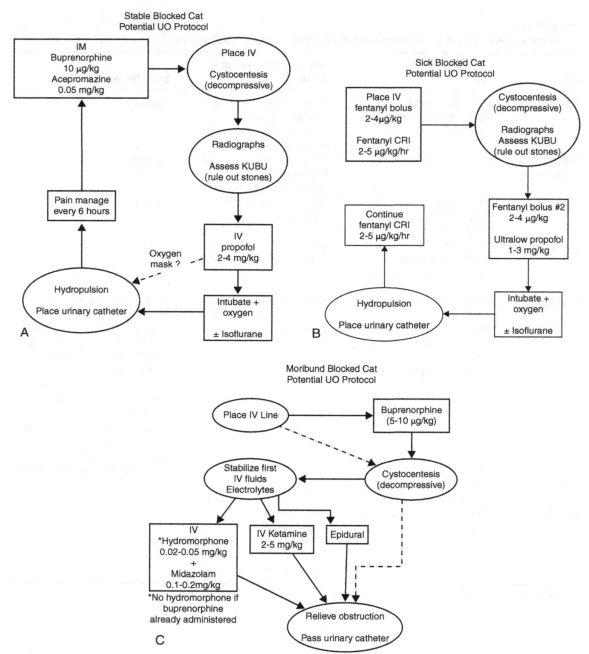

FIGURE 11-12 ■ **A, B**, and **C**, Examples of sedation/analgesia protocols for use in cats with urethral obstruction. *CRI,* Constant rate of infusion; *KUBU,* kidney, ureter, bladder, urethra.

H. Plain abdominal radiographs (including the perineal region) should be obtained after decompressive cystocentesis to identify mineralized plugs, urethral calculi, or cystic calculi. Some clinicians obtain radiographs after catheter passage, but the presence of an indwelling urinary catheter can make it easier to miss urethral calculi.

Anesthesia Protocols (see Figure 11-12)

1. Do not immediately anesthetize severely affected cats; they should be stabilized with IV fluids and decompressive cystocentesis first (as described earlier).
2. The goal is to administer sufficient anesthesia to provide immobilization and urethral relaxation, because less urethral trauma occurs under these conditions.
3. Ketamine and diazepam or ketamine and acepromazine generally are very safe protocols.
   a. These combinations have been used for many years by primary care veterinarians.
   b. The dosage of ketamine for IV use in combination with other drugs is 2 to 4 mg/kg.
   c. The dosage of acepromazine for IV use in combination with other drugs is 0.02 to 0.05 mg/kg.
   d. A fixed dose combination protocol works well: Combine 0.1 mL of a 100 mg/mL solution of ketamine (10 mg) with 0.01 mL of a 10 mg/mL solution of acepromazine (0.1 mg) in a 1.0 mL syringe for IV injection.
   e. An additional dose of 10 mg ketamine (0.1 mL of a 100 mg/mL solution) can be given if more time is needed or if the cat is very large.
   f. Ketamine (100 mg/mL) plus diazepam (5 mg/mL) may be better in cats that are very sick because diazepam is less likely to cause hypotension than is acepromazine.
      (1) Give 2 to 4 mg/kg ketamine and 0.1 to 0.2 mg/kg diazepam in the same syringe IV.
      (2) A fixed dose combination protocol using equal volumes can be used: 0.25 mL of a 100 mg/mL ketamine solution (25 mg) and 0.25 mL of a 5 mg/mL diazepam solution (1.25 mg). Give 0.25 mL of the combined solution, and give the other 0.25 mL only if needed.
   g. Some cats are not relaxed enough with these ketamine combination protocols, and adding inhalational anesthesia may be necessary.
4. Propofol can be useful, but severe hypotension can occur.
   a. It is best to intubate the cat even if it appears to be ventilating adequately.
   b. This protocol is only recommended for personnel highly skilled in the relief of UO over a short period of time.
5. Inhalation of isoflurane via endotracheal tube can be used after premedication and induction with acepromazine and ketamine or diazepam and ketamine. This protocol provides the most complete relaxation and affords time that may be needed by less experienced personnel.

! Isoflurane may be the agent of choice to provide excellent relaxation and adequate time for inexperienced personnel to relieve UO.

6. Epidural.
   a. This procedure is not recommended for routine use by primary care veterinarians.
   b. The operator requires special training and skill to make the injection properly.
   c. This procedure is especially useful in cats that are metabolically unstable.

    d. Up to 12 to 18 hours of postprocedure analgesia can be provided depending on the amount of local anesthetic and opioid used. A combination of ropivacaine hydrochloride and morphine sulfate has been most commonly employed at The Ohio State University Veterinary Teaching Hospital.

    e. Hypotension occasionally is encountered with this technique.

Plug Retrieval

1. Plug retrieval should be attempted so as to document the cause of UO. Determining the mineral composition of the plug provides potentially useful information for future management to prevent recurrent plug formation.

    a. Spontaneous expulsion.

        (1) Gentle penile massage. Gentle massage of the penis may dislodge a urethral plug located in the penile urethra, especially when the plug is near the external urethral orifice. Gentle pulsatile bladder palpation after penile massage may cause a plug to be expelled.

        (2) Gentle bladder massage.

        (3) Cystocentesis and gentle bladder massage.

        (4) Massage of the pelvic urethra by means of rectal palpation also may contribute to plug dislodgment.

        (5) Gentle but persistent urethral lavage.

        (6) Aspiration using a urethral catheter.

    b. Submit urethral plugs for quantitative analysis of crystal and matrix content to a veterinary urolithiasis laboratory.

    c. Alternatively, make a coverslip wet mount of the plug and examine microscopically to identify crystal type or types.

Hydropulsion and Placement of a Urinary Catheter (Retrograde Technique)

1. Place cat in dorsal or lateral recumbency depending on operator preference. Sometimes one position or the other facilitates extrusion and stabilization of the penis (especially in obese cats).

2. Gentle, aseptic technique should be used while placing a urethral catheter. Clip the perineal area of hair and cleanse the region. Wear sterile gloves.

3. Extrude the penis.

    a. Place "stay" sutures at the junction of the penile and preputial epithelia to allow greater control of the penis.

    b. Alternatively, grasp the loose tissue at the base of the penis with a small mosquito hemostat. Do not grasp the penis with the forceps.

    c. The primary operator can maintain extrusion of the penis or have an assistant maintain extrusion.

4. Ensure that the penis is maximally retracted caudally to allow straightening of the urethra, otherwise the catheter cannot navigate the normal anatomic configuration of the distal urethra.

    a. One technique that may facilitate straightening of the urethra is to pull the prepuce caudally once the urinary catheter has been advanced into the external urethral orifice.

    b. Another technique is to push the prepuce cranially and then pull the prepuce and penis together caudally.

5. A well-lubricated urinary catheter is advanced into the urethra to the site of the obstruction.

    a. This often is best accomplished using a relatively rigid urinary catheter such as 10 cm polypropylene catheter (Figure 11-13).

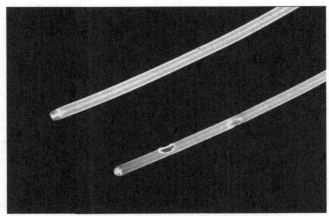

FIGURE 11-13 ■ Tomcat urinary catheters.

   b. Open-end catheters are better for the initial irrigation efforts than are catheters with side-holes because the latter tend to bend and become damaged.

   c. A 22-gauge "over-the-needle" catheter is preferred by some for use as a urinary catheter to advance and provide irrigation. These catheters, however, are not long enough to provide bladder drainage.

6. Urethral irrigation using a sterile physiologic solution (e.g., lactated Ringer's solution, 0.9% saline) may allow the urethra to be dilated and the obstructing plug irrigated and advanced distally between the catheter and urethral epithelium, and out the external urethral orifice.

7. Hydropulsion (reverse irrigation) via the urethra may be attempted at this point if the obstruction is not yet relieved. Sterile irrigating solution (e.g., 0.9% NaCl) is injected rapidly through the urinary catheter so as to advance plugs into the bladder or fatigue the urethra.

   a. Irrigating with a 50:50 mixture of water-soluble lubricant and sterile 0.9% NaCl through the catheter can facilitate catheter advancement and decrease urethral trauma by providing lubrication along the entire length of the urethra as the catheter advances.

   b. The increased viscosity of the solution associated with the presence of the lubricant will increase the irrigation pressure generated and promote hydropulsion.

8. Advance the urethral catheter into the bladder.

   a. Do not force the urethral catheter through the site of the obstruction.

   b. Irrigate at the site of the obstruction.

   c. The catheter should advance easily if enough irrigation of the urethra has already occurred.

   d. Remember to extend the penis and prepuce caudally.

   e. A combination of "pushing" the catheter and "pulling" the penis will facilitate advancement of the catheter.

   f. Do not attempt to force the catheter through the site of obstruction. It should advance easily after adequate irrigation.

   g. The urethra is thoroughly irrigated to be certain all debris in the lumen has been moved retrograde into the bladder or antegrade out the urethral orifice.

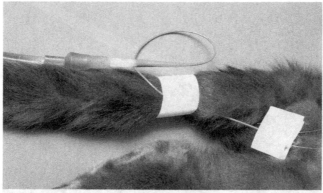

FIGURE 11-14 ■ A flexible polyvinyl urinary catheter has been secured using sutures through a butterfly piece of tape and the prepuce.

    h. Replace the shorter, stiffer (polypropylene) open end urinary catheter used to relieve the obstruction with a longer, softer (polyvinyl) catheter to leave in place as an indwelling urinary catheter and maintain bladder drainage. A urinary catheter that is at least 5 to 6 inches long is needed to adequately empty the bladder of most cats.

    i. The bladder is then immediately drained to relieve pressure if previous drainage by cystocentesis was not performed.

    j. Failure to adequately remove debris from the bladder and urethra is an important cause of re-obstruction soon after catheter removal.

    k. Place a 2-inch piece of adhesive tape over the urinary catheter near the prepuce in a butterfly fashion. Make sure no lubricant is on the catheter and that it is dry before affixing the tape to the catheter (Figure 11-14).

    l. Place one suture on each side of the tape butterfly and through the prepuce on each side; make sure excessive traction is not placed on the prepuce by the sutures (do not penetrate the mucosa with a needle).

    m. Attach a sterile urine collection system.

    n. Tape the collection line or long urinary catheter to the cat's tail. Make sure the cat can lift its tail without putting excessive traction on the prepuce.

  9. Do not use dental Cavitron attachments designed to vibrate putative plugs and facilitate relief of obstruction. These devices may overheat and injure the urethra and penis. We have observed thermal necrosis in some cats with use of these devices.

  10. Causes of resistance to passage of the urethral catheter.

    a. Inadequate penile extrusion caudally.

    b. Intraluminal urethral plug.

    c. Urethrolith.

    d. Urethritis with swelling and erosions.

    e. Urethral tears.

    f. Urethral spasm.

    g. Urethral stricture.

    h. Extraluminal compression of urethra (e.g., peri-urethral swelling).

❗ Resistance to passage of the urinary catheter is not synonymous with the presence of a urethral plug or stone.

    i. Urethral foreign body (e.g., catheter fragment from previous attempts at catheterization).

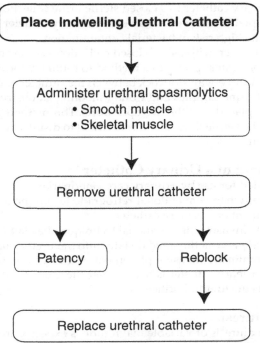

FIGURE 11-15 ■ Use of muscle-relaxing drugs with indwelling urinary catheter.

11. The urinary catheter is left in place to allow continuous urine drainage and allow inflammation and urethral spasm to subside. A urinary catheter is always left in place until resolution of azotemia occurs in cats that initially were azotemic.
   a. Remove the catheter as soon as possible to minimize complications associated with indwelling catheters (e.g., ascending UTI) (Figure 11-15).
   b. The goal is to leave a urinary catheter in place for no more than 24 to 72 hours. Leave the catheter in place until the urine has become clear, azotemia has resolved, and diuresis has subsided.
   c. Despite use of Elizabethan collars and sedation, many cats manage to remove their urinary catheters within 24 to 36 hours.
   d. Studies in cats have shown that indwelling polyvinyl catheters create less urethral trauma and inflammation than do indwelling polypropylene catheters. Silicone urinary catheters have not been specifically studied in cats.
   e. Do not administer glucocorticoids to a cat while an indwelling urinary catheter is in place.

! Do not administer glucocorticoids to a cat with an indwelling urinary catheter.

   (1) The risk for bacterial pyelonephritis is great in this setting.
   (2) Glucocorticoids are unlikely to control urethritis in this setting (i.e., continuous trauma from an indwelling catheter).

12. Connect the urinary catheter to a closed sterile urine collection system.
    a. It is not acceptable to leave an indwelling urinary catheter exposed to the environment because of the high risk of bacterial contamination.
    b. UTI can occur even with use of closed collection systems but less frequently.
    c. The collection system provides a method to routinely measure urine output.
    d. Insertion of a three-way stopcock between the catheter and collection line is useful for collection of urine samples and troubleshooting an obstructed urinary catheter. Injection caps are placed over the two open ports. This method potentially compromises the integrity of the sterile lines, and it is essential to disinfect the injection ports during any manipulations.

Antegrade Placement of a Urinary Catheter

1. Not recommended for use by primary care veterinarians.
2. Consider referral when conventional retrograde technique (described earlier) is not successful in placement of a urinary catheter.
3. In this minimally invasive interventional technique, the bladder is penetrated with a small trocar and a guide wire is threaded distally into the urethra under fluoroscopic guidance. Alternatively, minimally invasive placement of the cystoscope through the bladder wall can be used. A urinary catheter is placed over the guide wire and advanced into the urethra until it exits the urethral orifice.

Postobstructive Diuresis

1. Postobstructive diuresis of variable magnitude is expected in cats with substantial azotemia at the time of relief of UO.
2. The magnitude of diuresis often is proportional to the magnitude of azotemia at presentation.
3. Marked postobstructive diuresis can lead to hypovolemia and hypokalemia. Some cats produce up to 20 mL/kg/hr of urine initially.
4. Much of the diuresis is attributed to retention of osmotically active solutes (e.g., urea, electrolytes) that have accumulated before relief of obstruction and then are excreted when GFR is restored.
5. Other factors contributing to postobstructive diuresis include:
    a. Transient insensitivity of the distal nephron to antidiuretic hormone (ADH).
    b. Decreased renal tubular reabsorption of sodium.
    c. Excretion of previously retained water (especially after fluid therapy).
    d. Hemodynamic changes favoring blood flow to nephrons that do not contribute to elaboration of highly concentrated urine.
6. Postobstructive diuresis usually decreases as azotemia resolves.
7. Often it lasts 2 to 5 days in cats with substantial azotemia at presentation.
8. Some cats experience a delayed onset of diuresis until after hypovolemia has been corrected.
9. A poor prognosis may be warranted in cats with initially severe azotemia that do not undergo postobstructive diuresis after relief of obstruction and rehydration.
10. Minimal to no postobstructive diuresis is expected in cats with minimal to no azotemia at the time UO is relieved.

IV Fluids After Relief of Obstruction

1. Continue IV fluids as indicated by assessment of hydration and monitor urine output as a guide to the volume of fluids to be replaced. Use of an "ins and outs" protocol is helpful to ensure proper hydration for cats that undergo marked postobstructive diuresis.

2. The "ins and outs" protocol is started a few hours after correction of hypovolemia.
3. The goal of the "ins and outs" protocol is to generate an mL/hr fluid prescription.
   a. Consider a 5 kg cat with urine output of 320 mL for the past 4 hours (i.e., 80 mL/hr).

> **!** Consider using the "ins and outs" protocol to determine how much IV fluids to administer after relief of UO.

   b. For the next 4 hours, the cat should receive IV fluids at a rate of 80 mL/hr to replace urine output plus its insensible needs for that time period. The maintenance fluid needs of a 5 kg cat would be approximately 450 mL ($132 \times kg\ 0.75$) and approximately one third of the maintenance need would represent insensible losses (150 mL). Thus, to replace insensible losses, 25 mL would be required over a given 4-hour period or approximately 6 mL/hr. Thus, 86 mL/hr would be administered during the upcoming 4-hour period.
   c. During the next 4 hours the cat produces 160 ml of urine (i.e., 40 mL/hr).
   d. Thus, for the next 4 hours the cat will receive fluids at a rate of 46 mL/hr.
   e. Using this method to replace urine losses prevents development of dehydration in cats with substantial postobstructive diuresis.
4. Usually an alkalinizing polyelectrolyte crystalloid fluid (e.g., lactated Ringer's, Normosol-R, Plasmalyte-R) will be given for the first 12 to 24 hours. After 12 hours, most cats will no longer have appreciable metabolic acidosis and the fluid may be changed to a less alkalinizing fluid if desired.
5. Potassium supplementation of IV fluids usually is needed after 12 to 24 hours, especially when postobstructive diuresis is substantial.
   a. The extent of potassium supplementation should be based on serial measurement of serum potassium concentration, at least twice daily for the first 24 to 48 hours.
   b. If serial serum potassium concentrations cannot be determined and the cat is undergoing appropriate postobstructive diuresis, add 10 to 20 mEq of potassium per liter of infused crystalloid fluid as an estimate.
   c. More aggressive potassium supplementation is needed for some cats during postobstructive diuresis, but access to serial measurements of serum potassium concentration is necessary to make these decisions (Table 11-3).

Failure of Postobstructive Diuresis to Resolve

1. A spontaneous decrease in urine output typically accompanies resolution of azotemia.
2. Occasionally, the large volume of IV fluids being administered actually is driving the diuresis.

■ TABLE 11-3
■ ■ **Scott's Sliding Scale: Guidelines for Supplementation of IV Fluids With Potassium**

Serum K+ (mEq/L)	mEq KCl to add to 250 mL	mEq KCl to add to 1000 mL	Maximal infusion rate (mL/kg/hr)*
<2.0	20	80	6
2.1-2.5	15	60	8
2.6-3.0	10	40	12
3.1-3.5	7	28	18
3.6-5.0	5	20	25

*Do NOT exceed 0.5 mEq/kg/hr.
Courtesy of Richard C. Scott, Animal Medical Center, New York.

3. To determine whether or not this is the case, taper IV fluids by 25%. If the urine output decreases, continue to taper the fluid volume infused further. If the urine volume does not decrease, increase the fluid infusion to its previous rate and try again to taper the fluid infusion after 24 to 48 hours.

Additional Medical Management During Hospitalization

1. Continue analgesics and antispasmodics while the cat is in the hospital and for 5 to 7 days after release. We treat most UO cats with a combination of acepromazine and buprenorphine.

> **!** The combination of acepromazine and buprenorphine is recommended during hospitalization of cats with UO and for 5 to 7 days after discharge from the hospital.

2. Do not prescribe antibiotics while a urinary catheter is in place (unless you have documented by bacterial culture that a UTI already is present).
   a. Antibiotics do not prevent development of UTI in patients with indwelling urinary catheters.
   b. Antibiotic use may promote development of resistant isolates when UTI does develop.
   c. Consider culturing the urine when the urinary catheter is removed.

> **!** The use of antibiotics does not prevent the development of UTI in patients with indwelling urinary catheters.

3. The cat should be housed in a low stress environment (i.e., quiet, dark, away from dogs and frequent intrusions by humans) so as to limit activation of the sympathetic nervous system that otherwise may have adverse effects on the urethra (e.g., increased urethral spasm).
4. Serially measure BUN, serum creatinine, and serum potassium concentrations at least daily for the first 2 days after relief of UO.

Failure to Obtain Much Urine From the Indwelling Urinary Catheter

1. Mechanical problems are most common.
   a. Kinked outflow lines.
   b. Twisted or kinked urinary catheter.
   c. Disconnected or improperly connected outflow lines; air bubbles in the line may be an indication of this problem.
   d. Urinary catheter is not long enough to reach the bladder.
   e. Urinary catheter has passed through a tear in the urethra.
   f. Obstruction of the catheter or lines by clots, inflammatory debris, or crystals.
   g. Urinary catheter looped and tied into a knot after having been advanced too far into the bladder.
2. Large blood clots in the bladder may cause intermittent obstruction of the catheter by a ball-and-valve effect (Figure 11-16).
3. Ruptured bladder.
4. Low urine volume due to hypovolemia or dehydration.
5. Low urine volume due to acute renal failure (acute tubular necrosis) from renal ischemia (rare).

Failure to Urinate Adequately After Removal of the Urinary Catheter (Figure 11-17)

1. Recurrent UO from the same process initially identified.
2. Recurrent UO from a different process than initially identified (e.g., swelling, infection, clots, urethral tear, stricture).

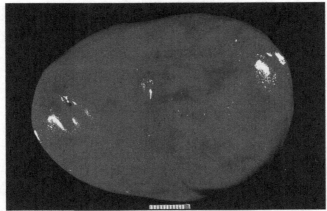

FIGURE 11-16 ■ Large blood clot surgically removed from the bladder of a cat with recurrent urethral obstruction.

! Inability to urinate after removal of the urinary catheter may be caused by a problem different from the problem that initially caused UO.

    3. Bladder atony.
    4. Conventional management is to replace the indwelling urinary catheter.
    5. An alternative management strategy is to begin decompressive cystocentesis for the next 24 to 48 hours without replacing the urinary catheter and continue antispasmodic and analgesic therapy (e.g., acepromazine and buprenorphine).

TREATMENT OF THE CAT WITH AN OVERDISTENDED URINARY BLADDER AND BLADDER ATONY

    A. Keep the bladder empty so as to decrease hydrostatic pressure and avoid bladder distension. An indwelling urinary catheter will facilitate this goal.
    B. Avoid manual expression of the bladder, which can exacerbate separation of the urothelial tight junctions.

! Avoid manual expression of an overdistended urinary bladder.

    C. Consider repeated decompressive cystocentesis as an alternative to replacing the urinary catheter.
    D. Consider the use of parasympathomimetic drugs (e.g., bethanechol) to stimulate detrusor contractions after relief of UO. Make certain no outflow obstruction is present when the detrusor muscle is stimulated.

! Make certain no urinary outflow obstruction is present when detrusor contraction is being stimulated by drugs.

COMPLICATIONS AFTER RELIEF OF URETHRAL OBSTRUCTION IN MALE CATS

    A. Persistent UO (ongoing episode has not resolved).
        1. Original urethral plug or debris has not been adequately cleared.
        2. A urethral calculus has been bypassed by the catheter and still remains in the urethra.
        3. Urethral spasm.

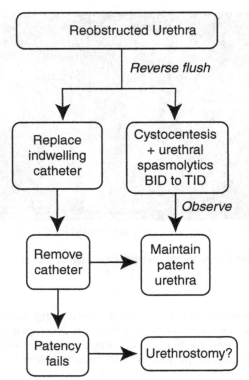

FIGURE 11-17 ■ Potential management approach following removal of an indwelling urethral catheter.

   B. New episode of UO.
      1. Additional urethral plug formation due to accumulation of some combination of RBCs, protein, and crystals.
      2. Bladder outflow obstruction due to intraluminal blood clots.
      3. Recurrent urethral spasm or swelling.
   C. Ongoing or recurrent episodes of urethritis/cystitis (Figure 11-18).
   D. Bacterial UTI as a consequence of previous indwelling urethral catheterization.
   E. Catheter-associated bladder or urethral trauma.
      1. Mechanical.
      2. Associated with irrigating agents.
      3. Bacterial UTI.
      4. Iatrogenic urethral rupture.
         a. Bruising and edema of the leg and cutaneous necrosis may be observed.
   F. Bladder rupture.
      1. Spontaneous (rare).
      2. Iatrogenic (especially after palpation).
   G. Bladder atony due to overdistension.
   H. Urethral stricture.
   I. Prerenal or postrenal azotemia.
   J. Primary renal disease or failure due to pyelonephritis (ascending) or acute tubular necrosis (rare).
   K. Persistent postobstructive diuresis (usually resolves within 2 to 5 days.)

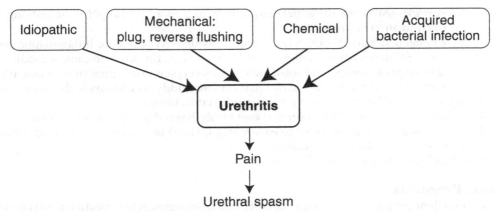

FIGURE 11-18 ■ Possible causes for urethritis and subsequent urethral pain and spasm following removal of a urinary catheter.

MANAGEMENT AT HOME

A. Decreased GFR and RBF that occur during UO will persist for a variable time despite return of BUN and serum creatinine concentrations to normal. Ability to maximally acidify the urine also may be impaired after relief of UO. Submaximal urinary concentrating ability may persist for 1 to 2 weeks after relief of UO.
   1. Dosages of drugs that are excreted by the kidneys may need to be decreased for a week or more after relief of UO.
   2. Acidifying diets should not be fed in the first 1 to 2 weeks after relief of UO.
B. Continue antispasmodics and analgesics (e.g., acepromazine and buprenorphine) for 5 to 7 days.
C. Try to transition the cat's diet to one that has more water (e.g., canned food) as would be done in management of idiopathic cystitis.
D. Stress reduction and environmental enrichment are warranted because cats with UO likely have underlying idiopathic cystitis (see Chapter 10, Nonobstructive Idiopathic or Interstitial Cystitis in Cats).
E. Administration of subcutaneous fluids is recommended to increase urine flow, but this approach has not been specifically studied. We often give a subcutaneous bolus of fluids at the time of discharge from the hospital.
F. Owners should be advised about the normal volume of urination to be expected for their cat.
G. Most cats will have stranguria and pollakiuria for several days after the urinary catheter has been removed. Some hematuria may persist and potentially will be visible to the owner.

MEDICAL RE-EVALUATION AND PREVENTION OF RECURRENT URETHRAL OBSTRUCTION

A. Bladder size should be assessed by gentle palpation whenever the owner is not sure if the cat is urinating an adequate volume of urine.
B. If the cat shows systemic signs of illness in the first few weeks after relief of UO, recurrence of UO or development of pyelonephritis should be considered.
C. Routine re-evaluation is recommended 7 to 14 days after discharge from the hospital. Factors to consider include:
   1. Has USG decreased (ideally to < 1.030)?
   2. What is urine pH and are crystals present in the absence of UO?

a. A previously high urine pH may return to a more acidic pH if underlying sterile inflammation has resolved.
   b. Crystalluria may diminish or disappear as underlying sterile inflammation resolves and USG decreases from dietary intervention (e.g., transition to canned food).
   c. If urine pH is not low and substantial struvite crystalluria is present with inactive urine sediment, change the diet to one that is more acidifying and has higher water content.
3. Is the extent of hematuria and proteinuria less than before?
4. Is pyuria now present? Or, if present previously, has it diminished or resolved?
5. Urine culture is recommended to ensure that UTI did not become established during and after removal of the urinary catheter.
D. Schedule 1- and 3-month reevaluations.

Acute Prognosis
1. Excellent prognosis with high survival rate is expected when treatment is started soon enough. In a recent study, almost 94% of affected cats survived initial treatment and were discharged from the hospital (Lee, Drobatz, 2003). Mortality of 16% was reported in an older study (Bovee, Reif, Maguire, et al., 1979).
2. Good prognosis for being able to urinate voluntarily after removal of the urinary catheter. Approximately 14% of affected cats re-obstructed soon after removal of the urinary catheter in one study (Drobatz, 2003). Approximately 25% of affected cats in our hospital are not able to adequately empty the bladder after removal of the urinary catheter.
3. Depending on severity of the episode of UO, hospitalization may last 1 to 6 days.
   a. The mean hospital stay was 1.8 days in one study (Lee, Drobatz, 2003).
   b. In another study, median hospitalization was 4.5 days (Gerber, Eichenberger, Reusch, 2008).
   c. Urinary catheters were in place a median of 2 days (and up to 6 days) in one study (Gerber, Eichenberger, Reusch, 2008) and for a median of 1 day (and up to 7 days) in another study (Lee, Drobatz, 2003).
4. Acute bacterial UTI develops in a small number of cats.

Chronic Prognosis
1. Eight of 22 (36%) cats with idiopathic UO re-obstructed after a median of 17 days in one study (Gerber, 2007).
2. Three of seven (43%) cats with UO associated with urethral plugs re-obstructed within 7 months (Gerber, Eichenberger, Reusch, 2008).
3. Recurrent obstruction was the cause for euthanasia in 21% of cats in this study (Gerber 2007).
4. In an older study, the recurrence rate was 35% within 6 months (Bovee, Reif, Maguire, et al., 1979).
5. No studies on recurrence rates for UO have been reported prospectively after implementation of environmental modification. Recurrence rates may be lower in cats for which environmental modification can be adequately implemented.
6. A small number of cats develop urethral strictures. This complication occurred in 11% of affected cats in one study (Barsanti, Brown, Marks, et al., 1996).
7. Some cats develop bacterial UTI after instrumentation of their urinary tract (i.e., catheterization), and this complication may occur as late as 6 months after relief of UO.
8. Signs of ongoing idiopathic cystitis are expected in 30% to 50% of cats that have had an episode of UO. In one study, 50% of cats with idiopathic UO developed lower urinary tract signs after relief of obstruction (Gerber, Eichenberger, Reusch, 2008).

Perineal Urethrostomy

1. Although discouraged by some veterinarians as a "mutilating procedure," judicious use of perineal urethrostomy may make the difference between survival and euthanasia in some cats. It should be considered as an option when medical management fails to prevent recurrences.

> **!** Recurrent UO is a common reason for euthanasia.

> **!** Cats that experience a second episode of UO are likely to have additional episodes, and should be considered candidates for perineal urethrostomy.

2. This surgery is performed less commonly now than in past years, possibly due to advances in the medical management of idiopathic cystitis in cats.
3. Perineal urethrostomy saves the lives of many cats that have failed diligent attempts at medical management.
4. Perineal urethrostomy may be necessary after a first episode of UO if severe trauma to the penis and urethra occur during relief of obstruction.
5. Considerable expense is associated with treatment of each episode of UO. Many owners are not willing or able to endure these costs. Perineal urethrostomy is a reasonable option for owners of such cats.
6. Urethrostomy also is indicated for cats that develop distal urethral strictures.
7. The option of perineal urethrostomy should be discussed with the owner during the first presentation of a cat with UO.
8. We usually recommend a perineal urethrostomy for a cat that is experiencing its third episode of UO. Some owners are unwilling to endure another episode of UO in their cat, and will request perineal urethrostomy after the second recurrence.
9. Perineal urethrostomy prevents future episodes of UO.
10. Although recurrent UO is prevented, signs of lower urinary tract disease still may be observed due to underlying idiopathic cystitis. Such signs usually are less severe than before.
11. Some cats will develop bacterial UTI up to a year after perineal urethrostomy despite minimal or no signs of lower urinary tract disease. Urine culture should be performed at 1, 3, and 6 months after surgery to identify asymptomatic UTI.
12. A very small number of cats will develop stricture at the site of the urethrostomy. Most often, stricture is the result of poor surgical technique, but it can occur even with excellent surgical technique.
13. Antepubic urethrostomy can be used successfully in some cats to rescue them from a failed perineal urethrostomy.
14. Antepubic urethrostomy is an option for cats in which perineal urethrostomy cannot be performed because of severe damage to the urethra or obstruction that is too far proximal in the urethra.

MANAGING URETHRAL OBSTRUCTION IN MALE CATS WITHOUT URETHRAL CATHETERIZATION USING HOSPITALIZATION FOR 3 DAYS

A. This treatment is proposed only as an alternative to euthanasia due to financial constraints of owners.

> ❗ As an alternative to euthanasia when owners cannot afford standard care, consider a protocol of decompressive cystocentesis, drug treatment, and a quiet environment for 3 days.

   B. Conventional treatment with passage of a urinary catheter and IV fluid infusion in the hospital should be offered as the first choice.
   C. We have used this protocol with success in some cats over the past 20 years, and this approach as an alternative to euthanasia recently was reported (Cooper, Owens, Chew, et al., 2010).
   D. This approach is not meant for cats with urethral calculi or those with severe metabolic derangements.
   E. The severity of azotemia does not determine use of this protocol.
   F. A plain lateral abdominal radiograph is taken to exclude calculi.
   G. Decompressive cystocentesis is performed initially and then as needed up to every 8 hours.
   H. The urethra is not irrigated or catheterized.
   I. No IV catheter is placed, and IV fluids are not administered.
   J. Drug treatments include:
      1. Acepromazine (0.25 mg IM or 2.5 mg PO every 8 hours).
      2. Buprenorphine (0.075 mg PO every 8 hours).
      3. Medetomidine (0.1mg IM every 24 hours if no urinations are noted in the first 24 hours).
   K. Place the cat in a quiet, low stress environment.
   L. Some fluids may be given subcutaneously as needed, but the goal is to avoid excessive urine production from full hydration.
   M. Treatment success was defined as spontaneous urination within 72 hours and subsequent discharge from the hospital.
      1. Treatment success occurred in 11 of 15 cats (73%).
      2. Treatment failure occurred in 4 of 15 cats (27%) due to uroabdomen (3) or hemoabdomen (1).
      3. Cats that experienced treatment failure had significantly higher serum creatinine concentrations.
      4. At necropsy, severe bladder inflammation was found, but there was no evidence of bladder rupture.

Alternative Rescue Protocol

   1. Another rescue protocol can be tried as an alternative to euthanasia for clients who cannot afford to hospitalize a cat with UO.
   2. This protocol is less expensive than that described above because it does not involve hospitalization.
   3. Outcomes from this protocol have not been specifically evaluated.
   4. A lateral abdominal radiograph is taken to rule out the presence of cystic or urethral calculi.
   5. Drug therapy includes:
      a. Buprenorphine (10 µg/kg) intramuscularly.
      b. Dexmedetomidine (4-5 µg/kg) intramuscularly.
   6. Decompressive cystocentesis is performed.
   7. A urinary catheter is passed, the urethra irrigated, the bladder emptied, and the catheter removed.
   8. A bolus of subcutaneous fluids is administered.

9. The cat is released to the owner with instructions to give buprenorphine (10-20 μg/kg) PO every 8 hours and acepromazine (2 mg, total dose) PO every 8 hours for 5 days. A convenient method that treats an average-sized cat is to combine both medications in a syringe using 0.25 mL (75 μg) buprenorphine and 0.20 mL (2 mg) acepromazine.
10. Environmental modification and enrichment recommendations are discussed should the cat survive this episode of UO.

Amitriptyline

1. A recent report suggests amitriptyline may be useful in relief of UO in male cats caused by urethral plugs (Achar, Achar, Paiva, et al., 2003).
2. Obstructed cats had serum creatinine concentrations of >4.0 mg/dL and BUN concentrations of >120 mg/dL before treatment.
3. Treatment details were not provided in this report. More details were given by the author by personal communication (2009).
   a. Some cats had decompressive cystocentesis performed.
   b. All were given IV 0.9% NaCl.
   c. No cats had urethral flushing or placement of an indwelling urinary catheter.
   d. No other drugs or anesthetic agents were administered besides ampicillin for prevention of UTI.
   e. This protocol has been used in the author's practice as the standard of care for several years.
4. Amitriptyline (1 mg/kg) was given orally for 30 days.
   a. This time period was chosen to decrease the likelihood of recurrence of UO.
   b. Amitriptyline should never be abruptly discontinued because of possible development of "abrupt withdrawal syndrome."
5. Urethral plugs were spontaneously eliminated and urinary flow was restored in all cats within 72 hours.
6. Urethral plugs were analyzed and found to contain varying proportions of struvite, calcium oxalate, and ammonium urates.
7. Transient somnolence was attributed to the use of amitriptyline, an effect that lessened as azotemia resolved. This effect has been described when amitriptyline is used in cats without azotemia.
8. All cats had normal BUN and serum creatinine concentrations when measured 30 days later.
9. No cats experienced recurrent UO during the 30 days of treatment.
10. The beneficial effects of amitriptyline in cats with UO appear to be mediated by relaxation of urinary tract smooth muscle through mechanisms that involve voltage-dependent potassium channels.

Tube Cystostomy

1. Minimally invasive surgical technique for emergency treatment of 5 cats with UO or urethral rupture (Bray, Doyle, Burton, 2009).
2. An inguinal approach with muscle splitting and minimal soft tissue dissection facilitates rapid placement of cystostomy tubes in metabolically unstable patients.
3. The catheter is secured into the bladder with a purse-string suture.
4. Cystopexy is performed to provide peritoneal protection should the cystostomy tube dislodge prematurely.
5. May be considered as an alternative to placement of a urinary catheter in a metabolically unstable patient.

Urethral Obstruction in Dogs

I. The principles for diagnosis and management of UO in dogs are similar to those outlined for cats.
II. The frequency and causes of UO in dogs differ from those in cats.
III. UO can be acute, subacute, or chronic depending on the completeness of obstruction. Dogs are subject to many more causes of chronic UO than are cats.
   A. Idiopathic obstruction due to urethral plugs is not a specific syndrome in dogs.
   B. Outflow obstruction due to bladder or urethral neoplasia is relatively common in older dogs (more often in females) as discussed in Chapter 14, Tumors of the Urinary System.
   C. Obstruction from prostatic neoplasia is an occasional cause of UO in both intact and neutered male dogs.
   D. Proliferative (granulomatous) urethritis is an occasional cause of UO in female dogs.
   E. Detrusor-urethral-dyssynergia is an occasional cause of functional UO, especially in large breed male dogs (see Chapter 13, Disorders of Micturition and Urinary Incontinence).
   F. Urethral stricture occurs occasionally in dogs that have previously passed urinary calculi, those that have had indwelling urinary catheters, and in those that have previously had urethral surgery.
   G. Urethral stones are the most common cause of UO in dogs and cause obstruction almost exclusively in male dogs.

HISTORY

   A. Stranguria.
   B. Pollakiuria.
   C. Hematuria.
   D. Paradoxical overflow incontinence.
   E. Urine stream initially may be normal and then dramatically diminish in dogs with detrusor-urethral-dyssynergia.

PHYSICAL EXAMINATION

   A. An enlarged, potentially painful, bladder is palpable.
   B. A mass in the bladder may be palpable if obstruction is related to bladder neoplasia.
   C. Rectal examination.
      1. A thickened, irregular urethra may be identified in dogs with urethral neoplasia or with proliferative urethritis.
      2. Urethral stones may be palpated in the pelvic portion of the urethra.
   D. Bradycardia and hypothermia may be present if the UO has been long-standing and the dog is hyperkalemic.
   E. Dehydration may be present if the dog is uremic.

DIAGNOSTIC TESTING

   A. Serum chemistry findings (abnormalities detected will depend on the duration and completeness of UO).
      1. Azotemia.
      2. Hyperphosphatemia.
      3. Hyperkalemia.
      4. Hyponatremia.

     5. Hypochloremia (especially if there is a history of vomiting).
     6. Metabolic acidosis.
  B. Urinalysis.
     1. Variable USG.
     2. Proteinuria.
     3. Hematuria.
     4. Pyuria.
     5. Increased numbers of epithelial cells or rafts of epithelial cells.
     6. Bacteriuria.
  C. Imaging.
     1. Survey radiographs may reveal urolithiasis, masses, or prostatic enlargement (in male dogs).
     2. Contrast urethrography may identify radiolucent urethral calculi, urethral mass, or urethral stricture.
     3. Ultrasonography may identify mass lesions in the bladder or bladder neck that may be contributing to UO but generally is not helpful for identifying urethral lesions.
     4. Urethroscopy can identify urethral stones, proliferative urethritis, urethral tumors or strictures.
  D. Histopathology.
     1. Necessary to differentiate neoplasia from proliferative urethritis in dogs with multiple mass lesions in the urethra.
     2. Necessary to differentiate bladder neoplasia (e.g., transitional cell carcinoma) from polypoid cystitis.

RELIEF OF OBSTRUCTION

  A. Perform decompressive cystocentesis as described above for male cats with UO.
  B. If available, consider lithotripsy for urethral calculi followed by basket retrieval or voiding urohydropulsion of fragments.
  C. Perform retropulsion of urethral calculi with reverse irrigation.
     1. Perform cystotomy to retrieve urethral calculi that were retropulsed into the bladder by reverse irrigation.
     2. Alternatively, consider medical dissolution for calculi that were retropulsed into the bladder.
  D. Pass a urethral catheter to empty the bladder whenever possible. Leave catheter in place to maintain bladder decompression.
  E. Consider tube cystostomy if a urethral catheter cannot be successfully advanced into the bladder.
  F. Consider temporary urethrotomy in male dogs if a urethral catheter cannot be successfully advanced into the bladder. A temporary opening in the urethra is created at a site proximal to the UO.
  G. Permanent urethrostomy may be needed in some dogs.
     1. Scrotal urethrostomy.
     2. Perineal urethrostomy.
     3. Prescrotal urethrostomy.
  H. Urinary diversion surgery can be considered in dogs with distal urethral masses.
  I. Treatment with nonsteroidal anti-inflammatory drugs (NSAIDs) (e.g., piroxicam) with or without adjunctive chemotherapy should be considered for dogs with transitional cell carcinomas that are causing UO.
  J. Long-term treatment with antibiotics, glucocorticoids, or NSAIDs (e.g., piroxicam) should be considered in dogs with proliferative urethritis.

Upper Urinary Tract Obstruction

PATHOPHYSIOLOGY

A. Return of renal function after correction of complete unilateral renal obstruction.
   1. 70% to 100% return of GFR after 1 to 2 weeks of obstruction.
   2. 20% to 30% return of GFR after 4 weeks of obstruction.
   3. No return of GFR after 6 to 8 weeks of obstruction.
B. Acute to subacute obstruction.
   1. Mild dilatation of renal pelvis and diverticula.
   2. Dilatation of renal tubules.
   3. Interstitial edema may occur due to backleak of tubular fluid.
C. Chronic obstruction (unilateral, complete).
   1. Moderate to marked enlargement of kidney (Figure 11-19).
   2. Marked dilatation of renal pelvis with radiating fibrous septa visible.
   3. Tubular dilatation.
   4. Interstitial fibrosis.
   5. Loss of cortical and medullary tissue (atrophy) secondary to ischemia associated with decreased RBF and pressure atrophy.
   6. Pyonephrosis may develop if fluid in the obstructed kidney is infected.
D. Pathophysiology of decreased GFR and RBF during obstruction.
   1. Increased pressure is transmitted up the ureters and causes renal tubular pressure to increase.
   2. Increased renal tubular pressure opposes hydrostatic forces within the glomeruli that normally favor filtration.
   3. RBF is decreased.
   4. Backleak of fluid across renal tubules occurs when renal tubular pressure is high.
   5. Decreased permeability of glomerular capillaries may occur.
   6. Afferent arteriolar vasoconstriction decreases glomerular capillary plasma flow in obstructed nephrons (the mediator of vasoconstriction is unknown).
   7. Pressure within the ureter decreases and actually may fall to zero as GFR ceases.
   8. Anatomic structures dilate with continuing obstruction, but pressure with the collecting system decreases.
   9. Decreased RBF parallels decreased GFR during obstruction, but the decrease in RBF is most severe in the medulla.

HISTORY AND CLINICAL SIGNS

A. Unilateral renal obstruction.
   1. Animal may be asymptomatic (i.e., renal obstruction is an incidental finding).
   2. Azotemia will not be present if the contralateral kidney is normal.
   3. Abdominal distension may be present if hydronephrosis is severe.
   4. The enlarged kidney may be readily palpable.
   5. Increased renal size on radiography.
   6. Hydronephrosis can be confirmed by ultrasonography or excretory urography.
   7. Fever may occur if urine or renal tissue proximal to the obstruction becomes infected.
   8. Urine volume will be unchanged if the unilateral obstruction is complete, because the contralateral kidney will compensate.
   9. Urine volume may increase if unilateral obstruction is partial because partial obstruction impairs concentrating ability in the obstructed kidney.

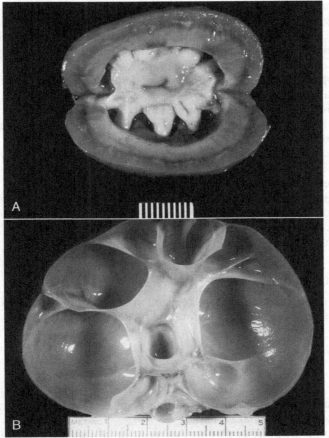

FIGURE 11-19 ■ **A,** Moderate hydronephrosis secondary to a sponge granuloma causing obstruction to one ureter in a dog. **B,** Severe hydronephrosis with complete atrophy of renal parenchyma in a cat. Only fibrous tissue bands remain. Both images are gross specimens, seen on necropsy.

     10. Urinalysis is normal if outflow is completely obstructed.
     11. Urinalysis may reflect the underlying cause if the obstruction is partial (e.g., hematuria, proteinuria, pyuria, bacteriuria).
     12. Urine may be more dilute with unilateral partial obstruction due to admixture of dilute urine from the obstructed kidney with urine from the unobstructed kidney.
  B. Bilateral renal obstruction.
     1. Complete.
       a. Resembles oliguric acute intrinsic renal failure in many ways.
       b. Uremia and death result after 3 to 5 days of complete bilateral obstruction.
       c. Anorexia.
       d. Vomiting.
       e. Lethargy.
       f. Hyperkalemia and metabolic acidosis become severe and lead to death.
       g. Progressive increases in BUN and serum creatinine concentrations.
       h. Moderate to marked hyperphosphatemia.

      i. Mild to moderate hypocalcemia.
      j. Enlarged, turgid bladder if the obstruction is in the urethra.
      k. Rectal examination may be abnormal if obstruction is in the urethra.
      l. A bladder or urethral mass causing outflow obstruction may be palpable or visible on ultrasonography or contrast radiography.
     m. Radiography may identify bilateral ureteral stones or stones within urethra causing obstruction.
      n. USG remains high during complete bilateral obstruction.
      o. Urinalysis often shows hematuria and proteinuria due to distension of the bladder from the process causing obstruction.
      p. Bacteriuria and pyuria may be seen if the process is associated with infection.
  2. Partial. (Figure 11-20).
      a. Can resemble polyuric chronic renal failure in many ways.
      b. Azotemia may or may not develop, depending on the extent of obstruction. Total GFR (i.e., sum total of both kidneys) must decrease to 25% of normal or less for azotemia to develop.
      c. Hydronephrosis.
      d. Dilute urine may be detected.

Ureterolithiasis in Cats

I. Ureterolithiasis has been increasingly recognized in cats since the early 1990s.
II. Ureterolithiasis is unilateral 75% of the time and bilateral 25% of the time.
III. Clinical findings are nonspecific.
  A. Inappetence.
  B. Vomiting.
  C. Lethargy.
  D. Weight loss.
IV. About 75% of cats with unilateral ureterolithiasis are azotemic suggesting contralateral renal parenchymal disease or prerenal azotemia.
  A. Azotemia commonly persists after surgical removal of a unilateral ureterolith.
  B. Chronic renal failure is a common reason for death or euthanasia later in the clinical course.
  C. Progressive renal damage may result from recurrent intermittent obstruction and relief of obstruction (ball-and-valve effect).
    1. Antegrade movement of the calculus causes it to lodge in the ureter with obstruction and proximal ureteral dilatation.
    2. Retrograde movement of the calculus into the dilated proximal ureter and relief of obstruction may occur with gravity when cat jumps down from a high place.
    3. This sequence of events may lead to big kidney-little kidney syndrome (i.e., one kidney is enlarged due to acute obstruction and the other kidney is chronically diseased from previous episodes of intermittent obstruction and relief of obstruction by retrograde movement of a ureterolith) (Figure 11-21).

IMAGING FINDINGS

  A. Ureteroliths are identified by plain abdominal radiography (high specificity, low sensitivity) or ultrasonography (high sensitivity, low specificity) in 90% of cases (Figure 11-22).
  B. Dilatation of the renal pelvis and ureter commonly are observed on ultrasonography indicating obstructive disease (Figure 11-23).
  C. These two imaging procedures complement one another in the diagnosis of feline ureterolithiasis.

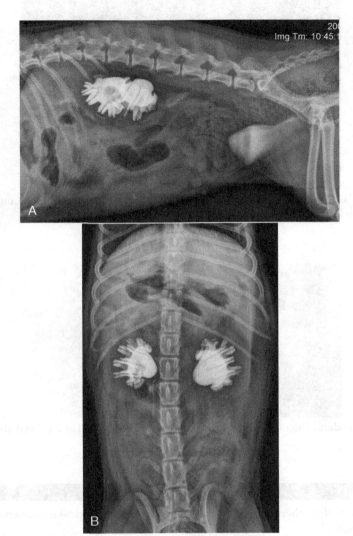

FIGURE 11-20 ■ **A, B**, Bilateral renal obstruction due to bilateral congenital uretero-pelvic stricture. Note marked dilatation of renal pelves and diverticula, but no dilatation of the ureter on this intravenous pyelogram (IVP). (Courtesy of Drs. Aimee Kidder, Joao Galvao, and Brian Scansen, The Ohio State University, Columbus, Ohio.)

D. The contralateral kidney is observed to be smaller than normal in approximately 50% of affected cats (see earlier explanation of big kidney-little kidney syndrome).
E. The majority of affected cats also have nephroliths.
 I. Nearly all of the retrieved uroliths are composed of calcium oxalate.
 II. <10% of affected cats have concomitant bacterial UTI.
III. Occasionally dried solidified blood clots occur in the upper urinary tract of cats.
A. Not visible on plain radiographs.
B. May be a cause for otherwise unexplained renal pelvic and proximal ureteral dilatation on abdominal ultrasonography.
C. No mineral content.

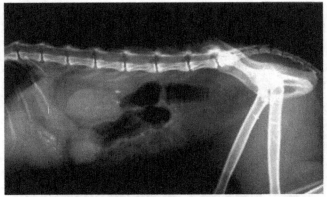

FIGURE 11-21 ■ Big kidney-little kidney syndrome. Lateral abdominal radiograph (Courtesy of Drs. Aimee Kidder, Joao Galvao, and Brian Scansen, The Ohio State University, Columbus, Ohio.)

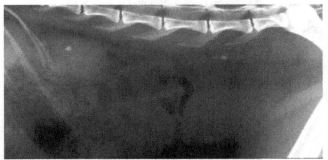

FIGURE 11-22 ■ Radiodense calculus overlying the kidneys and two calculi in the distal ureter, seen on a lateral radiograph.

MANAGEMENT

A. Factors to consider when deciding upon medical versus surgical management.
   1. Urolith size.
   2. Urolith location.
   3. Duration of clinical signs.
   4. Presence or absence of renal colic.
   5. Severity of serum biochemical abnormalities.
   6. Evidence of renal damage.
   7. Evidence of obstruction.

Conservative Medical Management
   1. Fluid therapy to promote antegrade movement of the ureterolith.
   2. Diuretics (e.g., furosemide) to promote antegrade movement of the ureterolith.
   3. Tamsulosin (alpha-A1 adrenoceptor antagonist).
   4. Ureteroliths can be expected to move into the bladder in 30% to 60% of cats managed medically.
   5. Twelve-month survival with conservative medical management is approximately 70%.

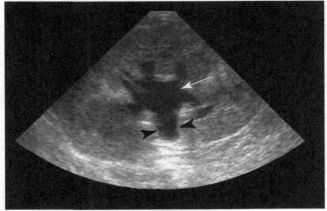

FIGURE 11-23 ■ Dilatation of the proximal ureter (black arrowheads) and renal pelvis (white arrow) secondary to ureteral obstruction demonstrated on renal ultrasonography. (Courtesy of Dr. Paul Barthez, European School for Advanced Veterinary Studies, Université du Luxembourg.)

Surgical Management

1. Ureterotomy recommended for calculi in the proximal ureter.
2. Ureteroneocystostomy recommended for calculi in the distal ureter.
3. Twelve-month survival with surgery (performed by a board-certified veterinary surgeon) is approximately 90%.
4. Postoperative complications can be expected in approximately 30% of cases.
   a. Uroabdomen.
   b. Recurrence of obstruction (especially with ureteroneocystostomy).
   c. Recurrence of ureterolithiasis.
5. Complications are especially high when nephrostomy tubes are used in management.
   a. Uroabdomen.
   b. Tube dislodgment.

A. Lithotripsy can be considered on a referral basis if expertise and equipment is available and expense is acceptable to the client.
B. Ureteral stenting can be considered on a referral basis if expertise and equipment is available and expense is acceptable to the client (Figure 11-24).
C. Clinical evidence justifying conservative medical management.
   1. Minimal compromise of renal function.
   2. Absence of infection.
   3. No apparent renal colic.
   4. Lack of progressive renal pelvic and ureteral dilatation (as documented by serial abdominal ultrasonography).
D. Clinical evidence justifying surgical intervention, lithotripsy, or ureteral stenting.
   1. Progressive azotemia.
   2. Infection (may require nephropyelocentesis to identify).
   3. Suspicion of complete obstruction.
   4. Ureterolith is not observed to be moving distally on serial imaging studies.
   5. Retrograde movement of ureterolith on serial imaging studies.

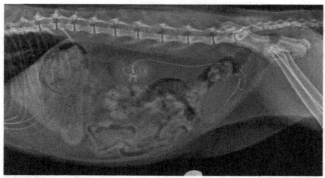

FIGURE 11-24 ■ A stent has been placed from the renal pelvis to the bladder along the ureter bypassing a ureteral obstruction. (Courtesy of Dr. Allyson Berent, The Animal Medical Center, New York, N.Y.)

    E. Challenges in clinical decision-making.
        1. Usually the clinician will not know how long the kidney has been obstructed.
        2. Often one cannot determine with certainty if obstruction is complete or partial.
        3. It is common to wait for 2 weeks in human patients when the onset of obstruction and renal colic (i.e., passage of calculus into ureter) is known, and most calculi of <5 mm will pass into the bladder.
        4. The trend in affected cats has been for early surgical intervention (i.e., after a few days of medical management).

WHAT DO WE DO?

- Place an IV catheter in all cats with UO soon after presentation.
- Provide sufficiently deep anesthesia to allow passage of a urinary catheter with minimal trauma in male cats with UO.
- Inject sterile dilute aqueous lubricant through the urinary catheter before it is advanced.
- Use a gentle touch when attempting to introduce and advance a urinary catheter.
- Make sure the urinary catheter is long enough and has been advanced far enough to be in the bladder and not the proximal urethra.
- Attach a closed sterile collection system to the urinary catheter.
- Prescribe drugs for analgesia (e.g., buprenorphine) and antispasmodic drugs (e.g., acepromazine) to decrease urethral spasm while the urinary catheter is in place and for several days after the cat has been discharged from the hospital.
- Avoid the use of NSAIDs in cats with UO, especially dehydrated cats and those in renal failure.
- Make sure the cat can urinate adequately after removing the indwelling urinary catheter and before discharging it from the hospital.
- Consider treatment protocols that do not require urethral catheterization or IV fluids in cats with UO as an alternative to euthanasia.
- Perform abdominal ultrasonography on all patients when ureteral calculi have been detected on abdominal radiography to determine if the calculi are causing obstruction or not (i.e., rule out hydroureter or hydronephrosis).
- Perform rectal examination on all dogs with UO to evaluate the urethra for mass lesions (e.g., neoplasia, proliferative urethritis) that could be causing obstruction.

THOUGHTS FOR THE FUTURE

- The underlying role of idiopathic cystitis in the development of UO in male cats will be better understood.
- Percutaneous tube cystostomy techniques will be further developed for use in cats with UO at initial presentation (as opposed to urethral catheterization).
- Pharmacologic management and decompressive cystocentesis will be offered as the initial treatment for cats with idiopathic UO or UO caused by plugs, instead of placement of a urinary catheter.
- Minimally invasive medical protocols using amitriptyline to provide relief of idiopathic UO or UO caused by urethral plugs in male cats will be further developed.
- Minimally invasive protocols using drugs that decrease ureteral smooth muscle tone and facilitate passage of ureteral stones (e.g., amitriptyline, tamsulosin) will be developed.
- Better drugs to manage visceral pain arising from the bladder and urethra in cats after relief of UO will be developed.
- Stenting procedures to relieve ureteral obstruction due to calculi will become more widely available.
- Urethral stenting for relief of UO will become more widely used in animals with urethral neoplasia, proliferative urethritis, and detrusor-urethral-dyssynergia.
- Techniques for laser ablation of urethral transitional cell carcinoma in dogs will become more widely available.

COMMON MISCONCEPTIONS

- Cystocentesis in cats with UO is dangerous. Actually, in the hands of a skilled operator, it is quite safe. An argument has been advanced that the bladder under pressure will rupture if a needle is passed through it. This is almost never true. It is safer to perform decompressive cystocentesis prior to the passage of a urinary catheter and backflushing of fluids.
- It is necessary to pass a urinary catheter to determine if the urethra is really obstructed or not. Obstruction is defined when there are signs of dysuria and increased urinary frequency with an easily palpable bladder.
- Crystalluria causes UO. Crystalluria may contribute to UO but in itself does not cause UO.
- Urethral plugs are the most common cause of UO in male cats. The cause of urethral obstruction is most often idiopathic or functional.
- A serum creatinine concentration >15 mg/dL or serum phosphorus concentration >20 mg/dL warrants a grave prognosis for survival in cats with UO. Absolutely not true. The degree of azotemia at the time of obstruction does not predict survival at all. Most cats with this degree of azotemia associated with urethral obstruction survive to be discharged from the hospital if adequate fluid therapy is given following relief of the obstruction.
- Use of a sterile collection system for attachment to a urinary catheter is an unnecessary expense. Acquired bacterial urinary infections are quite common when a sterile collection device is not employed.
- Abdominal radiographs are not necessary in cats with UO. It is imperative to take abdominal radiographs to know whether stones are in the urethra or not, as prognosis and treatment are altered. Also, it is important to know if there are stones in the kidneys, ureters, or bladder that may be contributing to the obstructing process.
- Ultrasonography (ULS) can be used instead of radiographs in cats with UO. ULS is complementary to radiographs as different information is gained. Urethral stones are routinely missed if only ULS is performed, whereas these stones are easily seen with radiographs.
- Antibiotics are useful in treatment of male cats experiencing their first episode of UO. Cats that have never had urethral obstruction or instrumentation of the urinary tract with catheters have an incredibly low chance of having a bacterial UTI at the time the urinary obstruction is relieved. UTI does occur with some frequency following the presence of an indwelling urinary catheter.

- Glucocorticoids are useful to decrease urethral inflammation in cats with idiopathic UO or UO due to urethral plugs. There is no evidence that glucocorticoid decrease urethral inflammation over placebo.
- Potassium supplementation of IV fluids in cats after relief of UO is dangerous. Although some cats with urethral obstruction will have hyperkalemia at the time of presentation, hyperkalemia rapidly resolves and hypokalemia emerges in those with intense postobstructive diuresis. Potassium supplementation is needed for most cats by 24 hours post relief of urethral obstruction, otherwise hypokalemia develops.
- Rectal examination is of limited value in dogs with UO. Rectal examination sometimes discloses the presence of obstructing urethral stones or masses.
- Ureteral calculi in cats and dogs, whether causing obstruction or not, are extremely painful, as they are in humans. Actually, dogs and cats do not often exhibit intense ureteral pain or colic, as do humans. Subtle pain is sometimes elicited during palpation of the affected kidney. It is possible that some malaise can be attributed to pain from the ureteral obstruction.

SUMMARY TIPS

- Perform decompressive cystocentesis before attempting to pass a urinary catheter into the bladder in male cats with UO.
- Extend the penis caudally to facilitate advancement of the urinary catheter.
- Take abdominal radiographs that include the entire urinary tract (i.e., including the perineal region) in cats with UO. Urinary calculi sometimes are found in several sites besides the urethra.
- Perform a positive contrast urethrogram if plain abdominal radiographs do not reveal the cause for UO. The urethra is not well evaluated using ultrasonography.
- If necessary, adjust the rate of IV fluid administration using the "ins and outs" protocol for the first 24 to 48 hours after relief of UO due to the unpredictable magnitude of postobstructive diuresis.
- Do not administer glucocorticoids while an indwelling urinary catheter remains in place. Such treatment will not resolve traumatic urethritis but increases the likelihood that bacterial UTI will develop.
- Do not administer antibiotics while an indwelling urinary catheter remains in place unless bacterial UTI has already been documented by bacterial culture of the urine.
- Do not manually express urine from the bladder after removal of a urinary catheter because doing so may promote additional injury to a bladder already traumatized by overdistension.
- Attempt to limit recurrent episodes of UO in male cats by implementing environmental enrichment (see Chapter 10, Nonobstructive Idiopathic or Interstitial Cystitis in Cats).
- Culture urine 1 to 2 weeks after discharge from the hospital to identify bacterial UTI that may have been acquired as a consequence of an indwelling urinary catheter.
- Avoid ureteral surgery in cats with ureterolithiasis unless clear evidence of obstruction (i.e., proximal hydroureter, hydronephrosis) is present.
- Consider ureteral stenting as treatment for obstructive ureteral calculi instead of ureteral surgery, especially in cats and small dogs.
- Consider tube cystostomy in dogs with transitional cell carcinoma of the bladder or urethra that is causing obstruction to urine outflow.

FREQUENTLY ASKED QUESTIONS

Q: **When do you recommend perineal urethrostomy in cats?**

A: We suggest this possibility during consultation at the first visit, and recommend it after the second or third obstruction.

Q: How often does serious renal injury occur in cats with UO?

A: Very uncommonly. The azotemia (which can be severe) typically is postrenal and prerenal. Azotemia resolves in nearly all affected cats after relief of UO and medical management.

Q: How do you handle UO in a cat owned by clients who cannot afford standard medical care?

A: First we offer such clients standard care including hospitalization, IV fluids, anesthesia, passage of an indwelling urinary catheter, and monitoring in intensive care. If the owner cannot afford this approach, we offer a less expensive protocol as an alternative to euthanasia. This approach includes decompressive cystocentesis, analgesic and antispasmodic drugs, and up to 3 days of hospitalization in a quiet environment.

Q: Can relief of UO be carried out under sedation alone?

A: No. This is a painful procedure and full anesthesia facilitates nontraumatic passage of a urinary catheter.

Q: Do you add lidocaine to the irrigating fluid used for hydropulsion?

A: No. Substantial amounts of lidocaine can be absorbed across the mucosa, especially in the presence of trauma and high hydrostatic pressure.

Q: How do you prevent a cat from removing its indwelling urinary catheter?

A: An Elizabethan collar prevents the cat from licking excessively at its urethra. Care should be taken to insure that the collar is wide enough–the cat's nose must not be able to extend beyond the edge of the collar. Also, the urinary catheter must be properly secured in place. The use of acepromazine also facilitates management by sedating the cat and also decreasing urethral tone by alpha-adrenergic blockade.

Q: Is there concern about re-obstruction of the urethra in the 12 to 24 hours after the urinary catheter has been removed?

A: Yes. The cat should remain in the hospital and be carefully observed for 24 hours after removal of the urinary catheter. Use of antispasmodic drugs (e.g., acepromazine) during this time also may be helpful.

Q: What about the use of glucocorticoids or NSAIDs after an indwelling urinary catheter is placed?

A: There is little evidence that these drugs actually lessen urethral inflammation during an episode of UO. The immunosuppressive effects of steroids may cause increased risk of development of bacterial UTI and ascension to the kidneys (i.e., pyelonephritis). NSAIDs impair renal blood flow in dehydrated animals and pose a risk for development of acute intrinsic renal failure.

Q: Do you clip and cleanse the perineal region before attempting to relieve UO?

A: Yes. Although contamination commonly occurs at some point during the procedure, we try to minimize its occurrence by clipping and cleansing the area and wearing sterile gloves during the procedure.

Q: Postobstructive diuresis sometimes continues even after BUN and serum creatinine concentrations have returned to normal. What role does fluid therapy play in the duration of post-obstructive diuresis?

A: Sometimes more fluids are given than actually are needed, and in these instances the clinician is driving the diuresis. After the cat is feeling better and its renal function has improved, try tapering the volume of fluid administered and monitoring urine output. If urine output decreases, the fluid therapy has actually been driving the diuresis. If diuresis continues and the cat begins to get dehydrated, the postobstructive diuresis has not yet resolved and fluid administration again must be increased.

Q: Do you prescribe prophylactic antibiotics after relief of UO?

A: No, not while the urinary catheter is in place. However it is appropriate to culture the urine when the catheter is removed and prescribe antibiotics as necessary to treat bacterial UTI that has developed as a consequence of the indwelling urinary catheter.

Q: How long should an indwelling urinary catheter be left in place after relief of UO?

A: This time can be quite variable. We often try to keep the catheter in place for 24 to 48 hours, but some cats manage to dislodge their catheters within this time frame. In general, the urinary catheter is removed when the cat is feeling better, hematuria is resolving, and azotemia has resolved.

Q: Does the volume of urine removed when UO is first relieved predict bladder atony?

A: Possibly, but this has not been specifically studied. It seems logical that bladders with very large volumes would be most likely to be stretched and possibly have damage to intercellular junctions.

Q: How important in the pathogenesis is the alkaline urine pH that I find in many cats with UO? Is this a primary event leading to urethral plug formation?

A: Anorexia and exudation of plasma proteins into urine from an inflamed and hemorrhagic bladder both may contribute to neutral somewhat alkaline urine pH. As urine pH increases, struvite crystals become less soluble and can precipitate out of solution. This effect is independent of the type of food that has been fed to the cat. Finding a persistently alkaline urine pH after resolution of the present episode of UO, however, is an appropriate reason to recommend a change to a more acidifying diet.

Q: Is amitriptyline effective in relief of UO in male cats?

A: One experimental study showed resolution of UO in 20 cats with urethral plugs within 3 days of starting treatment with amitriptyline. This result has not been verified and this approach cannot be recommended yet for standard treatment of cats with UO.

Q: The parasympathomimetic agent bethanechol recently has become difficult to find. Are there alternative drugs that may stimulate contraction of the detrusor muscle of the bladder in cats with persistent bladder atony?

A: Cisapride may stimulate detrusor contraction and could be considered for this purpose.

Q: Is laser ablation of urethral transitional cell carcinoma helpful in relieving UO caused by this tumor?

A: Laser ablation can provide relief of UO in dogs with urethral obstruction caused by urethral neoplasia, thus preventing the need for tube cystostomy. However the procedure is not curative for transitional cell carcinoma, and multiple laser ablation procedures will be needed over time as the tumor recurs.

Q: What is the role of urethral stenting in dogs with UO due to urethral transitional cell carcinoma?

A: Urethral stenting under these circumstances can relieve UO, but the procedure does not prevent local tumor growth and some dogs will develop urinary incontinence after urethral stenting.

Q: What quality of life can be expected after placement of a cystostomy tube in a dog with UO due to transitional cell carcinoma?

A: Some dogs do well after cystostomy tube placement. The owners must be trained how to manage urinary drainage in a sterile manner and how to bandage the catheter to protect it from being removed by the dog. Development of bacterial UTI is inevitable, and treating UTI becomes an ongoing issue. Often, the infecting organisms become highly resistant to commonly used antibiotics.

SUGGESTED READINGS

Lower Urinary Tract Obstruction

Achar E, Achar RA, Paiva TB, et al: Amitriptyline eliminates calculi through urinary tract smooth muscle relaxation, *Kidney Int* 64:1356–1364, 2003.

Barsanti JA, Brown J, Marks A, et al: Relationship of lower urinary tract signs to seropositivity for feline immunodeficiency virus in cats, *J Vet Intern Med* 10:34–38, 1996.

Barsanti JA, Shotts EB, Crowell WA, et al: Effect of therapy on susceptibility to urinary tract infection in male cats with indwelling urethral catheters, *J Vet Intern Med* 6:64–70, 1992.

Bray JP, Doyle RS, Burton CA: Minimally invasive inguinal approach for tube cystostomy, *Vet Surg* 38:411–416, 2009.

Bovee KC, Reif JS, Maguire TG, et al: Recurrence of feline urethral obstruction, *J Am Vet Med Assoc* 174:93–96, 1979.

Burrows CF, Bovee KC: Characterization and treatment of acid-base and renal defects due to urethral obstruction in cats, *J Am Vet Med Ass* 172:801–805, 1978.

Cooper ES, Owens TJ, Chew DJ, Buffington CAT: A novel approach to treatment of urethral obstruction in male cats, *J Am Vet Med Ass* (in press).

Corgozinho KB, HJMd Souza, Pereira AN, et al: Catheter-induced urethral trauma in cats with urethral obstruction, *J Feline Med Surg* 9:481–486, 2007.

Drobatz KJ, Cole SG: The influence of crystalloid type on acid-base and electrolyte status of cats with urethral obstruction, *J Vet Emerg Crit Care* 4:355–361, 2008.

Drobatz KJ, Hughes D: Concentration of ionized calcium in plasma from cats with urethral obstruction, *J Am Vet Med Assoc* 211:1392–1395, 1997.

Drobatz KJ, Ward C, Graham P, Hughes D: Serum concentrations of parathyroid hormone and 25-OH vitamin D_3 in cats with urethral obstruction, *J Vet Emerg Crit Care* 15:179–184, 2005.

Finco DR: Induced feline urethral obstruction: Response of hyperkalemia to relief of obstruction and administration of parenteral electrolyte solution, *J Am Anim Hosp Assoc* 12:198–202, 1976.

Finco DR, Barsanti JA: Diet-induced feline urethral obstruction, *Vet Clin North Am: Small animal practice* 14:529–536, 1984.

Finco DR, Barsanti JA, Crowell WA: Characterization of magnesium-induced urinary disease in the cat and comparison with feline urologic syndrome, *Am J Vet Res* 46:391–400, 1985.

Finco DR, Cornelius LM: Characterization and treatment of water, electrolyte, and acid-base imbalances of induced urethral obstruction in the cat, *Am J Vet Res* 38:823–830, 1977.

Gerber B, Boretti FS, Kley S, et al: Evaluation of clinical signs and causes of lower urinary tract disease in European cats, *J Small Anim Pract* 46:571–577, 2005.

Gerber B, Eichenberger S, Reusch CE: Guarded long-term prognosis in male cats with urethral obstruction, *J Feline Med Surg* 10:16–23, 2008.

Hostutler RA, Chew DJ, Eaton KA, et al: Cystoscopic appearance of proliferative urethritis in 2 dogs before and after treatment, *J Vet Intern Med* 18:113–116, 2004.

Kruger JM, Osborne CA, Goyal SM, et al: Clinical evaluation of cats with lower urinary tract disease, *J Am Vet Med Assoc* 199:211–216, 1991.

Lee JA, Drobatz KJ: Characterization of the clinical characteristics, electrolytes, acid-base, and renal parameters in male cats with urethral obstruction, *J Vet Emerg Crit Care* 13:227–233, 2003.

Lee JA, Drobatz KJ: Historical and physical parameters as predictors of severe hyperkalemia in male cats with urethral obstruction, *J Vet Emerg Crit Care* 16:104–111, 2006.

Loeb WF, Knipling GD: Glucosuria and pseudoglucosuria in cats with urethral obstruction, *Mod Vet Pract* 52(13):40–41, 1971.

Malouin A, Milligan JA, Drobatz KJ: Assessment of blood pressure in cats presented with urethral obstruction, *J Vet Emerg Crit Care* 17:15–21, 2007.

Marks SL, Straeter-Knowlen IM, Moore M, et al: Effects of acepromazine maleate and phenoxybenzamine on urethral pressure profiles of anesthetized, healthy, sexually intact male cats, *Am J Vet Res* 57:1497–1500, 1996.

Mawby DI, Meric SM, Crichlow EC, Papich MG: Pharmacological relaxation of the urethra in male cats: A study of the effects of phenoxybenzamine, diazepam, nifedipine and xylazine, *Can J Vet Res* 55:28–32, 1991.

Reif JS, Bovee K, Gaskell CJ, et al: Feline urethral obstruction: A case-control study, *J Am Vet Med Assoc* 170:1320–1324, 1977.

Straeter-Knowlen IM, Marks SL: Use of muscle relaxants in feline obstructive lower urinary tract disease, *Feline Pract* 25:26–33, 1997.

Straeter-Knowlen IM, Marks SL, Rishniw M, et al: Urethral pressure response to smooth and skeletal muscle relaxants in anesthetized, adult male cats with naturally acquired urethral obstruction, *Am J Vet Res* 56:919–923, 1995.

Straeter-Knowlen IM, Marks SL, Speth RC, et al: Effect of succinylcholine, diazepam, and dantrolene on the urethral pressure profile of anesthetized, healthy, sexually intact male cats, *Am J Vet Res* 55:1739–1744, 1994.

Upper Urinary Tract Obstruction

Adin CA, Herrgesell EJ, Nyland TG, et al: Antegrade pyelography for suspected ureteral obstruction in cats: 11 cases (1995-2001), *J Am Vet Med Assoc* 222:1576–1581, 2003.

Block G, Adams LG, Widmer WR, Lingeman JE: Use of extracorporeal shock wave lithotripsy for treatment of nephrolithiasis and ureterolithiasis in five dogs, *J Am Vet Med Assoc* 208:531–536, 1996.

Dalby AM, Adams LG, Salisbury SK, Blevins WE: Spontaneous retrograde movement of ureteroliths in two dogs and five cats, *J Am Vet Med Assoc* 229:1118–1121, 2006.

Kyles AE, Hardie EM, Wooden BG, et al: Clinical, clinicopathologic, radiographic, and ultrasonographic abnormalities in cats with ureteral calculi: 163 cases (1984-2002), *J Am Vet Med Assoc* 226:932–936, 2005.

Kyles AE, Hardie EM, Wooden BG, et al: Management and outcome of cats with ureteral calculi: 153 cases (1984-2002), *J Am Vet Med Assoc* 226:937–944, 2005.

Kyles AE, Stone EA, Gookin J, et al: Diagnosis and surgical management of obstructive ureteral calculi in cats: 11 cases (1993-1996), *J Am Vet Med Assoc* 213:1150–1156, 1998.

Westropp JL, Ruby AL, Bailiff NL, et al: Dried solidified blood calculi in the urinary tract of cats, *J Vet Intern Med* 20:828–834, 2006.

12 Urinary Tract Trauma and Uroperitoneum

INTRODUCTION

A. Types of trauma to the urinary tract (Figure 12-1).
  1. Kidney: Renal trauma is not commonly recognized in dogs or cats, possibly because the kidneys are protected by a fibrous capsule and embedded in perirenal fat. Absorption of shock also is facilitated by the fact that both kidneys are relatively mobile in the dog and cat. Further protection of the kidneys is provided by the ribs, epaxial musculature, and spine.
    a. Contusion: Subcapsular bruising and ecchymosis.
      (1) Hemorrhage stops spontaneously.
      (2) Microscopic hematuria can be observed.
    b. Hematoma: Blood accumulates in the perinephric region between the renal capsule and fascia.
      (1) Hemorrhage may stop spontaneously.
      (2) Perinephric cyst or abscess may form as hematoma is liquefied.
      (3) Microscopic hematuria can be observed.
    c. Fissure: Renal parenchymal tear that extends through the renal capsule resulting in a perinephric hematoma (Figure 12-2).
    d. Rupture: Tear that is extensive enough to allow blood to accumulate in the retroperitoneal space or peritoneal cavity.
      (1) Laceration: Sharp line of demarcation.
      (2) Fracture or pulpifaction (Figure 12-3).
      (3) Tear through renal pelvis: Extravasation of blood and urine.
    e. Pedicle injury.
      (1) Vascular avulsion: Severe and rapid loss of blood.
      (2) Ureteral avulsion: Extravasation of urine.
  2. Ureter.
    a. Avulsion from kidney or bladder.
    b. Rupture along its length.
  3. Urinary bladder.
    a. Rupture: More likely in males due to anatomy of urethra.
    b. Contusion.
  4. Urethra.
    a. Avulsion from the bladder.
    b. Rupture.
  5. Periurethral: Swelling and compression may result in obstruction.

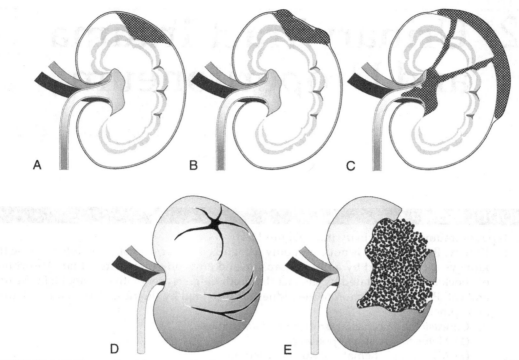

FIGURE 12-1 ■ Types of renal trauma. **A,** Contusion. **B,** Contusion with some bleeding into subcapsular space. **C,** Bleeding into retroperitoneal space and into renal pelvis. **D,** Laceration of renal parenchyma. **E,** Pulpifaction of renal parenchyma. (Drawn by Tim Vojt.)

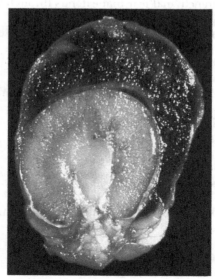

FIGURE 12-2 ■ Perinephric hematoma. Note the degree of retroperitoneal hemorrhage surrounding this kidney.

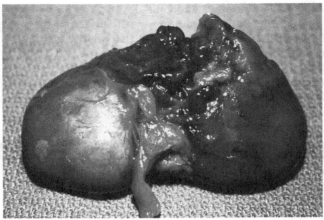

FIGURE 12-3 ■ Pulpifaction of renal tissue following severe renal trauma. (Courtesy of Dr. William DeHoff, Med Vet, Worthington, Ohio.)

PATHOGENESIS AND PATHOPHYSIOLOGY

Causes of Urinary Tract Trauma

1. Blunt abdominal trauma (e.g., hit by a car, fall from height, kicked) is most common.
2. Penetrating injury (e.g., knife, bullet wound).
3. Iatrogenic.
   a. Improper urinary catheterization technique.
   b. Accidental tear of urinary tissues during surgery.
   c. Improper cystotomy closure or breakdown of closure.
   d. Overzealous attempts to manually express urine from the bladder.
   e. Cystocentesis performed on a severely distended and devitalized bladder associated with urethral obstruction.
   f. Cystostomy tube leakage (very uncommon).
   g. Cystoscopy technique errors.
4. Rupture of bladder, urethra, or ureter secondary to obstruction or erosion by a calculus.
5. Urethral obstruction with secondary bladder rupture (rare).
6. Breakdown of friable neoplastic or infected tissue anywhere along the urinary tract.
7. Spontaneous rupture of large intrarenal cysts (i.e., pre-existing cystic renal disease).

Syndromes Caused by Urinary Tract Trauma or Rupture

1. Direct tissue injury (hemorrhage, swelling, inflammation, necrosis).
2. Blood loss.
3. Urine extravasation into body cavity.
   a. Uroperitoneum is the accumulation of urine in the peritoneal or retroperitoneal spaces due to a rupture of the urinary tract anywhere along its course (i.e., kidney, renal pelvis, ureter, urinary bladder, urethra).
   b. Urinary bladder rupture is the most common traumatic disruption of the urinary tract and source of urine leakage.
4. Urine extravasation into subcutaneous tissues from a tear in the urethra causes swelling, bruising, and sloughing of tissues.

5. Postrenal azotemia and failure. Azotemia develops as nitrogenous waste products accumulate in the peritoneal cavity and are absorbed across the semipermeable peritoneal membranes. Absorption of waste products also can occur from the subcutaneous tissues when urine accumulates there.
6. Peritonitis.
   a. Chemical peritonitis can occur from urine irritation in dogs and cats.
   b. Bacterial peritonitis can occur from urinary tract infection or contamination of ischemic tissue or blood.

HISTORY
A. Known trauma (e.g., observed as hit by a car).
B. Recent abdominal surgical procedure, especially cystotomy.
C. Recent attempts at manual bladder expression.

CLINICAL SIGNS
A. Increasing abdominal girth may be noted if enough time has elapsed since the rupture.
B. Lack of observed urinations or decreased volume of urine produced if rupture is in the lower urinary tract.
   1. Urine volume is variable in animals with ruptured bladder.
   2. Observation of voiding does not rule out ruptured bladder.

! Some animals continue to urinate despite the accumulation of urine in the abdomen due to ruptured bladder.

C. Dysuria, stranguria, and pollakiuria may occur with rupture of the bladder or urethra.
D. Hematuria may be observed, but is not specific or sensitive for rupture of the urinary tract.
E. Increased thirst sometimes is noted as a consequence of fluid shifts that occur as urine accumulates in the peritoneal cavity.
F. Reluctance to walk.
G. As uroperitoneum persists, the signs of uremia including vomiting, lethargy, and dehydration become more apparent.
H. Because uroperitoneum frequently is associated with trauma, additional signs often will be present due to other systemic injuries (e.g., musculoskeletal injuries).
I. Trauma associated with a fractured pelvis or femur increases the likelihood of bladder or urethral rupture, especially in dogs.

PHYSICAL EXAMINATION
A. Pain near the site of rupture may be noted during palpation.
B. Abdominal fluid may be detected, especially after fluids are administered.
C. Evidence of extensive abdominal injury (e.g., bruising) or fractures (e.g., pelvis, femur) in small animals (Figures 12-4 and 12-5).
D. A small urinary bladder may be palpable in dogs and cats with ruptured bladder.
   1. Bladder fails to fill during fluid therapy because fluid continues to leak into the abdomen.
   2. If the tear is in one kidney or ureter, the bladder still may fill adequately from urine formed by the intact kidney.

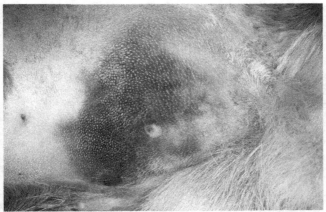

FIGURE 12-4 ■ Deep bruising of caudal abdomen. This type of bruising should raise suspicion for the possibility for severe damage to underlying organs, especially for rupture of the bladder or urethra.

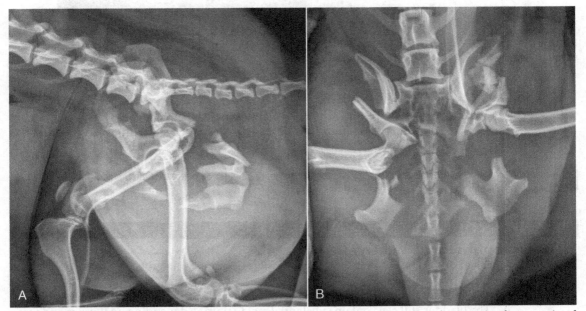

FIGURE 12-5 ■ Radiogram showing severe trauma to the boney pelvis. This type of trauma is often associated with rupture of the urethra or bladder. **A,** Lateral view of pelvis. Note multiple fractures. **B,** Ventrodorsal (VD) view of pelvis. Note multiple fractures. (Courtesy of The Ohio State University Veterinary Medical Center Orthopedics Program and Dr. Jon Dyce.)

3. If a bladder tear is small, a substantial volume of urine can distend the bladder and render it palpable despite ongoing leakage of urine into the peritoneum.
E. Distal urethral rupture can result in urine accumulation in the soft tissues of the perineum, caudal thighs, and inguinal region (Figure 12-6). Bruising, cellulitis, and sloughing of tissues may be detected after 12 to 36 hours.

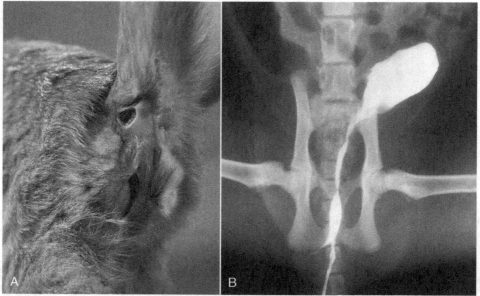

FIGURE 12-6 ■ **A,** Sloughing of perineal skin in two areas due to urethral rupture in a cat and urine accumulation in the subcutaneous tissues. **B,** Urethrogram showing communication of lateral urethra with lateral thigh.

F. Rectal examination.
1. May reveal pain as a ruptured urethra or bladder neck is palpated.
2. May reveal fragments of fractured pelvis that can be associated with or have caused the ruptured bladder.

> **!** Retrieval of a substantial volume of urine after passage of a urinary catheter does not exclude the possibility of a ruptured bladder or urethra.

DIAGNOSIS OF UROPERITONEUM

Passage of Urethral Catheter
1. Retrieval of a substantial volume of fluid after urethral catheterization does not rule out ruptured bladder.
   a. The catheter may pass through the ruptured bladder and collect abdominal fluid.
   b. The bladder still can contain substantial residual urine depending on the size and location of the leak.
2. It may be difficult to pass a catheter if the urethra is ruptured.

Abdominocentesis
1. The ratio of the abdominal fluid creatinine concentration to the serum creatinine concentration (both in mg/dL) provides evidence that the suspect abdominal fluid is urine.
2. The concentrations of creatinine and urea in urine entering the peritoneal cavity from a ruptured bladder are very high. Having a higher molecular weight than urea, creatinine does not move across the peritoneal membranes into blood as rapidly as urea, and thus accumulates to a greater degree in the abdominal fluid.

3. The concentration of creatinine in a sample of the abdominal fluid can be compared with the serum creatinine concentration. For example, the concentration of creatinine in the abdominal fluid may be 16.0 mg/dL and serum creatinine concentration may be 4.0 mg/dL. This ratio of 4:1 is definitive evidence that the fluid is urine (a ratio of >2:1 is expected in most cases of ruptured bladder).

4. Simultaneous determination of the abdominal fluid urea nitrogen concentration as compared to blood urea nitrogen (BUN) concentration also can be performed but is not as helpful. Urea has a lower molecular weight than creatinine and equilibrates across the peritoneal membranes more rapidly, resulting in a lower ratio of abdominal fluid urea concentration to BUN concentration. For example, the fluid urea nitrogen concentration may be 90 mg/dL as compared with a BUN concentration of 80 mg/dL (ratio of 1.1).

> **!** The ratio of peritoneal fluid creatinine concentration to serum creatinine concentration decreases over time as equilibration with blood occurs across the peritoneum.

5. Also due to molecular size differences, phosphate will be retained in the abdominal fluid longer than potassium.

6. In a study of 13 dogs with ruptured bladder, abdominal fluid creatinine concentration was at least four times greater than the upper limit of normal serum creatinine concentration in all cases.

   a. The median abdominal fluid creatinine concentration to serum creatinine concentration ratio was 4.0 (range, 1.4 to 19.2). A ratio of >2.1 identified 86% of dogs with uroperitoneum. The median abdominal fluid creatinine concentration was 16 mg/dL (range, 7.5 to 22.5 mg/dL) and median serum creatinine concentration was 4.4 mg/dL (range, 0.6 to 11.4 mg/dL).

   b. As expected, the largest gradients were seen in animals that had minimal azotemia and the smallest gradients were seen in animals with overt azotemia.

   c. The median abdominal fluid potassium concentration to serum potassium concentration ratio was 2.7 (range, 1.4 to 3.3). A ratio of >1.4 predicted uroperitoneum accurately in all of the dogs.

   d. Dogs with ascites of other cause had a median abdominal fluid creatinine concentration to serum creatinine concentration ratio of 1.1 and an abdominal fluid potassium concentration to serum potassium concentration ratio of 1.0.

   e. Specificity and sensitivity were 100% for the diagnosis of uroperitoneum in dogs when the abdominal fluid creatinine concentration was at least 4 times the upper limit of the laboratory reference range for normal serum creatinine concentration, the abdominal fluid potassium concentration to serum potassium concentration ratio was >1.4, and the abdominal fluid creatinine concentration to serum creatinine concentration ratio was >2.1.

   f. Serum potassium concentration was >6.0 mEq/L in 31% of dogs with ruptured bladder.

7. In a study of 26 cats with uroperitoneum, abdominal fluid chemistry was available in 5 affected cats.

   a. Abdominal fluid creatinine concentration was 12.5 ± 4.9 mg/dL (range, 5.5 to 15.6 mg/dL). Mean abdominal fluid creatinine concentration to serum creatinine concentration ratio in 4 cats was 2.0 (range, 1.1 to 4.1).

   b. Abdominal fluid potassium concentration was 9.3 ± 7.4 mEq/L (range, 4.1 to 22.2 mEq/L). Mean abdominal fluid potassium concentration to serum potassium concentration ratio was 1.9 (range, 1.2 to 2.4).
   c. Fifty-two percent of the affected cats had hyperkalemia at time of diagnosis and 95% were azotemic.
8. Abdominocentesis is performed with the patient in lateral recumbency. The ventral abdomen is clipped and aseptically prepared. A syringe with a 20-gauge needle, a 19-gauge butterfly catheter, or an over-the-needle intravenous catheter is inserted into the abdominal cavity slightly to one side of ventral midline and 2 to 3 cm caudal to the umbilicus (i.e., a site cranial to the bladder and distal to the falciform fat). Fluid can be readily removed using this technique if a moderate volume of peritoneal fluid is present. If difficulty is encountered when attempting to retrieve fluid, a 4-quadrant abdominal paracentesis can be performed. Alternatively, drainage with a percutaneous dialysis catheter can be attempted. Ultrasound guidance to locate small pockets of fluid for aspiration can be very helpful when trauma has been recent.

Injection Through a Urinary Catheter
1. Injection of methylene blue through a urinary catheter and subsequent retrieval of blue-colored fluid during abdominocentesis confirms a tear in the urinary tract.
2. Hissing of air leaking from a ruptured bladder usually can be heard during pneumocystography (it was heard in all experimental dogs in one study).

Imaging
1. Plain radiographs may show loss of abdominal detail due to fluid accumulation.
   a. A *ground glass* appearance may be observed if a large amount of fluid (urine) has accumulated (Figure 12-7).
   b. Loss of retroperitoneal detail and inability to clearly identify the kidneys occurs when rupture involves the renal parenchyma, renal pelvis, or ureter(s) and the retroperitoneal space has not been disrupted by the trauma (Figure 12-8).
2. Ultrasound examination may disclose small amounts of abdominal and retroperitoneal fluid soon after injury, but blood and urine cannot be differentiated.

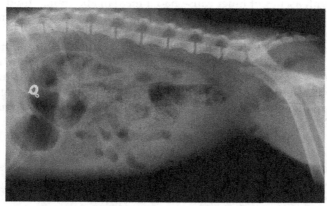

FIGURE 12-7 ■ Survey abdominal radiograph showing *ground glass* appearance of abdominal effusion, in this case due to uroperitoneum from ruptured bladder.

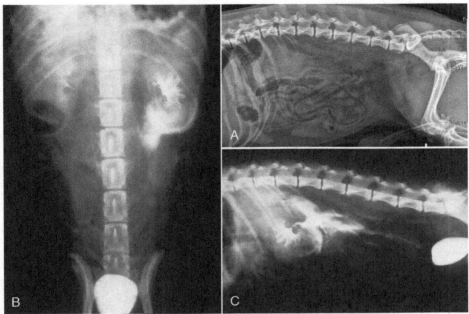

FIGURE 12-8 ∎ **A,** Survey abdominal radiographs showing loss of retroperitoneal detail. Note streaking within the retroperitoneal space and loss of ability to clearly see the kidneys. This dog was hit by a car and was leaking urine from one kidney into this area. **B,** VD and lateral projections. **B** and **C,** Excretory urography from a different dog with renal trauma. Note extravasation of contrast into the retroperitoneal space confirming that loss of detail in this region is from urine. (**A,** Courtesy of The Ohio State University Department of Radiology.)

      a. May disclose hematomas and abnormal shapes or echoes associated with renal trauma.
      b. Often will disclose a collapsed bladder in patients with ruptured bladder.
      c. May disclose an irregular structure of mixed echogenicity due to lesions from trauma to the bladder.
      d. Site of bladder rupture or urine leakage cannot always be determined.
   3. Contrast radiography or ultrasound examination usually is required to localize the site of urinary tract rupture. Demonstration of continuity between the urinary bladder and surrounding fluid accumulation is conclusive.
      a. Positive-contrast cystography is the procedure of choice in bladder rupture (Figure 12-9).
      b. Radiographic images are much more difficult to interpret if a negative contrast (air or CO_2) study or pneumocystography is used.
      c. Inability to distend the bladder adequately may be noted during contrast infusion.
      d. False negative results may occur if insufficient contrast is injected to achieve adequate bladder distention because leakage of contrast agent will not be demonstrated unless the tear is large.
      e. Ultrasound contrast cystography (contrast cystosonography) can be useful at times instead of positive contrast cystography, because the ultrasound equipment can be brought to the cage. Rapid infusion of microbubbles (3 mL air and 32 mL sterile saline mixed using a 3-way stopcock just before infusion) allows easy visualization of swirling bubbles as they escape the bladder.

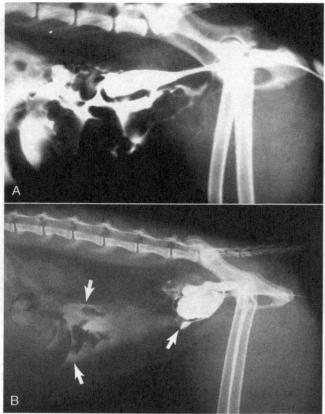

FIGURE 12-9 ■ **A,** Positive contrast cystogram—ruptured bladder in a dog. Notice that the bladder fails to distend during contrast infusion because there is a large leak of contrast into the abdominal cavity. **B,** Positive contrast cystogram—ruptured bladder in a cat. The bladder tear in this cat is considerably smaller than that in **A.**

    f. Positive contrast urethrography is necessary to identify the site of urethral rupture (Figure 12-10).
    g. Excretory urography is required to demonstrate rupture of the kidney or ureter.
    h. Caution must be exercised in patients with dehydration or underlying renal insufficiency because excretory urography can result in acute renal injury in rare instances.
  4. Urethrocystoscopy also can be used to determine the site of bladder rupture or urethral tear (Figure 12-11).

Serum Biochemistry
  1. BUN concentration is the first biochemical variable to become abnormal. Increases in BUN start as early as 5 hours after bladder rupture in experimental uroabdomen in dogs.
  2. Serum creatinine concentration also increases but not as rapidly as BUN due to previously discussed differences in molecular weight.

> **!** Calculation of abdominal fluid to serum creatinine concentration ratios and contrast radiography are the most reliable methods for definitive diagnosis of uroperitoneum.

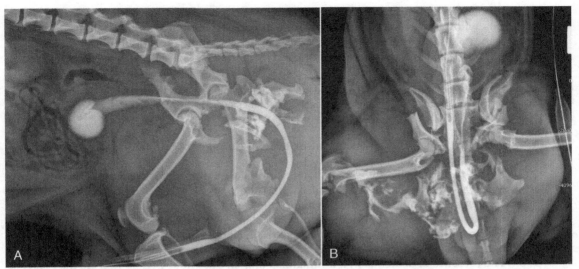

FIGURE 12-10 ■ Urethrogram. Positive contrast urethrography to localize the site of urethral rupture. Notice extravasation of infused contrast agent into the soft tissues in both the lateral (**A**) and ventrodorsal (**B**) views. (Courtesy of The Ohio State University Veterinary Medical Center Orthopedics Program and Dr. Jon Dyce.)

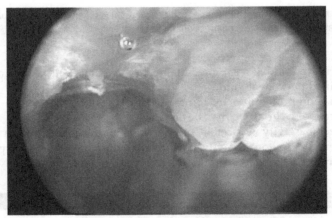

FIGURE 12-11 ■ Cystoscopic view of ruptured bladder. Note the ragged edges of the bladder wall tear and the abdominal cavity in the distant view. This bladder rupture occurred during cystoscopy when an assistant squeezed on the bag of infusing fluids to clear the view but the bladder was already fully distended.

3. The magnitude and rapidity of increase in BUN and serum creatinine concentrations may be increased by concomitant prerenal factors that commonly accompany trauma (e.g., shock, hypotension).
4. Increased serum potassium concentration is a relatively late finding (2 to 3 days post-rupture) in uroperitoneum cases, but can occur earlier if shock and severe metabolic acidosis are present.
5. Serum sodium and chloride concentrations decrease progressively in experimental dogs with bladder rupture. Similar changes occur in dogs with naturally occurring

uroperitoneum but hyponatremia and hypochloremia are less consistently observed in cats with naturally occurring uroperitoneum. Urine concentrations of sodium and chloride typically are low compared with serum concentrations, and equilibration results in hyponatremia and hypochloremia.

> ! The combination of hyperkalemia, hyponatremia, and azotemia in uroperitoneum can be confused with hypoadrenocorticism, especially when there is no clear history of trauma.

6. Progressive hyperphosphatemia also develops during uroperitoneum due to the high urinary concentration of phosphorus.
7. Blood gases usually show metabolic acidosis with respiratory compensation. In some instances, the pH is relatively normal and the pco_2 is lower than expected for normal compensation suggesting the possibility of a mixed disorder such as combined primary metabolic acidosis and primary respiratory alkalosis, the latter possibility associated with hyperventilation due to pain. The extent of metabolic acidosis may be much more severe in animals with major trauma and shock (i.e., possible contribution of lactic acidosis).
8. The presence of azotemia in a traumatized animal does not by itself indicate the presence of uroperitoneum. Furthermore, the absence of azotemia in a traumatized animal does not exclude the possibility of uroperitoneum if the animal has been presented soon after the trauma.

> ! Azotemia in a recently traumatized animal could be a result of prerenal (e.g., shock, dehydration), ischemic acute renal, or postrenal (e.g., uroabdomen, obstruction) factors.

Urinalysis
1. It is difficult to know if a sample obtained by catheter is urine or a combination of urine and modified peritoneal fluid.
2. Hematuria and proteinuria are common.
3. Some degree of pyuria also may be observed.
4. Urine specific gravity is variable and depends on the concentration of the urine that initially enters the peritoneal cavity, how long the fluid has been in the peritoneal cavity, and the response of the body to modify the fluid.

CLINICAL CASES OF UROABDOMEN IN SMALL ANIMALS
A. Twenty-six dogs and 14 cats were diagnosed with uroperitoneum over a 5-year period at the University of Pennsylvania.
B. The cause of uroperitoneum was trauma in 84.6% of cases.
C. Mortality was 42.3%.
D. Pelvic fractures were identified in 46.2%.

SUMMARY OF EXPERIMENTAL UROABDOMEN IN DOGS (Burrows, 1974)
A. Average survival was 65 hours (range, 47 to 90 hours).
B. Within 12 hours, central nervous system (CNS) depression, anorexia, reluctance to walk, abdominal pain on palpation, increased water intake, increased packed cell volume (PCV), stranguria, and hematuria were noted.

C. Vomiting was noted within 15 hours.
D. BUN was increased by 5 hours and was the first biochemical variable to become abnormal.
  1. Mean BUN of 52 mg/dL at 21 hours.
  2. Mean BUN of 75 mg/dL at 29 hours.
  3. Mean BUN of 140 mg/dL at 69 hours.
E. Serum creatinine concentration (SCr) was clearly increased by 21 hours.
  1. Mean SCr of 2.2 mg/dL at 21 hours.
  2. Mean SCr of 2.8 mg/dL at 29 hours.
  3. Mean SCr of 6.0 mg/dL at 69 hours.
F. Hyperkalemia is a relatively late finding. Serum potassium (K) concentration was slightly increased at 53 hours and clearly increased by 69 hours.
  1. Mean serum K of 5.9 mEq/L at 53 hours (range, 4.1 to 7.8 mEq/L).
  2. Mean serum K of 6.4 mEq/L at 69 hours (range, 4.9 to 8.4 mEq/L).
G. Serum sodium (Na) concentration progressively decreases (hyponatremia).
  1. Mean serum Na of 139 mEq/L at 29 hours.
  2. Mean serum Na of 136 mEq/L at 45 hours.
  3. Mean serum Na of 129 mEq/L at 53 hours.
  4. Mean serum Na of 129 mEq/L at 69 hours.
H. Serum chloride (Cl) concentration progressively decreases (hypochloremia).
  1. Mean serum Cl of 92 mEq/L at 29 hours.
  2. Mean serum Cl of 83 mEq/L at 45 hours.
  3. Mean serum Cl of 80 mEq/L at 53 hours.
  4. Mean serum Cl of 76 mEq/L at 69 hours.
I. Serum phosphorus (Pi) concentration progressively increases (hyperphosphatemia).
  1. Mean serum Pi of 6.5 mg/dL at 21 hours.
  2. Mean serum Pi of 8.1 mg/dL at 29 hours.
  3. Mean serum Pi of 10.7 mg/dL at 45 hours.
  4. Mean serum Pi of 11.4 mg/dL at 53 hours.
  5. Mean serum Pi of 12.8 mg/dL at 69 hours.
J. Blood gases.
  1. Minimal acidemia at 69 hours, similar to changes seen at 5 hours.
  2. Relatively mild acidosis with respiratory compensation.
K. Abdominal fluid chemical analysis at 45 hours:

Factor	Abdominal Fluid	Serum
Creatinine	11.6 mg/dL	4.3 mg/dL
Urea nitrogen	107 mg/dL	113 mg/dL
Sodium	127 mEq/L	136 mEq/L

TREATMENT OF URINARY TRACT TRAUMA AND UROPERITONEUM

Renal Hemorrhage
1. Maceration and hemorrhage into the retroperitoneal space makes gross inspection and evaluation of the renal pedicle difficult.
2. Nephrectomy for ongoing hemorrhage, severe fractures or pulpifaction of renal tissue.
3. Partial nephrectomy if parenchymal injury involves one pole of the kidney.
4. Suture over area of hemorrhage if hemorrhage is not too severe.
5. Pressure or Gelfoam applied to area of hemorrhage.

Ruptures
Urethra
a. Use of a stent with an indwelling urethral catheter for 7 days may suffice if the tear is small.
b. Tube cystostomy to allow some urethral healing and resolution of swelling.
c. Primary closure is required if the tear is large.
d. Fair to guarded prognosis for long-term success because urethral stricture and surgical site breakdown can be a problem.

Urinary Bladder
a. Requires primary closure if the tear is large.
b. Good to excellent prognosis in most cases.
c. Some small tears can be managed by catheterization of the urinary bladder for several days until bladder healing can begin.

Ureteral Rupture Repair Depends on Location (Proximal or Distal)
a. Use of stent for 7 days.
b. Primary re-anastomosis is associated with a guarded prognosis because of stricture formation and urinary leakage.
c. Ureteral transposition into new bladder location for more distal rupture location also is associated with a guarded to fair prognosis.
d. Ureteronephrectomy if none of the other procedures is feasible or as a salvage procedure. A guarded to good prognosis is warranted when ureteronephrectomy is performed if the remaining kidney is functioning well.

Kidney
a. Renal pelvic tears are very difficult to close and nephrectomy usually is required.
b. Partial nephrectomy may be possible if leakage is occurring from one pole of the kidney.

Stabilization of the Patient Before Surgery – Uroperitoneum
Patient Concerns
a. Dehydration and volume depletion.
b. Hyperkalemia.
c. Metabolic acidosis.
d. Azotemia.

> ❗ Repair of the site of urine leakage is not a surgical emergency but drainage of urine from the peritoneal cavity is an emergency.

Anesthetic Risks Are a Concern When Anesthetizing Patients With Urinary Tract Trauma
a. Hypovolemia.
b. Arrhythmias due to acidosis and electrolyte disturbances.

Stabilization Before Surgery Is Necessary
a. Determine if bacterial peritonitis is present using cytology as well as bacterial culture and sensitivity of abdominal fluid. Broad spectrum antibiotics are warranted as appropriate based on gram stain and expected pathogens.
b. Fluid replacement to correct hypovolemia and dehydration.
   (1) Balanced electrolyte solution (lactated Ringer's solution, Plasmalyte 148, Normosol-R).
   (2) Consider addition of synthetic colloids if total protein concentration is low or colloid osmotic pressure (COP) is low.
   (3) Blood products may be indicated if PCV is <20%.

(4) Fresh frozen plasma (FFP) may be helpful in patients at risk for systemic inflammatory response syndrome (SIRS) or when hemostatic dysfunction is present or anticipated.

c. Acidosis should resolve with appropriate fluid therapy.

   (1) Bicarbonate therapy is indicated if acidosis is persistent and as long as concurrent respiratory acidosis is not present.

   (2) Investigation of underlying reasons for persistent acidosis may be indicated.

d. Life-threatening hyperkalemia (e.g., bradycardia, shock).

   (1) Fluid therapy will have a dilutional effect on serum potassium concentration ("dilution is the solution to pollution").

   (2) Protect the myocardium by administering 2 to 10 mL of a 10% calcium gluconate solution intravenously.

   (3) Intravenous regular insulin (0.25 to 0.5 U/kg) and dextrose (1 to 2 g per U of insulin administered) if life-threatening hyperkalemia is unresolved with the above treatment.

   (4) Bicarbonate therapy (1 to 2 mEq/kg) if life-threatening hyperkalemia is unresolved with the above treatment.

e. Azotemia and hyperkalemia.

   (1) Partial resolution of azotemia and hyperkalemia may be accomplished with abdominal fluid drainage.

      (a) Urinary catheter may be placed into abdominal cavity through the ruptured bladder.

      (b) A dialysis catheter may be placed into the abdominal cavity.

   (2) More complete resolution of azotemia and hyperkalemia is accomplished with peritoneal dialysis.

Drainage of Urine From the Abdomen

1. Pass a urinary catheter into the bladder–bladder decompression can decrease passage of more urine into the abdominal cavity.

2. Pass a urinary catheter through the bladder tear into the abdominal cavity. This will allow drainage of urine that has already accumulated in the peritoneal space. This can happen by chance while passing a urinary catheter if the defect in the bladder is large. Fluoroscopy can assist passage of the urinary catheter.

3. Place a commercially available percutaneous dialysis catheter through the abdominal wall into the peritoneal cavity. These catheters contain multiple fenestrations that help prevent catheter occlusion and facilitate drainage.

4. Balloon-tipped or latex Penrose drains can be surgically placed into the abdominal cavity to drain urine. The abdominal incision is closed around these drains. Penrose drains are not optimal for abdominal fluid drainage because fluid cannot be collected in a sterile manner. These drains should be covered with sterile bandaging to decrease the risk of ascending infection into the abdominal cavity.

5. Drainage of urine in addition to parenteral fluid therapy support usually results in resolution of azotemia within 24 to 48 hours (depending on the severity of azotemia at the outset with more severe azotemia taking longer to resolve).

6. Dialysis can be started if the patient is severely azotemic. Dialysis is only necessary for a few days. Resolution of azotemia occurs more rapidly that it does with passive drainage of urine from the abdomen.

   a. Many kinds of catheters are available (e.g., Tenckhoff, T-fluted).

b. Nonsurgical placement is important in patients with uroperitoneum due to their frequently unstable condition.
c. Dialysate solution can be commercially purchased or formulated by addition of dextrose to a balanced electrolyte solution (lactated Ringer's solution, Plasmalyte-148 or Normosol-R).
d. Typically peritoneal dialysis is begun using a 1.5% dextrose solution.
e. A range of 10 to 40 mL/kg of dialysate fluid at body temperature (or 2 to 3 degrees higher to enhance vasodilatation) is infused rapidly and allowed to dwell for 30 to 45 minutes and then drained by gravity. Hourly exchanges are recommended initially.
f. A closed system of delivery and collection is ideal to prevent infection.
g. A 90% to 100% recovery of infused dialysate is the goal.
h. Volume of infusate and dwell times can be modified as needed.
i. Tenckhoff catheters typically are occluded by omentum within 12 to 72 hours, but this usually is enough time to control azotemia and hyperkalemia.

WHAT DO WE DO?

- Always rule out diaphragmatic hernia and ruptured urinary bladder or urethra in dogs and cats that have experienced severe blunt abdominal trauma (e.g., hit by car).
- Always rule out ruptured bladder or urethra in dogs and cats with fractured pelvis.
- Analyze fluid retrieved by abdominocentesis using cytology, bacterial culture and sensitivity, and serum biochemistry.
- Choose positive contrast cystography over pneumocystography in cases of suspected bladder rupture because it is easier to interpret the results of positive contrast studies.

THOUGHTS FOR THE FUTURE

- Ultrasonographic techniques will become more refined and this imaging modality will be used routinely to conclusively identify bladder rupture much earlier after blunt abdominal trauma.
- Percutaneous transabdominal catheters will be used more extensively to drain urine from the peritoneal cavity of animals with uroabdomen.
- Better techniques will become available for placing stents in ruptured ureters and urethras.

COMMON MISCONCEPTIONS

- If a dog or cat can urinate a reasonable volume after blunt abdominal trauma, it cannot have a ruptured bladder. No. Depending on the size and location of the rupture in the bladder, the bladder may partially fill and some urine may be voided.
- A palpable bladder on physical examination after blunt abdominal trauma excludes the possibility of rupture and uroabdomen. No. With small tears in the bladder, a substantial volume of urine may still be retained in the bladder.
- A ruptured bladder must be repaired within a few hours after diagnosis. There is no hurry to effect surgical closure of a bladder tear as long as the metabolic consequences of uroabdomen can be adequately managed (urine drainage through a urinary catheter or through abdominal drain tubes along with IV fluid therapy). It is better to stabilize the patient metabolically before anesthesia and surgery.

SUMMARY TIPS

- Calculate the abdominal fluid creatinine concentration to serum creatinine concentration ratio to determine if an abdominal effusion represents uroabdomen or not. The ratio is usually >2:1 if the fluid is urine.
- If the abdominal fluid creatinine concentration to serum creatinine concentration ratio is equivocal (i.e., ≤2:1), calculate the abdominal fluid potassium concentration to serum potassium concentration ratio. Patients with uroperitoneum will have a ratio of >1.4 (dogs) or >1.9 (cats).
- Because ruptured bladder is the most common cause of uroperitoneum in dogs and cats, start with a positive contrast cystogram to determine the site of the rupture. If positive contrast cystography is not definitive, excretory urography should be performed to determine if the kidneys or ureters are the source of the urine leakage.
- Stabilize the patient for up to 48 hours before definitive repa ir of the urinary tract rupture.

FREQUENTLY ASKED QUESTIONS

Q: Last week, I euthanized a 17-year-old cat that was presented for evaluation of anorexia and vomiting. Serum creatinine concentration was >20.0 mg/dL. The kidneys were slightly small on palpation and the cat was approximately 10% dehydrated based on skin turgor assessment. The cat was euthanized on the basis of a diagnosis of chronic renal failure. On necropsy, there was a considerable amount of abdominal fluid and a small hole in the bladder surrounded by a large bruise. Could all of these findings been the result of urine leakage from the bladder into the abdomen?

A: Yes. The magnitude of azotemia does not differentiate among prerenal, primary renal, or postrenal causes. Many older cats have chronic kidney disease, but older cats also may experience bladder rupture as was the case in this particular cat.

Q: I performed a dental prophylaxis on a 7-year-old female spayed Greyhound. I knew the dog had pre-existing renal disease with moderate azotemia and dilute urine. Intravenous fluids were administered before, during, and after the dental procedure for renoprotection. The dog was discharged later that same day but was returned early the next day in extreme pain. The dog was referred, and uroperitoneum was diagnosed. After one day of stabilization, the bladder rupture was repaired surgically. How did this happen?

A: At the time of referral, the dog's serum creatinine concentration was 7.0 mg/dL whereas it was 3.0 mg/dL before the dental procedure. Several possibilities were considered, including the possibility of acute-on-chronic renal disease with exacerbation of pre-existing chronic renal disease by anesthesia and possibly hypotension. Another possibility considered was that the sudden increase in serum creatinine concentration could have represented prerenal azotemia due to dehydration. Abdominal radiographs showed a slight loss of abdominal detail, and ultrasonography showed some free abdominal fluid. Biochemical analysis of the fluid showed the fluid creatinine concentration to be 37 mg/dL whereas the serum creatinine concentration was 7 mg/dL (i.e., fluid to serum creatinine concentration ratio of >5:1) supporting a diagnosis of uroabdomen. At surgery, the dog was observed to have a 2.5 cm tear in the dorsal bladder wall and the defect was closed. The dog did well after surgical repair. Review of the history determined that the dog's bladder had been manually expressed while it was recovering from anesthesia for the dental procedure. Urethral tone can be high during recovery and it is likely the bladder rupture occurred during this time. After recovery from anesthesia, the dog was noted to be panting and she assumed the "position of relief."

SUGGESTED READINGS

Aumann M, Worth LT, Drobatz KJ: Uroperitoneum in cats: 26 cases (1986-1995), *J Am Anim Hosp Assoc* 34:315–324, 1998.

Beck AL, Grierson JM, Ogden DM, et al: Outcome of and complications associated with tube cystostomy in dogs and cats: 76 cases (1995-2006), *J Am Vet Med Assoc* 230:1184–1189, 2007.

Burrows CF, Bovee KC: Metabolic changes due to experimentally induced rupture of the canine urinary bladder, *Am J Vet Res* 35:1083–1088, 1974.

Meige F, Sarrau S, Autefage A: Management of traumatic urethral rupture in 11 cats using primary alignment with a urethral catheter, *Vet Comp Orthop Traumatol* 21:76–84, 2008.

Schmiedt C, Tobias KM, Otto CM: Evaluation of abdominal fluid: Peripheral blood creatinine and potassium ratios for diagnosis of uroperitoneum in dogs, *J Vet Emerg Crit Care* 11:275–280, 2001.

Stiffler KS, McCrackin Stevenson MA, et al: Clinical use of low-profile cystostomy tubes in four dogs and a cat, *J Am Vet Med Assoc* 223:309–310, 2003:325-329.

Weisse C, Aronson LR, Drobatz K: Traumatic rupture of the ureter: 10 cases, *J Am Anim Hosp Assoc* 38:188–192, 2002.

13 Disorders of Micturition and Urinary Incontinence

INTRODUCTION

A. Micturition is the process of urinary storage (filling) and voiding (emptying). Approximately 99% of the time, the bladder and urethra are occupied in the storage of urine whereas only 1% of the time is occupied with voiding.

B. Incontinence is the involuntary passage of urine. The affected animal typically appears to be unaware of urine leakage, at least initially. Increased grooming of the perineum suggests awareness of the problem at some point in its clinical course.

C. Urinary incontinence is an important disorder encountered in primary care practice.

D. Urinary incontinence is much more common in dogs than in cats. When encountered in cats, urge incontinence from cystitis must be excluded as the most likely consideration.

E. Complex neurological input to the bladder and urethra are involved in coordinating the proper times for filling and storage of urine (see details later).

> **!** Bladder pressure exceeds urethral resistance in most forms of urinary incontinence.

F. Most forms of incontinence occur only when bladder pressure exceeds urethral resistance pressure. Incontinence may occur when bladder pressure is abnormally high (transiently or persistently), urethral pressure is low, or a combination of these factors. Exceptions to this rule occur when the incontinence is due to anatomical defects (e.g., ectopic ureter) that bypass the normal urethral sphincter mechanism.

PHYSIOLOGY OF URINATION

A. The normal physiology of urination involves both voluntary and involuntary (i.e., autonomic) components of the nervous system.

B. Stretch receptors in the bladder carry afferent information (general visceral afferent [GVA] and general proprioceptive [GP]) about bladder distension to the spinal cord.

C. This information is relayed to higher central nervous system (CNS) centers (e.g., brainstem, cerebral cortex) via the spinothalamic tract and general proprioceptive tract in the fasciculus gracilis allowing conscious perception of bladder distension.

D. If the circumstances are appropriate for urination, the emptying phase is initiated. The parasympathetic portion of the autonomic nervous system plays the dominant role in the emptying phase (Figure 13-1).

   1. Motor information descends from the higher CNS centers via the tectospinal and reticulospinal tracts to parasympathetic general visceral efferent lower motor neurons in the gray matter of the sacral spinal cord (S1-S2).

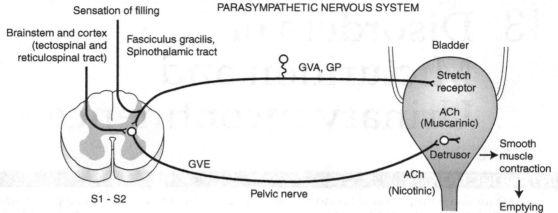

FIGURE 13-1 ■ Role of the parasympathetic nervous system in urination. ACh, acetylcholine; *GVE*, general visceral efferent; *GVA*, general visceral afferent; *GP*, general proprioceptive. (Drawn by Tim Vojt.)

2. These neurons reach the detrusor muscle of the bladder via the pelvic nerve and initiate detrusor contraction and bladder emptying.
3. This control is mediated by the parasympathetic nervous system and neurotransmission is cholinergic at both the preganglionic and postganglionic fibers. The receptors at the smooth muscle of the detrusor are muscarinic.
4. The GVA and GP afferent neurons from the bladder wall also synapse on the parasympathetic general visceral efferent (GVE) lower motor neurons in the sacral spinal cord. This is the basis for local spinal cord reflex voiding (see later).
5. At the same time, efferent fibers from higher centers inhibit transmission in the sympathetic nervous system, which normally facilitates bladder filling.
6. Also, there is inhibition of general somatic efferent (GSE) neurons located in the sacral spinal cord (S1-S2) that exit in the pudendal nerve and normally maintain tone in the striated muscle of the urethra (so-called *external* urethral sphincter). Failure of this inhibition contributes to increased urethral sphincter tone in patients with upper motor neuron (UMN) bladders.
7. GSE neurons to the striated muscle of the abdomen are stimulated and initiate abdominal wall contractions that increase intra-abdominal pressure and are important in the voiding response. This somatic component represents part of the voluntary control of urination.
8. Injury that results in a CNS lesion cranial to the sacral spinal cord is associated with detrusor areflexia and increased urethral sphincter tone (due in part to loss of UMN inhibitory influence).
   a. This results in loss of voluntary initiation of voiding.
   b. Manual expression of the bladder is difficult due to the high urethral tone.
   c. Within a few weeks of injury, local reflex voiding develops and is associated with incomplete bladder emptying and abnormally high residual volume.
   d. Such a bladder is called an *upper motor neuron* (UMN or automatic) bladder.
E. If the circumstances are inappropriate for urination, the filling phase continues. The sympathetic portion of the autonomic nervous system plays the dominant role in the filling phase (Figure 13-2).
   1. Efferent fibers descending from higher centers in the CNS inhibit the GVE lower motor neurons of the parasympathetic nervous system that are located in the sacral spinal cord (S1-S2).

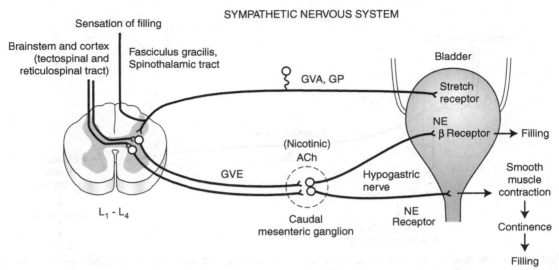

FIGURE 13-2 ■ Role of the sympathetic nervous system in urination. ACh, acetylcholine; *GVE*, general visceral efferent; *GVA*, general visceral aferent; *GP*, general proprioceptive; *NE*, norepine phrine. (Drawn by Tim Vojt.)

2. Sympathetic GVE neurons in the lumbar spinal cord (L2-L5) are stimulated and these preganglionic fibers synapse at the caudal mesenteric ganglion (cholinergic mediation). The postganglionic adrenergic fibers reach the bladder wall via the hypogastric nerve.

3. The postganglionic fibers that reach the body of the bladder terminate primarily on beta-adrenergic receptors. When these receptors (found primarily in the body of the bladder) are stimulated there is relaxation of the detrusor smooth muscle and bladder filling is facilitated.

4. The postganglionic fibers that reach the bladder neck and proximal urethra terminate mainly on alpha-adrenergic receptors. When these receptors (found primarily in the bladder neck and proximal urethra) are stimulated, contraction of smooth muscle in these regions occurs, which facilitates bladder filling and maintains continence. The smooth muscle in the proximal urethra is referred to as the *internal* urethral sphincter.

5. The distribution of beta- and alpha-adrenergic receptors in the bladder and proximal urethra (see earlier) establishes the role of the sympathetic nervous system in the regulation of urination.

6. Also during bladder filling, efferent fibers descending from higher CNS centers stimulate GSE neurons of the sacral spinal cord (S1-S2) that travel in the pudendal nerve to innervate the striated muscle of the urethra, the so-called *external* urethral sphincter. Neurotransmission at this striated muscle is cholinergic via nicotinic receptors. This somatic component represents part of the voluntary control of urination (Figure 13-3).

7. Simultaneously, GSE fibers that innervate the striated muscles of the abdomen are inhibited by higher CNS centers.

F. In summary, afferent information from the bladder about its state of distension ultimately reaches higher CNS centers in the brainstem and cerebral cortex. The higher CNS centers integrate this information with other afferent input and institute the appropriate efferent response with respect to urination.

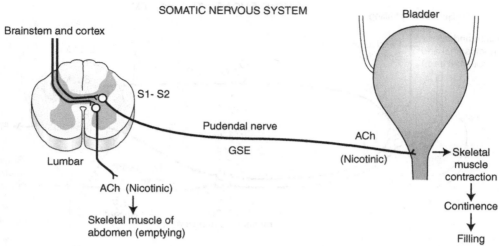

FIGURE 13-3 ■ Role of the somatic nervous system in urination. *ACh*, acetylcholine; *GSE*, general somatic efferent. (Drawn by Tim Vojt.)

G. It is important to understand how the GVE neurons of the parasympathetic and sympathetic components of the autonomic nervous system and the GSE neurons of the somatic nervous system interact in the control of bladder filling and emptying because the drugs that are used to manage animals with disorders of urination act on these systems.

H. Even a bladder that has lost its local sacral reflex arc consisting of the GVA and GVE parasympathetic neurons in the sacral spinal cord and pelvic nerve eventually can develop the ability to empty partially.
   1. This effect is due to the intrinsic ability of smooth muscle to contract.
   2. Urine overflow will occur when intravesical pressure exceeds the elasticity of the urethra.
   3. Such a bladder is called a *lower motor neuron* (LMN or autonomous) bladder and results from lesions in the sacral spinal cord, cauda equina, or pelvic nerves. The caudal vertebral and spinal cord malformations that occur in Manx cats represent a congenital condition causing a LMN bladder.
   4. The residual volume of urine in a LMN bladder usually exceeds that in an UMN bladder. Increasing the animal's intra-abdominal pressure by picking it up may initiate involuntary voiding.
   5. There is no ability to voluntarily initiate bladder emptying.
   6. Bladder contractions are weak and ineffective at bladder emptying.

DIFFERENTIAL DIAGNOSIS FOR URINARY INCONTINENCE (Box 13-1)

A. The causes of urinary incontinence classically are divided into neurogenic or non-neurogenic categories. Non-neurogenic causes are most common, and a thorough neurological examination is important in making this distinction.

B. Another approach is to divide causes of incontinence into those associated with small to normal-sized bladder and those associated with an enlarged bladder. Most cases of urinary incontinence (especially non-neurogenic causes) are associated with a small to normal-sized bladder at presentation.

■ BOX 13-1
■ **CAUSES OF URINARY INCONTINENCE**

Neurogenic
I. Upper motor neuron
   A. Brain/brainstem
      1. Neoplasia
      2. Dysautonomia
   B. Spinal cord
      1. Dysautonomia
      2. Intervertebral disk protrusion
      3. Fibrocartilaginous infarct
      4. Neoplasia
      5. Infectious
      6. Trauma
II. Lower motor neuron
   A. Trauma
   B. Congenital anomaly (e.g., Manx cat)
III. Reflex dyssynergy (detrusor-urethral dyssynergia)

Non-neurogenic
I. Primary sphincter mechanism incompetence
II. Anatomic abnormalities
   A. Ectopic ureter
   B. Patent urachus
   C. Bladder exstrophy
   D. Urethrorectal fistula
   E. Ureterovaginal fistula (e.g., after spaying)
   F. Female pseudohermaphrodism
   G. Urethral diverticulum
   H. Ureterocele
   I. Other
III. Paradoxical (obstructive)
IV. Urge incontinence associated with UTI or inflammation
V. Post-prostatectomy incontinence (dogs)
VI. Post-perineal urethrostomy incontinence (cats)
VII. Feline leukemia virus (FeLV) or feline immunodeficiency virus (FIV)-associated incontinence (cats)
VIII. Idiopathic detrusor hyperactivity (*overactive bladder*)

Clinical Approach to Patients Presented for Evaluation of Abnormal Micturition

SIGNALMENT

A. Congenital disorders are most commonly recognized in young animals. Certain large breed dogs are at increased risk for ectopic ureters. Manx cats have urinary incontinence associated with congenital vertebral and spinal cord anomalies.

B. Hormone-responsive incontinence and urethral sphincter incompetence usually occur in middle-aged, medium to large breed female dogs; certain breeds are at increased risk for this disorder (see later).

C. Reflex dyssynergy (detrusor-urethral-dyssynergia) occurs more frequently in large breed male dogs.

HISTORY

A. It is important to differentiate loss of voluntary control from behavioral changes or recent onset of polyuria and polydipsia.
   1. Development of polyuria as a result of an underlying disease such as chronic renal failure may result in the animal urinating in the house because it is not being allowed outdoors frequently enough.
   2. Some owners may misinterpret this situation as the animal losing control of urinations.
B. It is important to question the owner about the presence of dysuria or hematuria suggestive of urinary tract infection (UTI), inflammation or partial urinary tract obstruction.
C. It is important to identify any previous episodes of trauma or surgery adjacent to or involving the urinary tract that could have affected micturition.
D. Previous response to (or lack of response to) antibiotics or anti-inflammatory drugs may suggest the nature of an underlying condition.

PHYSICAL EXAMINATION

A. Observe the animal urinating. Characterize the animal's ability to initiate a urine stream, the diameter of the stream, any interruptions of the stream, and any apparent pain.
B. Observe the perineal region of females for wetness or foul odor.
C. Palpate the bladder, urethra, and the prostate gland in males.
   1. Determine the size (i.e., small, normal, enlarged) and position of the bladder before voiding.

> ❗ Rectal examination and determination of anal tone is an important first step in ruling out neurogenic causes of urinary incontinence.

   2. Determine the presence or absence of pain associated with palpation of the bladder (and prostate gland in males).
   3. Determine bladder size after voiding. An enlarged bladder after attempts to void suggests urine retention.
   4. Identify any masses in the bladder or prostate gland in males that could be associated with outflow obstruction, inflammation, or altered function.
   5. Evaluate the urethra on rectal examination in both males and females.
D. Depending on the clinical circumstances, digital vaginal examination in female dogs can be performed to evaluate for presence of a mass in the region of the vestibule or external urethra.
E. Perform a complete neurologic examination to assess the cerebrum, brainstem, and spinal cord. Pay special attention to the local sacral reflex arc including:
   1. *Anal tone* on rectal examination. Poor anal tone suggests the possibility of a LMN bladder.
   2. *Bulbocavernosus reflex* (manual compression of the bulbus glandis or clitoris causes contraction of the anal sphincter via the pudendal nerve).
   3. *Perineal reflex* (pricking or stroking the skin of the perineum) causes ventroflexion of the tail and contraction of the anal sphincter).
F. In animals with incontinence and an enlarged bladder, passage of a urethral catheter to rule out intraluminal obstruction can be helpful. Extramural masses may not be identified by this procedure.

G. Collect and measure residual urine in the bladder after the animal has voided. Residual urine volume of >0.4 ml/kg body weight suggests partial obstruction to urine outflow or functional inability to empty the bladder.

LABORATORY FINDINGS

A. A minimal database for animals with incontinence should include a urinalysis and urine culture.
B. If indicated by other findings, a hemogram and serum biochemical profile may be performed to identify systemic disease processes.

URINARY TRACT IMAGING

A. Urinary tract imaging is performed if the diagnosis is not apparent after initial evaluation or if empirical treatment has not been effective.
B. Survey abdominal radiography.
   1. Determine the position of the bladder (i.e., intra-abdominal or intrapelvic).
   2. Determine the size of the bladder (i.e., small, normal-sized, enlarged).
   3. Determine the shape of the bladder: Is there a distinct vesicourethral junction or not?
   4. Are radiopaque calculi present?
C. Contrast radiography is helpful to rule out anatomic abnormalities or radiolucent calculi.
   1. Excretory urography can be used to evaluate for the presence of ectopic ureters (see later), ureteral dilatation, or dilatation of the renal pelvis.
   2. Cystography and urethrography can be used to evaluate for the presence of anatomic abnormalities (e.g., urachal remnant, urethral diverticulum) and masses or radiolucent calculi in the bladder or urethra.
D. Ultrasonography can help exclude anatomical abnormalities, masses, and calculi.
E. Urethrocystoscopy is helpful to evaluate the vestibule, vagina, urethra, and bladder and to identify abnormal ureteral openings, masses, and other anatomic abnormalities (e.g., urachal diverticulum).
F. Contrast-enhanced excretory urography combined with computed tomography can be considered when a definitive diagnosis has not been obtained by other imaging procedures.

SPECIAL STUDIES

A. The *cystometrogram* (CMG) is a pressure-volume recording of the bladder's response to filling with fluid or CO_2 (Figure 13-4).
B. The *urethral pressure profile* (UPP) is a pressure tracing of the urethra as a catheter is slowly withdrawn from the bladder at a constant speed (Figures 13-5 and 13-6).
C. The UPP and CMG are diagnostic procedures that typically are performed on a referral basis. They require special equipment and technical expertise, and specific anesthetic regimens must be followed in order for results to be valuable.

! Urodynamic studies are not necessary for the diagnosis and management of most dogs with urinary incontinence seen in primary care practice.

D. The UPP and CMG are not needed to establish a presumptive diagnosis in most dogs with urinary incontinence.
E. Important parameters for UPP evaluation (see Figures 13-5 and 13-6):

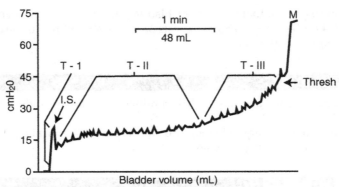

FIGURE 13-4 ■ Cystometrogram showing bladder pressure (cm H_2O) as the dependent variable (y-axis) and bladder volume (mL) as the independent variable (x-axis). During the T-II phase the bladder accommodates the accumulation of volume by relaxing (no significant increase in pressure). The bladder approaches its maximal capacity during the T-III phase (pressure begins to rise). The detrusor contracts to initiate voiding at the end of the T-III phase (thresh). *I.S.*, Initial spike; *M,* maximal contraction. (From Oliver JE, Young WO: Air cystometry in dogs under xylazine-induced restraint. *Am J Vet Res* 34:1433-5, 1973.)

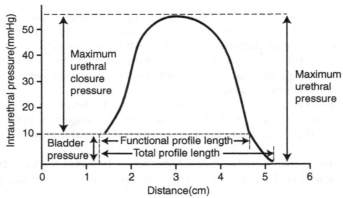

FIGURE 13-5 ■ An idealized urethral pressure profile (UPP) from a female dog. Maximum urethral closure pressure (MUCP) and functional profile length (FPL) are the two most reliable and widely used parameters in assessment of the UPP. (From Rosin A, Rosin E, Oliver J: Canine urethral pressure profile. *Am J Vet Res* 41:1114, 1980.)

1. Maximum urethral pressure (MUP): Highest pressure recorded during the profile.
2. Maximum urethral closure pressure (MUCP): Difference between MUP and intravesical pressure.
3. Functional profile length (FPL): Length of urethra over which urethral pressure exceeds intravesical pressure.

F. FPL is the most consistent parameter on the UPP. MUCP is more variable. MUCP occurs in the middle to distal urethra of female dogs and cats and in the postprostatic urethra of male dogs and cats.

G. The urodynamic tests described above are confirmatory for urethral sphincter incompetence, detrusor hyporeflexia, and detrusor hyperreflexia but typically are performed under chemical restraint and not during voiding. Consequently, they do not confirm or rule out reflex dyssynergia.

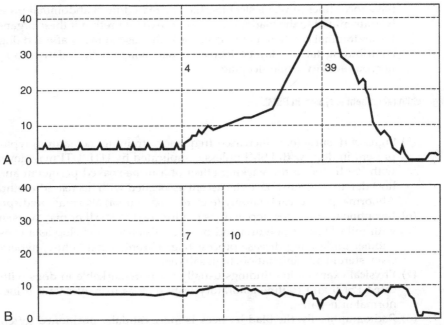

FIGURE 13-6 ■ Urethral pressure profile from a normal spayed female (**A**), and from a spayed female dog with primary sphincter incompetence (PSMI) (**B**). (Courtesy of Dr. Susi Arnold, Zurich, Switzerland.)

> ! Primary sphincter mechanism incompetence (PSMI) is the most common cause of urinary incontinence in adult dogs seen in primary care practice.

ABNORMAL URINATION (DISORDERS OF MICTURITION)

Non-neurogenic Causes of Urinary Incontinence
Primary Sphincter Mechanism Incompetence (PSMI)

a. PSMI is the most common non-neurogenic cause of urinary incontinence in dogs.
   (1) Incontinence in spayed female dogs previously was called hormone-responsive, or estrogen-responsive, incontinence.
   (2) Occurs approximately 3 years after ovariohysterectomy in approximately 20% of female dogs neutered between their first and second heat cycles.
   (3) More common in large dogs (more than 20 kg). May occur in any breed of dog or in mixed breed dogs but some breeds are over-represented:
      (a) Doberman pinscher.
      (b) Giant Schnauzer.
      (c) Old English sheepdog.
      (d) Rottweiler.
      (e) Boxer.
   (4) Urine leakage while the dog is sleeping or lying down is the most common historical finding in dogs with uncomplicated PSMI. Intra-abdominal pressure increases when dogs lie on their sides and this factor may explain why many affected dogs

have incontinence while sleeping (i.e., increased intra-abdominal pressure cannot be transmitted to the bladder neck and proximal urethra if these organs lie outside the abdominal cavity in pelvic canal as is the case in many affected dogs). Another contributing factor may be increased parasympathetic (relative to sympathetic) nervous activity while sleeping.

> **!** Urine leakage while recumbent is typical in PSMI.

(5) Signs of dysuria (e.g., increased frequency, straining, hematuria) typically are not present in dogs with PSMI unless complicated by UTI. UTI may develop in dogs with PSMI due to the wicking effect of a urine-soaked perineum and decreased host defenses against bacterial ascent associated with decreased urethral pressure. Abnormal perivulvar anatomy (e.g., recessed vulva) also may predispose to UTI.

(6) Incontinence may develop in dogs predisposed to PSMI or may worsen in animals with mild PSMI if polyuria and bladder distension develop as a consequence of another underlying disease process (e.g., chronic renal failure, hyperadrenocorticism, steroid administration, high salt diet).

(7) Physical examination findings usually are unremarkable in dogs with uncomplicated PSMI and routine laboratory tests such as urinalysis and urine culture are normal or negative.

(8) Radiographically, the bladder neck is more caudally positioned (often within the pelvic canal) in some female dogs with sphincter mechanism incompetence as compared with continent female dogs. This radiographic feature has been referred to as a *pelvic bladder* (Figures 13-7).

(9) MUCP is significantly lower and FPL significantly shorter on UPP in affected female dogs as compared with continent female dogs (see Figure 13-6).

(10) Incontinence is controlled in 75% to 90% of female dogs with PSMI treated with the alpha-adrenergic agonist phenylpropanolamine (PPA).

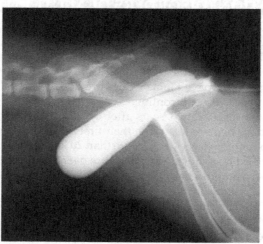

FIGURE 13-7 ■ Pelvic bladder (lateral abdominal radiograph). Note abnormal shape of bladder (lack of caudal tapering) and displacement of bladder into pelvic canal. This abnormality of positioning can predispose the dog to urinary incontinence.

! Phenylpropanolamine is the initial treatment of choice to restore urinary continence in dogs with PSMI.

    (a) PPA is used at a dosage of 1.0 to 1.5 mg/kg PO every 12 hours or every 8 hours (standard preparation).

    (b) PPA is also available as a sustained release product (Cystolamine, 75 mg capsule). Once daily administration may be desirable for many owners. The recommended dosage of Cystolamine is ½ capsule PO every 24 hours for dogs weighing <18 kg, 1 capsule PO every 24 hours for dogs 19 to 45 kg, and 1 ½ capsules PO every 24 hours for dogs weighing more than 45 kg.

    (c) MUCP is increased on the UPP after treatment with PPA.

    (d) Virtually all affected dogs have some improvement in continence after treatment with PPA.

    (e) The largest dose should be given at night to control incontinence while the dog is sleeping. In dogs with incontinence only at night, dosing only at night can be effective.

    (f) PPA may become less effective with prolonged use (so-called tachyphylaxis). Occasionally, simply increasing the dosage of PPA is sufficient to regain control of continence.

    (g) Potential adverse effects include restlessness and hypertension.

    (h) Relative contraindications to use include known underlying cardiac disease, chronic kidney disease, or systemic hypertension.

    (i) Although systemic hypertension did not develop after months of PPA exposure to young dogs in an experimental setting, we have observed client-owned dogs with PSMI on PPA that have developed systemic hypertension.

    (j) We recommend systemic blood pressure be measured before beginning PPA treatment and periodically thereafter to identify the development of systemic hypertension.

(11) Incontinence is controlled in 60% to 65% of affected dogs treated with estrogens alone for PSMI.

    (a) Estrogen increases the sensitivity of urethral alpha-adrenergic receptors to catecholamines; it also may increase the number of receptors.

! Estrogens are an effective treatment for PSMI in many dogs and can be given much less frequently than PPA.

    (b) MUCP is increased on the UPP after treatment with estrogens.

    (c) Estrogen preparations.

        (i) Diethylstilbestrol (DES).

            (•) Dosage: 0.1 to 1.0 mg per dog PO for 3-5 days followed by 0.1 to 1.0 mg PO every 3 to 7 days.

            (•) DES has become more difficult to obtain because it is no longer used in human patients.

        (ii) Premarin (conjugated estrogens).

            (•) Dosage: 20 µg/kg PO every 3 or 4 days.

            (•) Obtained from pregnant mare's urine.

            (•) Contains sodium estrone sulfate (50% to 65%), and sodium equilin sulfate (20% to 35%).

            (•) Estrone is converted to estradiol.

(•) Although published information on the use of Premarin in dogs with PSMI is lacking, we have had success with this product in our hospital.
(iii) Oestriol (Incurin).
  (•) Dosage: 2 mg per day for 1 week followed by reduction to minimally effective daily dose (0.25 to 2.0 mg) and finally alternate day dosing (dose not related to body weight).
  (•) Naturally-occurring, short-acting estrogen.
  (•) Sixty-one percent of treated dogs achieved continence and 22% improved for overall response rate of 83%.
  (•) No hematologic abnormalities identified.
(iv) Potential complications of treatment with estrogens.
  (•) Clinical signs of estrus.
  (•) Perineal alopecia.
  (•) Bone marrow suppression (a life-threatening complication most often seen after use of long-acting injectable estrogens such as estradiol cypionate, or with overdose). We have not encountered bone marrow suppression in dogs receiving low dose intermittent estrogens.
(12) Combination of estrogens with PPA.
  (a) Clinical experience suggests that some dogs require both PPA and estrogens for optimal control of incontinence suggesting synergism of effect.
  (b) One study indicated that adding PPA to estradiol did not result in additional increases in urethral resistance.
(13) Combination of PPA with anticholinergic drugs. Some dogs that fail to respond to PPA alone respond with the addition of flavoxate or oxybutynin. This finding suggests that bladder detrusor instability may complicate PSMI in some dogs.
(14) Gonadotropin-releasing hormone (GnRH) analogues.
  (a) Decreased estrogen concentration after spaying lead to extremely increased concentrations of gonadotropins: Follicle-stimulating hormone (FSH) and luteinizing hormone (LH).
  (b) GnRH analogues decrease FSH and LH concentrations by downregulating gonadotropin receptors in the pituitary gland.
  (c) Treatment with GnRH analogues controlled incontinence in 60% of a small group of dogs with PSMI that had failed PPA treatment or were not able to take this medication due to side effects.
  (d) The original hypothesis that increased FSH and LH concentrations in spayed dogs affects urethral resistance has not been supported by further investigations.
    (i) No correlation between MUCP on UPP and plasma concentrations of FSH and LH was observed.
    (ii) Spayed incontinent female dogs actually had lower FSH and LH concentrations than did spayed continent female dogs.
    (iii) GnRH analogues (i.e., leuprolide) had no effect on MUCP or other UPP parameters regardless of clinical response observed.
  (e) GnRH analogues may have a direct effect on the bladder to cause detrusor muscle relaxation.
  (f) Leuprolide had no effect on UPP of spayed continent beagles before or 8 weeks after treatment.
  (g) Cystometrograms of treated dogs showed increased bladder threshold volume and increased compliance (i.e., increased volume without an increase in pressure).

(h) Dosage: 5 to 10 mg leuprolide (Lupron) intramuscularly.
(i) Advantages.
    (i) No known adverse effects.
    (ii) Single injection may last 6 to 8 months.
    (iii) May be useful when dog does not respond to PPA or when PPA is contra-indicated.
        (•) Systemic hypertension.
        (•) Underlying cardiac disease.
        (•) Nervousness on PPA.
(15) Dogs with refractory PSMI can be treated by submucosal urethral injections of collagen injections.
  (a) The goal is to create cystoscopically-visible 360-degree apposition of the urethral mucosa by submucosal implantation of collagen at three sites: The 12-o'clock position (0 degrees), 4-o'clock position (120 degrees), and 8-o'clock position (240 degrees) approximately 1 to 1.5 cm caudal to the vesicourethral junction (Figure 13-8).

> ❗ Submucosal urethral collagen injections improve continence in most dogs that have failed PPA treatment for PSMI.

  (b) 50% to 80% response rate with collagen alone as treatment.
  (c) Dogs that fail to respond to PPA can be treated with urethral collagen injections. If treated dogs are not completely continent after collagen injections, additional improvement in continence may be achieved by adding PPA to the treatment regimen.
  (d) In one study, collagen injections controlled incontinence in 27 of 40 dogs treated for an average of 17 months (range, 1-64 months).
  (e) Advantages: Avoids the need for daily medication.
  (f) Disadvantages.
    (i) Expensive and may not have long duration of effect in some dogs.
    (ii) Requires special equipment and technical expertise.

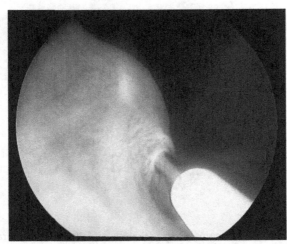

FIGURE 13-8 ■ Submucosal injection (endoscopic view) of collagen in the urethra of a female dog to control urinary incontinence.

(16) Surgical colposuspension (Figure 13-9).
    (a) Distal aspect of the vagina is sutured to the pre-pubic tendon, which repositions the bladder neck and proximal urethra cranially into the abdominal cavity.
    (b) Facilitates transmission of intra-abdominal pressure to the bladder neck and proximal urethra.
    (c) Urethra is functionally lengthened and compressed against the pelvic brim.
    (d) Immediately improves FPL and MUCP on UPP postoperatively.
    (e) Response rate of approximately 50% is seen but relatively poor success rate when evaluated one year after surgery.
    (f) Medical treatment with PPA improved continence in dogs that relapsed after colposuspension.
    (g) Complications.
        (i) Transient dysuria and stranguria associated with obstruction.
        (ii) Suture breakdown and relapse.
(17) Sphincter mechanism incontinence occurs rarely in male dogs and is poorly responsive to medical therapy.
    (a) Long-acting testosterone injections may be tried.
        (i) Testosterone propionate 2.2 mg/kg IM 3 times/wk; or,
        (ii) Testosterone cypionate 5.5 mg/kg IM every 30 days.
        (iii) In a study of male dogs with PSMI a poor (20%) response to testosterone was observed.
    (b) PPA also may be tried but the response (40% to 50%) is much lower than the response of females with PSMI.

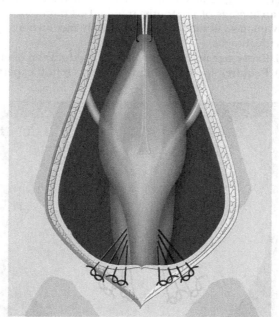

FIGURE 13-9 ■ Colposuspension. The vagina is repositioned cranially from the intrapelvic position to an intra-abdominal position by suture placement between the vagina and prepubic tendon. This procedure effectively increases the length of the urethra and its closure pressure. (Drawn by Tim Vojt.)

    (c) Vasopexy is a surgical alternative to increase urethral tone in intact male dogs with urinary incontinence.

    (d) Collagen injection performed antegrade using a cystoscope inserted into the bladder via cystotomy has been used in some male dogs with incontinence.

Anatomic Abnormality

  a. Ectopic ureter is the most common anatomic abnormality causing urinary incontinence in dogs; it is very rare in cats.

    (1) Usually young at presentation (less than 1 year of age; females tend to be presented at a younger age than males).

    (2) Females are diagnosed more often than males.

    (3) Ectopic ureters may be more common in males than appreciated because affected males frequently are not incontinent as a consequence of the length of urethra distal to the opening of ectopic ureter.

    (4) More common in certain breeds.

      (a) Siberian huskies.

      (b) Labrador retrievers.

      (c) Golden retrievers.

      (d) Soft coated Wheaten terriers.

      (e) Newfoundlands.

      (f) Poodles.

    (5) Bilateral involvement is detected more often than unilateral; early reports of primarily unilateral involvement likely were affected by limitations of imaging (i.e., lack of urethrocystoscopy).

    (6) Most ectopic ureters in female dogs terminate in the urethra after tunneling from more proximal locations (Figure 13-10).

    (7) Extramural ectopic ureters are reported rarely. Extramural ectopic ureters fail to attach and open at the bladder trigone. Extramural ectopic ureters bypass the

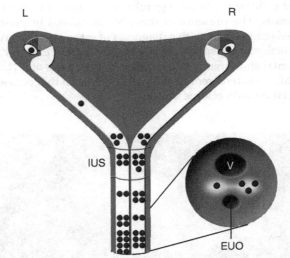

FIGURE 13-10 ■ Map of termination of ectopic ureteral openings. *EUO*, external urethral orifice; *IUS*, internal urethral sphincter; *V*, vagina. (From Cannizzo KL, McLoughlin MA, Mattoon JS, et al: Evaluation of transurethral cystoscopy and excretory urography for diagnosis of ectopic ureters in female dogs: 25 cases (1992-2000). *J Am Vet Med Assoc* 223:475-481, 2003.)

bladder and open directly into the urinary tract distal to the trigone or directly into the vagina or vestibule. We have observed this form of ectopic ureter only rarely.

(8) Ectopic ureters uncommonly terminate in the vestibule.

(9) Ectopic ureters may terminate in the vagina or uterus, but we have not encountered this presentation in our hospital.

(10) Ectopic ureters in male dogs usually are bilateral (15 of 16 dogs of which more than half were Labrador retrievers in a study recently completed at The Ohio State University). Four of the ectopic ureters were associated with ureteroceles. Three did not have urinary incontinence. Surgical correction produced a satisfactory outcome in 11 of 12 dogs.

(11) Positive results on excretory urography (Figure 13-11) can establish a diagnosis of ectopic ureter but negative results do not eliminate ectopic ureter as a possible diagnosis. Both false positive and false negative results may occur. Oblique positioning of the patient, concurrent negative contrast cystography, and fluoroscopy all can aid in identification of an ectopic ureter. Observing the typical "J" configuration of the ureter as it enters the trigone does not ensure that the ureter opens into the bladder at the normal location.

> **!** Excretory urography can establish a diagnosis of ectopic ureter but failure to identify an ectopic ureter on excretory urography does not eliminate the possibility of one being present.

(12) Computed tomography in combination with excretory urography is the gold standard for diagnosis of ectopic ureter in male dogs because ectopic ureteral openings can be missed during urethroscopy due to limitations of the procedure in males.

(13) Ectopic ureters occasionally can be identified on ultrasonography, especially if the ureter is dilated. Ultrasonography also is useful to identify hydroureter or hydronephrosis. The presence of these abnormalities in patients with urinary incontinence is compatible with a diagnosis of ectopic ureter. Hydroureter can result from obstruction of the submucosal segment of the ectopic ureter in the urethra, a developmental abnormality of the ureter, or the effects of UTI. Ultrasonography also can identify unilateral renal aplasia or hypoplasia that occasionally can be observed in association with ectopic ureter.

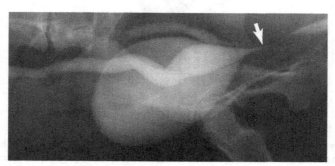

FIGURE 13-11 ■ Excretory urogram with oblique positioning of a dog with an ectopic ureter. Note contrast in the ectopic ureter passing beyond the trigone and terminating distally in the urethra (*arrow*).

(14) Color flow Doppler ultrasonography can identify jets of urine entering the bladder at the trigone. The presence of such urine jets usually excludes ectopic ureter as a diagnosis, but it is not always possible to obtain the necessary images.

(15) Urethrocystoscopy is the gold standard for the diagnosis of ectopic ureters in female dogs. Visualization of both ureteral openings in their normal position (i.e., two C-shaped openings facing each other) in the trigone conclusively rules out ectopic ureter (Figure 13-12).

> ❗ Urethrocystoscopy is the gold standard for diagnosis of ectopic ureters in female dogs

(16) A definitive diagnosis of ectopic ureter is made during urethrocystoscopy by visualization of additional openings in the urethra or vestibule. The ectopic ureter is classified as proximal, mid, or distal urethra (Figure 13-13). The ectopic ureteral openings in the urethra are always located dorsally or dorsolaterally as a consequence of the abnormal embryologic development.

(17) Other abnormalities that can accompany ectopic ureter include:
  (a) Hydronephrosis.
  (b) Renal hypoplasia.
  (c) Pyelonephritis.
  (d) Hydroureter.
  (e) Bladder hypoplasia (rare, associated with bilateral ectopic ureters).
  (f) Urethral sphincter mechanism incompetence.

(18) Surgical transposition of the ureter is helpful in controlling incontinence in approximately 50% of affected dogs. The owner must be warned that many affected dogs have coexisting sphincter mechanism incompetence and remain incontinent after surgical correction.

(19) Surgical excision of the intramural portion of the ectopic ureter may improve the surgical success rate to 70% to 80% (Figure 13-14).

(20) Endoscopic laser ablation of ectopic ureters has recently been reported. The laser can be used to ablate the submucosal tunnel and create a neo-ureterostomy in a more normal trigonal position.

(21) Submucosal urethral collagen injections can be used in some dogs with ectopic ureters that continue to have urinary incontinence after conventional surgery and can be considered instead of surgery for dogs with proximally located ectopic ureters.

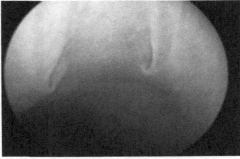

FIGURE 13-12 ■ Normal ureteral openings in the bladder observed during cystoscopy. The presence of two "C-shaped" ureteral openings facing one another in the trigone region rules out ectopic ureter.

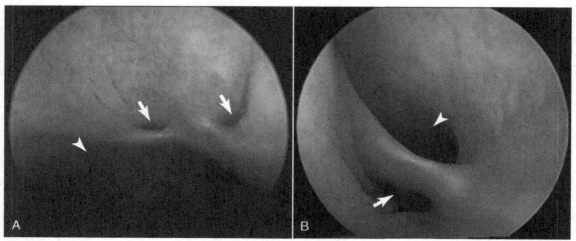

FIGURE 13-13 ■ **A,** Bilateral ectopic ureters (*arrows*) terminating in the proximal urethra. *Arrowhead* points to a dark region that represents the lumen of the bladder. **B,** Unilateral ectopic ureter opening in the middle section of the urethra (*arrowhead*). The arrow points to the urethra leading toward the bladder.

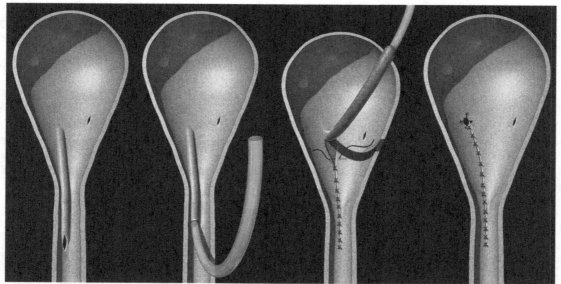

FIGURE 13-14 ■ Intraurethral ureterectomy. The distal ureteral opening first is catheterized, the ureteral wall is dissected, and the defect sutured closed. (Drawn by Tim Vojt.)

b. Vestibulovaginal stenosis has been described in association with urinary incontinence and recurrent UTI in female dogs. Historically, it has been defined on the basis of contrast radiographic measurements made during vaginography. Considerable variability in the width of this region exists in normal dogs, making establishment the diagnosis by radiography difficult. Measurements also are affected by reproductive status (i.e., intact or spayed) and can vary depending on the stage of estrus in intact female dogs. Cystoscopy rarely confirms narrowing that would be considered stenotic. We do not believe so-called vestibulovaginal stenosis plays a causative role in urinary incontinence in dogs. Procedures designed to enlarge this region are not recommended.

> **!** Vestibulovaginal stenosis does not play a causative role in urinary incontinence in dogs. Procedures to enlarge this region are not recommended.

c. Other anatomic abnormalities that have been associated with urinary incontinence in dogs and cats are rare.
   (1) Patent urachus.
   (2) Bladder exstrophy.
   (3) Urethrovaginal fistulas.
   (4) Ureterovaginal fistula (e.g., after spaying).
   (5) Female pseudohermaphroditism.
   (6) Urethral diverticulum.
   (7) Ureterocele.

Paradoxical (Obstructive) Incontinence

a. Overflow incontinence occurs when intravesical pressure exceeds urethral tone. This type of incontinence occurs in male cats with urethral obstruction and in dogs with urethral stones or outflow obstruction caused by tumors.
   (1) Incontinence has been reported after prostatectomy in male dogs with prostatic disease. It can also be encountered after castration for treatment of prostatomegaly
   (2) Idiopathic incontinence in feline leukemia virus (FeLV)-positive cats and feline immunodeficiency virus (FIV)-positive cats.
   (3) Idiopathic incontinence in FIV-positive cats.
   (4) Incontinence after perineal urethrostomy in cats is thought to be a consequence of neurological damage related to the surgical procedure.
   (5) Urge incontinence associated with UTI (a form of detrusor hyperactivity or *spastic bladder*).
   (6) Idiopathic detrusor hyperactivity (involuntary smooth muscle contractions during the filling phase).

Neurogenic Causes of Urinary Incontinence
Upper Motor Neuron (UMN or Automatic Bladder)

a. CNS lesions located cranial to sacral spinal cord segments S1-S2 can cause urinary incontinence.
b. Partial voiding may be observed because the local reflex arc is intact but the reflex only is initiated at high bladder volume.
c. A high residual volume typically is noted in the bladder.
d. It is difficult to express the bladder because the external urethral sphincter lacks UMN inhibition.

    e. Inability to initiate voluntary voiding.

    f. The underlying neurologic disease responsible for the incontinence should be identified and treated if possible.

    g. Training the owner to perform intermittent catheterization at least twice per day in males and temporary or permanent tube cystostomy are options for patients with neurologic disorders not amenable to correction.

Lower Motor Neuron (LMN or Autonomous Bladder)

    a. Due to a spinal cord lesion that interrupts the local reflex arc in sacral spinal cord segments S1-S2.

    b. Partial emptying is observed when intravesical or intra-abdominal pressure exceeds the elasticity of urethra.

    c. Residual volume usually is higher than that observed in an UMN bladder.

    d. It is easy to manually express the bladder because the external urethral sphincter provides minimal to no resistance.

    e. Inability to initiate voluntary voiding.

    f. The underlying neurologic disease responsible for the incontinence should be identified and treated if possible.

    g. Training the owner to perform intermittent catheterization at least twice per day in males or teaching them to manually express the animal's bladder are options for patients with neurologic disorders not amenable to correction.

Reflex Dyssynergy

    a. Reflex dyssynergy or detrusor urethral dyssynergia occurs when detrusor muscular contraction is not synchronized with urethral relaxation (i.e., the detrusor muscle contracts but the urethra fails to relax).

    b. The diagnosis is made by excluding mechanical obstruction (e.g., radiographic studies, passing a urethral catheter) and by observation of urination. Dogs with reflex dyssynergy initiate urination normally but then urine flow stops abruptly and is followed by dribbling.

    c. After observing the dog attempt to urinate, passage of a urinary catheter demonstrates lack of mechanical obstruction and high residual urine volume. Residual volume in dogs normally is <0.4 ml/kg and dogs with reflex dyssynergy may have residual urine volumes of 20 mL/kg or more.

    d. Middle-aged large to giant breed male dogs typically are affected.

    e. Initial treatment traditionally has been to use the nonspecific alpha blocker phenoxybenzamine followed by bethanechol in a few days if impaired bladder contractility is suspected.

       (1) Phenoxybenzamine.

          (a) 0.25 to 0.5 mg/kg PO every 12 hours or every 8 hours.

          (b) Lowers preprostatic urethral tone but has limited to no effect on postprostatic and penile urethral tone in males (i.e., primary effect is on smooth muscle of urethra).

          (c) Primary adverse effect is hypotension.

       (2) Bethanechol.

          (a) 5 to 15 mg total dose PO every 8 hours in dogs; 1.25 to 5.0 mg total dose PO every 8 hours in cats.

          (b) Parasympathomimetic drug with primarily muscarinic effects used alone for detrusor hypoactivity (*bladder atony*) or in combination with phenoxybenzamine for reflex dyssynergy.

        (c) Adverse effects.
           (i) Mild nicotinic effects may cause norepinephrine release at sympathetic postganglionic terminals and result in increased urethral tone. Phenoxybenzamine will block this effect.
           (ii) Clinical signs of parasympathetic excess: Anorexia, salivation, lacrimation, abdominal cramping, vomiting, diarrhea.
        (d) Bethanechol has become difficult to obtain due to limited use in human medicine.
    (3) Intermittent catheterization to maintain low residual volume and encourage recovery of bladder contractility is recommended during the first few days of therapy.
    (4) Specific alpha-2 blockers have little effect on canine urethral tone and specific alpha-1 blockers may be preferable to nonspecific alpha blockers. The specific alpha-1 antagonist prazosin may be used at a dosage of 0.1 mg/kg/day PO divided every 8 hours. The main adverse effect of prazosin is hypotension.
  f. If alpha blockers fail to relax the urethra, striated muscle relaxants such as diazepam and dantrolene can be considered.
    (1) Diazepam.
      (a) Used for urethral striated muscle spasm.
      (b) Dosage in dogs: 2 to 10 mg PO every 8 hours.
    (2) Dantrolene.
      (a) Direct acting skeletal muscle relaxant used for urethral striated muscle spasm.
      (b) Recommended dosage in dogs is 1 to 5 mg/kg PO every 12 hours to every 8 hours.
      (c) Dantrolene potentially is hepatotoxic and liver enzyme activity should be monitored.
  g. Chronic bladder hyporeflexia and recurrent chronic UTI are long term complications of reflex dyssynergy. Some dogs require intermittent catheterization by owners at home.
  h. The condition can be frustrating to treat and may lead to euthanasia.
  i. When medical treatments fail, consider placement of permanent tube cystostomy or placement of a urethral stent if a focal area of urethral contraction can be identified.

WHAT DO WE DO?

- Make certain abnormal urine leakage is a result of incontinence rather than pollakiuria or polyuria.
- Perform a rectal examination to be sure masses of the urethra, pelvic canal, or caudal bladder are not contributing to the problem. At the same time, evaluate for sublumbar lymphadenopathy as well as critically evaluate anal tone and the bulbocavernosus reflex to be sure lower motor neuron disorders are not the cause of urinary incontinence.
- Evaluate for urine retention and overflow by estimating the size of the bladder before and after voiding. Catheterize the bladder after voiding to determine residual urine volume in animals suspected of incomplete voiding.
- Critically evaluate the urinalysis, especially urine specific gravity to rule out dilute urine and associated overflow incontinence and also the urine sediment to identify any associated inflammation.
- Obtain bacterial culture of a urine sample collected by cystocentesis in animals without an obvious diagnosis or in those not responding to treatment.
- Perform imaging of the urinary tract (e.g., plain and contrast radiography, ultrasonography) to identify calculi, anatomical abnormalities or tumors that may be contributing factors.

- Use urethrocystoscopy as the definitive method to diagnose ectopic ureters in female dogs.
- Treat PSMI with PPA as the initial drug of choice.
- Consider treatment of PSMI with low doses of estrogens in dogs with PSMI that do not respond to PPA or consider adding estrogen in addition to PPA.
- Measure blood pressure before and during treatment with PPA.
- Consider submucosal urethral collagen injections to increase urethral tone in dogs with PSMI that have not responded to PPA and estrogens.
- Consider submucosal urethral collagen injections as a treatment for proximal ectopic ureters (i.e., those terminating in the proximal one third of the urethra) as an alternative to conventional surgery.
- Use intraurethral ureteral remnant excision and reconstruction of the urethra and trigone as the procedure of choice to treat ectopic ureters (rather than conventional ureteral transposition).

THOUGHTS FOR THE FUTURE

- New and better materials will become available to replace collagen for submucosal urethral injections. Beneficial treatment effects will last longer.
- The role of high concentrations of FSH and LH in spayed female dogs with PSMI will be clarified and more effective GnRH analogues will be discovered and become available.
- Drugs without serious adverse effects will become available to control detrusor hyperactivity (over-active bladder).
- Urodynamics (UPP and CMG) will become more widely available as diagnostic tools to evaluate dogs with urinary incontinence.
- Hydraulic occluder devices implanted around the urethra will become widely available to increase urethral tone.

COMMON MISCONCEPTIONS

- Urinary incontinence from ectopic ureters is seen only in young dogs. Though this is generally true, we sometimes encounter those with proximal ectopic ureters that develop clinical signs as urethral closure pressure declines with aging.
- Urinary incontinence from ectopic ureters occurs constantly rather than intermittently. This is generally true, but some dogs with confirmed ectopic ureters (especially those with proximal urethral terminations) incontinence is intermittent, possibly due to varying urethral tone from sympathetic nervous system input.
- Ectopic ureter is usually a unilateral condition. Older literature states this to be the case but when cystoscopic imaging is used, nearly all of the cases have bilaterial ectopia.
- A positive urine culture is not expected in dogs with ectopic ureter(s). True in most cases. Some have a positive urine culture due to wicking of bacteria if the incontinence is severe..
- A positive urine culture almost never occurs in dogs with PSMI. True for most, but as discussed previously, wicking of bacteria from severe incontinence and perineal wetting can occur. Also in PSMI, mid-urethral pressure is decreased. High mid-urethral tone retards the ascent of bacteria in normal dogs.
- It is OK to treat for presumed PSMI in dogs without results of a urinalysis. No, since UTI and sub-maximally concentrated urine will be missed as factors contributing to the incontinence.
- PPA is safe for use in all dogs. Though reputed to be safe in young experimental dogs, it is not always safe in clinical dogs. Some dogs become aggressive, lose their sleep patterns, or otherwise act anxious. Some dogs develop systemic hypertension after PPA. PPA is not safe for use for dogs with pre-existing CKD, heart disease, or systemic hypertension.

- Low dose estrogen administration is dangerous as treatment for PSMI in dogs. Estrogens at low doses are usually quite safe – we have never encountered a case with bone marrow suppression related to low dose estrogen therapy when given for maintenance once or twice weekly.
- Imaging of the urinary tract is useless in those suspected with PSMI. Though many with PSMI will have normal abdominal radiographic findings, some will have the presence of a pelvic-bladder disclosed and others may reveal non-palpable urinary stones. Pelvic bladder can magnify the problems associated with PSMI and incontinence.
- Negative results for IVP for the presence of ectopic ureter(s) is enough to dismiss this diagnosis as the cause for the urinary dribbling. Not necessarily. It is difficult to know for certain that an ectopic ureter is present or not with this method of imaging. When an IVP is combined with fluoroscopy or with CT, it becomes far less likely to mess the presence of an ectopic ureter.
- A negative ultrasound exam is great evidence that an ectopic ureter is not present. Not true. Ultrasound can be suggestive for ectopic ureter when the presence of hydroureter is found but not when the ureter is normal in size.
- One does not need to perform a rectal exam routinely in dogs with urinary incontinence. Definitely not true. Sometimes this is the only way to know that there is urethral disease (tumor, proliferative urethritis) that may be contributing to urinary incontinence.

SUMMARY TIPS

- Obtain oblique views and perform negative contrast cystography at the time of excretory urography to increase the likelihood of identifying an ectopic ureter.
- When urine specific gravity is <1.025, consider polyuria and overflow as factors potentially contributing to urinary incontinence.
- Remember that computed tomography can be used in combination with excretory urography to confirm ectopic ureters in male dogs.

FREQUENTLY ASKED QUESTIONS

Q: I have a 1-year-old spayed female Doberman pinscher that has had urinary incontinence for at least 6 months. There is no history of dysuria or hematuria and the dog appears normal in all other ways. Urinalysis shows a specific gravity of 1.044, negative dipstrip reactions and inactive urine sediment. The dog was spayed at 6 months of age. Which is more likely, ectopic ureter or PSMI?

A: A female Doberman pinscher with incontinence is presumed to have PSMI until proven otherwise. In the United States, Dobermans have the highest frequency of PSMI, and some develop incontinence before they are spayed. Ectopic ureters are very rare in Doberman pinschers.

Q: I have a 6-year-old golden retriever that recently developed urinary incontinence when lying down and during sleep. Physical examination is normal and urinalysis is unremarkable. Baseline blood pressure is normal. I think she has PSMI. Should if treat her with PPA without further diagnostic evaluation?

A: That approach seems reasonable. Golden retrievers, however, are a breed commonly affected by ectopic ureter, and she could have both PSMI and ectopic ureter. If an ectopic ureter is present, it likely has a proximal urethral termination. After spaying and development of PSMI, urethral closure pressure may decrease to a level that allows urine to leak out rather than refluxing back into the bladder, as would occur when urethral pressure is higher. Thus, the decreased urethral pressure associated with PSMI has allowed the ectopic ureter to manifest itself. If the dog's response to PPA is inadequate, cystoscopy should be performed to determine if ectopic ureters are a complicating factor. If a proximal ectopic ureter is present, submucosal urethral collagen injections could be performed.

Q: When are submucosal collagen injections indicated in the treatment of PSMI?

A: Submucosal urethral collagen injections usually are used in dogs that have not responded adequately to PPA or estrogen treatment. Collagen injections also may be used in dogs that cannot tolerate PPA (i.e., those with systemic hypertension or cardiac disease and those that develop undesirable behavior changes on PPA).

Q: Submucosal urethral collagen injections for PSMI are expensive. My client wants to know how successful this procedure is likely to be.

A: Nearly all dogs experience an improvement in urinary continence after collagen injections. Not all dogs however will be completely continent after the procedure. Many dogs can achieve full continence when PPA treatment is added to the treatment regimen in addition to the collagen injections. Urinary continence was maintained for an average of 17 months in one study. In some dogs, the treatment effect lasts years, in others it only lasts months, and in some it doesn't work at all.

Q: I have a large breed dog with an UMN bladder related to intervertebral disk disease. The dog does not urinate on its own, and I put the dog on diazepam to make it easier to express the bladder. Despite the diazepam, the bladder remains difficult to express. What else can I do?

A: Diazepam relaxes skeletal muscle in the urethra. Urethral tone is maintained to a large extent by the input of the sympathetic nervous system to smooth muscle in the urethra. Thus, adding drugs such as acepromazine or prazosin can decrease urethral tone by virtue of their alpha-adrenergic receptor blocking effects.

Q: I have heard about gonadotropin-releasing hormone analogues such as leuprolide to treat urinary incontinence in dogs. How do these agents work?

A: GnRH analogues initially were thought to work by increasing urethral resistance but recent studies have shown that this original hypothesis may not be true. GnRH analogues had no effect on MUCP or other urethral pressure profile parameters regardless of clinical response. GnRH analogues may have a direct effect on the bladder to cause detrusor muscle relaxation. GnRH analogues may be useful in dogs with PSMI that do not respond to PPA or when PPA is contraindicated (e.g., high blood pressure, underlying cardiac disease).

Q: I have just examined a 3-year-old intact male Gordon setter with a history of occasionally being unable to urinate when the owner comes home from work. The dog is kenneled in the owner's absence and never urinates in its kennel. When taken out of the kennel, the dog sometimes dribbles urine and is only able to generate small spurts of urine when taken outside to urinate. The owners note that the dog is very uncomfortable when the posturing to urinate and abdomen is very tense. The growls when its abdomen is touched. Physical examination is normal. What should be done?

A: The history is classic for reflex dyssynergy. Reflex dyssynergy typically occurs in large breed male dogs. Urinalysis and urine culture should be performed to rule out UTI. Sometimes urine flow can be re-established by manual expression of the abdomen by the veterinarian or owner. If not, urinary catheterization should be performed to empty the bladder. The owner can be taught how to perform intermittent clean catheterization to empty the bladder and keep it relatively small until reflex dyssynergy resolves. Unfortunately, sometimes reflex dyssynergy is a permanent disorder. Treatment with drugs that reduce urethral tone such as acepromazine or prazosin can be helpful in allowing spontaneous voiding to occur. Longstanding dyssynergy may result in bladder atony, which makes long term management very difficult. Inadequate opportunity to urinate over an extended period of time may be a risk factor for development of intermittent reflex dyssynergy. Providing increased opportunities to void may decrease the occurrence of dyssynergy in these cases. Decreased water intake during periods of limited opportunity to urinate (such as during kenneling) also may be a useful maneuver. We have noticed increased risk for dyssynergy in male dogs that are kenneled for extended periods of time and in nervous dogs.

SUGGESTED READINGS

Angioletti A, De Francesco I, Vergottini M, Battocchio ML: Urinary incontinence after spaying in the bitch: incidence and oestrogen-therapy, *Vet Res Commun* 28(Suppl 1):153–155, 2004.

Arnold S, Hubler M, Lott-Stolz G, Rusch P: Treatment of urinary incontinence in bitches by endoscopic injection of glutaraldehyde cross-linked collagen, *J Small Anim Pract* 37:163–168, 1996.

Aaron A, Eggleton K, Power C, Holt PE: Urethral sphincter mechanism incompetence in male dogs: a retrospective analysis of 54 cases, *Vet Rec* 139:542–546, 1996.

Bacon NJ, Oni O, White RAS: Treatment of urethral sphincter mechanism incompetence in 11 bitches with a sustained-release formulation of phenylpropanolamine, *Vet Rec* 151:373–376, 2002.

Barth A, Reichler IM, Hubler M, et al: Evaluation of long-term effects of endoscopic injection of collage into the urethral submucosa for treatment of urethral sphincter incompetence in female dogs: 40 cases (1993-2000), *J Am Vet Med Assoc* 226:73–76, 2005.

Berent AC, Mayhew PD, Porat-Mosenco Y: Use of cystoscopic-guided laser ablation for treatment of intramural ureteral ectopia in male dogs: four cases (2006-2007), *J Am Vet Med Assoc* 232:1026–1034, 2008.

Cannizzo KL, McLoughlin MA, Mattoon JS, et al: Evaluation of transurethral cystoscopy and excretory urography for diagnosis of ectopic ureters in female dogs: 25 cases (1992-2000), *J Am Vet Med Assoc* 223:475–481, 2003.

Diaz Espineira MM, Viehoff FW, Nickel RF: Idiopathic detrusor-urethral dyssynergia in dogs: a retrospective analysis of 22 cases, *J Small Anim Pract* 39:264–270, 1998.

Gookin JL, Stone EA, Sharp NJ: Urinary incontinence in dogs and cats. Part 1. Urethral pressure profilometry, *Compend Contin Educ Vet* 18:407–418, 1996.

Hamaide AJ, Grand JG, Farnir F, et al: Urodynamic and morphologic changes in the lower portion of the urogenital tract after administration of estriol alone or in combination with phenylpropanolamine in sexually intact and spayed female dogs, *Am J Vet Res* 67:901–908, 2006.

Holt PE: Long-term evaluation of colposuspension in the treatment of urinary incontinence due to incompetence of the urethral sphincter mechanism in the bitch, *Vet Rec* 127:537–542, 1990.

Lamb CR, Gregory SP: Ultrasonographic findings in 14 dogs with ectopic ureter, *Vet Radiol Ultrasound* 39:218–223, 1998.

Lappin MR, Barsanti JA: Urinary incontinence secondary to idiopathic detrusor instability: cystometrographic diagnosis and pharmacologic management in two dogs and a cat, *J Am Vet Med Assoc* 191:1439–1442, 1987.

Mandigers RJ, Nell T: Treatment of bitches with acquired urinary incontinence with oestriol, *Vet Rec* 149:764–767, 2001.

Nickel RF, van den Brom W: Simultaneous diuresis cysto-urethrometry and multi-channel urethral pressure profilometry in female dogs with refractory urinary incontinence, *Am J Vet Res* 58:691–696, 1997.

Rawlings C, Barsanti JA, Mahaffey MB, et al: Evaluation of colposuspension for treatment of incontinence in spayed female dogs, *J Am Vet Med Assoc* 219:770–775, 2001.

Reichler IM, Jöchle W, Piché CA, et al: Effect of a long-acting GnRH analogue or placebo on plasma LH/FSH, urethral pressure profiles and clinical signs of urinary incontinence due to sphincter mechanism incompetence in bitches, *Theriogenology* 66:1227–1236, 2006.

Reichler IM, Hubler M, Jöchle W, et al: The effect of GnRH analogues on urinary incontinence after ablation of the ovaries in dogs, *Theriogenology* 60:1207–1216, 2003.

Richter KP, Ling GV: Clinical response and urethral pressure profile changes after phenylpropanolamine in dogs with primary sphincter incompetence, *J Am Vet Med Assoc* 187:605–611, 1985.

Scott L, Leddy M, Bernay F, Davot JL: Evaluation of phenylpropanolamine in the treatment of urethral sphincter mechanism incompetence in the bitch, *J Small Anim Pract* 43:493–496, 2002.

Stocklin-Gautschi NM, Hassig M, Reichler IM, et al: The relationship of urinary incontinence to early spaying in bitches, *J Reprod Fertil* (Suppl 57):233–236, 2001.

Weber UT, Arnold S, Hubler M, Kupper JR: Surgical treatment of male dogs with urinary incontinence due to urethral sphincter mechanism incompetence, *Veterinary Surgery* 26:51–56, 1997.

14 Tumors of the Urinary System

Renal Neoplasia

I. Primary renal tumors are uncommon, comprising approximately 1% of all neoplasms in dogs and 1% to 1.5% of all neoplasms in cats.
   A. Occur with equal frequency in the left or right kidney.
   B. Approximately 4% are bilateral.
II. Most are of epithelial origin (approximately 85%), metastasize, and are associated with a poor prognosis.
III. Problems at presentation:
   A. Renal hematuria (painless).
   B. Renal failure if bilateral involvement (e.g., as with lymphosarcoma [LSA]).
   C. Mass effect: Based on abdominal palpation or finding on imaging with ultrasound or radiographs (Figure 14-1).
   D. Paraneoplastic syndromes: Polycythemia, extreme leukocytosis, cachexia, hypoglycemia, hypertrophic osteopathy.
   E. Metastases: Bone, lung, lymph nodes.
IV. Definitive diagnosis requires biopsy in most instances.
   A. LSA frequently can be diagnosed by fine-needle aspiration cytology.
   B. Aspiration cytology can be highly suggestive for renal adenocarcinoma.

Renal Adenoma

I. Approximately 15% of primary renal epithelial tumors.
II. Usually an incidental finding on necropsy.
III. Typically solitary nodules <2 cm in diameter.
IV. Arise from the epithelium of the proximal convoluted tubule.

Renal Carcinoma

I. Most common primary renal tumor of dogs; occur sporadically in cats.
II. Usually occurs in older dogs (average age, 8 years), but can occur in dogs younger than 2 years of age. Affected cats typically are older than 9 years of age.
III. Male dogs are more commonly affected than female dogs; in cats there is no sex or breed predilections.

❗ Renal carcinoma is the most common primary renal tumor of dogs.

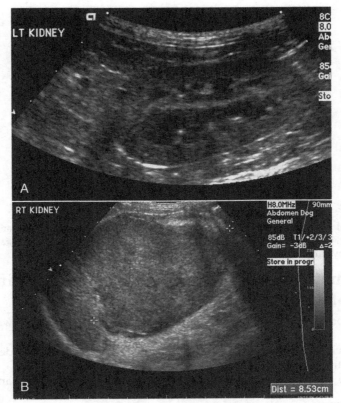

FIGURE 14-1 ■ Renal ultrasonography of normal and neoplastic kidney. Note normal left kidney in **A** (length of 5.2 cm) compared with the very enlarged (length 8.5 cm) and misshapen right kidney, **B.** The right kidney is also quite hyperechoic. The right kidney was enlarged due to a benign tumor (myxoma). (Courtesy of Dr. Lisa Zekas and the Radiology Section of The Ohio State University College of Veterinary Medicine, Columbus, Ohio.)

CLINICAL SIGNS

A. Include hematuria, palpable abdominal mass, and weight loss.
B. Polycythemia may be seen due to increased erythropoietin production.
C. Hypertrophic osteopathy may be present with or without pulmonary metastases.
D. Other paraneoplastic syndromes include disseminated intravascular coagulation, neutrophilic leukocytosis, and bone infarcts.
E. Metastases often are present by the time of presentation.

GROSS OR ULTRASONOGRAPHIC APPEARANCE

A. Spherical or ovoid mass, usually on one pole of the kidney.
B. Typically well demarcated; the remaining renal tissue is atrophic and compressed (Figure 14-2).
C. Usually gray or light yellow in color, with areas of necrosis and hemorrhage.
D. Can invade the renal pelvis, ureter, renal vein, and hilar lymphatics.

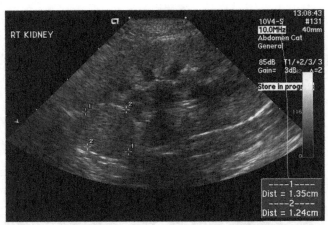

FIGURE 14-2 ■ Renal adenocarcinoma in an older cat. Note well-demarcated nodular region on the cranial pole of the right kidney of this ultrasound image (1.35 × 1.24 cm). The diagnosis was established by fine-needle aspiration (FNA) and by surgical removal that followed.

Nodular Dermatofibrosis With Renal Cystadenocarcinoma in German Shepherd Dogs

   I. Autosomal dominant syndrome; 6 % of German shepherd dogs in Norway are affected with renal tumors.

  II. Cystadenocarcinoma is usually bilateral and can metastasize to lymph nodes, peritoneum, liver, spleen, lung, and bone.

 III. All breeds are potentially at risk but most commonly reported in German shepherds. No sex predisposition.

 IV. Lesions of the skin and subcutis are the main reason for presentation. Some dogs are lame as a consequence of lesions on the paws that frequently are overlooked. Ulceration and inflammation can be associated with the skin lesions.

  V. Fibrosis may occur both in skin and kidney. Tubular obstruction and cyst formation occur in the kidneys. The lesion may progress from cyst to cystic adenomatous hyperplasia to cystadenoma and ultimately to cystadenocarcinoma.

 VI. Affected kidneys may be enlarged and abnormally shaped on abdominal radiographs. Cysts of varying size are identified on renal ultrasonography, which also confirms changes in renal size and shape.

 VII. Computed tomography identifies multiple cysts and tumor masses of varying size bilaterally. The earliest lesions have been detected between 4 and 5 years of age, with the smallest cysts being 2 to 3 mm in diameter. Small amounts of tumor tissue often can be identified inside the cyst wall or renal parenchyma.

VIII. In one study, mean age at first detection of nodular dermatofibrosis was 6.4 years, renal cystadenocarcinoma with nodular dermatofibrosis was 8.2 years, and death occurred at 9.3 years.

 IX. Most intact females also have multiple uterine leiomyomas at the time of diagnosis.

  X. Euthanasia usually results, as a consequence of extensive renal lesions and metastases.

Nephroblastoma (Wilms Tumor, Embryonal Nephroma)

  I. Occurs sporadically in dogs and cats.

 II. More common in adult dogs than in young dogs (Figure 14-3).

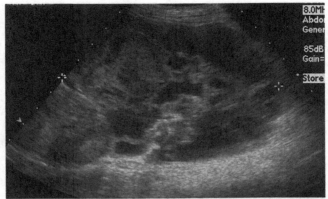

FIGURE 14-3 ■ Nephroblastoma. Ultrasonographic image from an 8-year-old dog with renal enlargement. Note irregular renal enlargement with both hyperechoic and hypoechoic regions within the kidney. Only the left kidney was involved.

III. Originate from nephrogenic blastema and may contain epithelial and mesenchymal components.
IV. Extremely large in size, causing abdominal enlargement. There may be multiple tumors in one kidney; occasionally they are bilateral.
V. Widespread metastasis to lung and liver is common in affected dogs.
VI. Prognosis is good if tubular or glomerular differentiation is observed; prognosis is poor if categorized as a sarcoma.

Other Tumors

I. Transitional cell papilloma and carcinoma of the renal pelvis are very rare.
II. Squamous cell carcinoma of the renal pelvis is uncommon, but has been associated with renal pelvic calculi.
III. Primary mesenchymal tumors have a poor prognosis.
   A. Hemangioma is most common; hematuria is the most consistent clinical sign.
   B. Hemangiosarcoma has been reported in the cat.
   C. Angiomyolipoma has been reported in the cat.
   D. Interstitial cell tumors occur in old dogs in the renal cortex and medulla.
   E. Benign cortical fibroma.
   F. Congenital mesoblastic nephroma.
   G. Renal oncocytomas originate from the collecting ducts.
IV. Metastatic tumors are common.
   A. Primary pulmonary adenocarcinomas are difficult to distinguish from primary renal adenocarcinoma with pulmonary metastases.
   B. LSA is common, and is the most common renal neoplasm in cats.
      1. Nodules are poorly defined and fatty in appearance at surgery or necropsy.
      2. If there is diffuse involvement, the kidney may appear fatty and enlarged.
      3. Hypoechoic nodules frequently are observed in cats with renal LSA during ultrasonography.
      4. A recent study showed that hypoechoic subcapsular thickening of the kidney is associated with renal LSA in the cat (Figure 14-4).
      5. Can occur in feline leukemia virus (FeLV)-negative or feline immunodeficiency virus (FIV)-negative cats, but retrovirus status still should be checked because these viral infections can be associated with LSA.

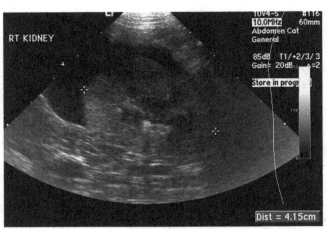

FIGURE 14-4 ■ Subcapsular lymphosarcoma (LSA) in a cat. Note the hypoechoic region outside the kidney parenchyma. This could be confused with a perinephric pseudocyst, but a fine-needle aspiration (FNA) of this region yielded a large population of malignant lymphocytes.

6. Renal LSA usually is bilateral in cats. It can be associated with renal failure if infiltration of the kidneys is extensive.
7. We have observed long-term remissions of renal LSA in some cats treated with chemotherapy. In some instances, dramatic improvement in renal function has accompanied chemotherapy.

Treatment

I. If renal neoplasia is unilateral with no metastases, nephrectomy is the treatment of choice. Efforts should be made before surgery to ensure adequate function of the contralateral kidney in patients with marginal renal function before surgery. Renal scintigraphy with determination of individual kidney glomerular filtration rate (GFR) is ideal to make this assessment.
II. Renal LSA is treated by chemotherapy.
III. Prognosis is not well defined. Survival time is usually short, but some have survived up to 4 years. Nephroblastoma is less metastatic, and nephrectomy can be curative. Benign tumors may also be cured with surgery.

Bladder Neoplasia

I. Bladder neoplasia accounts for approximately 2% of all reported malignancies in dogs.

! Bladder neoplasia accounts for approximately 2% of all malignancies in dogs.

II. Primary malignant bladder tumors.
   A. Epithelial.
      1. Transitional cell carcinoma (TCC) is the most common tumor of the bladder in dogs.
      2. Squamous cell carcinoma (SCC).
      3. Adenocarcinoma (ACA).
      4. Undifferentiated carcinoma.

! Transitional cell carcinoma (TCC) is the most common bladder tumor of dogs and cats.

        B. Mesenchymal.
            1. Fibrosarcoma.
            2. Leiomyosarcoma.
            3. Rhabdomyosarcoma.
  III. Primary benign tumors.
        A. Fibroma.
        B. Leiomyoma.
        C. Papilloma.
  IV. Secondary metastatic tumors of the bladder.
        A. Hemangiosarcoma.
        B. Lymphoma.
        C. Adenocarcinoma.
  V. Canine bladder neoplasia.
        A. TCC is most common.
        B. Papilloma.
        C. Benign mesenchymal.
        D. Unclassified carcinoma.
        E. SCC.
        F. ACA.
        G. Rhabdomyosarcoma.
            1. Young dogs.
            2. Often large breed.
            3. Sometimes associated with hypertrophic osteopathy (HO).
            4. Usually located at trigone and not usually surgically resectable.
            5. Often *botryoid* (grape-like cluster) in appearance (Figure 14-5).
            6. Special immunohistochemical staining may be needed to confirm the skeletal muscle origin of the tumor. Desmin, sarcomeric actin, and vimentin are likely to be positive, whereas cytokeratin and smooth muscle actin should be negative on immunohistochemistry. Cross-striations of skeletal muscle are sometimes seen on routine hematoxylin and eosin–stained specimens.

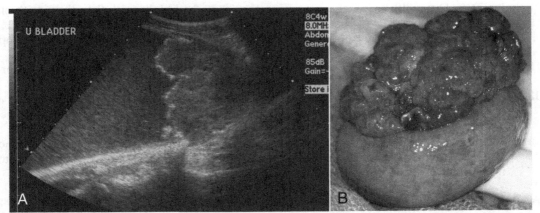

FIGURE 14-5 ■ Botryoid rhabdomyosarcoma. Note the ultrasonographic appearance of this tumor in a young Great Dane with significant obstruction to urinary outflow in **A**. Note the classic grape-like clusters of malignant tissue in the everted bladder following cystotomy in a young Bassett hound, **B**.

VI. Feline bladder neoplasia.
  A. TCC is most common, but much less common than in dogs.
  B. SCC.
  C. Benign mesenchymal.
  D. ACA.
  E. Lymphoma.
  F. Leiomyosarcoma.
  G. Hemangiosarcoma.
  H. Rhabdomyosarcoma.

Etiology and Risks

  I. Etiology is multifactorial. Risk factors are related to chemical carcinogen exposure. The bladder is the storage site for eliminated waste products, and chronic exposure of bladder tissue to carcinogenic compounds appears to play a role.
  II. Obesity. Fat tissue acts as a storage site for lipophilic chemicals and pesticides allowing for prolonged exposure in the body.
  III. Previous treatment with the chemotherapeutic agent, cyclophosphamide. Cyclophosphamide frequently causes sterile hemorrhagic cystitis. Chronic irritation of the bladder by this drug may play a role in development of neoplasia.
  IV. Bladder tumors are more common in industrialized parts of the world.
   A. A direct correlation was found between level of industrialization and manufacturing in the United States and parts of Canada and the occurrence of bladder cancer in dogs.
   B. Bladder neoplasms have been induced experimentally by administration of industrial chemicals containing aromatic amines (e.g., tryptophan, benzene, beta-naphthylamine) to dogs.
  V. Chemical Exposure.
   A. Topical flea and tick dips, shampoos, powders, sprays and collars, and the dose applied were directly correlated with disease in one study.
   B. The use of spot-on flea and tick control products containing fipronil and imidacloprid did not cause increased risk of TCC in Scottish terriers.
   C. Scottish terriers exposed to phenoxy herbicide lawn treatments had increased risk of developing TCC. Dogs with seasonal or year-round exposure had higher risk than those with only sporadic exposure.
   D. Dogs living near areas that are frequently sprayed with insecticides to control mosquito populations are more likely to develop TCC.
  VI. The incidence of bladder neoplasia is unrelated to second-hand cigarette smoke exposure or to chronic drinking of chlorinated water (known risk factors in humans).
  VII. Neutered female dogs are at higher risk for TCC than males, whereas neutered male cats are at increased risk as compared with females. Potential reasons for this association have been proposed.
   A. Females void less frequently than male dogs. Marking behavior in male dogs leads to more frequent urination. Prolonged urinary retention in female dogs increases contact time for toxins with the bladder epithelium.

❗ Female dogs and male cats are at a higher risk for development of bladder neoplasia.

   B. Females have a higher percentage of body fat than males.

VIII. Bladder neoplasia is more common in dogs than cats.
   A. Tryptophan metabolism differs between cats and dogs. Dogs metabolize this amino acid by forming ortho-amino-phenol, which is similar in structure to chemicals known to induce bladder tumors in dogs.
   B. Cats do not form the same metabolite from tryptophan and thus have less ortho-amino-phenol in their urine.
 IX. Vegetable Consumption.
   A. A study of TCC in Scottish terriers found a significant correlation between vegetable ingestion and risk of TCC.
      1. Consumption of any type of vegetable at least three times per week decreased the risk of developing TCC by 70%.
      2. Green, leafy vegetables and yellow-orange vegetables consumed at least three times weekly decreased risk of TCC by 70% to 90%.
      3. Consumption of cruciferous vegetables did not decrease the risk of TCC.
      4. A dose response relationship was identified: The higher the frequency of vegetable consumption, the greater the reduction in risk of TCC.
   B. Green, leafy vegetables and yellow-orange vegetables have antitumor activity.
      1. Plants contain phytochemicals or other bioactive compound that detoxify carcinogenic chemicals and remove oxidizing agents.
      2. These vegetables contain carotenoid and retinol that are hypothesized to control cell proliferation and differentiation and stabilize cell membranes, making them less susceptible to carcinogens.

Canine Transitional Cell Carcinoma (TCC)

 I. TCC is a primary malignant neoplasm arising from the transitional cells of the bladder and is the most common bladder tumor in dogs and cats.
   A. Epithelial neoplasms account for 90% of canine bladder cancer.
   B. Of the epithelial tumors, 75% to 90% are TCC.
   C. The prevalence of TCC in dogs increased more than 600% between 1975 and 1995.

SIGNALMENT

   A. Older dogs (average age, 11 years at the time of diagnosis).
   B. Females more commonly affected than males with a female to male ratio of 1.7:1.
   C. Breed predispositions have been identified (Table 14-1). The reason for these associations is unknown, but genetic predisposition is suspected. Differences in metabolic activation and detoxification pathways could account for increased risk in selected breeds.
      1. Scottish terriers have the highest prevalence of TCC and are 18 times more likely to develop TCC than mixed breed dogs.

! Scottish terriers have the highest prevalence of transitional cell carcinoma.

      2. West Highland white terrier.
      3. Airedale terrier.
      4. Beagle.
      5. Dachshund.
      6. Shetland sheepdog.

■ TABLE 14-1
■ ■ **Breed Risk for Diagnosis of Transitional Cell Carcinoma in Dogs**

Breed	Odds Ratio	95% Confidence Interval
Mixed breed	1.0	—
All purebreds	0.74	0.62-0.88
Scottish terrier	18.09	7.30-44.86
Shetland sheepdog	4.46	2.48-8.03
Beagle	4.15	2.14-8.05
Wirehaired fox terrier	3.20	1.19-8.63
West Highland white terrier	3.02	1.43-6.40
Miniature Schnauzer	0.92	0.54-1.57
Miniature poodle	0.86	0.55-1.35
Doberman pinscher	0.51	0.30-0.87
Labrador retriever	0.46	0.30-0.69
Golden retriever	0.46	0.30-0.69
German shepherd	0.40	0.26-0.63

Modified from Knapp DW, Glickman WN, DeNicola DB, et al: Naturally-occurring canine transitional cell carcinoma of the urinary bladder: A relevant model of human invasive bladder cancer. *Urol Oncol* 5:47-59, 2000. Data in this table provides a summary from 1290 dogs with transitional cell carcinoma (TCC) and 1290 institution and age-matched control dogs without TCC in the Veterinary Medical Data Base.

    7. Collie.
    8. German shepherd dogs are underrepresented.

CLINICAL SIGNS

  A. Lower urinary tract signs are most common.
    1. Dysuria (84%).
    2. Hematuria (50%).
    3. Pollakiuria (37%).
    4. Stranguria.
    5. Urinary incontinence.
  B. Polyuria and polydipsia may be associated with partial obstruction.
  C. Oliguria or anuria, vomiting, and anorexia may be associated with azotemia if acute or chronic obstruction is present.
  D. Lameness may be caused by bone metastasis or HO secondary to metastatic lung lesions.
    1. Bone metastases often are lytic on radiographs.
    2. Metastases from prostate neoplasia, mammary tumors, and bladder TCC are most commonly associated with lytic bone lesions.
  E. Respiratory difficulty caused by pulmonary metastasis.
  F. Lethargy.
  G. Weight loss.

HISTORY

  A. The history of treatment with antibiotics for chronic recurrent lower urinary tract infections (UTIs) is often reported by owners. Minimal long-term clinical improvement is observed in response to this therapy.

> ❗ Many dogs with transitional cell carcinoma have been treated for repeated urinary tract infections prior to diagnosis.

PHYSICAL EXAMINATION

A. Rectal examination may reveal a thickened urethra and enlarged sublumbar lymph nodes if the tumor has spread to the urethra and metastasis has already occurred.
B. A mass in the caudal abdomen may be palpated in smaller dogs and cats.
C. Spinal hyperpathia caused by metastasis to lumbar vertebral bodies.
D. Physical examination can be normal in up to 30% of dogs with bladder tumors.

DIFFERENTIAL DIAGNOSES

Benign Tumors
1. Fibroma.
2. Papilloma.
3. Leiomyoma.

Non-Neoplastic Lower Urinary Tract Disease
1. Chronic cystitis.
2. Polypoid cystitis.
3. Eosinophilic granuloma.
4. Proliferative (granulomatous) urethritis.
5. Prostatitis.
6. Benign prostatic hyperplasia.

DIAGNOSTIC TESTS

Laboratory Evaluation
1. A complete blood count (CBC) and biochemical profile should be performed to rule out other systemic diseases. The most common abnormalities recognized are azotemia and anemia of chronic disease.
2. Do not obtain urine samples by cystocentesis. TCC tumors are exfoliative and tumor cells can be seeded anywhere along the needle tract, including the skin (Figure 14-6).

> ❗ If urinary bladder neoplasia is suspected, do *not* obtain urine samples by cystocentesis because of the risk of tumor seeding.

3. Urinalysis.
   a. Proteinuria.
   b. Pyuria.
   c. Hematuria.
   d. Bacteriuria.
   e. Neoplastic transitional cells are identified in 30% of cases.
      (1) Rafts of epithelial cells.
      (2) Neoplastic cells are difficult to distinguish from reactive epithelial cells that result from chronic inflammation.
      (3) Results may be highly suggestive for TCC (e.g., anisocytosis, anisokaryosis, binucleate cells, mitotic figures, clumps or rafts of epithelial cells) (Figure 14-7).

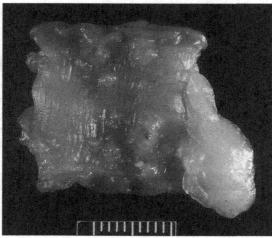

FIGURE 14-6 ■ Needle tract seeding of transitional cell carcinoma (TCC) from a cat that underwent multiple episodes of cystocentesis. Note multiple nodules of carcinoma along the peritoneum at necropsy.

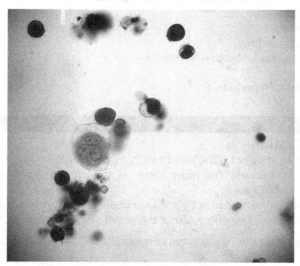

FIGURE 14-7 ■ Wet mount microscopy of urine sediment from a dog with transitional cell carcinoma (TCC). Note cellular atypia. Multinucleated epithelial cell is in the center of the field. The other large cells are also epithelial cells (Sedi-Stain, ×600).

(4) Clumps of epithelial cells may be clinically suggestive of TCC if they occur alone or with red blood cells especially in the absence of white blood cells or bacteria (Figure 14-8).

❗ Clumps of epithelial cells (rafts) in the urine sediment should raise suspicion for TCC.

4. Urine cultures should always be performed when bladder neoplasia is suspected. Secondary lower UTIs are extremely common in these patients due to disruption of normal host defenses.

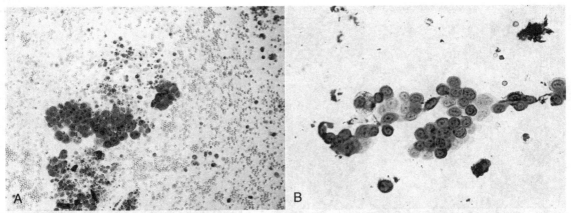

FIGURE 14-8 ■ Rafts of epithelial cells from a dog with transitional cell carcinoma (TCC)–wetmount urinary sediment microscopy. In panel **A,** only red blood cells and clumps of large epithelial cells are seen. This is very suggestive for TCC in the absence of pyuria. Panel **B** shows more detail of cellular atypia in clumps of epithelial cells (Sedi-Stain, ×400).

Radiographic and Ultrasonographic Findings

1. Thoracic radiographs should be obtained to evaluate pulmonary parenchyma for evidence of metastatic nodules. Metastases are identified in 10% to 30% of affected dogs at the time of diagnosis.

> **!** Thoracic radiograph should be obtained in all cases of TCC. Metastases (lung, bone, lymphnode) are found in 10% to 30% of affected dogs at the time of diagnosis.

2. Abdominal radiographs.
   a. Typically do not allow visualization of bladder tumors.
   b. May allow identification of sublumbar lymphadenopathy and metastatic lesions in lumbar vertebrae.
3. Abdominal ultrasound is the most commonly employed imaging tool (Figure 14-9).
   a. Determines the location of the tumor within the bladder.
   b. The urethra cannot be imaged adequately with this modality.
   c. Allows for evaluation of the kidneys and ureters, to identify enlargement or hydronephrosis caused by tumor obstruction of the ureteral openings.
   d. Imaging of the liver, spleen, and abdominal lymph nodes allows identification of metastatic lesions.
4. Contrast cystography.
   a. Allows visualization and localization of the lesion within the bladder and identification of any urethral involvement.
   b. A thickened bladder wall is a common finding.
   c. May show small lesions not seen on ultrasonography.
5. Excretory urography aids in identifying hydroureter arising as a consequence of ureteral obstruction by the tumor.

Cytology

1. Cytology can confirm the diagnosis of TCC but alone is not ideal because chronic inflammation can create dysplastic changes in epithelial cells that often are confused with evidence of neoplasia (Figure 14-10).

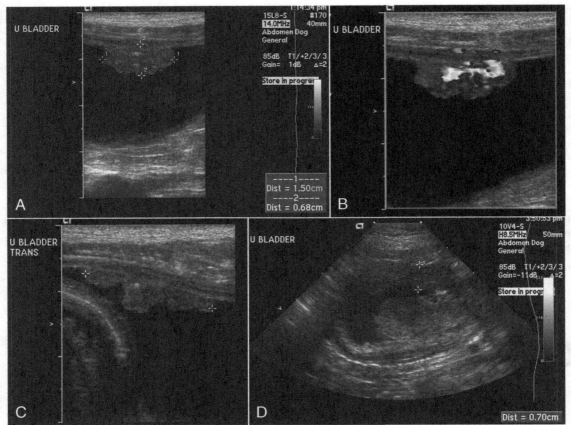

FIGURE 14-9 ■ Ultrasonographic appearance of transitional cell carcinoma (TCC) in the bladder of dogs. Panel **A** shows a 1.5 × 0.7 cm mass along the ventral wall of the bladder from a female dog. Another mass emanating from the trigone is not so clearly seen. Panel **B** shows blood flow through this mass using Doppler. Panel **C** shows multiple fronds of TCC with the linear ultrasound probe from the same dog. Panel **D** shows extensive tumor mass of TCC at the trigone and along the ventrum of the bladder wall, this is from a male dog, and this tumor extended into the prostate.

    a. Biopsy by so-called *traumatic catheterization* approaches 80% accuracy compared with surgical biopsy.

    b. Fine-needle aspiration through the abdominal wall. This technique yields a small sample and aspiration may lead to the seeding of tumor cells anywhere along the needle tract, including the skin.

Diagnosis

  1. Definitive diagnosis requires histologic examination of biopsy specimens. Samples can be obtained by the following techniques:

    a. Full thickness biopsy at exploratory laparotomy (Figure 14-11).

> ❗ Definitive diagnosis of TCC requires histologic examination of tissue. Cytology alone is not definitive because chronic inflammation can create dysplastic changes that mimic neoplasia.

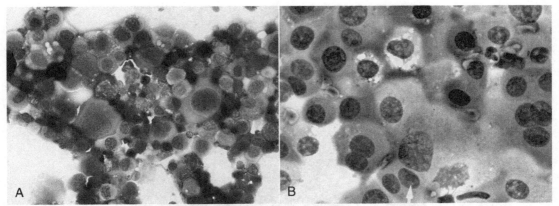

FIGURE 14-10 ■ Cytology performed on dry mounts from urinary sediment of two different dogs affected with transitional cell carcinoma (TCC). Cytology reveals more cytoplasmic and nuclear detail than is possible from evaluation of wet mount microscopy of urinary sediment. Note wide variation in cell size as well as that for nuclear size. Panel **B** has one multinucleated cell (Wright-Giemsa stain, ×1,000).

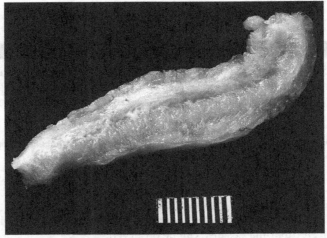

FIGURE 14-11 ■ Full thickness bladder biopsy from a dog with invasive transitional cell carcinoma (TCC). Note the degree of bladder wall thickening due to protrusion of TCC mass from the mucosa and also due to TCC invasion into the submucosa.

      (1) Bladder incision should be made farther than 1 cm from the tumor.
      (2) Seeding of the abdomen or the incision with tumor cells can be a complication. Change surgical packs and use new instruments during closure to limit tumor seeding.

! Seeding of the biopsy tract occurs much more often with TCC than with other tumors.

    b. Forceps biopsy of the urothelium.
      (1) Ultrasound-guided.
      (2) By cystoscopy.

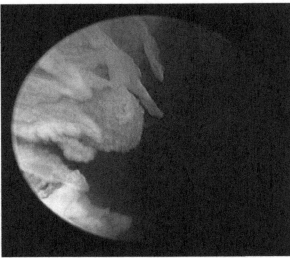

FIGURE 14-12 ■ Cystoscopic findings from dog with bladder transitional cell carcinoma (TCC). Note typical fronds projecting into the bladder lumen.

CYSTOSCOPY

A. Cystoscopy provides direct visualization of the entire bladder and urethra that may aid in identifying the location and extent of tumor growth and in diagnosing other abnormalities of the lower urinary tract. Other imaging modalities tend to underestimate the extent of disease.

> **!** Cystoscopy often reveals much more extensive disease than initially suspected from ultrasonography or contrast urography.

B. Small tissue samples are easily obtained for histologic examination.
C. The technique requires special equipment and training.
D. Single fronds or groups of fronds are the most characteristic cystoscopic appearance of TCC (Figure 14-12). Nodular masses also can be observed.

BLADDER TUMOR ANTIGEN TEST (BTA)

A. The BTA is a qualitative latex agglutination test using human antibodies that recognize a bladder tumor-associated glycoprotein complex present in the urine of animal patients with TCC. Two theories concerning the origin of the glycoprotein complexes have been proposed:
   1. Degradation of the urothelial basement membrane caused by tumor cell growth and attachment leads to the release of the glycoprotein antigen.
   2. Tumor cells produce the antigen autonomously.
B. The BTA urine dipstick test originally was created as a screening test for TCC in humans. The basement membrane of the glycoprotein complex may be similar among species allowing human antibodies to recognize canine TCC antigens.
C. The BTA test should be used as a screening test rather than a diagnostic test in patients with suspected TCC.

1. The specificity of the veterinary BTA test was 94% and the sensitivity was 90% when comparing normal dogs to those with lower urinary tract neoplasia. However, the specificity decreased to 35% when comparing dogs with neoplasia to dogs with non-neoplastic lower urinary tract disease.
2. False-positive results are obtained in patients with proteinuria, pyuria, and glucosuria. Diagnosis of TCC typically occurs late in the course of the disease when hematuria and pyuria are common secondary complications making interpretation of the results difficult.
D. The other diagnostic tests and imaging methods mentioned above are more helpful in the diagnosis of TCC than is the BTA urine test.

Urine Telomerase

1. Telomerase activity has been detected in urothelial cells of carcinomas, but not in the urothelium of healthy humans.
2. The telomeric repeat amplification protocol (TRAP) assay can measure telomerase activity in urine.
3. In studies in humans, the specificity was 88% and sensitivity was 90%.
4. This test may be useful in the future as a screening test for dogs at a high risk of developing TCC and as a diagnostic test in dogs in which TCC is suspected. The usefulness of this test in dogs has not yet been studied.
5. Early diagnosis may improve treatment success and long-term prognosis.

Basic Fibroblastic Growth Factor (bFGF) Urinary Marker

1. bFGF is an angiogenic peptide involved in promoting tumor growth that has been detected in the urine of humans with urinary tract and other malignancies.
2. An enzyme-linked immunosorbent assay (ELISA) test kit containing an anti-bFGF human antibody is available to quantify the amount of bFGF in the urine.
3. Dogs with bladder cancer had significantly higher urinary concentrations of bFGF compared with normal dogs and dogs with lower UTIs.
4. May be useful in deciding if dogs with lower urinary tract signs need additional diagnostic tests for bladder neoplasia.
5. More research is needed to determine if detection of bFGF will lead to earlier diagnosis of TCC and improved prognosis in dogs.

Recognition of Transitional Cell Carcinoma by Canine Olfaction of Urine Samples

1. Tumors produce substances that may have recognizable odors that dogs can detect with their exceptional sense of smell.
2. Dogs can be trained to recognize a characteristic odor in the urine of human patients with TCC as described in a 2004 study.
   a. Dogs correctly identified 41% of patients with TCC by the smell of their urine independent of the presence of glucosuria, pyuria, proteinuria, and hematuria.
   b. The success rate was statistically significant and greater than success expected by chance alone.
3. Research into this phenomenon is preliminary. Continued work with this concept and training of dogs for olfactory detection of TCC may lead to improved success rate in the future.

❗ TCC usually is diagnosed at an advanced stage in dogs and cats as compared with humans, who often have very superficial and less invasive disease at presentation.

■ TABLE 14-2
■ ■ **TNM Classification Scheme for Stages of Canine Bladder Cancer**

Classification	Characteristics
T: PRIMARY TUMOR	
Tis	Carcinoma in situ
T0	No evidence for primary tumor
T1	Superficial papillary tumor
T2	Tumor invading the bladder wall, with induration
T3	Tumor invading neighboring organs (prostate, uterus, vagina, and pelvic canal)
N: REGIONAL LYMPH NODE (INTERNAL AND EXTERNAL ILIAC LYMPH NODE)	
N0	No regional lymph node involved
N1	Regional lymph node involved
N2	Regional lymph node and juxta regional lymph node involved
M: DISTANT METASTASES	
M0	No evidence of metastasis
M1	Distant metastasis

At diagnosis about 80% of dogs are classified as T2, and 20% as T3. About 16% are classified as either N1 or N2 at diagnosis and 40% at time of death. Approximately 14% are M1 at diagnosis and 50% at death. Classifications defined by the World Health Organization (WHO). TNM, tumor, node, metastasis.

STAGING

A. Confirm the diagnosis of TCC with histopathology.
B. Thoracic radiography and abdominal imaging should be performed to identify metastases.
C. The tumor/node/metastasis (TNM) classification scheme created by the World Health Organization (WHO) is used to stage bladder cancers (Table 14-2).
   1. Classifies the degree with which the tumor has invaded the bladder wall and surrounding structures.
   2. Takes into account surrounding lymph node involvement as well as metastasis to other parts of the body.
D. Other staging schemes have been used in dogs. These include histologic classification, growth pattern, extent of infiltration, histologic grade, vascular invasion, lymphoid reactivity around the tumor, and lymphoid reactivity within the tumor. Most dogs with TCC have papillary infiltrative TCC of intermediate to high grade.

BIOLOGICAL BEHAVIOR

A. Tumors occur most often (66%) at the trigone of the bladder in dogs. There is no such preference for tumor location in cats, in which TCC occurs with nearly equal frequency in various part s of the bladder.

❗ Tumors occur most often in the trigone of the bladder in dogs. Local invasion of the urethra, prostate, and ureters is common.

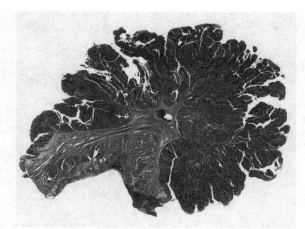

FIGURE 14-13 ■ Histopathology of bladder showing papillary transitional cell carcinoma (TCC). (Courtesy of Dr. Paul Stromberg, The Ohio State University, Columbus, Ohio.)

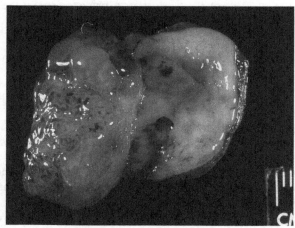

FIGURE 14-14 ■ Bladder polyp. Notice the large mass attached by a single stalk to the bladder mucosa. This specimen was derived from a cystotomy and partial cystectomy.

    B. Growth patterns.
       1. Papillary projections that protrude into the bladder lumen (Figure 14-13). This lesion must be distinguished from that of a bladder polyp (Figure 14-14).
       2. Flat, plaque-like lesions.
       3. Infiltrating lesions.
         a. Most common form of TCC (90%) in dogs and cats.
         b. Invades the bladder wall and may involve the submucosa and muscularis layers (Figure 14-15). In more severe cases, surrounding structures can be involved.
       4. Non-infiltrating tumors do not penetrate the bladder wall.
    C. Metastasis eventually occurs in more than 50% of cases.
       1. Regional lymph nodes (sublumbar, inguinal).
       2. Bone.

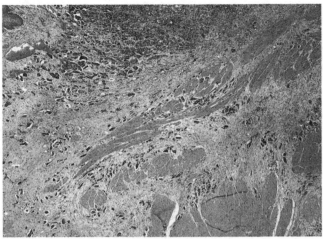

FIGURE 14-15 ■ Infiltrating transitional cell carcinoma (TCC) of canine bladder. This tumor exhibits local tissue invasion into the mucosa of the bladder wall. There are islands of tumor cells infiltrating from the base of the tumor into the stroma and lymphatics often stimulates desmoplasia (×100) (Courtesy of Dr. Paul Stromberg, The Ohio State University, Columbus, Ohio.)

     3. Lung.
     4. Abdominal organs.
  D. Local invasion of the urethra, prostate, and ureters is common. The urethra is involved in 56% of affected dogs.
  E. At the time of diagnosis, the lesions often are advanced.
     1. Tumor may be found invading the muscular layer of the bladder wall or fixed to surrounding structures.
     2. Metastasis has already occurred in 37% of affected dogs at presentation.
  F. Growth of the tumor can lead to ureteral obstruction and hydronephrosis or urethral outflow obstruction (Figure 14-16).
     1. Owners must be educated about the clinical signs associated with obstruction and monitor their pet's urinations on a daily basis.
     2. Urinary obstruction by the primary tumor causes death before metastases become lethal.
  G. Survival with no therapeutic intervention averages 3 months.
  H. Occasionally, the diagnosis is made fortuitously in dogs without clinical signs or cytologic changes in urine. This scenario may occur when ultrasound is performed for some other reason and a bladder mass is detected incidentally.

TREATMENT

Surgical Options Depend on the Location and Extent of the Tumor

     1. Tumors located at the apex or body of the bladder offer the best chance for surgical resection.
       a. Partial cystectomy can be performed in these cases. Local or distant recurrence of tumor growth occurs in 80% of patients that undergo this surgery.
       b. More than 80% of the bladder can be removed with eventual return to near-normal capacity.

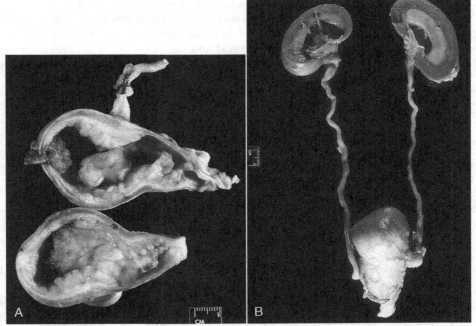

FIGURE 14-16 ■ Transitional cell carcinoma (TCC) and effects on ureters and kidneys. **A,** Extensive TCC in bladder wall and lumen of dog. **B,** Note that the tumor mass is obstructing both ureters resulting in bilateral hydroureter and hydronephrosis.

2. TCC located at the trigone is difficult to remove and the likelihood of urethral involvement is great.
   a. Surgical removal is impossible without performing total cystectomy and ureteral diversion.
   b. Palliative surgery and medical management to relieve obstruction are the best options.
3. At best, surgery only provides local control of tumor growth; curative surgical removal is rare.

> ❗ Surgery for tumor removal is rarely curative.

   a. TCC may have multiple foci within the bladder.
   b. Tumor size and stage usually are advanced at the time of diagnosis.
   c. If surgical removal is attempted, clean margins are difficult to achieve.
4. The primary surgical goal should be to alleviate obstruction.
5. Total cystectomy with or without urethrectomy and ureteral diversion has been performed with limited success.
   a. Ureterocolonic diversion is an invasive procedure with multiple, serious complications including hyperammonemia, hyperchloremic metabolic acidosis, uremia, and pyelo-nephritis.
   b. This procedure is not a realistic surgical option in small animals.
   c. Survival is approximately 5 months without other forms of treatment.
6. Partial resection alone is associated with median survival of 4 months.

7. Total resection alone is associated with median survival of 12 months.
8. Surgical debulking has been helpful in some but not other studies as adjunctive therapy.
9. In one study, cystoscopically directed laser ablation surgery alleviated clinical signs in affected dogs but did not increase survival time.
   a. Laser ablation can effectively remove masses that impinge on the ureters and would otherwise result in hydroureter and hydronephrosis.
   b. This technique also is helpful for patients with outflow obstruction from bladder masses projecting into the proximal urethra.
   c. Laser ablation surgery is not curative by itself or with chemotherapy.
   d. Repeated ablation is required as the tumor returns.

Chemotherapy

1. TCC generally are poorly responsive to chemotherapy.

> **!** TCC generally are poorly responsive to chemotherapy. A response rate of 15% to 20% can be expected in dogs.

2. Cisplatin.
   a. A cell cycle phase nonspecific heavy-metal compound that binds within and between DNA strands, inhibiting transcription and protein synthesis.
   b. Cisplatin is highly nephrotoxic. Treatments should be given concurrently with a 0.9% NaCl diuresis. Renal function tests should be monitored before each treatment.
   c. Progressive azotemia and renal dysfunction are observed in 22% to 50% of treated dogs.
   d. Vomiting is observed in 86% of dogs during cisplatin administration. Butorphanol should be given 30 minutes before cisplatin administration to suppress vomiting.
   e. Cisplatin is given at a dosage of 50 to 70 mg/m^2 intravenously over 20 minutes every three weeks.
   f. Average survival was 132 days in one study.
   g. Cisplatin treatment provided partial remission in 20% of patients.
3. Carboplatin.
   a. Similar mode of action to cisplatin with less nephrotoxicity.
   b. Carboplatin exhibited cytotoxic effects on TCC cells during in vitro studies.
   c. In vivo clinical studies did not provide complete or partial remission in any of the 11 dogs that received carboplatin.
   d. The suggested dose of 300 mg/m^2 should be administered intravenously every 3 weeks.
   e. Average survival was 132 days.
   f. Myelosuppression was observed in 50% of dogs but clinical signs associated with myelosuppression were not observed.
   g. Gastrointestinal toxicity was observed in 48% of dogs.
4. Mitoxantrone: Partial remission is achieved in 17% of dogs.
5. Adriamycin: Partial remission is achieved in 20% of dogs.
6. Actinomycin D: Partial remission is achieved in 17% of dogs.

Piroxicam

> **!** Piroxicam is considered the standard of care for TCC in dogs and may have specific advantages over other NSAIDs.

1. Inducible cyclooxygenase 2 (COX-2) enzymes are not expressed in the normal urinary bladder but are upregulated in tumors including TCC.

    a. COX-2 is expressed in both primary and metastatic TCC.

    b. COX-2 enzymes and their product, prostaglandin E_2 (PGE_2), a potent immunosuppressive compound, promote tumor growth by preventing apoptosis, stimulating tumor cell proliferation, and promoting angiogenesis.

    c. PGE_2 concentrations are increased in the bladder mucosa of patients with TCC growth as compared with normal bladder mucosa.

2. Piroxicam, a COX enzyme inhibitor, has antitumor activity and decreases the size of tumors when used in dogs with TCC.

    a. The mechanism of action is not based on cytotoxicity.

    b. COX inhibition may provide some immunomodulation by suppressing PGE_2 and thereby inducing apoptosis, inhibiting angiogenesis, and decreasing tumor cell proliferation.

    c. Decreased inflammation alone cannot account for the partial and complete remissions achieved in vivo.

3. Piroxicam provides good control of clinical signs and improves quality of life in some patients. Owners usually note increased activity and improvement in the attitude of their pet while the dog is receiving piroxicam.

4. Clinical studies of piroxicam in dogs with TCC indicate an overall response rate of 16%.

> ❗ Piroxicam provides good control of clinical signs, improving the quality of life in many dogs with TCC.

    a. Complete remission is achieved in 4% of treated dogs.

    b. Partial remission is observed in 13%.

    c. Disease remained stable in 58%.

    d. Progressive disease was noted in 25%.

5. Gastrointestinal toxicity occurred in 17% of treated dogs.

    a. Signs of toxicity included anorexia, melena, and vomiting.

    b. Gastroprotectants may be used in combination with piroxicam.

        (1) H_2 receptor blockers.

        (2) Proton pump inhibitors.

        (3) Sucralfate.

        (4) Misoprostol (prostaglandin E_1 analogue).

6. Acute renal failure is a potential complication of nonsteroidal anti-inflammatory drugs (NSAIDs). Renal function should be monitored regularly while prescribing this medication for dogs with TCC.

7. Piroxicam is used at a dosage of 0.3 mg/kg orally once daily if tolerated. It is given every other day to limit adverse effects in some patients.

    a. Only 10 mg and 20 mg capsules are available.

    b. Compounding pharmacies can reformulate this medication into varying concentrations to accommodate smaller animals.

8. Median survival with piroxicam as the sole form of treatment is approximately 6 months. About 20% of treated dogs survived for one year.

9. Piroxicam may have unique effects against TCC as compared with other NSAIDs. This possibility has not been studied in TCC, but it is well known that each NSAID has its own profile of effect against a variety of other tumors in experimental studies in mice.

Combination of Mitoxantrone and Piroxicam

> The highest reported success rate for treatment of TCC has been with a combination of mitoxantrone and piroxicam.

1. A dose of 5 mg/m^2 IV every 3 weeks of mitoxantrone with 0.3 mg/kg PO once daily of piroxicam has produced the best results.
2. Partial remission was observed in 35% of dogs.
3. Median survival was 9 to 10 months.
4. 75% of owners reported a subjective improvement in clinical signs and quality of life.

Radiation Therapy
1. Difficult to perform without including other internal organs in the radiation field.
2. Curative doses decrease quality of life and can even lead to perforation of the colon; the target dose is the highest tolerated dose.
3. Intraoperative radiation has been performed in combination with partial cystectomy to minimize effects on other organs.
4. Adverse effects include pollakiuria, urinary incontinence, cystitis, stranguria, and irreversible bladder fibrosis.
5. External beam radiation requires daily treatment for a total of 15 to 18 doses.
6. Treatment with intraoperative and external beam radiation provides a median survival time of 4 months.
7. Radiation only provides local control. Metastatic lesions still progress.
8. Best results are achieved when used in conjunction with chemotherapy to treat both primary and metastatic disease.

Palliative Treatment to Manage Urethral Obstruction
1. Temporary urethral catheterization until stent or cystostomy tube can be placed or until piroxicam becomes effective.
2. Permanent cystostomy catheter.
   a. Should not be performed in animals with ureteral obstruction or hydroureter.
   b. A mushroom tip or Foley urinary catheter is placed in the bladder via a ventral midline incision and passed outside of the body through a paramedian body wall incision.
   c. Owners must drain the bladder with a syringe 3 to 4 times per day.
   d. Secondary bacterial cystitis is common and urine cultures should be performed every 2 to 4 weeks.
   e. Continued growth of the tumor will eventually block the catheter.
   f. A median survival time after catheter placement of 106 days has been reported.
   g. Can be performed whether or not the owners elect to pursue further treatment.
   h. Cystostomy catheters can be placed in dogs with outflow obstruction while monitoring the response to other forms of medical management (Figure 14-17).
3. Urethral stenting.
   a. Balloon-expanding or self-expanding metallic stents are placed into the urethra with the assistance of a guide wire and are seated across areas of obstruction using fluoroscopy to visualize placement (Figure 14-18).
   b. Stent size should be 10% wider than the maximal urethral diameter to allow for a secure fit and decrease the chance of stent migration.

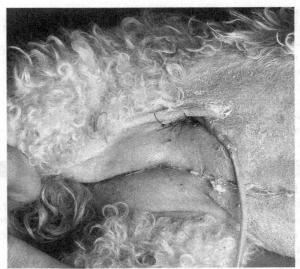

FIGURE 14-17 ■ Cystostomy tube in place in dog. Note tube exiting from caudal lateral abdominal wall. This type of tube is secured around the dog's body and urine is aspirated four to six times daily. This dog also has sutures along the ventral midline following a celiotomy.

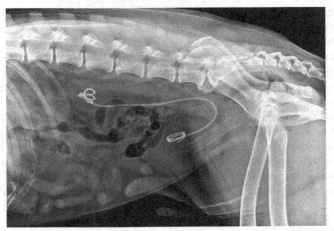

FIGURE 14-18 ■ Radiograph of urethral and ureteral stent in place in a male dog. The urethral stent was deployed to bypass transitional cell carcinoma (TCC) in the urethra that was creating obstruction to urinary outflow. The ureteral stent was placed to bypass obstruction of the ureteral opening into the bladder from the TCC. (Courtesy of Dr. Allyson Berent, Animal Medical Center, New York.)

  c. The stent should extend no more than 1 cm on either side of the obstruction to prevent damage to the surrounding healthy urethra with the intent of maintaining urinary continence.
  d. The procedure requires special equipment and training.
  e. Stent placement has been successful at relieving obstruction.
  f. Complications.

(1) Persistent obstruction.
(2) Atonic bladder (inability to urinate despite resolution of obstruction) caused by detrusor muscle dysfunction.
(3) Incontinence.
(4) Stranguria.
(5) Stent displacement and migration.
4. Surgical tumor debulking. This procedure is controversial with regard to how helpful it can be in combination with chemotherapy.
5. Antibiotic therapy to control secondary bacterial UTI.

THERAPIES ON THE HORIZON

Photodynamic Therapy (PDT)

1. A photosensitive agent that concentrates and localizes within tumor tissue is used.
   a. A photosensitizer is a compound that can be excited by light to induce cell damage.
   b. The exact mechanism by which the photosensitizing agent localizes in tumor tissue is unknown.
   c. The more hydrophobic the drug, the better it localizes in the tissue of interest.
   d. Several different kinds of agents are available that target different components of the cell.
2. Light of the appropriate wavelength is directed at the tumor with a laser light source.
   a. The wavelength of light is chosen based on the photosensitive agent.
   b. The depth to which the light penetrates is directly proportional to its wavelength.
   c. The correct fluence (amount of light or number of photons measured in joules [J]/cm^2) and power density (rate at which light is delivered measured in watts [W]/cm^2) are chosen for the tumor.
   d. Superficial, interstitial, or intraoperative irradiation can be performed.
3. Tumor cells undergo necrosis and apoptosis by several mechanisms induced by PDT.
   a. Activation of the photosensitizer by the light source generates oxidizing radicals that overwhelm tumor cell repair mechanisms leading to cell death.
   b. Oxidative damage to tumor vasculature causes ischemic death.
   c. Cytokines and inflammatory mediators are released by damaged tissue creating an immune response leading to nonspecific death of tumor cells.
4. Photosensitive agents are systemically absorbed despite preferential concentration in tumor tissue. Damage to healthy tissue therefore occurs.
   a. Necrosis, fibrosis, and decreased bladder capacity can occur as a result of full bladder PDT.
   b. After PDT, patients will experience lower urinary tract irritation.
5. New research has focused on inducing tumor cells to produce an intracellular photosensitizer to prevent damage to surrounding healthy tissue and minimize unwanted effects.
   a. 5-Aminolevulinic acid (ALA), a component of heme biosynthesis, is converted to protoporphyrin IX (PpIX), a photosensitizer, by malignant cells.
   b. An in vitro study reported promising results after incubating cultured canine TCC cells with ALA. TCC cells converted ALA into enough PpIX to cause cell death when exposed to 635 nm light.
   c. ALA was well tolerated when given orally.
   d. In the bladder, ALA allowed for fluorescence only within the mucosa, sparing the muscularis and serosa from damaging effects.
6. PDT has been used with success to treat TCC in human medicine.
7. Additional research to determine clinical effectiveness in animals is needed.

Calcitriol (Activated Vitamin D)
1. Canine TCC cells express many vitamin D receptors (VDR).
2. Calcitriol may act as an antiproliferative agent by inducing cell cycle arrest and apoptosis of TCC cells via alteration in tumor cell receptors and signaling pathways.
3. The effects of calcitriol were improved when combined with dexamethasone, which improves binding of calcitriol to VDR.
4. Doses required to cause antineoplastic activity are substantially higher than physiologic doses; systemic hypercalcemia and its associated adverse effects are therefore a concern.
   a. Direct delivery of calcitriol into the bladder may prevent systemic hypercalcemia.
   b. Intermittent dosing may decrease adverse effects.
   c. Co-administration of dexamethasone prevents binding of calcitriol to the receptors in the intestinal tract that normally allow for vitamin D absorption.

PROGNOSIS
A. Regardless of the form of treatment, median survival is 1 year.
B. Factors not affecting prognosis:
   1. Age and breed did not correlate with survival.
   2. Histologic and immunohistochemical tumor variables did not correlate with prognosis.
C. Factors associated with a negative prognosis include hydronephrosis and hydroureter.

Urethral Neoplasia
I. Most urethral tumors are malignant epithelial tumors (TCC or squamous cell carcinoma) (Figure 14-19).
   A. Fifty-six percent of dogs with bladder TCC also have TCC in the urethra.
   B. Twenty-nine percent of male dogs with bladder TCC also had prostatic involvement.
II. Chondrosarcoma has been reported.

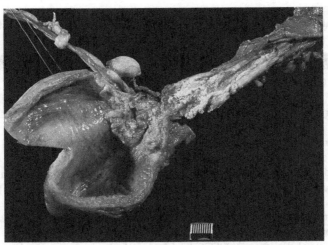

FIGURE 14-19 ■ Transitional cell carcinoma (TCC) in the urethra of a female dog. Note extensive tumor masses in the urethra and also in the area of the junction of the bladder with the urethra. The bladder is thickened due to the chronic effects of partial obstruction to outflow of urine.

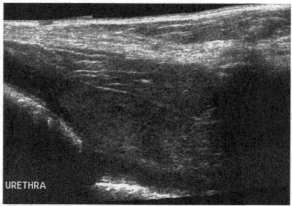

URETHRA

FIGURE 14-20 ■ Ultrasonography of urethra of a female dog. Notice large intraluminal mass due to transitional cell carcinoma (TCC). This mass could also have been from lesions of proliferative urethritis, a nonmalignant condition.

DIFFERENTIAL DIAGNOSIS

A. Urethral tumors (Figure 14-20) must be distinguished from proliferative (granulomatous) urethritis

TREATMENT

A. Most are not resectable.
B. Vaginourethroplasty, urethral reconstruction, and urethral stents have been used.
C. Urethral TCC responds to chemotherapy or piroxicam treatment in a manner similar to TCC of the bladder.
D. Cystoscopically directed laser ablation has been helpful in decreasing clinical signs and urinary obstruction. Laser ablation is not curative by itself and requires repeated treatments as the tumor regrows.
E. Urethral stents and tube cystostomy can be used to bypass urethral obstruction.

WHAT DO WE DO?

- Always consider TCC as a possible diagnosis in an older dog that develops what appears to be a bacterial UTI.
- Especially consider TCC in an older dog that has been treated for UTIs but clinical signs have not abated.
- Evaluate the urinary sediment carefully to look for rafts of epithelial cells in the absence of white blood cells as supportive for a diagnosis of TCC.
- Perform cytologic dry mount evaluation of urinary sediment with routine hematology stains. Much greater cellular detail will be gained compared with wet-mount microscopy at lower power magnification.
- Consider botryoid rhabdomyosarcoma in young dogs with bladder masses, especially if the masses are grape-like in appearance on diagnostic imaging.
- Confirm the cytological diagnosis of TCC by histopathology on tissue obtained by catheter aspiration biopsy (so-called *traumatic catheterization*), cystoscopic guidance of biopsy instruments, or surgical biopsy (full thickness biopsy of bladder wall during surgically attempted excision).

- Avoid cystocentesis in dogs with known bladder masses likely to be TCC to avoid the possibility of bladder tumor seeding along the cystocentesis tract.
- Perform fine-needle aspiration of nodules or masses of the kidney, especially in cats. This procedure often is rewarding in the diagnosis of LSA.

THOUGHTS FOR THE FUTURE

- We will learn how to diagnose TCC in dogs and cats before the tumor is advanced and invasive.
- Biomarkers in the urine are likely to be identified that indicate the presence of urinary neoplasia. These biomarkers will be positive long before clinical signs are obvious and could become part of wellness screening examinations.
- Present tests that detect bladder tumor antigens are often falsely positive—new technology will be developed to overcome these false-positive test results.
- Photodynamic therapy to eradicate TCC will become popular when we learn to diagnose TCC at an earlier stage of the disease.
- We will learn how to successfully treat TCC using local installation of drugs into the bladder.
- Calcitriol or calcitriol analogues will be increasingly used for their anti-proliferative effects. They will be given either systemically using methods that avoid hypercalcemia or locally within the bladder.
- Protocols for bladder installation of paclitaxel nanoparticles to coat TCC will become widely available.
- Newer NSAIDs will be identified that have greater activity against TCC.
- Local radiation therapy as a form of palliation will receive more attention as methods to decrease local tissue damage become available.
- Practical methods of laser surgery to decrease the size of tumors will become available.
- Immunotherapy with injections delivered via cystoscopy will become feasible when TCC can be diagnosed earlier in its clinical course.
- Urethral stenting technology will become more advanced and widely available to relieve urinary tract obstruction in patients with TCC.
- It will become clearer whether or not debulking surgery is helpful as an adjunctive treatment for TCC.

COMMON MISCONCEPTIONS

- Documentation of UTI in an older dog with lower urinary tract is not unusual and does not raise particular concern for bladder cancer. Actually, many older dogs with bladder cancer do have a bacterial UTI in addition to or because of the tumor.
- Surgery can be curative for TCC. Surgery can be helpful to decrease clinical signs in some patients, but recurrence is very common even in cases in which apparently complete resection has been performed. Surgical cure is very rare.
- Failure to find a mass lesion on double-contrast cystography or ultrasonography of the lower urinary tract rules out bladder or urethral neoplasia. Sometimes early bladder neoplasia is missed with these imaging techniques—they would however be seen with the use of cystoscopy. Ultrasonography is not expected to disclose urethral neoplasia unless it is extensive and extends cranially toward the bladder.

SUMMARY TIPS

- Always culture the urine of dogs with TCC because bacterial UTI is common either at time of diagnosis or later during the course of the disease and its treatment.
- Always consider the possibility that lower urinary tract signs in older dogs could be a consequence of underlying, undetected cancer of the bladder or urethra.

- Always perform a careful rectal examination in older dogs with signs of lower urinary tract disease. This procedure may be the best way to identify potential urethral invasion in a dog with a thickened urethra.
- Remember that ultrasonographic studies can be negative in patients with early TCC of the bladder. Double-contrast radiographic imaging studies also can be negative. Cystoscopic examination should be considered in such patients.
- Ultrasonography often is negative in patients with urethral tumors. The urethra is not well visualized with ultrasonography because of its location.
- Use cystoscopy to find small lesions of TCC because the magnification associated with this procedure facilitates identification of small lesions on the mucosal surface.
- Always consider that rafts of transitional epithelial cells indicate TCC and follow up with other diagnostic tests.
- Consider cancer of the bladder and urethra as a possibility in dogs with lower urinary tract signs, negative urine culture, and no evidence of urinary stones.
- Painless hematuria is the hallmark of upper urinary tract bleeding, and renal neoplasia must be considered in these instances.
- Consider renal cell carcinoma as the diagnosis for patients with polar masses or nodules of the kidney seen on ultrasonography.
- Perform fine-needle aspiration and cytology study of renal nodules or masses because results from this procedure are very helpful in determining a diagnosis for renal neoplasia in many instances (especially LSA).
- Remember that undetected bladder TCC may be the reason for unilateral or bilateral hydronephrosis if sufficient tumor mass is present at the vesicoureteral junction.

FREQUENTLY ASKED QUESTIONS

Q: I just removed a histopathologically confirmed TCC from the apex of the urinary bladder of a dog. The pathologist says the margins are "clean." Is surgical removal sufficient or should I consider some kind of chemotherapy?

A: Even when it appears that the TCC has been completely removed based on inspection at surgery and reports from histopathology, recurrence often occurs near the site of excision. For this reason, we recommend chemopreventive treatment with mitoxantrone and piroxicam.

Q: I have a confirmed diagnosis of TCC in a female dog in which resection is not possible. I know that NSAIDs can have some antitumor effect. Is any single NSAID better than the others?

A: Most of our experience is with piroxicam, an NSAID that is a nonselective COX inhibitor. Some oncologists believe that piroxicam has more effect against TCC than other newer generation NSAIDs that are "COX-sparing." Experimentally, the antitumor effect of NSAIDs can vary considerably by the NSAID employed. We continue to recommend piroxicam at this time.

Q: I have clients who want to do everything possible to keep their female dog with obstructive TCC alive as long as possible. The dog is already being treated with piroxicam and has had three courses of mitoxantrone chemotherapy. The dog has improved somewhat, but still has urgency during voiding and her bladder remains relatively full after attempts to void.

A: This dog is a candidate for placement of a transurethral stent to bypass the obstructing tumor, although this treatment is very costly. The stent doesn't do anything specific to treat the tumor, but it does relieve the urinary obstruction. However, urinary incontinence may become a problem with this approach. Laser ablation surgery can be considered as a means to mitigate clinical signs, but typically doesn't prolong the life of the dog. Permanent tube cystostomy could be used to relieve obstruction, but bacterial UTI is a common complication of this procedure. Unfortunately, there are complications associated with all of these palliative treatments.

Q: I just diagnosed a dog with TCC. She had 3 days of hematuria and some urgency before we established the diagnosis. The tumor mass is large on ultrasonography. There are no signs of distant metastasis. How can the tumor be so extensive and yet only be associated with clinical signs for a few days?

A: Unfortunately, this scenario is relatively common. Humans present much earlier in the course of their disease because they identify hematuria earlier. Dogs usually present with advanced invasive disease from TCC.

Q: I have heard that local instillation of various chemicals into the bladder can "cure" bladder cancer in humans. Why don't we consider this type of treatment in dogs with TCC?

A: Local instillation of chemical agents into the bladder can be successful in humans with TCC when there is only superficial involvement of the bladder mucosa with the neoplastic process. If the tumor is superficial, the infused drugs can make sufficient contact with and be effective against the tumor. Unfortunately, veterinarians do not often get the opportunity to diagnose dogs with superficial TCC. In addition, even though it may appear that TCC is only in the bladder, it often is in the urethra as well and this becomes apparent when urethrocystoscopy is performed.

Q: We just evaluated an 11-month-old spayed female Great Dane dog. Her owners brought her in with the complaint of limping and some straining to urinate. Physical examination showed thickening of the distal long bones of all limbs and both rectal and abdominal palpation identified a bladder mass. What can explain all of these findings?

A: Young, large breed, dogs can be predisposed to develop botryoid rhabdomyosarcoma. Some of these tumors are associated with hypertrophic osteopathy, and that is the likely explanation for the lameness and thickening of the distal extremities in this dog. Radiographs of the extremities and ultrasonography or contrast urography of the bladder will determine if this clinical suspicion is correct or not.

SUGGESTED READINGS

Upper Urinary Tract Tumors

Borjesson DL: Renal cytology, *Vet Clin North Am Small Anim Pract* 33:119–134, 2003.

Bryan JN, Henry CJ, Turnquist SE, et al: Primary renal neoplasia of dogs, *J Vet Intern Med* 20:1155–1160, 2006.

Henry CJ, Turnquist SE, Smith A, et al: Primary renal tumours in cats: 19 cases (1992-1998), *J Feline Med Surg* 1:165–170, 1999.

Moe L, Lium B: Computed tomography of hereditary multifocal renal cystadenocarcinomas in German shepherd dogs, *Vet Radiol Ultrasound* 38:335–343, 1997.

Moe L, Lium B: Hereditary multifocal renal cystadenocarcinomas and nodular dermatofibrosis in 51 German shepherd dogs, *J Small Anim Pract* 38:498–505, 1997.

Mooney SC, Hayes AA, Matus RE, MacEwen EG: Renal lymphoma in cats: 28 cases (1977-1984), *J Am Vet Med Assoc* 191:1473–1477, 1987.

Valdes-Martinez A, Cianciolo R, Mai W: Association between renal hypoechoic subcapsular thickening and lymphosarcoma in cats, *Vet Radiol Ultrasound* 48:357–360, 2007.

Lower Urinary Tract Tumors

Andreasen CB, White MR, Swayne DE, Graves GN: Desmin as a marker for canine botryoid rhabdomyosarcomas, *J Comp Pathol* 98:23–29, 1988.

Backer LC, Coss AM, Wolkin AF, et al: Evaluation of associations between lifetime exposure to drinking water disinfection by-products and bladder cancer in dogs, *J Am Vet Med Assoc* 232:1663–1668, 2008.

Bae IH, Kim Y, Pakhrin B, et al: Genitourinary rhabdomyosarcoma with systemic metastasis in a young dog, *Vet Pathol* 44:518–520, 2007.

Beck AL, Grierson JM, Ogden DM, et al: Outcome of and complications associated with tube cystostomy in dogs and cats: 76 cases (1995-2006), *J Am Vet Med Assoc* 230:1184–1189, 2007.

Dettlaff-Pokora A, Matuszewski M, Schlichtholz B: Telomerase activity in urine sediments as a tool for noninvasive detection of bladder cancer, *Cancer Lett* 222:83–88, 2005.

Erdem E, Dikmen G, Atsu N, et al: Telomerase activity in diagnosis of bladder cancer, *Scand J Urol Nephrol* 37:205–209, 2003.

Glickman LT, Raghavan M, Knapp DW, et al: Herbicide exposure and the risk of transitional cell carcinoma of the urinary bladder in Scottish Terriers, *J Am Vet Med Assoc* 224:1290–1297, 2004.

Henry CJ, McCaw DL, Turnquist SE, et al: Clinical evaluation of mitoxantrone and piroxicam in a canine model of human invasive urinary bladder carcinoma, *Clin Cancer Res* 9:906–911, 2003.

Kaewsakhorn T, Kisseberth WC, Capen CC, et al: Effects of calcitriol, seocalcitol, and medium-chain triglyceride on a canine transitional cell carcinoma cell line, *Anticancer Res* 25:2689–2696, 2005.

Khan KN, Knapp DW, Denicola DB, Harris RK: Expression of cyclooxygenase-2 in transitional cell carcinoma of the urinary bladder in dogs, *Am J Vet Res* 61:478–481, 2000.

Knapp DW, Glickman NW, Mohammed SI, et al: Antitumor effects of piroxicam in spontaneous canine invasive urinary bladder cancer, a relevant model of human invasive bladder cancer, *Adv Exp Med Biol* 507:377–380, 2002.

Knapp DW, Glickman NW, DeNicola DB, et al: Naturally-occurring canine transitional cell carcinoma of the urinary bladder. A relevant model of human invasive bladder cancer, *Urologic Oncology* 5:47–59, 2000.

Knapp DW, Richardson RC, Chan TC, et al: Piroxicam therapy in 34 dogs with transitional cell carcinoma of the urinary bladder, *J Vet Intern Med* 8:273–278, 1994.

Mohammed SI, Bennett PF, Craig BA, et al: Effects of the cyclooxygenase inhibitor, piroxicam, on tumor response, apoptosis, and angiogenesis in a canine model of human invasive urinary bladder cancer, *Cancer Res* 62:356–358, 2002.

Mohammed SI, Craig BA, Mutsaers AJ, et al: Effects of the cyclooxygenase inhibitor, piroxicam, in combination with chemotherapy on tumor response, apoptosis, and angiogenesis in a canine model of human invasive urinary bladder cancer, *Mol Cancer Ther* 2:183–188, 2003.

Mutsaers AJ, Widmer WR, Knapp DW: Canine transitional cell carcinoma, *J Vet Intern Med* 17:136–144, 2003.

Norris AM, Laing EJ, Valli VE, et al: Canine bladder and urethral tumors: A retrospective study of 115 cases (1980-1985), *J Vet Intern Med* 6:145–153, 1992.

Raghavan M, Knapp DW, Bonney PL, et al: Evaluation of the effect of dietary vegetable consumption on reducing risk of transitional cell carcinoma of the urinary bladder in Scottish Terriers, *J Am Vet Med Assoc* 227:94–100, 2005.

Raghavan M, Knapp DW, Dawson MH, et al: Topical flea and tick pesticides and the risk of transitional cell carcinoma of the urinary bladder in Scottish Terriers, *J Am Vet Med Assoc* 225:389–394, 2004.

Ridgway TD, Lucroy MD: Phototoxic effects of 635-nm light on canine transitional cell carcinoma cells incubated with 5-aminolevulinic acid, *Am J Vet Res* 64:131–136, 2003.

Stiffler KS, McCrackin Stevenson MA, et al: Clinical use of low-profile cystostomy tubes in four dogs and a cat, *J Am Vet Med Assoc* 223:309–310, 2003:325-329.

Upton ML, Tangner CH, Payton ME: Evaluation of carbon dioxide laser ablation combined with mitoxantrone and piroxicam treatment in dogs with transitional cell carcinoma, *J Am Vet Med Assoc* 228:549–552, 2006.

Van Rhijn BW, van der Poel HG, van der Kwast TH: Urine markers for bladder cancer surveillance: A systematic review, *Eur Urol* 47:736–748, 2005.

Vignoli M, Rossi F, Chierici C, et al: Needle tract implantation after fine needle aspiration biopsy (FNAB) of transitional cell carcinoma of the urinary bladder and adenocarcinoma of the lung, *Schweiz Arch Tierheilkd* 149:314–318, 2007.

Weisse C, Berent A, Todd K, et al: Evaluation of palliative stenting for management of malignant urethral obstructions in dogs, *J Am Vet Med Assoc* 229:226–234, 2006.

Willis CM, Church SM, Guest CM, et al: Olfactory detection of human bladder cancer by dogs: Proof of principle study, *BMJ* 329:712, 2004.

Wilson HM, Chun R, Larson VS, et al: Clinical signs, treatments, and outcome in cats with transitional cell carcinoma of the urinary bladder: 20 cases (1990-2004), *J Am Vet Med Assoc* 231:101–106, 2007.

15 Approach to Polyuria and Polydipsia

■■■

NORMAL PHYSIOLOGY

Polydipsia

1. Polydipsia (PD) is defined as consumption of a larger than normal amount of water per day.
   a. Normal water intake in dogs can be as high as 90 mL/kg/day (40 mL/lb/day) but often is 60 mL/kg/day (30 mL/lb/day) or less.
   b. As a general rule of thumb, normal dogs drink an average of about 1 ounce of water per pound of body weight per day.

> ! Normal water intake in the dog is about 1 ounce of water per pound of body weight per day.

   c. Normal water intake is more variable than urine output because of variations in environmental conditions, dietary water intake, fecal water content, respiratory evaporative losses, age, and physiologic status (e.g., pregnancy, lactation).
   d. Cats typically drink less water than dogs, and maximal water intake for normal cats is 45 mL/kg/day (20 mL/lb/day).
   e. Measurement of water intake at home by the owner can be helpful to determine if PD is really present. This approach is practical primarily in dogs.
   f. In most instances, PD occurs in association with increased urine production (see later).
   g. A history of isolated polyuria (PU) or PD usually means the owner has observed one abnormality and not the other or that the owner's initial impression was incorrect.

Polyuria

1. PU is defined as excretion of a larger than normal volume of urine per day.
2. Normal urine production in dogs and cats is 26 to 44 mL/kg/day (10 to 20 mL/lb/day).
3. As a general rule of thumb, normal urine production in dogs and cats is 0.5 to 1.0 mL per pound of body weight per hour (i.e., approximately 12 to 24 mL/lb/day).

Thirst

1. Osmoreceptors in the hypothalamus are responsible for stimulating or inhibiting thirst.
   a. Hypertonicity stimulates thirst.
   b. Hypotonicity inhibits thirst.
2. Dryness of the mucous membranes of the mouth and pharynx causes increased thirst.
3. Increased temperature of blood perfusing the hypothalamus increases thirst.
4. Hypotension and decreased effective extracellular fluid volume stimulate thirst.

PATHOPHYSIOLOGY

General Features

1. Increased urine output (PU) and increased water intake (PD) usually occur together in the animal.
2. In most instances, PU occurs first and is followed by compensatory PD.
3. Occasionally, PD will be the primary problem with compensatory PU, as occurs in animals with psychogenic polydipsia (PPD).
4. Any derangement in the normal production of urine or the thirst mechanism can result in PU/PD.

Mechanisms of Polyuria/Polydipsia

Four Organ Systems Must Be Considered in the Pathogenesis of Polyuria/Polydipsia

a. Nervous: Cerebral cortex, hypothalamus.
b. Endocrine: Pituitary gland, adrenal glands, pancreas, thyroid gland, paraneoplastic syndromes (Figure 15-1).
c. Renal: Primary renal disease or secondary influences on renal function from disease in other organ systems.
d. Hepatic.

Psychogenic Factors

a. Acquired habit that may represent a form of neurosis.
b. Primary PD with secondary PU.
c. No recognizable organic brain lesions.
d. Also may occur as a result of stimulation of thirst centers by various metabolites, chemicals or hormones produced in non-neurologic diseases (e.g., hepatic encephalopathy).

Hypothalamic Lesions

a. May affect thirst control centers.
b. Stimulation of dipsic or drinking neurons or inhibition of satiety neurons may result in primary PD.
c. Decreased synthesis or release of antidiuretic hormone (ADH, vasopressin) by the supraoptic and paraventricular nuclei may impair concentrating ability and lead to PU, as occurs in primary or central diabetes insipidus (CDI).

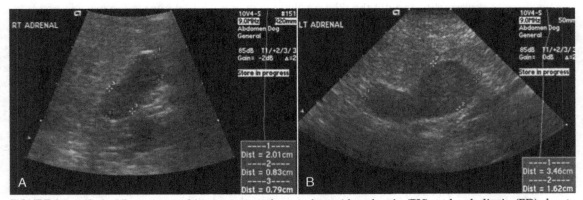

FIGURE 15-1 ■ **A**, Ultrasonographic appearance from a dog with polyuria (PU) and polydipsia (PD) due to pituitary dependent hyperadrenocorticism. Note increased width of adrenal gland. **B**, Ultrasonographic appearance of adrenal dependent hyperadrenocorticism. Note polar enlargement of the adrenal gland.

Antidiuretic Hormone (ADH)
    a. Pituitary lesions that interfere with the release of ADH.
        (1) CDI (see section "Hyposthenuric Disorders").
        (2) Drugs.
            (a) Ethanol (in humans consuming alcoholic beverages).
            (b) Phenytoin (an anticonvulsant not commonly used today).
            (c) Glucocorticoids.
        (3) Reset osmoreceptor (osmostat) sensitivity so that higher plasma osmolality is required before ADH is released.
    b. Interference with the action of ADH on the collecting ducts of the kidneys.
        (1) Congenital nephrogenic diabetes insipidus (NDI).
        (2) Acquired NDI (see section on hyposthenuric disorders).
            (a) Functional.
            (b) Structural.

Loss of Renal Medullary Hypertonicity
    a. The normal hypertonicity of the renal medulla is crucial for elaboration of highly concentrated urine. When medullary hypertonicity is decreased, the osmotic gradient necessary for movement of water from the collecting ducts into the interstitium and back into the bloodstream is disrupted, causing inappropriately dilute urine.
    b. Although the major cause of impaired concentrating ability in chronic renal disease is the necessity to excrete the daily solute load with a decreased number of functional nephrons, several renal diseases are associated with structural (i.e., histopathologic) abnormalities that also can contribute to impaired concentrating ability.
    c. Renal medullary washout of solute.
        (1) Long-standing PU/PD of any cause can result in loss of medullary solutes (e.g., NaCl, urea) necessary for normal urinary concentrating ability.
        (2) Structural lesions need not be present for impaired concentrating ability to occur.
        (3) Increased medullary blood flow associated with long-standing PU/PD can accelerate removal of solutes by the systemic circulation.
        (4) Decreased plasma osmolality associated with long-standing PPD impairs ADH release and the relative lack of ADH impairs reabsorption of urea by the inner medullary collecting ducts of the kidney.
        (5) Aldosterone deficiency in hypoadrenocorticism impairs NaCl reabsorption in the collecting ducts and contributes to medullary washout of solute. This effect explains why dogs with hypoadrenocorticism often have impaired urinary concentrating ability at presentation despite having structurally normal kidneys.
    d. Impaired production of urea can contribute to inadequate renal medullary hypertonicity.
        (1) Urea normally accounts for approximately half of the osmolality of the medullary interstitium.
        (2) The liver is the primary site of urea synthesis in the body.
        (3) Severe liver disease or portosystemic shunting can result in decreased urea production and less urea available to maintain normal medullary hypertonicity.
1. Lack of adequate physiologic stimuli for ADH release.
    a. Chronic hypotonicity of body fluids (e.g., PPD).
    b. Volume expansion (e.g., prolonged intravenous fluid therapy).
2. Obligatory solute diuresis in the kidneys.
    a. The filtered load of glucose in hyperglycemic diabetic patients exceeds the reabsorptive capacity of the renal tubules and results in an osmotic diuresis and glucosuria.

Infusion of 5% or 10% dextrose in water can result in hyperglycemia and glucosuria. Rarely, a defect in renal tubular reabsorption of glucose (i.e., renal glucosuria) can be the cause.

b. To maintain fluid balance, the decreased number of functional nephrons in patients with chronic renal disease must excrete the normal daily solute load and thus function under conditions of solute diuresis which results in PU and impaired urinary concentrating ability.

c. Increased excretion of low molecular weight radiocontrast agents can result in a transient osmotic diuresis.

3. Iatrogenic factors.
   a. Glucocorticoids.
   b. Diuretics (e.g., furosemide, thiazides).
   c. Intravenous or subcutaneous fluid administration.
   d. Some inhalation anesthetics (e.g., halothane, methoxyflurane) and drugs (e.g., lithium, demeclocycline) interfere with ADH action in the collecting ducts.
   e. Nephrotoxic drugs (e.g., aminoglycosides).
   f. High salt diets or treats.

DIFFERENTIAL DIAGNOSIS OF POLYURIA/POLYDIPSIA

A. There are many causes of PU/PD in dogs and cats including renal disease and several endocrine diseases.

B. Diseases associated with PU/PD, the mechanisms of PU/PD in these diseases, and useful diagnostic tests are listed in Table 15-1. An eponym to remember the causes of PU/PD is presented in Table 15-2.

1. The most common causes for PU/PD in the dog are:
   a. Chronic renal disease (CRD) or chronic renal failure (CRF).
   b. Diabetes mellitus.
   c. Hyperadrenocorticism.

2. The most common causes for PU/PD in the cat are:
   a. CRD or CRF.
   b. Diabetes mellitus.
   c. Hyperthyroidism.

> **Most common causes of PU/PD:**
> DOG: CRF, diabetes mellitus, hyperadrenocorticism.
> CAT: CRF, diabetes mellitus, hyperthyroidism.

HISTORY

A. The problem of PU/PD may be foremost in the client's mind or may only be elicited after careful questioning when PU/PD occurs as part of a more complicated disease process.

B. PU and PD most often are recognized together in an individual animal.
   a. It is usually impossible to determine which came first, PU or PD.
   b. The owner may recognize only one or the other, often the PD.

C. Recognition of PD by the owner tends to be more reliable than recognition of PU.
   1. A change in the number of times the water bowl needs to be filled often is noticed by the owner.

■ TABLE 15-1
■ ■ **Causes of Polyuria and Polydipsia With Mechanisms and Confirmatory Diagnostic Tests**

Disease	Mechanism of Polyuria and Polydipsia	Confirmatory Tests
Chronic renal disease* (S)	Osmotic diuresis in remnant nephrons Disruption of medullary architecture by structural disease	ECC CBC Profile Urinalysis Radiography Ultrasonography
Hyperadrenocorticism* (W)	Defective ADH release and action Psychogenic	LDDST, HDDST Plasma ACTH Ultrasonography
Diabetes mellitus* (S)	Osmotic diuresis caused by glucosuria	Blood glucose Urinalysis
Hyperthyroidism* (W)	Increased medullary blood flow and MSW Psychogenic Hypercalciuria	T_4 Technetium scan
Pyometra (W)	Escherichia coli endotoxin Immune complex glomerulonephritis	History Physical CBC Abdominal radiographs
Postobstructive diuresis (S)	Elimination of retained solutes Defective response to ADH Defective sodium reabsorption	History Physical examination Urinalysis
Hypercalcemia (W)	Defective ADH action Increased medullary blood flow Impaired NaCl transport in loop of Henle Hypercalcemic nephropathy Direct stimulation of thirst center	Serum calcium
Liver disease (W)	Decreased urea synthesis with loss of medullary solute Decreased metabolism of endogenous hormones (e.g., cortisol, aldosterone) Psychogenic (hepatic encephalopathy) Hypokalemia	Liver enzymes Serum bile acids Liver biopsy Blood ammonia
Pyelonephritis (W)	E. coli endotoxin Increased renal blood flow MSW Renal parenchymal damage	Urinalysis Urine culture CBC Excretory urography Ultrasonography
Hypoadrenocorticism (W)	Renal sodium loss with MSW	Serum Na and K ACTH stimulation
Hypokalemia (W)	Defective ADH action Increased medullary blood flow and loss of medullary solute	Serum K

Continued

■ TABLE 15-1
■ ■ **Causes of Polyuria and Polydipsia With Mechanisms and Confirmatory Diagnostic Tests—cont'd**

Disease	Mechanism of Polyuria and Polydipsia	Confirmatory Tests
Diuretic phase of oliguric ARF (S)	Elimination of retained solutes Defective sodium reabsorption	History CBC Profile Urinalysis Ultrasonography Renal biopsy
Partial urinary tract obstruction (S)	Redistribution of renal blood flow Defective sodium reabsorption Renal parenchymal damage	History Physical examination
Drugs (W)	Various mechanisms depending on drug	History
Salt administration (S)	Osmotic diuresis caused by excess sodium administered	History
Excessive parenteral fluid administration (W) (polyuria only)	Water diuresis caused by excess water administered	History
Central diabetes insipidus (CDI) (W)	Congenital lack of ADH (rare) Acquired lack of ADH (idiopathic, tumor, trauma)	Water deprivation test Exogenous ADH test ADH assay
Nephrogenic diabetes insipidus (NDI) (W)	Congenital lack of renal response to ADH (very rare) Acquired lack of renal response to ADH	Water deprivation test Exogenous ADH test ADH assay ECC
Psychogenic polydipsia (PPD) (W)	Neurobehavioral disorder (anxiety?) Increased renal blood flow MSW	Water deprivation test Exogenous ADH test Behavioral history
Renal glucosuria (S)	Solute diuresis caused by glucosuria	Blood glucose Urinalysis
Primary hypoparathyroidism (W)	Unknown (psychogenic?)	Serum calcium Serum phosphorus Serum PTH
Acromegaly (W, S)	Insulin antagonism Glucose intolerance Diabetes mellitus in affected cats	Neuroradiography Insulin-like growth factor
Polycythemia (W)	Unknown (increased blood viscosity?)	CBC
Multiple myeloma (W)	Unknown (increased blood viscosity?)	Serum electrophoresis
Renal MSW (W)	Depletion of medullary interstitial solute (urea, sodium, potassium)	Gradual water deprivation (3-5 days) Hickey-Hare test

Adapted from Bruyette DS, Nelson RW: How to approach the problems of polyuria and polydipsia, *Vet Med* 81:112-128, 1986.
*Most common causes of polyuria and polydipsia.
ACTH, adrenocorticotropic hormone; ADH, antidiuretic hormone; ARF, acute renal failure; CBC, complete blood count; ECC, endogenous creatinine clearance; HDDST, high dose dexamethasone suppression test; LDDST, low dose dexamethasone suppression test; MSW, medullary washout of solute; PTH, parathyroid hormone; (S), solute diuresis; (W), water diuresis.

■ TABLE 15-2
■ ■ Differential Diagnoses to Be Considered With Polyuria/Polydipsia

C	Calcium, Cushing, Cancer, Corticosteroids
L	Liver insufficiency, Leptospirosis (subacute)
A	Adrenal (hyperadrenocorticism and hypoadrenocorticism)
M	Metabolic, Mellitus (Diabetes), Malignancy, Medullary washout
P	Psychogenic, Pituitary, Polycythemia, Pyometra, Portosystemic shunt, Partial urinary obstruction, Paraneoplastic (hypoglycemia), Postictal
E	Endocrine, Electrolytes (increased or decreased calcium, decreased potassium)
D	Drugs, Diabetes, Diuresis (post-obstructive, hypertension-induced)
R	Renal insufficiency/failure
I	Insipidus (nephrogenic, central)
B	Brain
S	Salty treats, Salty diets

2. It can be helpful to ask the owner to estimate how much water the animal drinks in terms they can easily visualize (e.g., bowls, cups, quarts).
3. Less obvious sources of water (e.g., toilet bowls for large dogs, dripping faucets for cats) also must be considered. These sources often will not be considered by owners.
4. Owners usually do not observe cats drinking more water, and measuring the actual amount provided to the cat may be necessary.
5. Multiple animal households pose a challenge to identify PD in an individual animal. If necessary, the suspected animal may need to be isolated with its own water source for a few days to identify PD.

D. Rarely, PD may be present without PU (often transiently).
1. High ambient temperature (i.e., increased respiratory loss).
2. Excessive exercise.
3. Third space distribution of consumed water (e.g., sequestration of consumed water into the gastrointestinal tract, peritoneal space, or pleural space).
4. Large atonic bladder with increased residual capacity masking the observation of PU.
5. Correction of previous dehydration.

E. Owners may or may not be able to assess the volume of urine their pet is producing.
1. A negative history does not exclude the possibility that PU/PD exists.
2. Owner recognition of PU/PD is more common in dogs than cats.

! Owner recognition of PU/PD is more common in dogs than in cats.

3. Increased amounts of saturated litter in the litter box or increased odor may be clues suggesting PU/PD in a cat.
F. The volume of water consumed often is not helpful in determining the cause, however PU/PD tends to be most severe with PPD, CDI, and NDI, and urine specific gravity (USG) in these situations is typically in the hyposthenuric range (1.001 to 1.007).
G. Pollakiuria (i.e., increased frequency of urinations) may be confused with PU by the owner (i.e., owners sometimes assume that the animal is producing more urine if it is urinating more frequently than usual). Pollakiuria must be clearly differentiated from PU when the history is obtained.
1. Pollakiuria indicates inflammation in the lower urinary tract (i.e., bladder, urethra) regardless of any change in urine volume. The causes of pollakiuria are very different from the causes of PU.

2. Animals with PU may have a history of increased frequency of urinations because of their need to eliminate a larger volume of urine, but this increase in frequency usually is associated with passage of large volumes of urine whereas animals with pollakiuria pass small amounts of urine often with straining and sometimes with hematuria (depending on the underlying cause).

H. Nocturia (i.e., urinating during sleeping hours) often accompanies PU.

1. Nocturia may be the first sign detected by the owner of a dog with PU because urine is found in the house in the morning.

2. Sometimes nocturia is the presenting complaint because PU/PD during the day is not appreciated (e.g., outdoor dog with free access to water).

I. In the history, it is important to make sure that drugs (e.g., glucocorticoids, diuretics) that impair the urinary concentrating mechanism are not being administered. Glucocorticoids, administered either systemically or even topically (skin, eye, or ear), can cause marked PU/PD in dogs. This effect is less pronounced in cats.

❗ Make sure that drugs that impair urinary concentrating ability (steroids) are not being administered.

II. Physical examination findings can provide helpful clues about the cause of PU/PD.

A. Identification of small irregular kidneys on abdominal palpation suggests underlying chronic renal disease.

B. A neck mass in a cat suggests hyperthyroidism.

III. Diagnostic evaluation in animals with PU/PD is directed at identifying the underlying disease rather than focusing on the urinary concentrating defect.

DIAGNOSTIC TESTING

A. A minimum database should be obtained in all animals in which PU/PD has been verified or is strongly suspected (see Table 15-1).

1. Complete blood count (CBC).

2. Serum biochemistry profile.

3. Routine urinalysis.

4. Assessment of thyroid function should be included as part of the minimum data base for cats with PU/PD.

B. If the animal's urine USG is low (<1.025 in a dog or <1.035 in a cat), clinicians often proceed directly to obtaining a minimum database, whereas if the USG is higher than expected (i.e., >1.025 in a dog or >1.035 in a cat) they may recommend that the owner quantitate the animal's water consumption at home for several days before proceeding with an extensive diagnostic evaluation.

C. Often, clinically important underlying disorders are identified by evaluation of the minimum data base.

1. Renal failure.

2. Liver disease.

3. Hypercalcemia.

4. Hyperthyroidism.

5. Diabetes mellitus.

D. If the diagnosis is not clear after evaluation of the history, physical examination, and minimum database, further diagnostic evaluation is indicated. In dogs this evaluation includes diagnostic tests to exclude hyperadrenocorticism. See Table 15-1 for a list of the confirmatory tests to establish various causes of PU/PD.

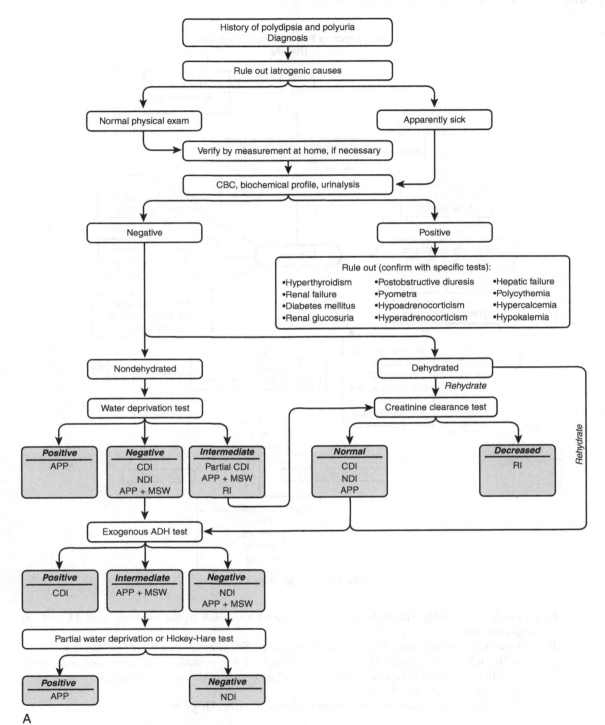

A

FIGURE 15-2 ■ Algorithm for polyuria/polydipsia (PU/PD). *APP,* apparent psychogenic polydipsia; *CBC,* complete blood count; *CDI,* central diabetes insipidus; *MRI,* magnetic resonance imaging; *MSW,* medullary washout of solute; *NDI,* nephrogenic diabetes insipidus; *RI,* renal insufficiency; *ULS,* ultrasound; *UPC,* urine protein-creatin ratio; *USG,* urine specific gravity. (**A,** From Fenner WR: *Quick reference to veterinary medicine,* ed 2, Philadelphia, 1991, JB Lippincott.)

Approach to Polyuria and Polydipsia
History

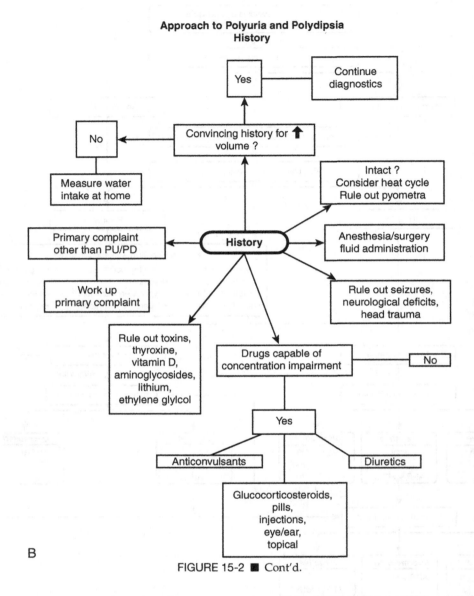

B

FIGURE 15-2 ■ Cont'd.

E. Figure 15-2 is an algorithm depicting our clinical approach to the evaluation of PU/PD in dogs and cats.
F. Urine concentration most often is evaluated using USG as estimated by refractometry.
   1. Although urine osmolality is the gold standard for evaluation of urine concentration, excellent correlation has been reported in dogs between USG as determined by refractometry and urinary osmolality.
   2. Dipstrip tests to estimate USG are not reliable in either dogs or in cats.

❗ Urine specific gravity should be evaluated by refractometry. Dipstrip tests to estimate USG are not reliable.

**Approach to Polyuria and Polydipsia
Based on Initial USG**

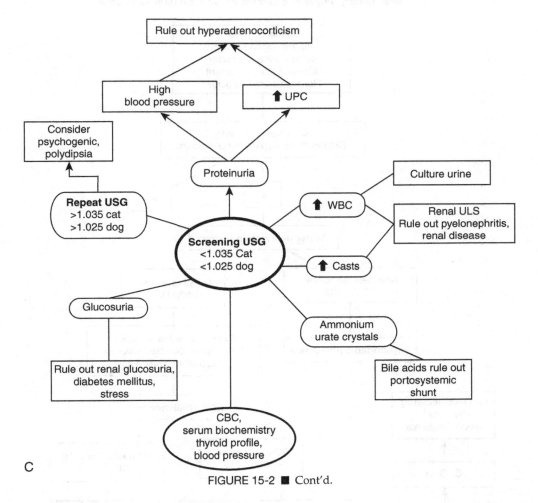

C

FIGURE 15-2 ■ Cont'd.

3. Estimates of USG determined by refractometry may differ depending on several factors.
   a. Type and brand of refractometer used.
   b. Temperature compensation.
   c. Scale used to make the reading on the refractometer.
4. Refractometers that use temperature compensation and scales calibrated specifically for dogs or cats should be used.
G. The USG of normal animals (i.e., normal hypothalamic-pituitary-renal axis) depends on dietary intake (food and water), hydration status, ambient temperature and humidity, and activity level.
H. Dogs can produce urine of widely varying concentration throughout the day. Urine should be collected in the morning before eating and drinking, because this urine sample is likely to have the highest USG obtained during the day.
   1. USG was 1.035 ± 0.010 (range, 1.009 to >1.050) in one study of 62 normal dogs.

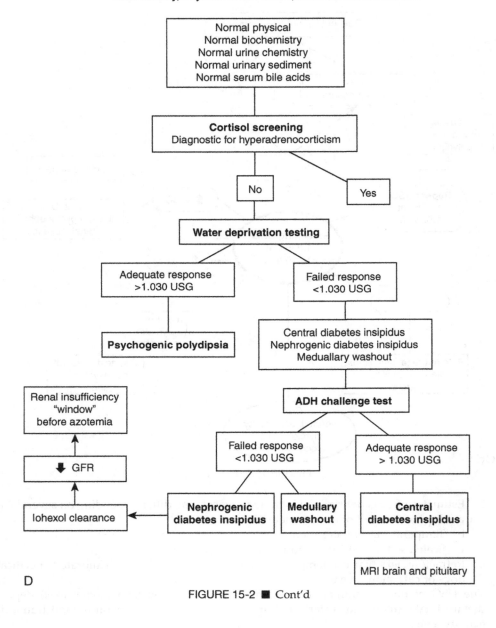

**Approach to Polyuria and Polydipsia
When Cause is Not Obvious
After History, Physical Examination, and Minimum Data base**

D

FIGURE 15-2 ■ Cont'd

2. USG was higher in morning urine samples than in those collected in the evening.
3. USG decreased with advancing age.
4. Median USG was 1.042 and mean USG was 1.038 in 51 urine samples taken weekly from 13 apparently normal dogs eating a variety of foods. In that study, USG ranged from 1.003 to 1.068 and 37 of the 51 samples had USG >1.030. (Chew, unpublished observations.)
5. Pooled 24-hour urine samples from normal dogs usually have USG of 1.020 or more.
6. USG can vary from as low as 1.006 to more than 1.040 in the same dog during a 24-hour period.
7. The USG of normal cats varies much less throughout the day than does the USG of normal dogs. Normal cats housed under laboratory conditions in our hospital usually produce urine with a minimum USG of 1.035 when eating dry food and a minimum USG of 1.025 when eating canned food.
8. Submaximal concentration of urine is expected in patients with PU/PD. The USG of normal dogs that are water-deprived should be 1.050 to 1.076 and USG of 1.047 to 1.087 is expected for normal cats.
9. A USG of 1.040 is considered the minimum expected value in dehydrated sick dogs or cats. Although healthy dogs and cats can have USG values as low as 1.001, this is extremely uncommon.

I. In dogs with PU/PD, water deprivation testing (WDT) is the next step after hyperadrenocorticism has been ruled out. Responses to water deprivation testing are presented in Figure 15-3.

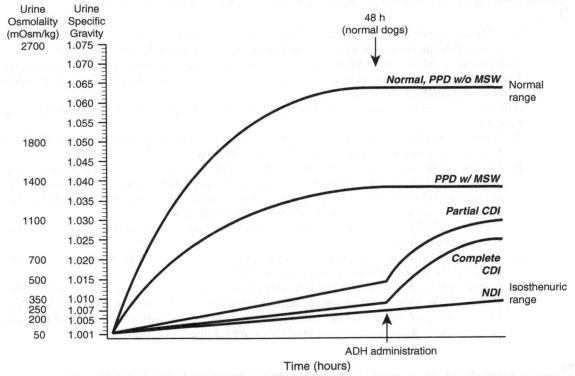

FIGURE 15-3 ■ Hypothetical response to water deprivation testing and ADH testing. *ADH,* antidiuretic hormone: *CDI,* central diabetes insipidus; *NDI,* nephrogenic diabetes insipidus; *MSW,* medullary solute washout; *PPD,* psychogenic polydipsia. (From Disorders of sodium and water: hypernatremia and hyponatremia. In DiBartola SP, editor: *Fluid, electrolyte and acid-base disorders in small animal practice,* ed 3, St Louis, 2006, Saunders-Elsevier.)

> ❗ Water deprivation testing is often performed in dogs with apparent psychogenic polydipsia (PPD), central diabetes insipidus (CDI), or NDI.

1. WDT establishes the patient's physiologic response to the hypertonicity of plasma perfusing the hypothalamus, which normally stimulates release of ADH from the neurohypophysis.
2. Mild dehydration causes release of ADH into the peripheral circulation, where it can exert its effects on the collecting ducts of the kidney to concentrate urine and increase USG.
3. Empty the animal's bladder and weigh the animal accurately at the beginning of the study.
4. USG should be determined by the same operator using the same refractometer to ensure consistency of reported readings.
5. Carefully monitor the progress during WDT so the patient does not become too dehydrated (i.e., lose more than 5% of body weight).
6. WDT should not be performed in patients that are already dehydrated, because they have already failed the challenge to concentrate their urine.
7. WDT also should not be performed in animals with azotemia, because dehydration may cause further injury to the kidneys.
8. WDT should not be performed in animals with hypercalcemia because the severity of the hypercalcemia will be increased.

> ❗ Do not perform water deprivation testing if the patient is already dehydrated, azotemic, or hypercalcemic.

9. Although not contraindicated, it is not necessary to perform WDT in animals with other organ system dysfunctions or metabolic disorders that readily explain the presence of PU/PD.
J. Unfortunately, ADH is not routinely measured, because of issues with method and handling. Even if this measurement were readily available, pulsatile secretion of ADH in dogs could make its interpretation difficult.
K. Abrupt WDT involves sudden removal of all water from the patient and is performed in the hospital.
   1. We recommend no food be fed during this time because moisture content and solute load for renal excretion will influence urinary concentration.
   2. The patient is weighed accurately before the start of the test and the bladder is completely emptied by urinary catheterization. It is important to empty the bladder at the start of the study to avoid confusion in the event that concentrated urine were to be elaborated by the kidneys and added to a bladder containing very dilute urine.
   3. The abrupt WDT is stopped if the patient loses 5% of body weight or if adequately concentrated urine is produced.
   4. Body weight and USG should be evaluated every 2 hours in patients with severe PU/PD or every 4 hours in patients with less severe PU/PD.
   5. During WDT, achievement of USG of >1.040 indicates adequate concentrating ability. USG of >1.030 may indicate adequate concentrating ability in patients with long-standing PU/PD because prolonged PU/PD will cause renal medullary washout, which will impair concentration of urine until renal medullary hypertonicity has been restored.

> ❗ Water deprivation testing is terminated if USG remains unchanged, when mild dehydration develops, or if 5% of body weight is lost.

   6. Obtaining serial USG measurements is facilitated by placement of an indwelling urinary catheter.

7. The effects of WDT and ADH administration in patients with common hyposthenuric disorders (e.g., PPD, CDI, NDI) are presented in Figure 15-3.
8. If USG increases to >1.030 during WDT, the diagnosis is PPD. PPD may be a neurobehavioral disorder, but also can occur secondary to portosystemic shunting, advanced liver disease, polycythemia, paraneoplastic hypoglycemia, hypoparathyroidism with hypocalcemia, or hyperadrenocorticism.
9. WDT is terminated when the USG is relatively unchanged over sequential USG determinations or when mild dehydration develops (assessed based on loss of 5% of body weight). Presence of 5% dehydration assures maximal stimulation of ADH release. A lack of sequential change in USG is defined as a <10% increase in USG on three consecutive urine samples taken at 2- to 4-hour intervals.
10. The WDT also is terminated if 5% or more of body weight has been lost, regardless of USG.
11. Failure to adequately respond to WDT occurs in patients with CDI, NDI, and in patients with renal medullary washout of solute.

L. In patients that fail to produce concentrated urine after WDT, exogenous ADH is administered to differentiate failure of the kidneys to respond to ADH (NDI) from failure of the pituitary gland to release ADH (CDI).
1. ADH testing begins immediately after WDT fails to result in production of concentrated urine based on lack of change in three sequential USG determinations.
2. Desmopressin (1-desamino-8-D-arginine vasopressin; DDAVP) is an aqueous form of synthetic ADH with minimal vasopressor activity and enhanced antidiuretic properties compared with native ADH.
3. One to 5 μg of the nasal formulation of DDAVP is given subcutaneously and USG evaluated at 30, 60, 90, and 120 minutes after administration to determine response.
4. A marked increase in USG typically occurs in patients with CDI after exogenous administration of DDAVP. Failure to respond to WDT followed by failure to respond to DDAVP is consistent with a diagnosis of NDI or severe renal medullary washout of solute.

M. When a patient has very dilute urine and the suspicion is high for CDI, ADH testing instead of WDT can be performed while the animal is at home with the owner.
1. DDAVP (either a 100 or 200 μg tablet) can be given PO every 8 hours for 3 to 7 days. A 100 μg tablet provides approximately 5 μg of DDAVP because orally administered DDAVP has limited bioavailability compared with the nasal spray formulation.
2. The owner should collect urine samples several times throughout the day for measurement of USG and to determine the effect of exogenous ADH.
3. Some renal medullary washout likely exists initially, however, so USG determinations should be performed after a few days of treatment with DDAVP.
4. Alternatively, 1 to 4 drops of the nasal spray (1 drop provides 1.5 to 4 μg of DDAVP) can be placed in the conjunctival sac every 12 hours and USG monitored. Although the nasal spray is not sterile, 2 to 5 μg (100 μg/mL; 0.05 mL = 5 μg) can be administered by subcutaneous injection twice daily (ideally after filtration through a Millipore filter), and the effects monitored.
5. All forms of DDAVP are expensive. Twice daily treatment with DDAVP is needed to adequately increase USG and minimize PU, but it can be given once daily in the evening to minimize cost. Also, larger doses may increase the magnitude of urinary concentration and its duration of effect.
6. Treatment with DDAVP is not required if the animal has free access to water, stays hydrated, and is allowed to urinate large volumes frequently in spaces acceptable to the owners (e.g., outdoor dog). Water restriction in the absence of DDAVP treatment and ongoing large losses of water in the urine can lead to severe hypernatremia and hyperosmolality that may have severe neurologic consequences for the patient.

N. In patients that fail both abrupt WDT and ADH testing, renal medullary solute washout must be considered in addition to NDI.

1. In these instances, gradual WDT, either alone or in conjunction with DDAVP administration, should allow restoration of normal renal medullary hypertonicity.
2. Gradual water deprivation involves progressive water restriction over several days. Water intake is decreased over several days from its current level to approximately 100 mL/kg/day.
3. Gradual WDT is discontinued if body weight decreases by 5% or if the animal shows clinical signs of illness.
4. After this gradual WDT, abrupt WDT again is performed. If the patient fails to adequately concentrate its urine during the second WDT, renal medullary solute washout is excluded from further consideration.
5. Animals that concentrate their urine on abrupt WDT after gradual WDT are likely to have either CDI or PPD.

CLINICAL FINDINGS, DIAGNOSIS, AND TREATMENT OF HYPOSTHENURIC DISORDERS

A. PU and PD are not diagnoses but rather clinical signs of an underlying disease process. Treatment depends upon establishing an accurate diagnosis and instituting appropriate treatment for the causative disease (see Table 15-1).

Psychogenic Polydipsia

> ! PU/PD are not a diagnoses but rather clinical signs of an underlying disease process.

1. PPD is an uncommon but not rare disorder that usually occurs in large breed dogs. German shepherds may be over-represented.
2. The owner may report that the dog has a nervous disposition or that PD developed after some stressful event.
3. Some hyperactive dogs placed in an exercise restricted environment have developed PPD, and some dogs seem to have developed it as a learned behavior to get attention from the owner.
4. Rarely, PPD will be encountered in dogs with primary brain lesions.
5. Some dogs with PPD lower their water intake dramatically as a result of the stress of hospitalization, and this is sometimes a useful diagnostic observation.
6. In one study, dogs with PPD had daily water consumption of 150 to 250 mL/kg, USG of 1.001 to 1.003, urine osmolality of 102 to 112 mOsm/kg, plasma osmolality of 285 to 295 mOsm/kg, and serum sodium concentration of 131 to 140 mEq/L. Although not consistently present, slightly low serum sodium concentration in a dog with PU/PD and marked hyposthenuria supports a diagnosis of PPD.
7. In the same study, approximately 67% of dogs with PPD had a normal response to water deprivation, whereas the others had some degree of renal medullary washout of solute, but responded to gradual water deprivation.
8. PPD appears to be extremely rare in cats (if it exists at all in this species).
9. PPD is treated by gradual water restriction into the normal range over several days. This approach should correct any renal medullary washout of solute that is present. The owner must be careful to eliminate other less obvious sources of water such as toilet bowls or dripping faucets.

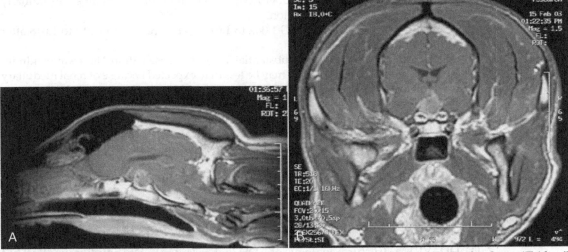

FIGURE 15-4 ■ Magnetic resonance imaging (MRI) of the cranium of an 11-year-old male Gordon Setter, "Fridge," with severe polyuria (PU) and polydipsia (PD) and average urinary specific gravity of 1.004. This dog failed water deprivation testing and immediately responded to exogenous ADH administration with concentrated urine. MR shows a large pituitary mass on both the axial (**A**) and sagittal (**B**) views. "Fridge's" pituitary tumor was treated with radiation therapy and he lived another year but required DDAVP tablets to allow him to control the degree of PU and PD.

Central Diabetes Insipidus (Figure 15-4)

1. CDI, or pituitary diabetes insipidus, is due to a partial or complete lack of ADH (vasopressin) production and release from the neurohypophysis.

> ❗ Central diabetes insipidus is due to a partial or complete lack of ADH production and release from the neurohypophysis.

2. Causes of CDI.
   a. Congenital (rare).
   b. Idiopathic.
   c. Neoplasia.
   d. Trauma (may be transient).
   e. Neuroanatomic abnormality (e.g., cystic craniopharyngeal duct).
   f. Hypophysectomy for treatment of hyperadrenocorticism (often transient).
   g. Visceral larval migrans (rare).
3. Diagnosis.
   a. Animals with CDI have severe PU/PD.
   b. Severe hyposthenuria (urine osmolality 60-200 mOsm/kg) is common. Urine osmolality may reach 400 to 500 mOsm/kg if the animal is severely dehydrated.
   c. Variability in USG and urine osmolality at the time of presentation is related to hydration status and severity of ADH deficiency.
   d. In one study, dogs were classified as having complete or partial CDI based on the magnitude of increase in USG and urine osmolality after induction of 5% dehydration.

(1) Dogs with complete CDI had USG 1.001 to 1.007 that did not change substantially after induction of 5% dehydration.

(2) Dogs with partial CDI had USG 1.002 to 1.016 that increased to 1.010 to 1.018 after induction of 5% dehydration.

(3) ADH administration leads to a substantial increase in USG within 2 hours after administration, but the initial response may be less than expected because of renal medullary washout of solute. In one study, USG increased to 1.018 to 1.022 after ADH administration in dogs with complete CDI and to 1.018 to 1.036 in dogs with partial CDI.

  e. Increased plasma osmolality and hypernatremia may occur in dogs and cats with CDI. These results suggest that some affected dogs and cats do not obtain enough water to maintain water balance and are presented in a hypertonic state.

4. Treatment.

  a. Treatment with ADH restores medullary hypertonicity and normal urinary concentrating ability in animals with CDI.

❗ Daily administration of DDAVP (desmopressin) is the treatment for CDI.

(1) DDAVP is a structural analogue of ADH that has more potent antidiuretic effect but minimal vasopressive effect and is relatively resistant to metabolic degradation.

(2) DDAVP is available as a nasal spray (0.1 mg/mL), injectable solution (4 μg/mL), or tablet for oral administration (100 and 200 μg).

  (a) The injectable solution is much more expensive than the nasal spray, and the nasal spray has been used subcutaneously in dogs and cats with CDI at a dosage of 1 μg/kg every 12 hours without adverse effects.

  (b) The nasal spray can be administered in the conjunctival sac at a dosage of 1.5 μg/kg every 8 hours. One drop of the nasal spray contains 1.5 to 4 μg of desmopressin, and duration of effect varies from 8 to 24 hours.

  (c) In humans, the bioavailability of DDAVP after oral administration is 0.1% as compared with 3% to 5% after intranasal administration, and gastrointestinal absorption is improved when it is given in a fasted state. In dogs, an antidiuretic effect was observed even after oral doses as low as 50 μg.

  b. Chlorpropamide is a sulfonylurea hypoglycemic agent that potentiates the renal tubular effects of small amounts of ADH and may be useful in management of partial CDI.

    (1) The recommended dosage of chlorpropamide is 10 to 40 mg/kg/day orally and hypoglycemia is a potential adverse effect.

    (2) It has been useful in the management of CDI (up to 50% reduction in urine output) in some reports but not in others, possibly because some animals have partial and some have complete CDI.

  c. The prognosis in animals with CDI depends on the underlying cause (e.g., idiopathic versus neoplasia). Many older dogs with CDI have tumors in the region of the pituitary gland and eventually develop neurologic signs.

Nephrogenic Diabetes Insipidus
Congenital Nephrogenic Diabetes Insipidus

  a. Rare in dogs and cats.

    (1) Affected animals are presented at a very young age for severe PU/PD.

    (2) Urine osmolality and USG are in the hyposthenuric range.

    (3) Affected animals show no response to WDT, exogenous vasopressin administration, or hypertonic saline infusion.

    (4) Plasma ADH concentration was markedly increased in one case report in a dog.
    (5) Low affinity V_2 receptors were thought to be responsible for NDI in a family of Siberian huskies.
  b. Congenital NDI is caused by mutations in the V_2 receptor (X-linked recessive) or aquaporin 2 (AQP2) channel (autosomal recessive) in humans.

Acquired Nephrogenic Diabetes Insipidus

  a. Acquired NDI includes a diverse group of disorders in which structural or functional abnormalities interfere with the ability of the kidneys to concentrate urine.

FUNCTIONAL

    (1) Glucocorticoids (endogenous or exogenous).
    (2) Diuretics.
    (3) Hypercalcemia and hypercalciuria.
    (4) Hypokalemia.
    (5) Sepsis and endotoxemia (e.g., *Escherichia coli* urinary tract infection [UTI], pyelonephritis, pyometra).

Pyometra should be ruled out when PU/PD is present in an intact female.

    (6) Altered medullary tonicity (e.g., hypoadrenocorticism).
    (7) Nephrotoxic drugs (e.g., aminoglycosides).
    (8) Postobstructive diuresis.
    (9) Acromegaly.

STRUCTURAL

    (1) Renal medullary interstitial amyloidosis.
    (2) Polycystic kidney disease.
    (3) Chronic pyelonephritis.
    (4) Chronic interstitial nephritis.

Thiazide Diuretics

  1. Thiazide diuretics (chlorothiazide 20 to 40 mg/kg PO every 12 hours or hydrochlorothiazide 2.5 to 5.0 mg/kg PO every 12 hours) have been used to treat animals with CDI and NDI.
    a. Diuretic administration results in mild dehydration, enhanced proximal renal tubular reabsorption of sodium, decreased delivery of tubular fluid to the distal nephron, and reduced urine output.
    b. Thiazides have been reported to result in a 20% to 50% reduction in urine output in dogs with NDI and in cats with CDI.
    c. In other reports, thiazides were reported to be ineffective in decreasing urine output in a dog and a cat with CDI.
    d. Restriction of dietary sodium and protein reduces the amount of solute that must be excreted in the urine each day and thus further reduces obligatory water loss and polyuria. A low salt diet and hydrochlorothiazide (2 mg/kg PO every 12 hours) were used successfully to manage a dog with congenital NDI for 2 years.

WHAT DO WE DO?

• Perform water deprivation testing in patients with confirmed PD and PU when the diagnosis is not apparent after a diagnostic evaluation that has included a CBC, serum biochemistry, urinalysis, and urine culture.

- Weigh the animal every few hours during water deprivation testing and conclude testing if 5% of body weight is lost during testing.
- Determine iohexol clearance in patients in which PU is suspected to be a consequence of underlying nonazotemic renal disease (i.e., all other likely diagnoses have been excluded by other diagnostic tests).
- Consider psychogenic PD, especially in puppies and in young large breed dogs.
- Never perform water deprivation testing in an azotemic animal.
- Rule out hypercalcemia and hypokalemia as potential causes of impaired urinary concentrating ability and polyuria before performing water deprivation testing.
- Administer exogenous ADH (DDAVP) to rule out CDI when the patient has failed to concentrate urine during water deprivation testing.

THOUGHTS FOR THE FUTURE

- Assays for ADH will become more widely available, facilitating the diagnostic approach to PU and PD and overcoming difficulties in interpretation associated with pulsatile secretion of ADH will be developed.
- Measurement of urinary aquaporins will become available and will facilitate the diagnostic evaluation of patients with PU and PD.
- Estimation of glomerular filtration rate (GFR) by iohexol clearance will become routine in primary care practice and will help in the evaluation of nonazotemic patients with PU and PD in which primary renal disease is suspected of being the underlying cause.

SUMMARY TIPS

- Tailor water deprivation testing to each patient based on individual response rather than any set time period.
- Make sure occult urinary tract infection and pyelonephritis have been ruled out by negative urine culture in patients in which an obvious cause for PU and PD has not been identified.
- Perform abdominal imaging (i.e., abdominal radiographs, ultrasonography) to further evaluate the adrenal glands, kidneys, gastrointestinal tract, and liver in patients in which the initial diagnostic evaluation has not identified the cause of the PU and PD.
- Consider water deprivation testing primarily as a tool to distinguish among central diabetes insipidus, nephrogenic diabetes insipidus, and apparent psychogenic PD.
- Always rule out corticosteroid administration as a cause of PU and PD and remember that topical corticosteroids (i.e., those used on the skin and in the ears and eyes) also can result in PU and PD.
- Ask the owner to measure their pet's water intake at home over several days when the existence of PD and PU is questionable.

COMMON MISCONCEPTIONS

- Water deprivation testing should be done for 12 or 24 hours. Actually, water deprivation should not be carried out for any predetermined period of time. The duration of testing is determined by the patient's response to water deprivation (i.e., changes in body weight, skin turgor, hematocrit, total plasma proteins, and urine specific gravity).
- Water deprivation testing is needed to assess patients with hypercalcemia on routine serum biochemistry testing. No. Water deprivation would be hazardous for a hypercalcemic patient, and other procedures (e.g., evaluation of peripheral lymph nodes, rectal palpation, parathyroid hormone determination) are more likely to yield valuable diagnostic information.

- Most older dogs with PU and PD without obvious cause have hyperadrenocorticism or central diabetes insipidus. Such dogs may well have underlying chronic renal disease that has resulted in impaired urinary concentrating ability but not azotemia (i.e., between 67% and 75% loss of functional nephrons).

FREQUENTLY ASKED QUESTIONS

Q: I have an 11-year-old neutered male German shepherd dog. Hyperadrenocorticism has been definitively diagnosed and treated with mitotane leading to a hypoadrenal crisis in the past (pre- and post- adrenocorticotropic hormone (ACTH) cortisol concentrations currently are within the normal range). Persistent severe PU and PD developed in the last month. Serum biochemistry results, including BUN and serum creatinine concentrations are normal. Urinalysis was normal, with the exception of a USG of 1.010. The USG was still 1.010 after water restriction to 30 mL/lb/day. Results of abdominal radiographs and abdominal ultrasound imaging are normal. The dog was given 0.2 mg DDAVP orally twice a day which resulted in a USG of 1.040. The USG returned to 1.010 shortly after the DDAVP tablets were discontinued. Does this dog have CDI?

A: Apparently so. The dramatic response to the DDAVP followed by a rapid return to much more dilute urine in the absence of DDAVP supplementation supports a diagnosis of CDI.

Q: In the previous case, why wasn't the USG in the hyposthenuric range if the diagnosis is CDI?

A: Animals with complete CDI typically have hyposthenuria (USG 1.001-1.006), but some dogs with complete CDI can concentrate into this range despite complete absence of ADH if they are dehydrated (but usually not above USG 1.017). An alternate explanation is that the dog has partial CDI. If available, brain imaging (magnetic resonance imaging [MRI] or computed tomography [CT]) can be performed to evaluate the hypothalamus and pituitary gland for diseases that could interrupt production or secretion of ADH.

Q: The owners of a 13-week-old male Labrador retriever are having difficulty housebreaking the puppy. The dog seems to drink constantly and urinates while walking around the house. Urinalysis was normal except for a USG of 1.003. Could this dog have CDI?

A: CDI is possible, but psychogenic PD is far more common in puppies. Some puppies drink water in excess of their physiological need. They usually outgrow this tendency by the time they are 4 to 5 months old. If necessary, psychogenic PD can quickly be differentiated from CDI by during water deprivation testing. This dog's USG was >1.040 after approximately 6 hours of water deprivation, confirming normal urinary concentrating ability. If the dog had CDI, its USG would have remained low and certainly would not have increased to more than 1.015.

Q: We anesthetized an 11-year-old spayed female mixed breed dog for dental extractions. Her history indicated no problems, and she was normal on physical examination before the dental procedure. CBC and serum biochemistry results also were normal before the procedure, but no urinalysis was performed. Anesthesia and the dental procedure lasted approximately one hour and she received some intravenous fluids during this time. The nonsteroidal anti-inflammatory drug (NSAID) carprofen and the antibiotic enrofloxacin were prescribed for one week after the procedure. A few days after release from the hospital, the owners reported that the dog was drinking quite a bit of water and urinating large volumes. Urinalysis at this time was normal except for a USG of 1.010 and trace proteinuria, and urine culture showed no growth. Serum biochemistry results at this time were still normal. A low dose dexamethasone test to evaluate for hyperadrenocorticism was normal. What can I tell the owner?

A: More information is needed. It would have been helpful to have urinalysis results (including USG) before anesthesia. In dogs with underlying renal disease, urinalysis results (especially USG) are likely to be abnormal long before changes in serum biochemistry become apparent. Some dogs with chronic nonazotemic renal disease decompensate after anesthesia. NSAID administration could have transiently affected urine concentration. Some dogs develop renal medullary washout (which can persist for several weeks) after anesthesia and IV fluid administration. Determination of iohexol clearance would identify if GFR is decreased despite normal BUN and serum creatinine concentrations. If GFR is decreased, the dog likely has nonazotemic chronic renal disease. If GFR is normal, gradual water deprivation could be performed to determine if renal medullary washout has occurred. This procedure also will correct renal medullary washout if it is present.

SUGGESTED READINGS

Baas JJ, Schaeffer F, Joles JA: The influence of cortisol excess on kidney function in the dog, *Vet Q* 6:17–21, 1984.

Breitschwerdt EM, Verlander JW, Bribernik TN: Nephrogenic diabetes insipidus in three dogs, *J Am Vet Med Assoc* 179: 235–238, 1981.

Dossin O, Germain C, Braun JP: Comparison of the techniques of evaluation of urine dilution/concentration in the dog, *J Vet Med A Physiol Pathol Clin Med* 50:322–325, 2003.

George JW: The usefulness and limitations of hand-held refractometers in veterinary laboratory medicine: An historical and technical review, *Vet Clin Pathol* 30:201–210, 2001.

Harb MF, Nelson RW, Feldman EC, et al: Central diabetes insipidus in dogs: 20 cases (1986-1995), *J Am Vet Med Assoc* 209:1884–1888, 1996.

Hardy RM, Osborne CA: Aqueous vasopressin response test in clinically normal dogs undergoing water diuresis: technique and results, *Am J Vet Res* 43:1987–1990, 1982.

Hardy RM, Osborne CA: Repositol vasopressin response test in clinically normal dogs undergoing water diuresis: technique and results, *Am J Vet Res* 43:1991–1993, 1982.

Hardy RM, Osborne CA: Water deprivation test in the dog: Maximal normal values, *J Am Vet Med Assoc* 174:479–483, 1979.

Hendriks HJ, de Bruijne JJ, van den Brom WE: The clinical refractometer: a useful tool for the determination of specific gravity and osmolality in canine urine, *Tijdschr Diergeneeskd* 103:1065–1068, 1978.

Joles JA, Rijnberk A, van den Brom WE, Dogterom J: Studies on the mechanism of polyuria induced by cortisol excess in the dog, *Tijdschr Diergeneeskd* 105:199–205, 1980.

Kraus KH: The use of desmopressin in diagnosis and treatment of diabetes insipidus in cats, *Compend Contin Educ Pract Vet* 9:752–755, 1987.

Lage AL: Apparent psychogenic polydipsia. In Kirk RW, editor: *Current veterinary therapy VI*, Philadelphia, 1977, WB Saunders Co, p 1098.

Luzius H, Jans DA, Grunbaum EG, et al: A low affinity vasopressin V2-receptor in inherited nephrogenic diabetes insipidus, *J Recept Res* 12:351–368, 1992.

Mulnix JA, Rijnberk A, Hendriks HJ: Evaluation of a modified water deprivation test for diagnosis of polyuric disorders in dogs, *J Am Vet Med Assoc* 169:1327–1330, 1976.

Nichols R: Polyuria and polydipsia. Diagnostic approach and problems associated with patient evaluation, *Vet Clin North Am Small Anim Pract* 31:833–844, 2001.

Ross LA, Finco DR: Relationship of selected clinical renal function tests to glomerular filtration rate and renal blood flow in cats, *Am J Vet Res* 42:1704–1710, 1981.

Takemura N: Successful long-term treatment of congenital nephrogenic diabetes insipidus in a dog, *J Small Anim Pract* 39:592–594, 1998.

Van Vonderen IK, Kooistra HS, de Bruijne JJ: [Evaluation of a test strip for the determination of urine specific gravity in the dog.], *Tijdschr Diergeneeskd* 120:400–402, 1995.

Van Vonderen IK, Kooistra HS, Rijnberk A: Intra- and interindividual variation in urine osmolality and urine specific gravity in healthy pet dogs of various ages, *J Vet Intern Med* 11:30–35, 1997.

Vilhardt H, Bie P: Antidiuretic response in conscious dogs following peroral administration of arginine vasopressin and its analogues, *Eur J Pharmacol* 93:201–204, 1983.

16 Miscellaneous Syndromes

Benign Essential (Idiopathic Renal) Hematuria In Dogs

INTRODUCTION AND PATHOPHYSIOLOGY

A. Bleeding originates in the kidney, but its cause is obscure.
B. The renal hemorrhage usually is unilateral, but occasionally it may be bilateral. Either kidney may be affected but some reports suggest the left side is affected more frequently. At initial presentation, hemorrhage typically originates from one kidney. Nephrectomy resolves the clinical signs, but hemorrhage can develop in the remaining kidney at a later time.

DIAGNOSIS

Signalment

1. Any age, but usually young dogs. Most affected dogs have been younger than 5 years of age.
2. Often large breed dogs (i.e., Weimaraners, boxers, and Labrador retrievers have been most commonly reported). Five of 15 reported cases have been immature (<1 yr).
3. Male or females may be affected.

History

1. The owner typically reports severe macroscopic hematuria that does not appear to cause any discomfort to the dog (i.e., no dysuria or increased frequency). Occasionally, however, a history of stranguria may be obtained.
2. Hematuria occurs throughout urination.
3. Blood clots may be present in the urine.

The typical history in benign idiopathic renal hematuria is one of painless, macroscopic hematuria.

4. Bleeding may be intermittent. It may occur for days or weeks and then disappear for months only to return at a later time.
5. There is no history of trauma.

PHYSICAL FINDINGS

A. No abnormalities are detected on physical examination.
B. No other sites of hemorrhage are detected and there is no petechiation or bruising.

LABORATORY FINDINGS

A. Complete blood count (CBC) may show moderate to severe regenerative anemia. The anemia may be acute (i.e., macrocytosis, polychromasia, reticulocytosis) or chronic with evidence of iron deficiency (i.e., microcytosis, hypochromasia). Mild to moderate leukocytosis may be present.

B. Serum creatinine and blood urea nitrogen (BUN) concentrations are normal and urine specific gravity shows moderately concentrated urine (i.e., renal function is normal).

C. Coagulation tests and platelet counts are normal.

D. Urine culture is negative.

IMAGING FINDINGS

A. Hydronephrosis and hydroureter have been observed by excretory urography on the affected side. These abnormalities are a result of ureteral obstruction by blood clots.

B. Filling defects caused by blood clots can be observed on contrast cystography.

C. Hydronephrosis, hydroureter, and blood clots in the bladder also may be observed on ultrasonography.

CYSTOSCOPY

A. In female dogs, cystoscopy allows identification of the affected side by observation of normal urine flowing from one ureteral opening as compared with blood coming from the contralateral ureteral opening (Figure 16-1). If cystoscopy is not available, the affected side can be identified at surgery by passing catheters into each of the ureteral openings in the trigone region and determining from which side the hemorrhage arises.

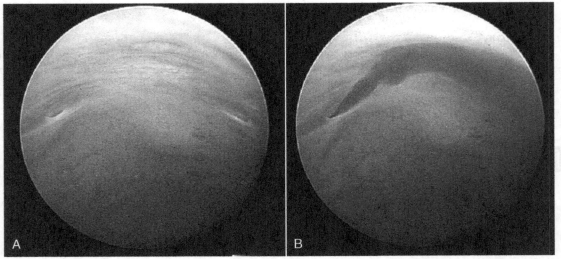

FIGURE 16-1 ■ **A,** Cystoscopic appearance of two normal ureteral openings in a dog before ureteral urine is observed. **B,** Cystoscopic appearance of hemorrhage from one ureteral orifice into the bladder and not the other in a dog with benign renal hematuria originating from one kidney. Furosemide can be given IV during the procedure to increase urine flow to allow visualization of hematuria.

GROSS AND MICROSCOPIC PATHOLOGY

A. Examination of removed kidneys shows blood clots in renal pelvis, ureter, or both. No other gross or histologic abnormalities typically are observed.

B. One affected dog was reported to have histologic evidence of chronic pyelitis, but urine culture was negative.

C. Abnormal small blood vessels below the urothelial surface of the renal pelvis were observed histologically in two affected dogs. These lesions resembled hemangiomas.

D. In one study, occasional small electron dense deposits were identified by electron microscopy in the glomerular mesangium in 5 of 9 affected dogs. The clinical relevance of these deposits is unknown.

E. In one other case, wedge-shaped mature infarcts were observed histologically in the resected kidney. These lesions were chronic (i.e., characterized by fibrosis) and not thought to have contributed to the renal hemorrhage.

DIFFERENTIAL DIAGNOSIS

A. Renal neoplasia.

B. Renal trauma.

C. Urolithiasis.

D. Renal vascular anomalies (e.g., renal telangiectasia of Welsh corgis).

TREATMENT

A. Nephrectomy should be considered if bleeding is documented to be unilateral and has been intractable and severe with development of severe anemia.

B. Nephrectomy resolves hematuria in dogs with unilateral renal hemorrhage, but some dogs have been reported to develop hemorrhage from the contralateral kidney some time after nephrectomy. Thus, the decision to perform nephrectomy should be weighed carefully.

C. Some affected dogs have intermittent periods of hemorrhage that are interspersed with long asymptomatic time periods. Thus, if there is no anemia or if anemia is mild, observation of the patient over time with monitoring of hematocrit may be preferable to nephrectomy.

D. In dogs with unilateral hemorrhage and severe anemia and in those with severe bilateral renal hemorrhage, symptomatic treatment with transfusions may be necessary.

E. Hydronephrosis or hydroureter due to obstruction of the distal ureter by a blood clot is another indication for surgery. In dogs with unilateral disease that have severe anemia and ureteral obstruction by blood clots, nephrectomy may be warranted.

F. Renal function typically does not deteriorate in affected dogs and consequently ureteral obstruction and severe anemia are the primary indications for nephrectomy in dogs with unilateral disease.

G. Selective infarction following catheterization of renal arteries is being explored as a less invasive treatment.(Dr. Larry Adams, Purdue University.)

PROGNOSIS

A. Good in dogs with severe bleeding due to unilateral disease that have undergone nephrectomy. The owner should be advised before surgery that hemorrhage from the contralateral kidney may occur in the future.

B. Fair to good in dogs with mild intermittent hematuria due to unilateral or bilateral disease with clinical monitoring. Long periods of remission may occur between episodes of hematuria.

C. Guarded in dogs with bilateral disease and severe hemorrhage.

Perinephric Pseudocysts (PNP)

INTRODUCTION AND PATHOPHYSIOLOGY

A. Perinephric diseases are uncommon and consist of perinephric abscesses, hematomas, and pseudocysts.

B. A PNP is a fluid-filled fibrous sac surrounding the kidney. A transudative fluid accumulates between the renal capsule and the renal parenchyma. The term *pseudocyst* is used because the structure does not have the epithelial lining typical of a true cyst. The cyst is attached at the renal hilus (most commonly) or poles (less commonly) of the kidney.

C. The transudative fluid within the pseudocyst is characterized by a low cell count and low total protein content. The urea nitrogen and creatinine concentrations of the cyst fluid are similar to those of the peripheral blood.

> ❗ Many cats with perinephric pseudocysts also have underlying mild to moderate chronic renal failure.

D. The pseudocysts may be unilateral (approximately 60%) or bilateral (approximately 40%). Either kidney may be affected. Cats with unilateral pseudocysts may later develop a pseudocyst in the contralateral kidney.

E. Many affected cats also have mild to moderate chronic renal failure (CRF).

F. Pseudocysts can be identified first with CRF occurring months to years later or cats can be diagnosed with CRF and develop pseudocysts 1 to 3 years later. Approximately 80% to 90% of cats with pseudocysts have at least mild CRF at the time of diagnosis. The relationship between PNP and CRF is unclear and may be incidental, as both are diseases of geriatric cats. Up to 25% to 30% of cats that live beyond 10 years of age are thought to develop CRF, and PNP are a rare complication even in this population of geriatric cats with CRF.

G. In rare instances, PNP have been associated with prior trauma or with an underlying renal neoplasm (e.g., renal adenocarcinoma). Most are idiopathic, however.

DIAGNOSIS

Signalment

1. Typically, very old (geriatric) cats are affected (mean age 9 years). Approximately 80% are older than 8 years of age at presentation.

2. Early reports suggested male cats (80%) were more commonly affected than females (20%), but later studies indicated that both males (60%) and females (40%) may be affected.

3. No breed predilection.

History

1. Progressive abdominal distension over weeks to months.

2. Often affected cats have minimal clinical signs and the first abnormality detected by the owner is the abdominal distension.

3. Systemic signs of illness if present often are related to the presence and severity of accompanying CRF.
   a. Polyuria (PU), polydipsia (PD), or both.
   b. Lethargy.
   c. Weight loss.
   d. Anorexia.
   e. Vomiting.
4. Occasionally, vomiting has been reported in cats with PNP without evidence of CRF, and it is speculated that pressure on or displacement of abdominal organs by the pseudocyst may lead to vomiting.
5. Some owners believe their cats are in pain based on increased vocalizations or difficulty finding a comfortable resting posture.

PHYSICAL FINDINGS

A. Abdominal distension.
B. A large mass or masses can be detected on abdominal palpation. It typically seems that one or both kidneys are extremely enlarged (i.e., 8 to 12 cm). It is impossible to differentiate a pseudocyst from renomegaly on the basis of palpation alone.
C. In cats with unilateral pseudocysts, the contralateral kidney may be small and irregular suggesting the presence of chronic renal disease.
D. Other physical findings (e.g., emaciation, dehydration, poor hair coat) are attributable to the presence of CRF.
E. Systemic blood pressure should be measured because hypertension is common in cats with CRF.
F. Presence of a thyroid nodule should prompt evaluation for hyperthyroidism but CRF and PNP are systemic nonthyroidal illnesses that can cause serum thyroxine concentrations to be only mildly increased or within the normal reference range. Pertechnetate scanning may be indicated to definitively diagnose hyperthyroidism.

LABORATORY FINDINGS

A. The hemogram usually is normal. Nonregenerative anemia may be present if advanced CRF is present.
B. Serum biochemistry often shows evidence of mild to moderate CRF (i.e., mild to moderate increases in BUN and serum creatinine concentrations). Occasionally CRF may be severe.
C. Urinalysis shows urine specific gravity (USG) in the isosthenuric range (average USG of 1.016).
D. Results of cytological analysis of fluid from the cysts almost always are typical of a transudate or, rarely, of a modified transudate.
   1. Cell count <400/μL.
   2. Specific gravity 1.010 to 1.034.
   3. Protein concentration <2.5 g/dL.
   4. BUN or creatinine concentration similar to or slightly higher than that of peripheral blood.
E. Urinary tract infection (UTI) may be present in 40% or more of cats with PNP, and urine culture should be performed routinely as lower urinary tract signs typically are not present.
F. Bacterial culture of the cyst fluid yields no growth.

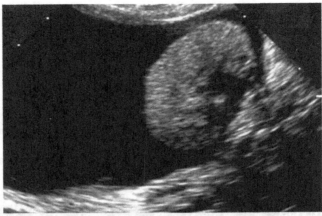

FIGURE 16-2 ■ Ultrasound appearance of perinephric pseudocyst. Note anechoic fluid surrounding the kidney.

IMAGING FINDINGS

A. Plain abdominal radiographs demonstrate what appears to be a severely enlarged kidney or kidneys.

B. Excretory urography can be used to identify the PNP.

C. Abdominal ultrasonography is the diagnostic imaging procedure of choice and allows rapid diagnosis of PNP (i.e., the kidney is seen to be separated from the renal capsule and surrounded by anechoic fluid; the cyst typically occupies an area twice the size of the kidney; Figure 16-2). The presence of perinephric fluid of mixed echogenicity should prompt concern about the possibility of a perinephric abscess, perinephric hematoma, or neoplasia. Occasionally, cats with renal lymphoma will have small accumulations of perinephric fluid, as well as hypoechoic nodules in the renal parenchyma.

DIFFERENTIAL DIAGNOSIS

A. Differential diagnosis includes other perinephric diseases (e.g., perinephric abscess or hematoma) and causes of renomegaly (e.g., hydronephrosis, polycystic kidney disease, renal lymphoma, granulomatous nephritis due to feline infectious peritonitis, pyonephrosis).

TREATMENT

A. Resection of the cyst wall is the most definitive treatment and allows any additional fluid accumulation into the peritoneum to be reabsorbed into the general circulation (Figure 16-3). In some cases, fluid accumulation may be mild to moderate and nonprogressive with minimal or no apparent discomfort to the cat. In such situations, medical surveillance and periodic ultrasound-guided drainage of the cyst as necessary may be a reasonable approach to management. In extremely rare instances, fluid accumulation may be so severe that detectable ascites may occur after cyst wall resection.

! Resection of the cyst wall is the most definitive treatment for perinephric pseudocysts. The kidney on the affected side must be preserved.

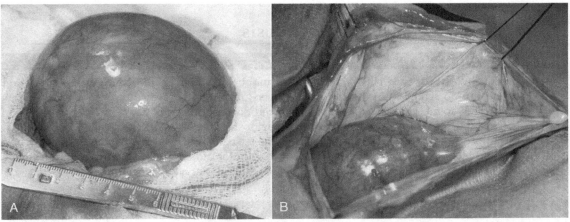

FIGURE 16-3 ■ Appearance of perinephric pseudocyst at surgery. The perinephric pseudocyst before incision (**A**) and the opened cyst after fluid has been drained (**B**) are shown. Note presence of underlying chronic renal disease in the kidney itself.

B. Do not remove the kidney on the affected side. Most of these cats have mild to moderate CRF with interstitial fibrosis and lymphoplasmacytic interstitial nephritis. Removal of one kidney predisposes to rapid progression of renal disease in the contralateral kidney.

C. The pseudocysts may be drained under ultrasound guidance but fluid re-accumulates over the course of weeks to months. Drainage of the perinephric cyst has not been shown to improve glomerular filtration rate (GFR) in the affected kidney. Rarely, repeated ultrasound-guided drainage of a PNP will be associated with resolution of the cyst.

PROGNOSIS

A. Most cats respond well to surgical removal of the cyst wall, as long as the kidney is preserved.

B. The limiting factor in prognosis appears to be the rate of progression of the underlying chronic renal disease.

Renal Tubular Acidosis (RTA)

INTRODUCTION

A. RTA is uncommonly recognized in small animal practice.

B. It is characterized by hyperchloremic (normal anion gap) metabolic acidosis caused by either decreased bicarbonate reabsorption (proximal RTA) or defective acid excretion (distal RTA) in the presence of a normal GFR.

❗ Unexplained hyperchloremic metabolic acidosis should prompt consideration of renal tubular acidosis.

Distal (Type I) Renal Tubular Acidosis

PATHOPHYSIOLOGY

A. In distal (classic or type 1) RTA, the urine cannot be maximally acidified because of impaired hydrogen ion secretion in the collecting ducts, and urine pH typically is above 6.0, despite moderately to markedly decreased plasma bicarbonate concentration.

B. Increased urine pH (>6.0) in the presence of acidosis is the hallmark of distal RTA.

C. Mutations in cytosolic carbonic anhydrase, the basolateral Cl^-/HCO_3^- anion exchanger, and luminal H^+-ATPase that affect function of the α-intercalated cells in the renal tubules have been associated with inherited forms of distal renal tubular acidosis in humans.

DIAGNOSIS

A. UTI by a urease positive organism (e.g., *Proteus* sp, *Staphylococcus aureus*) must be ruled out before considering distal RTA.

B. Urinary net acid excretion is decreased, but bicarbonaturia usually is mild because urinary bicarbonate concentration is only 1 to 3 mEq/L in the pH range of 6.0 to 6.5.

C. Urinary fractional excretion of HCO_3^- is normal (<5%) in distal RTA when plasma HCO_3^- concentration is increased to normal by alkali administration.

D. A diagnosis of distal RTA can be confirmed by an ammonium chloride tolerance test during which urine pH is monitored (using a pH meter) before and at hourly intervals for 5 hours after oral administration of 0.2 g/kg NH_4Cl. Under such conditions, the urine pH of normal dogs decreased to a minimum value of 5.16 at 4 hours after administration of ammonium chloride.

E. Nephrolithiasis (usually calcium phosphate stones), nephrocalcinosis (resulting from alkaline urine pH and decreased urinary citrate concentration), bone demineralization (resulting from loss of bone buffer stores during chronic acidosis), and urinary potassium wasting with hypokalemia are features of distal RTA in human patients.

F. Distal RTA has been reported in two cats with pyelonephritis caused by *Escherichia coli*. Clinical signs included PU, PD, anorexia, lethargy, enlarged kidneys, and isosthenuria. In one cat, urine pH was 5.0 at the time pyelonephritis was first diagnosed, but distal RTA was documented at a later time by the presence of hyperchloremic metabolic acidosis, alkaline urine pH, and failure to lower urine pH after oral administration of NH_4Cl. Findings were similar for the other cat, but hyperphosphaturia and persistent hypokalemia also were detected.

TREATMENT

A. The amount of alkali required to correct the acidosis in human patients with distal RTA is variable but typically less than that required in proximal RTA. The required dosage of alkali in distal RTA may be as little as 1 mEq/kg/day (i.e., that required to offset daily endogenous acid production) or more than 2 to 4 mEq/kg/day.

B. A combination of potassium and sodium citrate (depending on potassium balance) may be the preferred source of alkali.

C. Cats with distal RTA should be investigated for the possibility of UTI (specifically, pyelonephritis).

Proximal (Type 2) Renal Tubular Acidosis

PATHOPHYSIOLOGY

A. In proximal (type 2) RTA, renal reabsorption of bicarbonate is markedly reduced and urinary fractional excretion of HCO_3^- is increased (>15%) when plasma HCO_3^- concentration is increased to normal.

B. Bicarbonaturia is absent and urine pH is appropriately low when metabolic acidosis is present and plasma HCO_3^- concentration is decreased, because distal acidifying ability is intact.

C. When plasma HCO_3^- concentration is decreased, the filtered load of HCO_3^- is reduced, and almost all of the filtered HCO_3^- is reabsorbed in the distal tubules, despite the presence of the proximal tubular defect. Thus, proximal RTA can be viewed as a "self-limiting" disorder in which plasma HCO_3^- stabilizes at a lower than normal concentration after the filtered load falls sufficiently that distal HCO_3^- reabsorption can maintain plasma HCO_3^- at a new but lower steady state concentration.

D. Mutations in renal tubular transport proteins such as the electrogenic basolateral $Na^+/3HCO_3^-$ co-transporter and one of the five forms of the luminal Na^+/H^+ antiporter have been implicated in the pathogenesis of inherited forms of proximal renal tubular acidosis in humans.

E. Other abnormalities of proximal tubular function typically accompany impaired HCO_3^- reabsorption in proximal RTA, and these include defects in glucose, phosphate, sodium, potassium, uric acid, and amino acid reabsorption. This combination of proximal tubular defects is known as Fanconi syndrome (see later).

F. Serum potassium concentration usually is normal in affected human patients at the time of diagnosis, but alkali therapy may precipitate hypokalemia and aggravate urinary potassium wasting, presumably by increasing distal delivery of sodium and HCO_3^-.

DIAGNOSIS

A. The diagnosis of proximal RTA is made by finding an acid urine pH (<5.5 to 6.0) in the presence of hyperchloremic (normal anion gap) metabolic acidosis and normal GFR but increased urine pH (>6.0) and increased urinary fractional excretion of HCO_3^- (>15%) after plasma HCO_3^- concentration has been increased to normal by alkali administration.

! A high urine pH is expected in distal RTA but urine pH is low in proximal RTA in the presence of marked acidosis and low serum bicarbonate concentration.

B. If present, the detection of other defects in proximal tubular function (e.g., glucosuria with normal blood glucose concentration) establishes the diagnosis.

TREATMENT

A. Correction of metabolic acidosis by alkali therapy is more difficult in proximal RTA than in distal RTA because of the marked bicarbonaturia that occurs when plasma HCO_3^- concentration is increased to normal.

B. Alkali dosages in excess of 10 mEq/kg/day may be required to correct the plasma HCO_3^- concentration, and such therapy may result in hypokalemia. Thus potassium citrate may be the preferred source of alkali.

! The dosage of bicarbonate to control distal RTA usually is modest but the dosage required to control proximal RTA is very high.

Type 4 Renal Tubular Acidosis

I. Hyporeninemic hypoaldosteronism, characterized by hyperkalemia with decreased plasma renin and aldosterone concentrations, occurs in some human patients, notably those with diabetes mellitus who also have mild to moderate renal insufficiency.

II. The hyperchloremic (normal anion gap) metabolic acidosis observed in these patients has been called type 4 RTA.

III. This syndrome has not been characterized in veterinary medicine but should be considered in dogs and cats with hyperkalemia and mild to moderate hyperchloremic metabolic acidosis after hypoadrenoco rticism has been ruled out by an adrenocorticotropic hormone (ACTH) response test.

IV. The diagnosis may be established by finding an inappropriately decreased plasma aldosterone concentration in the presence of hyperkalemia.

Fanconi Syndrome

INTRODUCTION

A. Multiple renal tubular reabsorptive defects resembling Fanconi syndrome have been reported in young Basenji dogs.

B. The renal tubular disorder in affected Basenjis is thought to be the result of a metabolic or membrane defect that affects sodium transport and secondarily affects transport of other solutes that are cotransported with sodium in the proximal tubule (e.g., glucose, phosphate, amino acids, bicarbonate).

C. In one study, brush border membranes isolated from Basenji dogs with Fanconi syndrome had decreased sodium-dependent glucose transport but no abnormality of cystine uptake despite the observed reabsorptive defect for cystine.

DIAGNOSIS

A. Fanconi syndrome may affect 10% to 15% of Basenji dogs in the United States.

B. Most affected Basenji dogs are diagnosed between 4 and 8 years of age.

C. Clinical findings include PU, PD, weight loss, dehydration, and weakness.

D. Affected Basenji dogs have abnormal fractional reabsorption of glucose, bicarbonate, phosphate, sodium, potassium, and urate, and isolated cystinuria or generalized aminoaciduria.

E. Hyperchloremic (normal anion gap) acidosis of variable severity may be present.

F. The finding of normal blood glucose concentration and glucosuria in a Basenji dog is presumptive evidence of the diagnosis. Confirmation requires identification of amino aciduria. This can be accomplished by identifying cystine in the urine by an inexpensive screening test (available at the Medical Genetics Division of the School of Veterinary Medicine, University of Pennsylvania, Philadelphia) or by quantification of individual amino acids in the urine (an expensive procedure with limited availability).

❗ The finding of glucosuria with normal blood glucose concentration is not diagnostic of Fanconi syndrome. The presence of other abnormalities of tubular reabsorption (e.g., amino aciduria) must be documented.

G. Aminoaciduria and proteinuria are not synonymous. The finding of proteinuria is not diagnostic of Fanconi syndrome.

H. Hypokalemia may be observed late in the course of the disease.
I. Defective urinary concentrating ability leads to isosthenuria or hyposthenuria.
J. GFR may be normal initially but decreased later in the course of the disease.
K. A distinctive histopathologic renal lesion is hyperchromatic karyomegaly of renal tubular cells.
L. Fanconi syndrome has been observed sporadically in other breeds and has been reported in association with administration of some drugs.
1. In one case, Fanconi syndrome developed in association with primary hypoparathyroidism and resolved after treatment with calcium and calcitriol. Rickets in growing children and osteomalacia in adults are features of Fanconi syndrome in human patients that usually are not observed in affected dogs. However, congenital Fanconi syndrome and renal dysplasia were associated with histologic features of rickets in two Border terriers. The skeletal abnormalities in one of the affected dogs resolved after treatment with calcitriol and potassium phosphate.
2. Transient Fanconi syndrome and proximal renal tubular acidosis also have been reported in a dog with high liver enzyme activities, and toxin exposure was considered as a possible explanation.
3. Transient Fanconi syndrome has been reported in small breed dogs that have consumed chicken-based jerky treats manufactured in China. Clinical signs include vomiting, diarrhea, and lethargy. Liver enzymes are mildly elevated, with severe hypokalemia, acidosis, glucosuria, and granular casts in the urine. Affected animals are not consistently azotemic. Treatment is supportive, and most appear to recover, though some develop more permanent renal damage.

TREATMENT

A. A high quality diet that maintains good nutrition is recommended because affected dogs have aminoaciduria of variable severity.
B. Correction of metabolic acidosis by alkali therapy may be difficult because of the marked bicarbonaturia that occurs when plasma HCO_3^- concentration is increased to normal in patients with proximal RTA (as occurs in Fanconi syndrome).
C. Alkali dosages in excess of 10 mEq/kg/day may be required to correct the plasma HCO_3^- concentration, and such therapy may result in hypokalemia. Thus, potassium citrate may be preferred over sodium bicarbonate as a source of alkali in dogs with poor response to bicarbonate or those that develop hypokalemia.
D. Because of the presence of renal glucosuria, the dog should be monitored for development of UTI, and UTI that occurs should be treated with appropriate antibiotic therapy.

PROGNOSIS

A. Fanconi syndrome is due to a genetic disorder of renal tubular transport that cannot be corrected.
B. Its severity and rate of progression seem to vary considerably among affected Basenji dogs, making it difficult to give an accurate prognosis in an individual dog.
C. Careful management of metabolic acidosis, hypokalemia, UTI, and the patient's nutritional status offers the best chance of long-term survival.
D. Death usually results from acute renal failure and papillary necrosis or acute pyelonephritis.

Idiopathic Hypercalcemia (IHC) Of Cats

INTRODUCTION AND PATHOPHYSIOLOGY

> **!** IHC is the most common cause of ionized hypercalcemia in cats today.

A. Since 1990, unexplained hypercalcemia has been increasingly noted as an incidental finding on serum biochemistry profiles of cats. It is now the most common cause of ionized hypercalcemia in cats.

B. In early reports, hypercalcemia in cats was associated with calcium oxalate urolithiasis.

C. Dietary acidification and metabolic acidosis may increase glomerular filtration of calcium, decrease renal tubular reabsorption of calcium, and promote skeletal mobilization of calcium.

D. One hypothesis about the relationship between hypercalcemia and calcium oxalate urolithiasis in cats is that feeding magnesium-restricted, acidifying diets for the control of struvite urolithiasis is associated with increased bone turnover of calcium, hypercalcemia, hypercalciuria, and oxalate urolithiasis.

E. However, many cats are fed acidifying diets and presumably relatively few develop hypercalcemia and calcium oxalate urolithiasis. Consequently, other factors such as hyperabsorption of calcium or oxalate from the gastrointestinal tract or renal tubular dysfunction characterized by hypercalciuria or hyperoxaluria may contribute to development of hypercalcemia and calcium oxalate urolithiasis in susceptible cats.

F. IHC does not appear to be due to excessive parathyroid hormone (PTH), 25-hydroxyvitamin D, or calcitriol concentrations in most cats. Ionized magnesium concentrations are typically normal and thus PTH secretion does not seem to have been inhibited by alterations in serum ionized magnesium concentration.

DIAGNOSIS

Signalment

1. Cats of any age may be affected (mean age 10 years; range, 0.5 to 20 years).
2. No sex predilection.
3. Any breed and mixed breed cats may be affected. Long-haired cats may be over-represented (27% of affected cats in one retrospective study of 427 cats).

History

1. In a review of 427 cats with IHC, 46% had no clinical signs, 18% had mild weight loss with no other clinical signs, 6% had inflammatory bowel disease, 5% had chronic constipation, 4% had a history of vomiting, and 1% were anorexic. Uroliths were observed in 15%, with calcium oxalate stone identified in 10% of cases. Other clinical signs include dysuria, inappropriate urinations, hematuria, and lethargy.
2. PU and PD are not commonly reported in hypercalcemic cats.
3. Often there is a history of being fed an acidifying diet for control of struvite urolithiasis. However acidifying diets are widely fed to cats, and not all cats fed acidifying diets develop hypercalcemia. Also, not all cats with hypercalcemia have a history of having been fed an acidifying diet.

4. There is no history of exposure to excess vitamin D, however, owners should be questioned regarding the use of supplements and exposure to plants, antipsoriasis creams and other human anti-aging creams that can contain high concentrations of vitamins D and A.

PHYSICAL FINDINGS

A. Often unremarkable.
B. Kidneys may be normal-sized or small and irregular.

LABORATORY FINDINGS

A. Serum total calcium concentrations are mildly to moderately increased (average, 12.5 mg/dL).
B. Serum ionized calcium concentrations are moderately increased (average, 1.7 mmol/L or 6.8 mg/dL).
C. Serum PTH concentrations are in the lower part of the reference range (mean 1.1 pmol/L; reference range 0 to 4 pmol/L).
D. Serum parathyroid hormone-related polypeptide (PTHrP) concentrations are low (< 1.0 pmol/L)
E. Ionized magnesium concentration is within normal limits (mean 0.6 mmol/L; reference range 0.43 to 0.70 mmol/L).
F. Serum 25-hydroxyvitamin D concentrations are normal or slightly high (mean, 96 nmol/L; range, 22 to 198 nmol/L; reference range 65 to 170 nmol/L). Unlike calcitriol, serum 25-hydroxyvitamin D concentrations are not closely regulated and variability most likely reflects differences in dietary vitamin D intake.
G. Serum calcitriol concentration has been determined in a small number of cats with IHC, with a mean of 45 pmol/L (reference range 50 to 100 pmol/L).
H. Serum phosphorus concentrations are normal.
I. Venous blood gas analysis generally is normal in affected cats.
J. BUN and serum creatinine concentrations are normal in most cats with IHC.
   1. In most cats with IHC, CRF either does not develop during the course of their disease or develops after the onset of hypercalcemia. Thus, CRF is unlikely to be the cause of IHC.
   2. Occasionally, IHC and CRF with azotemia are identified concurrently.
   3. Occasionally, cats with IHC will develop CRF and azotemia 1 to 4 years later. Consequently, the role of hypercalcemia in producing renal injury in cats with IHC warrants further investigation.
K. Urinalysis findings.
   1. Urine of affected cats usually is moderately concentrated (mean, 1.036; range, 1.012 to 1.060).
   2. Urine pH ranges from 5.5 to 7.0.
   3. Hematuria occasionally is identified but pyuria is rare. Hematuria may be a consequence of traumatic cystocentesis in some cats in which urine has been collected by this method.
   4. Struvite or calcium oxalate crystalluria may be observed on urine sediment examination.
L. In the few cases in which it has been evaluated, the fractional excretion of calcium in the urine has been increased (range, 0.8 to 2.8%; normal, <0.2%). It is possible that this increase in urinary calcium excretion reflects an appropriate physiologic response to hypercalcemia.
M. No evidence of malignancy as a cause of hypercalcemia has been found in affected cats despite extensive diagnostic evaluations (i.e., negative feline leukemia virus [FeLV] and feline immunodeficiency virus [FIV] enzyme-linked immunosorbent assay [ELISA] test results, normal bone marrow cytology).

IMAGING FINDINGS

A. Abdominal radiographs and ultrasonography show normal-sized (67%) or small kidneys (33%).
B. Radiopaque uroliths may be observed in the kidneys, ureter, or bladder of more than 50% of affected cats on abdominal radiography. When analyzed, calculi have been composed of calcium oxalate.
C. Abdominal ultrasonographic findings include nephrocalcinosis and renal pelvic dilatation in some cats.
D. Ultrasonography of the neck has been normal in cats in which this procedure has been performed.

DIFFERENTIAL DIAGNOSIS

A. Hypercalcemia of malignancy (e.g., lymphoma, squamous cell carcinoma, multiple myeloma).
B. Primary hyperparathyroidism. Cats with this disorder should have decreased serum phosphorus concentration and increased serum PTH concentration. In many instances, a cervical mass may be detected on physical examination or ultrasonography.
C. Vitamin D toxicosis (e.g., rodenticide ingestion, excessive calcitriol administration, ingestion of antipsoriasis creams or other topical products containing vitamin D, diet formulation errors, or excessive ingestion of supplements). Serum phosphorus concentration is typically increased.
D. Calcitriol synthesis by mononuclear cells in cats with granulomatous disease.

TREATMENT

A. Increased dietary fiber has decreased serum calcium in some cats. Some clinicians have had success with low fat, high fiber diets such as Hill's w/d that have been used in an attempt to reduce the availability of calcium for intestinal absorption. However, most pet food manufacturers increase the quantity of calcium in high-fiber diets to offset this decreased absorption.

! Conventional treatment for IHC in cats consists of a high-fiber diet and oral administration of glucocorticoids if necessary.

B. Feeding veterinary renal diets may result in normocalcemia, possibly due to the reduced calcium content of these diets. Veterinary renal diets are alkalinizing, or at least less acidifying than maintenance diets, and are generally low in calcium and phosphorus. Renal diets have very different formulations compared with maintenance diets, and it is possible that other dietary factors play a role.
C. Glucocorticoids (prednisone, 5 to 20 mg PO per cat per day) have been effective in decreasing serum total and ionized calcium concentrations in many affected cats. In some cats, normocalcemia can be maintained after tapering and discontinuing treatment with glucocorticoids after an extended period of time.
    1. Glucocorticoids exert a modulating effect in hypercalcemia by reducing bone resorption, decreasing intestinal absorption of calcium, and increasing renal excretion of calcium.
    2. The increased urinary excretion of calcium could enhance the formation of calcium-containing calculi. However, the filtered load of calcium decreases as serum ionized calcium concentration decreases, which offsets the formation of calculi.

   3. Some cats become refractory to glucocorticoid therapy with a return of ionized hypercalcemia.
   D. Surgical removal of two to three of four parathyroid glands has resulted in only very transient improvement (i.e., a few days) of hypercalcemia. Excised parathyroid glands have shown no evidence of hyperplasia or neoplasia (e.g., adenoma, adenocarcinoma).
   E. If dietary modification and prednisone therapy are unsuccessful, bisphosphonates treatment should be considered. Pamidronate (1.3 to 2.0 mg/kg) diluted in 0.9% sodium chloride has been infused intravenously over at least 2 hours. Fluids should be given before, during, and after the infusion of pamidronate. In most cats, however, oral administration of bisphosphonates is adequate.
   F. Beneficial effects of chronic administration of SC fluids or furosemide have not been evaluated.
   G. In the future, treatment with other bisphosphonates (e.g., alendronate) or calciotropic agents (e.g., cinacalcet) may be possible if efficacy and safety can be documented in cats with IHC. Preliminary results from a small number of IHC cats treated with Alendronate for 6 months showed safety and efficacy. (Dr. Brian Hardy.)

PROGNOSIS

   A. Some cats with IHC may survive many years with limited consequences.
   B. Affected cats are likely at increased risk of calcium oxalate urolithiasis and its complications.
   C. CRF may occur in some affected cats but the relationship of IHC and CRF is unclear.

Hyperthyroidism And The Kidney

I. The clinical evaluation and management of geriatric cats with concurrent hyperthyroidism and chronic renal disease (CRD) are challenging.

> **!** Hyperthyroidism masks the presence of CRD, and CRD is a nonthyroidal illness that lowers serum thyroxine concentration and confounds the diagnosis of hyperthyroidism.

   A. The tendency of nonthyroidal illness (CRD) to decrease serum thyroxine concentration makes the diagnosis of hyperthyroidism difficult in a cat with CRD.
   B. At the same time, the presence of hyperthyroidism in a cat with CRD increases GFR, which decreases serum creatinine concentration and masks CRD.

PATHOPHYSIOLOGY

   A. Hyperthyroidism increases cardiac output and decreases peripheral vascular resistance, leading to increased renal plasma flow (RPF) and increased GFR.
   B. Increased GFR reduces serum creatinine concentration whereas increased body turnover of protein may increase BUN concentration slightly.
   C. Mild proteinuria may occur as a consequence of increased GFR, especially if accompanied by intrarenal or systemic hypertension.
   D. Reduction in muscle mass decreases total body stores of potassium, and muscle weakness due to hypokalemia may occur in some hyperthyroid cats before or during therapy. This may result from episodic translocation of potassium from extracellular to intracellular fluid.
   E. Progressive weight loss and reduction in muscle mass also contribute to lower serum creatinine concentrations in hyperthyroid cats which, in turn, may mask underlying renal disease in some affected cats.

F. Observed increases in serum creatinine concentration after treatment of hyperthyroidism may reflect unmasking of preexisting renal dysfunction, a decrease in GFR with correction of the hyperthyroid state, weight gain with increased muscle mass or some combination of these factors.

G. Whether the commonly observed simultaneous occurrence of hyperthyroidism and CRD in older cats is coincidental or the result of some pathophysiologic interaction between these two disorders is an intriguing but presently unanswered question.

H. Whereas most emphasis has been placed on the potentially adverse effects of treatment of hyperthyroidism on renal function, it also is possible that hyperthyroidism may contribute to development of CRD in older cats. In clinically normal cats, nearly 60% of renal perfusion pressure is transmitted to the glomerular capillary bed. Systemic hypertension may be present in some cats with hyperthyroidism. If failure of autoregulation occurs, a substantial portion of systemic hypertension may be transmitted to glomeruli, resulting in intraglomerular hypertension and glomerular hyperfiltration. These factors are recognized as contributing to glomerular sclerosis and progression of renal disease in rats.

I. The possible pathophysiologic relationship between hyperthyroidism and CRD raises important questions about the treatment of hyperthyroidism. It could be argued that reducing serum thyroxine concentrations in older cats with mild hyperthyroidism and CRD should be avoided because treatment may reduce GFR and allow emergence of azotemia and uremia. On the other hand, if increased GFR results in glomerular hyperfiltration in hyperthyroid cats, it may contribute to progression of renal disease. If so, hyperthyroidism in older cats actually may predispose to CKD, and early effective treatment of hyperthyroidism may be important to prevent pathophysiologic changes in the kidney that could lead to progressive renal disease.

DIAGNOSIS

A. Ideally, GFR should be measured in affected cats. The presence of lower than normal GFR in a hyperthyroid cat indicates increased risk for adverse clinical outcome after treatment of hyperthyroidism. Unfortunately, methods for measurement of GFR are not widely available or practical. Consequently, careful evaluation of routine serum chemistry and urinalysis results must suffice in most instances.

B. Cats with normal BUN, serum creatinine, and serum electrolyte concentrations, and highly concentrated urine are at minimal risk for adverse effects on renal function after treatment of hyperthyroidism. Serum creatinine concentration, however, should be evaluated in light of the cat's body condition and muscle mass. An emaciated cat is expected to have a somewhat lower serum creatinine concentration than a well-muscled cat with similar renal function. Availability of previous serum creatinine determinations in the cat in question may be helpful in making this evaluation.

C. Occasionally, cats with considerable renal disease retain considerable renal concentrating ability. Consequently, the clinician cannot assume that mild azotemia with concentrated urine in a geriatric cat necessarily is prerenal in origin.

D. In most cats, abdominal palpation of the kidneys is easily performed and yields considerable information about the presence or absence of renal disease. Small, firm, irregular kidneys suggest CKD.

E. Renal ultrasonography should be considered if questions remain about the cat's renal function after physical examination and routine laboratory testing.

F. More difficult yet is establishing a diagnosis of hyperthyroidism in geriatric cats with CRD. Chronic renal disease is one of several nonthyroidal illnesses that may decrease serum thyroxine concentrations to within the normal range, making the diagnosis of concurrent hyperthyroidism difficult. The extent to which serum thyroxine concentration is decreased in cats with nonthyroidal illness is related more to the severity than to the nature of the illness. The clinician must therefore rely on the presence of a palpable thyroid nodule and use alternate diagnostic methods (e.g., T3 suppression test, pertechnetate thyroid imaging) to establish a diagnosis of hyperthyroidism in some cats with CRD.

G. The ability to consistently palpate a thyroid nodule on physical examination is a very practical and valuable clinical tool, and its importance in diagnosis should not be ignored.

TREATMENT

A. The effects of methimazole on thyroid function are rapidly reversible, and it is prudent initially to treat azotemic hyperthyroid cats with methimazole until it can be determined whether correction of the hyperthyroid state will worsen azotemia and result in uremia.

> ❗ A methimazole challenge should be performed in any hyperthyroid cat that has any evidence whatsoever of underlying renal disease.

B. Affected cats can be treated with 2.5 mg methimazole PO every 24 hours for 7 to 10 days. If routine tests of renal function remain unchanged, the dosage is increased to 2.5 mg PO every 12 hours. If renal function tests remain stable after an additional 7 to 10 days, the dosage is increased to 7.5 mg PO divided into 2 doses and administered every 12 hours. If renal function tests remain stable after additional 7 to 10 days, the dosage of methimazole is increased to 5 mg PO every 12 hours. If the cat's renal function remains stable for several weeks on a dosage of methimazole that renders the cat euthyroid (i.e., serum thyroxine concentration of approximately 1.0 mg/dL), other treatments (e.g., surgery, radioiodine) may be considered. This procedure is referred to as a *methimazole challenge*. If renal function deteriorates at any point during this protocol, methimazole treatment is discontinued and the cat's clinical condition reassessed. Some increase in serum creatinine and BUN concentrations after correction of the hyperthyroid state may be an unavoidable consequence of effective treatment of hyperthyroidism in some cats. It is unknown what, if any, increase in serum creatinine concentration would be safe during treatment of feline hyperthyroidism. Many older cats with serum creatinine concentrations of 2.0 to 3.0 mg/dL do very well clinically over a course of several years. Provided their underlying CKD is nonprogressive or slowly progressive, cats with serum creatinine concentrations in this range seem to be at minimal risk for adverse clinical outcome.

WHAT DO WE DO?

- Use cystoscopy in female dogs with idiopathic renal hematuria to determine whether the left or right kidney is responsible for the hematuria.
- Drain perinephric pseudocysts and surgically remove the capsule, but preserve the kidney.
- Suspect and evaluate the animal for renal tubular acidosis if unexplained hyperchloremic metabolic acidosis is identified on serum biochemistry. Use blood gas analysis to facilitate the diagnosis.
- Use the University of Pennsylvania Division of Medical Genetics urine test for cystine as a method to identify dogs suspected of Fanconi syndrome based on presence of glucosuria with normal blood glucose and hyperchloremic metabolic acidosis.
- Use repeated determinations of both ionized and total serum calcium concentrations as well as calciotrophic hormones (e.g., PTH, calcitriol, 25-hydroxycholecaliferol, PTHrP) to identify cats with IHC. Evaluate cats with IHC for renal disease and the presence of urolithiasis.
- Perform a methimazole challenge in any hyperthyroid cat suspected of having underlying CKD before making a decision about radioiodine therapy.

THOUGHTS FOR THE FUTURE

- Increased usage of interventional radiology procedures will allow identification and ablation of small renal vessels responsible for hematuria in some dogs with idiopathic renal hematuria.
- Ultrasound-guided drainage of perinephric pseudocysts will be increasingly used as a less invasive procedure. Cysts can be expected to refill over weeks to months. Placement of a peritoneal-vascular shunt can be considered for cats that develop ascites from fluid accumulation even after the cyst capsule has been resected surgically.
- More animals with hyporeninemic hypoaldosteronism (type 4 RTA) will be identified as target populations (e.g., patients with diabetes mellitus and renal impairment) are evaluated.
- Mutations in cell membrane carrier proteins responsible for renal tubular acidosis will be identified.
- Mutations responsible for Fanconi syndrome in dogs will be identified.
- Newer drugs such as the calcimimetic cinacalcet and the bisphosphonate alendronate will be increasingly used to treat IHC in cats if safety can be demonstrated.
- Better understanding of the bioavailability of topically administered methimazole will facilitate medical treatment of cats with chronic renal failure and hyperthyroidism.

COMMON MISCONCEPTIONS

- The offending kidney always should be removed in dogs with idiopathic renal hematuria. Actually, in some dogs, hematuria may be intermittent with long periods of normalcy between episodes. The kidney should be removed only if the hematuria is severe and protracted with consequent severe blood loss anemia.
- Clinical signs in cats with perinephric pseudocysts usually are directly attributable to the cysts themselves. Actually, the presenting clinical signs often are a result of the underlying chronic renal disease and failure present in many cats with perinephric pseudocysts.
- The urine pH must be high to diagnosis RTA. A high pH is typical of distal RTA, but urine pH is appropriately low in animals with proximal RTA by the time metabolic acidosis is severe and the filtered load of bicarbonate is low.
- Proteinuria in the presence of glucosuria with normal blood glucose concentration is diagnostic of Fanconi syndrome. Proteinuria and amino aciduria are *not* synonymous! Diagnosis of Fanconi syndrome requires the presence of amino acids (e.g., cystine) in the urine, not protein.
- Malignancy is the most common cause of hypercalcemia in cats. Actually, IHC is the most common cause of hypercalcemia in cats. Hypercalcemia of malignancy is much less common in cats than in dogs.
- Hyperthyroidism in cats with chronic renal failure should not be treated because the increased renal blood flow and GFR are maintaining renal function. Actually, severe hyperthyroidism is a serious multisystemic disorder and it is possible that the increased GFR may contribute to progression of CKD by glomerular hyperfiltration. Thus, a "methimazole challenge" to determine how much control of hyperthyroidism can be safely achieved in a cat with CKD is warranted.

SUMMARY TIPS

- Painless macroscopic hematuria (often pronounced) without obvious explanation on routine diagnostic evaluation suggests the possibility of idiopathic renal hematuria.
- Make every attempt possible to save the kidney at the time of surgery to drain perinephric pseudocysts and resect the cyst wall. Many of these cats have underlying chronic renal disease and nephrectomy will hasten progression of renal disease in the contralateral kidney.
- Ultrasound examination is the most direct and simple way to diagnose perinephric pseudocysts in cats.

- Titrate the dosage of bicarbonate to achieve control of acidosis in patients with RTA. High dosages many be necessary in patients with proximal RTA. Address complicating disturbances such as hypokalemia as necessary.
- Pay careful attention to correction of acidosis and electrolyte abnormalities (e.g., hypokalemia) in dogs with Fanconi syndrome. Vigilance to detect and treat UTIs and close attention to nutrition also are important in long-term management of dogs with Fanconi syndrome.
- Recognize that the historical and physical findings in cats with IHC often are mild or vague.
- Perform a methimazole challenge in hyperthyroid cats with any evidence whatsoever of CRD to determine whether treatment of the hyperthyroidism can be safely achieved before resorting to irreversible forms of treatment of hyperthyroidism such as radioiodine or surgery.

FREQUENTLY ASKED QUESTIONS

Q: I have a 10-month-old female Weimeraner presented for a history of severe hematuria (identified when the dog urinated on a snow bank). Although shocking to the owner, the hematuria seems to be of no concern to the dog (no straining, no increased frequency, no apparent pain). Routine urinalysis shows too numerous to count red blood cells (TNTC RBC) in the sediment, but urine culture and imaging studies (plain radiographs, ultrasonography) are negative. Could this be a case of idiopathic benign hematuria?

A: Idiopathic benign hematuria is rare, and the diagnosis should always be approached with some skepticism. However, if no other cause for the hematuria can be identified, it should be considered. If possible, cystoscopy should be performed to evaluate the urine issuing from the ureteral orifices in the trigone region. In most dogs with idiopathic benign hematuria, the blood comes only from one kidney. The dog may be managed conservatively until it can be determined if the hemorrhage will be long-standing or severe enough to cause anemia. There is no rush to remove the kidney!

Q: I have performed ultrasound-guided drainage of a perinephric pseudocyst in an elderly cat on two occasions and both times the cyst refilled within a few weeks. Next, I resected the cyst wall surgically and preserved the kidney. Now the cat is accumulating fluid in its abdomen and presents for ascites. Is there anything else that can be done?

A: Advanced surgical procedures to place a shunt from the peritoneal space to the general circulation can be considered in this situation.

Q: I unexpectedly identified hyperchloremic metabolic acidosis in a cat with a urine pH of 8.0. I suspect distal RTA. Is there anything else I should consider?

A: RTA is rare in both dogs and cats. Blood gas analysis will help characterize the acid base status of the cat. A urine culture should be submitted and imaging studies to evaluate for pyelonephritis should be carried out because, although rare in cats, distal RTA has been reported in association with chronic pyelonephritis in this species.

Q: I have diagnosed Fanconi syndrome in a Basenji dog with a blood glucose concentration of 90 mg/dL, 3-plus glucosuria, and 1-plus proteinuria. Serum potassium is 3.4 mEq/L, serum chloride is 125 mEq/L, and serum bicarbonate is 12 mEq/L. How can I be sure the diagnosis is accurate?

A: Fanconi syndrome is likely in this dog. However, remember that proteinuria and amino aciduria are *not* synonymous. A good screening test for amino aciduria is to send a urine sample to the University of Pennsylvania Division of Medical Genetics to identify cystine. If the urine is positive for cystine the diagnosis of Fanconi syndrome in this Basenji is assured.

Q: A 10-year-old female spayed Persian cat is presented for routine geriatric evaluation. The owner reports no specific problems with the cat except for some mild weight loss. The cat has been fed a diet that has been marketed to "promote urinary health." Serum biochemistry shows a total serum calcium concentration of 12.1 mg/dL. Even after subcutaneous fluids overnight, the total serum calcium concentration still is 11.8 mg/dL. A plain abdominal radiograph shows a small radiopaque ureteral stone on the right side. Ultrasound examination of the kidneys shows them to be slightly small (3.0 cm in length) but otherwise normal without evidence of pyelectasia on either side. What other tests should be done, and how should the cat be managed?

A: Serum ionized calcium should be evaluated. The cat's neck should be carefully examined for any possible parathyroid masses, and the mouth should be examined carefully for squamous cell carcinoma. A panel of calciotrophic hormones (e.g., PTH, calcitriol, 25-hydroxycholcalciferol, PTHrP) should be determined. If the PTH and PTHrP are low and the vitamin D results normal, the cat should be presumptively diagnosed as having IHC. A high-fiber diet can be tried first, but many affected cats will also require prednisone therapy. The ureteral stone should be monitored for progression down the ureter and development of pyelectasia in the kidney on the affected side.

Q: I have a 14-year-old spayed female domestic shorthair cat presented for PU, PD, and severe weight loss, but with fairly normal appetite. A thyroid nodule is consistently palpable on the left side of the trachea. The kidneys are approximately 3.0 to 3.5 cm in length and feel smooth on palpation. Urine specific gravity is 1.019, serum creatinine is 2.0 mg/dL, and BUN is 38 mg/dL. Is it safe to proceed with radioiodine treatment of the hyperthyroidism?

A: Probably not. This cat should be managed initially with a methimazole challenge to determine the effect on renal function of rendering the cat euthyroid (i.e., serum thyroxine of approximately 1.0 mg/dL). In an institutional setting, renal scintigraphy can be used to determine the cat's GFR, but this procedure is not generally available in most practice settings. Iohexol clearance also may be used to estimate GFR and is available to practitioners by commercial diagnostic laboratories.

SUGGESTED READINGS

Idiopathic Renal Hematuria

Hitt ME, Straw RC, Lattimer JC, et al: Idiopathic hematuria of unilateral renal origin in a dog, *J Am Vet Med Assoc* 187:1371–1373, 1985.

Holt PE, Lucke VM, Pearson H: Idiopathic renal haemorrhage in the dog, *J Small Anim Pract* 28:253–263, 1987.

Mishina M, Watanabe T, Yugeta N, et al: Idiopathic renal hematuria in a dog: The usefulness of a method of partial occlusion of the renal artery, *J Vet Med Sci* 59:293–295, 1997.

Stone EA, DeNovo RC, Rawlings CA: Massive hematuria of nontraumatic renal origin in dogs, *J Am Vet Med Assoc* 183:868–871, 1983.

Perinephric Pseudocysts

Beck JA, Bellenger CR, Lamb WA, et al: Perirenal pseudocysts in 26 cats, *Aust Vet J* 78:166–171, 2000.

Ochoa VB, DiBartola SP, Chew DJ, et al: Perinephric pseudocysts in the cat: A retrospective study and review of the literature, *J Vet Intern Med* 13:47–55, 1999.

Renal Tubular Acidosis

Brown SA, Spyridakis LK, Crowell WA: Distal renal tubular acidosis and hepatic lipidosis in a cat, *J Am Vet Med Assoc* 189:1350–1352, 1986.

DiBartola SP, Leonard PO: Renal tubular acidosis in a dog, *J Am Vet Med Assoc* 180:70–73, 1982.

Drazner FH: Distal renal tubular acidosis associated with chronic pyelonephritis in a cat, *Calif Vet* 34:15–21, 1980.

Shaw DH: Acute response of urine pH following ammonium chloride administration to dogs, *Am J Vet Res* 50:1829–1830, 1989.

Watson AD, Culvenor JA, Middleton DJ, Rothwell TL: Distal renal tubular acidosis in a cat with pyelonephritis, *Vet Rec* 119:65–68, 1986.

Fanconi Syndrome

Bovee KC, Joyce T, Blazer-Yost B, et al: Characterization of renal defects in dogs with a syndrome similar to the Fanconi syndrome in man, *J Am Vet Med Assoc* 174:1094–1099, 1979.

Breitschwerdt EB, Ochoa R, Waltman C, et al: Multiple endocrine abnormalities in Basenji dogs with renal tubular dysfunction, *J Am Vet Med Assoc* 182:1348–1353, 1983.

Easley JR, Breitschwerdt EB: Glucosuria associated with renal tubular dysfunction in three Basenji dogs, *J Am Vet Med Assoc* 168:938–943, 1976.

Noonan CH, Kay JM: Prevalence and geographic distribution of Fanconi syndrome in Basenjis in the United States, *J Am Vet Med Assoc* 197:345–349, 1990.

Idiopathic Hypercalcemia

Midkiff AM, Chew DJ, Randolph JF, et al: Idiopathic hypercalcemia in cats, *J Vet Intern Med* 14:619–626, 2000.

Hyperthyroidism and the Kidney

Adams WH, Daniel GB, Legendre AM, et al: Changes in renal function in cats following treatment of hyperthyroidism using 131-I, *Vet Radiol Ultrasound* 38:231–238, 1997.

Adams WH, Daniel GB, Legendre AM: Investigation of the effects of hyperthyroidism on renal function in the cat, *Can J Vet Res* 61:53–56, 1997.

Becker TJ, Graves TK, Kruger JM, et al: Effects of methimazole on renal function in cats with hyperthyroidism, *J Am Anim Hosp Assoc* 36:215–223, 2000.

Broussard JD, Peterson ME, Fox PR: Changes in clinical and laboratory findings in cats with hyperthyroidism from 1983 to 1993, *J Am Vet Med Assoc* 206:302–305, 1995.

DiBartola SP, Broome MR, Stein BS, et al: Effect of treatment of hyperthyroidism on renal function in cats, *J Am Vet Med Assoc* 208:875–878, 1996.

Graves TK, Olivier NB, Nachreiner RF, et al: Changes in renal function associated with treatment of naturally-occurring hyperthyroidism in cats, *Am J Vet Res* 55:1745–1749, 1994.

Nemzek JA, Kruger JM, Walshaw R, et al: Acute onset of hypokalemia and muscular weakness in four hyperthyroid cats, *J Am Vet Med Assoc* 205:65–68, 1994.

Peterson ME, Becker DV: Radioiodine treatment of 524 cats with hyperthyroidism, *J Am Vet Med Assoc* 207:1422–1428, 1995.

Peterson ME, Gamble DA: Effect of nonthyroidal illness on serum thyroxine concentrations in cats: 494 cases (1988), *J Am Vet Med Assoc* 197:1203–1208, 1990.

Peterson ME, Graves TK, Gamble DA: Triiodothyronine (T3) suppression test: An aid in the diagnosis of mild hyperthyroidism in cats, *J Vet Int Med* 4:233–238, 1990.

Peterson ME, Melian C, Nichols R: Measurement of serum concentrations of free thyroxine, total thyroxine, and total triiodothyronine in cats with hyperthyroidism and cats with nonthyroidal disease, *J Am Vet Med Assoc* 218:529–536, 2001.

Index

9-Lives checklist, 315f–318f

Abdominocentesis, in uroperitoneum, 396–398
  procedure of, 398
Abyssinian cat, familial amyloidosis in, 198t–199t,
  202–203, 202f, 230
  papillary necrosis in, 203f
ACE (angiotensin-converting enzyme) inhibitors,
  in treatment of chronic kidney disease, 182b,
  185–187, 185b, 186f
Acepromazine
  for feline idiopathic cystitis, 326, 326b, 333t
  for feline urethral obstruction, 359t
Acid-base balance, in chronic kidney disease, 163
Activated vitamin D. *See* Calcitriol therapy.
Acute intrinsic renal failure (AIRF), 63, 65–73
  in animals with pre-existing renal disease, 69b
  causes of, 63, 65–66
    aminoglycoside nephrotoxicity, 114–117. *See
      also* Aminoglycoside nephrotoxicity
    ethylene glycol toxicity, 93–105. *See also*
      Ethylene glycol-induced renal failure
    food associated toxicity, 137–139. *See also*
      Melamine/cyanuric acid associated renal
      failure
    frequently asked questions on, 140–142
    grape or raisin toxicity, 118–120. *See also* Grape
      and raisin nephrotoxicity
    heatstroke, 134–137. *See also* Heatstroke-
      induced renal failure
    hypercalcemia, 126–131. *See also*
      Hypercalcemia-induced renal damage
    leptospirosis, 105–114. *See also* Leptospirosis-
      induced renal failure
    lily toxicity, 120–122. *See also* Lily
      nephrotoxicity
    Lyme nephritis, 131–134. *See also* Borreliosis-
      associated glomerulonephritis
    nonsteroidal anti-inflammatory drug (NSAID)
      toxicity, 122–125. *See also* NSAID-
      associated renal failure
  dehydration in, 74b
  diagnosis of, 75–78, 89, 139

Acute intrinsic renal failure *(Continued)*
    differential, 167–168
    hemogram in, 75
    renal imaging studies in, 77
    serum biochemistry in, 76–77
  frequently asked questions about, 91–92
  future treatment of, 89–90
  history and clinical signs of, 73
  hyperkalemia and treatment in, 80–81, 80f, 80b
  hyponatremia and hypocalcemia and
    treatment in, 81
  metabolic acidosis and treatment in, 81
  oliguria in, treatment of, 79, 79b
  pathophysiology of, 64, 66–73
  phases of, 71–73, 71f
  physical examination in, 74
  prognosis in, 87–88, 87b
  renal blood flow in, maintaining, 72b
  serum phosphorus control in treatment of, 81–82
  suggested readings on, 92
  treatment of, 78–87, 89, 139
    atrial natriuretic peptide in, 84–85
    dialysis, 86–87
    diuretic use in, 82–84
    failure in, 85–86
    future developments in, 89–90, 139–140
    goals in, 78, 78b
    initial stabilization in, 79–85
    misconceptions regarding, 90
    nutritional support in, 85
    rehydration fluids in, 80
    success in, 85
    systemic blood pressure control in, 85
    tips in, 90
  urine enzymology in, 77
  urine quality in diagnosis of, 72b
Acute renal failure (ARF), 63. *See also* Acute
    intrinsic renal failure (AIRF).
  classification of, 63, 64f
  diagnosis of, 74–78, 89
  history and clinical signs of, 63b, 73
  pathogenesis and pathophysiology of, 64–73
  physical examination in, 73–74

Acute renal failure *(Continued)*
  postrenal, 65. *See also* Postrenal acute renal
      failure
  prerenal, 64. *See also* Prerenal acute renal failure
  prognosis in, 87–88
  suggested readings on, 92
  treatment of, 78–87, 89
Acute tubular necrosis, 66–73, 67f
Alaskan malamute, suspected familial renal
    dysplasia in, 198t–199t, 203
Alpha agonists, in preventing urinary tract
    infection, 261
Aluminum hydroxide (Amphogel), as phosphorus
    binder, 176–177
Aminoglycoside nephrotoxicity, 114–117
  diagnosis of, 116, 116b
  pathophysiology of, 114–115
  prevention of, 117, 117b
  risk factors for, 115–116
  suggested readings on, 142
Aminoglycosides, for urinary tract infection, 257
Amitriptyline
  for feline idiopathic cystitis, 333t, 334
  for urethral obstruction in male cats, 313
Ammonium urate calculi, 282f
Amyloid syndromes, 228
Amyloidosis, 227–237. *See also* Glomerular disease.
  familial trait, 198t–199t, 210f
      in Abyssinian cat, 202–203, 202f
      in beagle, 204
      in English foxhound, 207
      in Shar-pei, 211
  histopathology of, in dog, 228f
  treatment of, 233–234
Anabolic steroids, in treatment of chronic kidney
    disease, 189
Anafranil. *See* Clomipramine.
Angiotensin II therapy, for chronic kidney disease,
    185–186, 185b
Antegrade urinary catheter placement, in male
    cats, 366
Anti-emetics, dosages for treatment in chronic
    kidney disease, 181
Antimicrobial agents, for urinary tract infections,
    255–257
  dosages and urine concentrations, in normal
      dogs, 255t
  response rate for appropriate treatment with, 257
  uropathogen susceptibility to, 257, 258t–259t
Antizol-Vet. *See* 4-Methylpyrazole.
Anuscopes, 2–3, 4f
Ash Advantage T-fluted peritoneal dialysis
    catheter, 86, 86f
Atrial natriuretic peptide (ANP), in treatment of
    acute intrinsic renal failure, 84–85
Automatic bladder, 427–428

Autonomous bladder, 428
Azodyl, for chronic kidney disease, 189
Azotemia, 32
  differentiation of types of, 33t

Bacteria, in urine specimen, 25–26, 25f
  culture of, 241–248. *See also* Urine culture
Basement membrane, of glomerulus, 218
Basement membrane disorder, familial trait,
    198t–199t, 206f
  in bull terrier, 204–205
  in Dalmatian, 207
  in English Cocker spaniel, 206
  in Newfoundland, 208
  in Samoyed, 210–211
  suspected
      in beagle, 204
      in bull mastiff, 205
      in Doberman pinscher, 207
      in Rottweiler, 209
Basenji, familial renal disease in, 198t–199t, 204,
    496–497
Basic fibroblastic growth factor (bFGF) urinary
    marker, 449
Baytril. *See* Enrofloxacin.
Beagle, familial renal disease in, 198t–199t, 204, 230
Benazepril, in treatment of chronic kidney disease
  in cats, 187
  in dogs, 187
Benign essential hematuria, in dogs, 487–490
  diagnosis of, 487–489, 487b
      cystoscopy in, 488, 488f
      differential, 489
      gross and microscopic pathology in, 489
  prognosis in, 489–490
  treatment of, 489
BENRIC study, 187
Bernese mountain dog, familial renal disease in,
    198t–199t, 204, 229
Bilirubin, in urine, 15
Bladder
  biopsy of, 57–58
  calculi of
      history in, 285
      physical findings in, 286–287
  digital palpation of, 2
  infection of. *See* Cystitis; Urinary tract infection
  neoplasia of, 438–441
      benign, 439, 443
      canine, 439, 439f. *See also* Canine transitional
          cell carcinoma
      common misconceptions about, 461
      diagnosis of, 460–461
      etiology of, 440–441
      feline, 440
      frequently asked questions about, 462–463

Bladder *(Continued)*
  future diagnosis and treatment of, 461
  incidence of, in dogs, 438b
  metastatic, 439
  primary tumors in, 438
  risk of
    in female dogs and male cats, 440, 440b
    vegetable consumption and, 441
  summary tips on, 461–462
  transitional cell carcinoma in, 438b
  overdistension of, in male cats, 369
  polyps of, 451f
  rupture of
    cystoscopy in, 401f
    positive contrast cystography in, 400f
    treatment of, 404
  ultrasonography of, 53–54
Bladder tumor antigen (BTA) test, 43, 448–449
Borreliosis-associated glomerulonephritis,
    131–134, 131b
  clinical signs and history in, 133
  diagnosis of, 134
  pathophysiology of, 131–133, 133f
  prognosis in, 134, 134b
  suggested readings on, 142
  treatment of, 134
Boxer, primary sphincter incompetence in, 417–427
Brittany spaniel, familial renal disease in,
    198t–199t, 204, 229
Bulbocavernosus reflex, 414
Bull mastiff, familial renal disease in, 198t–199t,
    205
Bull terrier, familial renal disease in, 198t–199t,
    204–205, 230
BUN concentration
  in acute intrinsic renal failure, 76
  in chronic kidney disease, 159
  and glomerular filtration rate, 37–39, 38t
  laboratory evaluation of, 36, 37b
Buprenorphine (Buprenex), for feline idiopathic
    cystitis, 326, 326b, 333t
Buspirone (Buspar), for feline idiopathic cystitis,
    333t
Butorphanol
  dosage, as anti-emetic, 181
  for feline idiopathic cystitis, 333t

Cairn terrier, familial renal disease of, 198t–199t,
    205
Calcitriol poisoning, 129, 129b
Calcitriol (activated vitamin D) therapy
  for canine transitional cell carcinoma, 459
  in chronic kidney disease, 183–185, 184f
Calcitriol trade-off hypothesis, 165–166, 165f
Calcium acetate, as phosphorus binder, 177
Calcium carbonate, as phosphorus binder, 177

Calcium oxalate calculi, 278
  formation of, 278f
Calcium oxalate crystalluria, 27, 28f
Calcium oxalate stone, management algorithm
    for, 295f
Calculus, 272
Canine olfaction, and detection of transitional cell
    carcinoma, 449–450
Canine transitional cell carcinoma, 441–459, 453f
  breed disposition to, 436, 441b, 442t
  clinical signs of, 442, 443b
  common misconceptions about, 461
  diagnosis of, 443–450, 449b, 460–461
    biopsy in definitive, 446–447, 447f, 447b
    cystocentesis in, contraindication to, 441b,
        443, 443b
    cystoscopy in, 448, 448f
    cytology in, 445–446, 447f
    definitive, 446–447, 446b
    differential, 443
    epithelial cell rafts in, 443–444, 444b, 445f
    laboratory findings in, 443–444, 444b
    radiography and ultrasonography in, 445,
        445b, 446f
  etiology of, 440–441
  frequently asked questions about, 462–463
  future diagnosis and treatment of, 461
  histopathology of, 451f–452f
  incidence of, in dogs, 438b
  location of tumors in, 450–452, 450b
  metastatic, 439
  physical findings in, 443
  primary tumors in, 438
  prognosis in, 459
  risk of
    in female dogs and male cats, 440, 440b
    vegetable consumption and, 441
  screening tests for, 448–449
  signalment of, 441–442
  staging of, 450, 450t
  summary tips on, 461–462
  treatment of, 452–458
    chemotherapy in, 454, 454b
    mitoxantrone and piroxicam in, 456, 456b
    new and future, 458–459
    palliative management of urethral obstruction
        in, 456–458, 457f
    piroxicam in, 454b, 455
    radiation in, 456
    surgical, 452–454, 453b
Casts, in urinary sediment, 20–25
  cellular, 22–25, 23f
  classification of, 21f
  granular, 24, 24f
  hyaline, 21–22, 22f
  waxy, 24–25, 24f

Catheterization, urinary, 2–5
  in female cats, 3
  in female dogs, 2–3, 4f
  in male cats, 3
  in male dogs, 2, 3f
Cefadroxil, 256
Cefovecin, for urinary tract infection, 257
Cefpodoxime, for urinary tract infection, 257
Ceftiofur sodium, for urinary tract infection, 257
Cellular casts, in urinary sediment, 22–25, 23f
Central diabetes insipidus, 466, 470t, 473f,
    481f, 481b
  treatment of, 482
Cephalexin, for urinary tract infections, 256
Cephalosporins, first generation, for urinary tract
    infections, 256
Chlamydia, in recurrent urinary infections, 262
Chlorpromazine, dosage, as anti-emetic, 181
Cholecalciferol poisoning, 127–128
Chow, familial renal disease of, 198t–199t, 206
Chronic kidney disease (CKD), 145
  avoiding stress in animals with, 190
  blood pressure and control in, 186b, 188–189
  causes of, 147–148
    in cats, 148
    in dogs, 147–148
  common misconceptions regarding, 192–193
  diagnosis of, 154–168, 191
    anorexia in, 155
    clinical history in, 154–156
    gastrointestinal signs in, 155
    lethargy, weakness, and neurological signs in,
        155–156
    physical signs in, 156–157
      abdominal palpation, 156
      abnormal auscultation, 156
      blindness, 157
      coat dullness and dryness, 156
      dehydration signs, 156
      hemostatic defects, 157
      oral lesions, 156
      osteodystrophy, 156–157
      subcutaneous edema, 157
      systemic or local infections, 157
      weight loss, 155–156
    polyuria and polydipsia in, 154–155
    serum biochemistry in, 159–163
    serum creatinine concentration cut-off values
        in, 146t, 147, 147b
    systemic hypertension in, 157–158
  diagnostic imaging in, 166–167, 167f
    differential, 167–168
  dietary management of, 171–181
    caloric needs in, 179
    home-made diet for cats, 172t
    home-made diet for dogs, 171t
Chronic kidney disease *(Continued)*
    home-made diet for either dogs or cats, 173t
    lipid supplementation in, 179
    phosphorus restriction in, 174–176, 174b, 175f
    potassium levels and, 180
    protein restriction in, 172–174
    reduction of intestinal phosphate absorption,
        176–179, 176b, 177f
    sodium bicarbonate in, 180
    sodium chloride restriction in, 179–180
    veterinary renal diets in, 180–181
    vitamin supplements in, 180
  frequently asked questions about, 193–195
  histopathology of, 152, 152f
  hormonal status in, 163–166
  hypertension and control in, 186b, 188
  IRIS staging of, 145–147, 146t
  laboratory findings in, 158–168
    acid-base balance, 163
    BUN concentration, 159
    hemogram, 158–159
    hormones, 163–166
    serum calcium concentration, 161–162, 161b
    serum creatinine concentration, 159
    serum phosphorus concentration, 161
    serum potassium concentration, 159–161
    serum sodium concentration, 159
    thyroid hormone concentration in, 166
    urinalysis, 166
  pathophysiology of, 148–154
    intraglomerular hypertension and
        hyperfiltration in, 148b, 149–150, 149f
    renal functional and morphologic changes in,
        151–152, 151b
    uremia in, 148
  progression of
    factors contributing to, 151–153, 151f, 152b
      dietary intake, 152
      hypertension, 188
      systemic complications, 153
    and prognosis, 190–191
    species differences in, 151
  renal secondary hyperparathyroidism in,
      164–165, 164f
  suggested readings on, 195
  thyroid hormone concentration in, 166
  treatment of, 168–191
    ACE inhibitors in, 187
    anabolic steroids in, 189
    benazepril in, 187
    blood pressure control in, 188–189
    dietary management in, 171–181, 171t–173t
    enalapril in, 186
    endocrine replacement therapy in, 182–186
    future developments in, 191–192
    general management principles in, 168–171

Chronic kidney disease *(Continued)*
    levels of, 169b
    new and emerging, 189–190
    patient status checklist in, 170b
    solute balance in, 153–154
    summary tips on, 193
    vomiting and inappetence, 181–182
    water balance in, 154
Chronic renal failure (CRF), 145–147. *See also*
    Chronic kidney disease (CKD).
Cinacalcet, for chronic kidney disease, 190
Ciprofloxacin (Cipro), 256
Citrate formation, 280
Clinical evaluation, of urinary tract, 32, 58
    approach to, 33–34
    bladder and urethral biopsy in, 57–58
    common misconceptions about, 58–59
    cystoscopy in, 54–55
    diagnostic imaging in, 49–54
    frequently asked questions about, 59–61
    future developments in, 58
    history in, 33–34
    laboratory evaluation of renal function in, 35–47.
        See also Laboratory evaluation
    microbiology in, 47–48
    physical examination in, 35
    questions to be answered in, 32
    renal biopsy in, 55–57
    suggested readings in, 61
Clomicalm. *See* Clomipramine.
Clomipramine, for feline idiopathic cystitis, 333t,
    334
Collagen injections, submucosal, for primary
    sphincter incompetence, 421, 421f, 421b
Color flow Doppler renal ultrasonography, 53
Colposuspension, in treatment of primary
    sphincter incompetence, 422, 422f
Congenital nephrogenic diabetes insipidus,
    482–483
Contrast urography, of lower urinary tract, 50–51
Convenia. *See* Cefovecin.
Corynebacterium urealyticum, in recurrent urinary
    infections, 262–264
Covalzin. *See* Kremezin.
Crystalloid components, of uroliths, 272, 273f
Crystalloid formation, 274, 275f
    urine pH and, 274
    urine volume and, 274
Crystalluria, as indicator of urolithiasis, 287b
Crystals, in urine, 26–27. *See also* Urolithiasis.
    as artifacts of storage, 27b
    calcium oxalate, 27, 28f
    cystine, 27, 29f
    hippurate, 98
    struvite, 27, 29f
    urate, 27, 30f

Cystatin C concentration, laboratory evaluation, 39
Cysteine solubility, in urine, compounds that
    increase, 300f
Cysteine urolithiasis, 27, 29f, 283–284
    medical treatment of, 300–301
        alkalinization of urine in, 301
    signalment in, 285
Cystic calculi
    history in, 285
    physical findings in, 286–287
Cystitis
    in dogs, 240. *See also* Urinary tract infection
    non-obstructive, in cats, 306. *See also* Feline
        idiopathic cystitis; Feline interstitial cystitis
Cystocentesis, 5–7
    blind technique for, with nonpalpable bladder, 5
    complications of, 6–7
    decompressive, 358–361
    for quantitative microbiology, 48, 48b
    standard technique for, with palpable bladder, 5
    techniques in cat and dog, 6f–7f
    techniques in male dog in dorsal recumbency,
        6f–7f
Cystography
    double contrast, 51
    negative contrast, 51
    positive contrast, 50–51
Cystometrogram (CMG), 415–417, 416f
Cystoscopy, 54–55

Dalmatian
    familial renal disease of, 198t–199t, 207
    urate urolithiasis in, 281–283
Dantrolene, for feline urethral obstruction, 359t
Darbepoetin (Aransep), 182
DDAVP, for hyposthenuric disorders, 482, 482b
Decompressive cystocentesis, 358–361
Dehydration, signs of
    in acute intrinsic renal failure, 74b
    in chronic kidney disease, 156
Detrusor contraction, medical stimulation of, 369,
    369b
Detrusor urethral dyssynergia, 428–429
Diagnosis, of disease. *See* Clinical evaluation, of
    urinary tract.
Diagnostic imaging, 49–54. *See also* Renal imaging
    studies.
    contrast urographic, 50–51
    double contrast cystographic, 51
    excretory urographic, 49–50
    negative contrast cystographic, 51
    radiographic, 49
    ultrasonographic, 51–54
Dialysis treatment
    of acute intrinsic renal failure, 86–87
    in chronic kidney disease, 190

Diazepam, for feline urethral obstruction, 359t
Dibenzyline. *See* Phenoxybenzamine.
Dietary intake, and progression of chronic kidney disease, 152
Dietary management
  of chronic kidney disease, 171–181
    home-made feed, for cats, 172t
    home-made feed, for dogs, 171t
    home-made feed, for either dogs or cats, 173t
    veterinary renal feed, advantages of, 180–181
  of urinary tract infections, 257, 260–261, 260b
Difloxacin (Dicural), 256
1,25-Dihydroxyvitamin D. *See* Calcitriol (activated vitamin D) therapy.
Dipstrip evaluation, of urine specimen, 11
  possible error sources in, 11b
Dipstrip screening, for urine protein, 41–42, 42b
Diuretics
  in treatment of acute intrinsic renal failure, 82–84
  types of, and sites of action, 82–84
Doberman pinscher
  familial renal disease of, 198t–199t, 207, 230
  primary sphincter incompetence in, 417–427
Dopamine, for acute intrinsic renal failure, 83–84
Double contrast cystography, 51
Duragesic. *See* Fentanyl.
Dynamic renal scintigraphy, 40–41

Ectopic ureter, 423–427, 423f
  abnormalities associated with, 425
  diagnosis of
    computed tomography in, 424
    excretory urography in, 424, 424f
    ultrasonography in, 424
    urethrocystoscopy in, 425, 425f–426f, 425b
  intraurethral ureterectomy in treatment of, 425, 426f
  submucosal collagen injections in treatment of, 425
Elavil. *See* Amitriptyline.
Electrolyte clearance, fractional, 47, 47t
Elmiron. *See* Pentosan polysulfate sodium.
Embryonal nephroma, 436–437
Enalapril, in stabilization of dogs with chronic kidney disease, 186
Endocrine replacement therapy, in chronic kidney disease, 182–186
  angiotensin II and angiotensin-converting enzyme inhibitors in, 185–186
  calcitriol in, 183–185
  recombinant human erythropoietin in, 182–183
Endothelium, of glomerulus, 218
English bulldog, urate urolithiasis in, 281–283
English Cocker spaniel, familial renal disease of, 198t–199t, 206, 230
English foxhound, familial renal disease of, 198t–199t, 207, 230

English sheepdog, primary sphincter incompetence in, 417–427
Enrofloxacin, 256
Enterococci, in recurrent urinary infections, 262
Epakitin, as phosphorus binder, 178
Epithelial cells, in urinary sediment, 18f, 19–20, 20f
Erythropoietin, recombinant human, (rhEPO; Epogen), for chronic kidney disease, 182–183, 182b
Erythropoietin concentration, in chronic kidney disease, 166
Esophagostomy, percutaneous, in treatment of chronic kidney disease, 182, 182b
Esophagostomy feeding tubes, in treatment of chronic kidney disease, 182, 182b
Estrogens, in preventing urinary tract infection, 261
Ethanol therapy, for ethylene glycol toxicity, 102
Ethylene glycol induced renal failure, 93–105
  clinical signs and history in, 96–97, 96b
    cardiopulmonary, 95
  diagnosis of, 96–101
    high anion gap and high osmolal gap in, 100b
    utility of renal ultrasonography in, 52–53
  laboratory findings in, 97–101
    measured urine output, 98
    radiography, 100
    renal ultrasonography, 100–101, 100f
    serum biochemistry, 98–100
    urinalysis, 97–98
  pathophysiology of, 93–96, 94f
  phases of syndrome of, 94–96
  physical examination findings in, 97
  prognosis for recovery from, 105
  renal histopathology in, 95f
  renal involvement in, 95–96
  suggested readings on, 142
  treatment of, 101–105, 101b
    4-methylpyrazole in, 103–104
    dialysis in, 104–105
    diuresis in, 104
    ethanol in, 102–103
Excenel. *See* Ceftiofur sodium.
Excretory urography, 49–50

Familial renal disease(s), 197, 198t–199t
  diagnosis of, 212
  frequently asked questions about, 213
  future genetic identification of, 213
  history and clinical signs of, 200
  laboratory findings in, 200–202
    hemogram, 200
    histopathology, 201–202
    imaging, 201
    serum chemistry, 201
    urinalysis, 201

Familial renal disease(s) *(Continued)*
  physical findings in, 200
  signalment of, 197–200
  specific, 198t–199t, 202–212
    in Abyssinian cat, 202–203
    in Alaskan malamute, 203
    in Basenji, 204
    in beagle, 204
    in Bernese mountain dog, 204
    in Brittany spaniel, 204
    in bull mastiff, 205
    in bull terrier, 204–205
    in Cairn and West Highland white terriers, 205
    in chow, 206
    in Dalmatian, 207
    in Doberman pinscher, 207
    in English Cocker spaniel, 206
    in English foxhound, 207
    in German shepherd, 207
    in golden retriever, 207–208
    in Lhasa apso, and Shih tzu, 208
    in miniature Schnauzer, 208
    in Newfoundland, 208
    in Norwegian elkhound, 209
    in Persian cat, 209
    in Rottweiler, 209
    in samoyed, 210–211
    in Shar pei, 211
    in soft-coated Wheaten terrier, 211–212
    in standard poodle, 212
    in Welsh corgi, 212
  suggested readings on, 213
Fanconi syndrome, 496–497
  diagnosis of, 496–497, 496b
  drug administration associated with, 497
  prognosis in, 497
  treatment of, 497
Feline idiopathic cystitis, 306
  chronic, 308
  clinical signs of, 313
  common misconceptions about, 336
  diagnosis of, 320–324, 335
    blood count and serum biochemistry in, 322
    cystoscopy in, 323, 324f
    environmental history and assessment form
      in, 315f–318f
    hematuria in, 320b, 322b
    histopathology in, 323–324
    history in, 314–319
    inappropriate urination pattern in, 319, 319b
    physical findings in, 319–320
    radiographic imaging in, 322, 322b, 323f
    ultrasonographic imaging in, 322, 323f
    urethroscopy in, 323
    urinalysis in, 320–321
    urine culture in, 321–322, 321b

Feline idiopathic cystitis (Continued)
  differential diagnosis of, 313
    in cats older than 10 years of age, 313
    in cats younger than 10 years of age, 313, 313b,
      314f
  frequently asked questions about, 337–339
  neurogenic inflammation in, 309, 309b, 310f
  pathophysiology of, 307–311, 307f–308f
    adrenal deficits in, 311, 312f
    alpha-2-adrenoreceptors in, 311
    environmental stressors in, 309, 310f, 311b
    HPA axis abnormalities in, 311
    sensory neuron abnormalities in, 308–309
  signalment of, 312–313
  suggested readings on, 339
  summary tips on, 336–337
  treatment of, 324–335, 325f
    behavioral, 335
    fluoxetine in, 334
    future, 335–336
    glucosaminoglycan supplementation in,
      334–335
    goals in, 324–335, 324b
    level(s) of, 326
      first, 326, 326b
      second, 327, 327b
    successful, 326
    tricyclic antidepressants in, 334
    unsuccessful, 335b
Feline interstitial cystitis, 306
Feline urological syndrome, 306
Feliway. *See* Pheromones.
Fentanyl, for feline idiopathic cystitis, 333t
Fetal glomerulus, 198f
Filtration barrier, of glomerulus, 218–219
Fluoroquinolones, for urinary tract infection, 256,
  256b
Fluoxetine, for feline idiopathic cystitis, 333t, 334
Fosrenol. *See* Lanthanum carbonate.
Fractional clearance of electrolytes, 47, 47t
Fungal urinary tract infections, treatment of, 262–263

Gastric acid production, suppression of, 181
Gastroprotectants, 182
German shepherd
  familial renal disease of, 198t–199t, 207
  renal cystadenocarcinoma in, 436
Giant Schnauzer, primary sphincter incompetence
  in, 417–427
Glomerular capillary barrier, schematic of, 220f
Glomerular disease, 218
  amyloidosis in, 227–237
  causes of, 227
  clinical findings in, 229–232
    history and possible presentations, 230
    signalment, 229–230

Glomerular disease *(Continued)*
  common misconceptions about, 238
  complications of, 234–237
    hyperlipidemia in, 236
    hypertension in, 236–237
    hypoalbuminemia in, 234
    sodium retention in, 234–235
    thromboembolism in, 235–236, 235f
  diagnosis of, 237
  frequently asked questions about, 238–239
  laboratory findings in, 230–232
    renal biopsy, 231–232
    serum biochemistry, 231
    urinalysis, 230–231
    urine protein-to-creatinine ratio, 231–232
  lesions of, 226, 226f
  pathogenesis of, 220
    in immune-mediated glomerulonephritis,
      221–222
    in nonimmune glomerulonephritis, 223
  physical examination findings in, 230
  prognosis in, 237
  progression of, 225
  resolution of, 225
  suggested readings on, 239
  treatment of, 232–234, 237
    future, 237
    summary tips in, 238
Glomerular filtration rate (GFR)
  decreased, in acute intrinsic renal failure, 64f, 73–75
  in laboratory evaluation, 35–39
  radioisotopic estimation of, 40–41
  sedative and anesthetic effects on, 40
  single injection estimation of, 40
Glomerular function, 35–39, 36t
Glomerulonephritis, 218. *See also* Glomerular
  disease.
  familial trait, 198t–199t
    in Bernese mountain dog, 204
    in Brittany spaniel, 204
Glomerulus, anatomy and function of, 218–220, 219f
Glucosuria, pathology indicated by, 13b
Glycosaminoglycans, in preventing urinary tract
  infection, 260
Golden retriever, familial renal disease of,
  198t–199t, 207–208
Gradual water deprivation test, 46–47
Granular casts, in urinary sediment, 24, 24f
Grape and raisin nephrotoxicity, in dogs, 118–120,
  118b
  diagnosis of, 119
  pathophysiology of, 118
  prognosis in, 119–120
  risk factors for, 118
  suggested readings on, 142
  treatment of, 119, 119b

H2-receptor antagonists, 181
Halo sign, at corticomedullary junction, 101
Hanging head posture, in hypokalemic cat, 153f,
  160
Heatstroke-induced renal failure, 134–137, 134b
  clinical signs of, 135–136
  diagnosis of, 136
  pathophysiology of, 135
  prognosis in, 137
  suggested readings on, 142
  treatment of, 136–137
Hematoma, perinephric, 392f
Hematuria, idiopathic renal, in dogs, 487–490. *See*
  also Benign essential hematuria.
Hemorrhage, in renal biopsy, 57
Husbandry, in clinical history, 34
Hyaline casts, in urinary sediment, 21–22, 22f
Hydronephrosis, in renal biopsy, 57
Hydropulsion. *See* Urohydropropulsion.
Hypercalcemia
  in chronic kidney disease, 162, 162b
  idiopathic, in cats, 498–501, 498b
    diagnosis of, 498–500
      differential, 500
    prognosis in, 501
    treatment of, 500–501, 500b
Hypercalcemia-induced renal damage, 126–131,
  126b
  canine mortality from, 128–129, 128b
  clinical signs of, 130, 130b
  diagnosis of, 130–131
  histopathology of, 126, 126f
  pathophysiology of, 126–130
    calcitriol poisoning in, 129, 129b
    cholicalciferol poisoning in, 127–129
  suggested readings on, 142
  treatment of, 131, 132f
Hyperkalemia
  and treatment, in acute intrinsic renal failure,
    80–81, 80f
  in urethral obstruction in male cats, 350,
    350b–351b
Hyperparathyroidism, in chronic kidney disease,
  163–166, 163b
Hyperphosphatemia, acute, causing acute intrinsic
  renal failure, 66
Hypertension, in dogs or cats
  dietary and medical treatment of, 188–189
  guidelines for treatment of, 188
Hypervitaminosis D, in hypercalcemic renal
  pathology, 127–128, 128b
Hypocalcemia
  in chronic kidney disease, 162
  and treatment, in acute intrinsic renal
    failure, 81
  in urethral obstruction in male cats, 352, 352b

Hypokalemia, in chronic kidney disease, 159–161, 160f, 160b, 180
Hyponatremia, and treatment, in acute intrinsic renal failure, 81
Hyporeninemic hypoaldosteronism, 496
Hyposthenuric disorders, treatment of, 480–483, 480b

Idiopathic glomerulonephritis, 223. *See also* Glomerular disease.
　treatment of, 232–233
Idiopathic hypercalcemia, in cats, 498–501, 498b
　diagnosis of, 498–500
　　differential, 500
　prognosis in, 501
　treatment of, 500–501, 500b
Idiopathic renal hematuria, in dogs, 487–490. *See also* Benign essential hematuria.
Immune-mediated glomerulonephritis, 221–222, 221f. *See also* Glomerular disease.
　causes of, in dogs and cats, 224b–225b
　mechanisms of immune injury in, 222–223
　treatment of, 232–233
Inherited diseases. *See* Familial renal disease(s).
International Renal Interest Society (IRIS), staging of chronic kidney disease, 145–147
　proteinuria, 146t
　serum creatinine concentrations, 146t
　systemic blood pressure, 146t
Intrinsic azotemia, 33t

Ketone concentration, in urine, 14
Kremezin, for chronic kidney disease, 189

Laboratory evaluation, of renal function, 35–47
　bladder tumor antigen test in, 43
　BUN concentration in, 36
　cystatin C concentration in, 39
　fractional clearance of electrolytes in, 47
　glomerular filtration rate in, 35–39, 36t. *See also* Glomerular filtration rate (GFR)
　gradual water deprivation test in, 46–47
　microalbuminuria in, 42–43
　renal clearance in, 39
　serum creatinine concentration in, 36–37
　serum phosphorus concentration in, 41
　tubular function in, 44–47
　urine protein in, 41–42
　water deprivation test in, 45–46
Lanthanum carbonate, as phosphorus binder, 178
Leptospirosis, 105–107
　hosts of organisms causing, 106, 106t
　public health significance of, 113
　serovars of, 105–107
　vaccination against, 113–114, 113b

Leptospirosis-induced renal failure, 107, 107b
　clinical course and prognosis in, 112–113, 112b
　clinical signs and history of, 109
　diagnosis of
　　imaging in, 110
　　laboratory findings in, 109–112, 110b
　　liver biopsy results in, 111
　　physical examination findings in, 109
　　renal biopsy results in, 111f
　　signalment in, 108–109
　pathophysiology of, 101b, 107–108
　suggested readings on, 142
　treatment of, 112
　　short-term dialysis in, 112b
Leukocyte esterase reaction, 15
Lhasa apso, familial renal disease of, 198t–199t, 208
Lily nephrotoxicity, in cats, 120–122, 120b
　diagnosis of, 121
　pathophysiology of, 120–121
　prognosis in, 121b, 122
　suggested readings on, 142
　treatment of, 121
Linear infarcts, in renal biopsy, 57
Lithotripsy, 291
Loop diuretics, 83
Lower motor neuron incontinence, 428
Lower urinary tract. *See also* Urinary tract disease.
　contrast urography of, 50–51
Lyme nephritis. *See* Borreliosis-associated glomerulonephritis.

Mannitol, precautions in use of, 82b
Marbofloxacin, 256
Matrix urolith, 272
Medical history, 34
Medullary rim sign, 53
Melamine/cyanuric acid–associated renal failure, 137
　clinical signs of, 138
　diagnosis of, 138
　pathophysiology of, 138, 138f
　prognosis in, 139
　suggested readings on, 142
　treatment of, 139
Membranoproliferative glomerulonephritis, familial trait, in soft-coated Wheaten terrier, 211–212
MEMO (multimodal environmental modification), 327, 327b
　level 1, 328–330
　　cat conflict management in, 331
　　feeding practice management in, 330
　　increasing space in, 331
　　litter box management in, 328–329
　　pheromone therapy in, 332

MEMO (multimodal environmental modification)
   (*Continued*)
      promoting wild behaviors in, 331
      salt intake increase in, 330
      water intake increase in, 329, 330b
   level 2, 332
      analgesia and sedation in, 333–335
      outdoor exposure in, 332, 332b
      safe haven provision in, 332–333
   treatment of
      drugs used in, 333t
Mesangial cells, 219, 220f
Mesenchymal tumors, primary, 437
Metabolic acidosis, and treatment
   in acute intrinsic renal failure, 81, 81b
   in chronic kidney disease, 163
Metastatic tumors, 437–438
Methimazole challenge, 503, 503b
4-Methylpyrazole (4-MP; fomepizole),
      in treatment of ethylene glycol toxicity, 101b,
      102–104
Metoclopramide, dosage, as anti-emetic, 181
Microalbuminuria
   as indication of glomerular damage, 42b
   laboratory evaluation of, 42–43
Microbiology. *See also* Urine culture.
   quantitative, in determining urinary tract
      infection, 47–48, 250–251
   in differential diagnosis of urolithiasis, 288
   in vitro susceptibility patterns,
         to antibiotics, 257
      for cats, 259t
      for dogs, 258t
Microorganisms, in urinary sediment, 25–26, 25f,
   250–251
Micturition disorders, 409, 409b
   common misconceptions about, 430–431
   diagnosis of
      differential, 412, 413b
      history in, 414
      imaging in, 415
      laboratory findings in, 415
      physical examination in, 414–415, 414b
      signalment in, 413–414
      special studies in, 415–417, 415b
   frequently asked questions about, 431–433
   suggested readings on, 433
   treatment of, 429–430
      in anatomic abnormalities, 423–427
      future, 430
      in neurogenic causes, 427–429
      in paradoxical (obstructive) incontinence, 427
      in primary sphincter incompetence, 417–427
      summary tips on, 431
   vestibulovaginal stenosis in, in female dogs, 427
Midstream voided sample, 1

Miniature Schnauzer
   familial renal disease of, 198t–199t, 208
   urate urolithiasis in, 281–283
Minipress. *See* Prazosin.
Mitoxantrone, and piroxicam, 456, 456b
Modified Wright stain, of urine sediment, 250
Mycoplasma, in recurrent urinary infections, 262

Naxcel. *See* Ceftiofur sodium.
Negative contrast cystography, 51
Nephritis, causing acute intrinsic renal failure, 66
Nephroblastoma, 436–437, 437f
Nephrogenic diabetes insipidus, 482–483
Nephrosis, pathophysiology of, 66–73
Nephrotic syndrome, 218
Nephrotoxicant, 69
Nephrotoxicity, renal, pathophysiology of, 64f,
   66–73
Nephrotoxins, causing acute intrinsic renal
   failure, 65
Newfoundland, familial renal disease of,
   198t–199t, 208
Nonimmune glomerulonephritis, 223. *See also*
   Glomerular disease.
   treatment of, 232–233
Norfloxacin (Noroxin), 256
Norwegian Elkhound, familial renal disease of,
   198t–199t, 209
NSAID-associated renal failure, 122–125
   diagnosis of, 124–125
   pathophysiology of, 67, 67b, 122–124
   prevention of, 125
   risk factors for, 124, 124b
   suggested readings on, 142
   treatment of renal damage in, 125

Obstructive uropathy, and nephropathy, 341
   bilateral, 379–380, 381f
   common misconceptions about, 385–386
   diagnosis of, 384
      history and clinical signs in, 378–380
   etiologies of, 342
   frequently asked questions about, 386–389
   future treatment of, 385
   lower tract, 342–343
      in cats, 342–343. *See also* Idiopathic urethritis;
         Urethral plugs
      in dogs, 342–343. *See also* Cystic calculi;
         Urethral calculi; Urolithiasis
   pathophysiology of, 378, 379f
   suggested readings on, 389
   summary tips on, 386
   upper tract, 378–380
      in cats. *See* Ureterolithiasis, in cats
      in dogs. *See* Renal calculi; Ureteral calculi
Occult blood, in urine, 14–15, 14b

Omega-3 and omega-6 fatty acid supplementation, in chronic kidney disease, 179, 179b

Ondansetron, dosage, as anti-emetic, 181

Orbifloxacin (Orbax), 256

Oriental short hair cat, familial renal disease of, 198t–199t, 230

Ormetoprim-potentiated sulfonamides, for urinary tract infections, 256

Oxalate calculi, 278
  formation of, 279f

Oxalate crystalluria, 27, 28f

Oxalate urolithiasis
  medical treatment of, 294–298, 295f
  pathophysiology of, 277–281
  prevention of
    citrate administration in, 297–298
    commercial diets in, 296–297
    dietary, 280–281, 294–296
    diuretic administration in, 298
  risk factors for
    in cats, 277–278
    dietary, 280–281
    in dogs, 277
  signalment in, 285
  urinary tract infection and risk of, 281

Oxybutynin, for feline urethral obstruction, 359t

Parathyroid hormone status, in chronic kidney disease, 163–166, 163b

Parietal epithelial cells, of glomerular capsule, 219

Pelvic bladder, 418, 418f

Penicillins, for urinary tract infections, 256

Pentosan polysulfate sodium, for feline idiopathic cystitis, 333t

Percutaneous esophagostomy (PEG), in treatment of chronic kidney disease, 182, 182b

Perineal reflex, 414

Perineal urethrostomy, for urethral obstruction in male cats, 373, 373b

Perinephric hematoma, 392f

Perinephric pseudocyst, 490–493, 490b
  diagnosis of, 490–492
    differential, 492
    imaging in, 492, 492f
    laboratory findings in, 491
    physical findings in, 491
  prognosis in, 493
  surgical resection of, 492–493, 492b, 493f

Persian cat, familial renal disease of, 198t–199t, 209

Phenoxybenzamine
  for feline idiopathic cystitis, 333t
  for feline urethral obstruction, 359t

Pheromones, for feline idiopathic cystitis, 333t

Phosphorus binders, in treatment of chronic kidney disease, 176, 176b, 177f

Phosphorus restriction, in managing chronic kidney disease, 174–176, 174b, 175f

Photodynamic therapy, for canine transitional cell carcinoma, 458

Physical examination, in clinical evaluation, 35

Piroxicam, 454, 454b–455b

Plasma clearance of isotopes, 40

Plasma cortisol concentration, in chronic kidney disease, 166

Polycystic kidney disease, familial trait, 198t–199t, 208f
  in bull terrier, 205
  in Cairn and West Highland white terriers, 205
  in Persian cat, 209

Polydipsia, 465
  psychogenic, treatment of, 480

Polyuria, 465

Polyuria, and polydipsia
  causes of, 468b, 469t–470t
  diagnosis of disorders causing, 473f–475f, 483–484
    ADH response testing in, 479
    adrenal ultrasonography in, 466f
    common misconceptions about, 484–485
    differential, 468–472, 471t
    frequently asked questions about, 485–486
    history in, 468–471
    laboratory tests in, 472–480
    renal medullary solute washout in, 480
    suggested readings on, 486
    summary tips on, 484
    urine specific gravity in, 474, 474b
    water deprivation testing in, 477, 477f, 478b
  pathophysiology of, 466–468
    antidiuretic hormone in, 467
    hypothalamic lesions in, 466
    organ systems involved in, 466
    psychogenic factors in, 466
    renal medullary hypertonicity decrease in, 467–468
  treatment of disorders causing, 480–483, 480b

Positive contrast cystography, 50–51

Positive contrast urethrography, 50

Postrenal acute renal failure, 63, 65. *See also* Obstructive nephropathy/uropathy; Urinary tract trauma; Uroabdomen.
  causes and pathogenesis of, 65
  history and clinical signs of, 73
  prognosis in, 87

Postrenal azotemia, 33t

Prazosin
  for feline idiopathic cystitis, 333t
  for feline urethral obstruction, 359t

Prerenal acute renal failure, 64
  causes and pathophysiology of, 64
  diagnosis of, 74–75

Prerenal acute renal failure *(Continued)*
  history and clinical signs of, 73
  physical examination in, 73
  prognosis in, 87
Prerenal azotemia, 33t, 63
Primary sphincter incompetence (PSMI), 417–427
  incidence of, 417b
  in male dogs, treatment of, 433
  refractory, treatment of
    collagen injections in, 421, 421f, 421b
    surgical colposuspension in, 422, 422f
  treatment of
    anticholinergics and phenylpropanolamine
      in, 420
    estrogens and phenylpropanolamine in, 420
    estrogens in, 419, 419b
    gonadotropin-releasing hormone analogues
      in, 420–421
    phenylpropanolamine in, 418, 419b
  urine leakage in, 418b
Primor. *See* Ormetoprim-potentiated
  sulfonamides.
PromAce. *See* Acepromazine.
Propantheline, for feline urethral obstruction, 359t
Prostate gland, ultrasonography of, 54
Protein restriction, in managing chronic kidney
  disease, 172–174
Proteinuria
  dipstrip evaluation of, 12–13
  pathologic processes indicated by, 12b
Proteus spp, in recurrent urinary infections, 262
Prozac. *See* Fluoxetine.
Pseudocyst, perinephric, 490–493, 490b
  diagnosis of, 490–492
    differential, 492
    imaging in, 492, 492f
    laboratory findings in, 491
    physical findings in, 491
  prognosis in, 493
  surgical resection of, 492–493, 492b, 493f
Pseudomonas, in recurrent urinary infections, 262
Psychogenic polydipsia, treatment of, 480
Purine metabolism, products of, 283f

Radiography, 49
Rapidly progressive glomerulonephritis, 131–134,
  131b
  clinical signs and history in, 133
  diagnosis of, 134
  pathophysiology of, 131–133, 133f
  prognosis in, 134, 134b
  suggested readings on, 142
  treatment of, 134
Recombinant human erythropoietin (rhEPO;
  Epogen), for chronic kidney disease, 182–183,
  182b

Recurrent urinary tract infections, 266–267
  urine culture scheduling in, 267t
Red blood cells, in urinary sediment, 16–18, 17f
Reflex dyssynergy, 428–429
Rehydration fluids, in acute intrinsic renal failure,
  80
Relative supersaturation, 280
Renagel. *See* Sevelamer HCl.
Renal adenocarcinoma, in cat, 436f
Renal adenoma, 434
Renal biopsy, 55–57
  in acute intrinsic renal failure, 77–78, 77b
  complications of, 57
  techniques of, 55–57, 56f
  utility of, 55
Renal blood flow, during hemodynamic insult, 70f
Renal calculi
  history in, 286
  physical findings in, 287
Renal carcinoma, 434–436, 434b
Renal clearance, 39
Renal cystadenocarcinoma, familial trait, in
  German shepherd, 198t–199t, 207
Renal disease, 32. *See also* Uropathy, and
  nephropathy.
  acute, 63. *See also* Acute intrinsic renal failure;
    Acute renal failure
  chronic, 145. *See also* Chronic kidney disease
  familial, 197. *See also* Familial renal disease(s)
  glomerular, 218. *See also* Glomerular disease
Renal dysplasia, familial trait, 198t–199t
  in soft-coated Wheaten terrier, 211–212
  suspected
    in Alaskan malamute, 203
    in chow, 206
    in golden retriever, 207–208
    in Lhasa apso and Shih tzu, 208
    in miniature Schnauzer, 208
    in Norwegian elkhound, 209
    in standard poodle, 212
Renal epithelial cell casts, in urinary sediment,
  22–23, 23f
Renal epithelial cells, in urinary sediment, 20
Renal failure, 32. *See also* Acute intrinsic renal
  failure; Chronic kidney disease.
Renal function, laboratory evaluation of, 35–47
  bladder tumor antigen test in, 43
  BUN concentration in, 36
  cystatin C concentration in, 39
  fractional clearance of electrolytes in, 47
  glomerular filtration rate in, 35–39, 36t. *See also*
    Glomerular filtration rate (GFR)
  gradual water deprivation test in, 46–47
  microalbuminuria in, 42–43
  renal clearance in, 39
  serum creatinine concentration in, 36–37

Renal function, laboratory evaluation *(Continued)*
  serum phosphorus concentration in, 41
  tubular function in, 44–47
  urine protein in, 41–42
  water deprivation test in, 45–46
Renal glucosuria, familial trait, in Norwegian
  elkhound, 198t–199t, 209
Renal hematuria, idiopathic, in dogs, 487–490. *See
  also* Benign essential hematuria.
Renal hemorrhage, treatment of, 403
Renal hyperthyroidism, in cats, 501–503, 501b
  diagnosis of, 502–503
  pathophysiology of, 501–502
  treatment of, 503, 503b
Renal ischemia
  causing acute intrinsic renal failure, 65–66
  pathophysiology of, 66–73, 70f
Renal length, and body weight, in adult dogs, 52t
Renal neoplasia, 434–438, 435f
  adenomas in, 434
  carcinomas in, 434–436
  clinical signs of, 435
  nephroblastomas in, 436–437
  other types of, 437–438
  treatment of, 438
  ultrasonography of, 435, 435f
Renal pulpifaction, 393f
Renal rupture, treatment of, 404
Renal secondary hyperparathyroidism
  development of, in chronic kidney disease,
    163–166, 164f–165f
  pathophysiology of, 148
Renal telangiectasia, familial trait, in Welsh corgi,
  198t–199t, 212
Renal transplantation, in chronic kidney disease, 190
Renal trauma, 391, 392f
  causes of, 393
  common misconceptions about, 406
  diagnosis of, 406
    history and clinical signs in, 394, 394b
    physical findings in, 394–396, 395f–396f
  diagnosis of uroperitoneum in, 396–403
    abdominocentesis in, 396–398
    differential, 402b
    imaging in, 398–400, 398f–400f
    methylene blue injection in, 398
    serum biochemistry in, 400–402
    urethral catheter passage in, 396, 396b
    urinalysis in, 402
  frequently asked questions about, 407
  future treatment of, 406
  syndromes resulting from, 393–394
  treatment of, 403–406
    stabilization before surgery in, 404–405
    summary tips about, 407
    urine drainage from abdomen in, 405–406

Renal tubular acidosis (RTA), 493–496
  distal (type I), 494
    treatment of, 494
  proximal (type II), 495, 495b
    treatment of, 495, 495b
  type 4, 496
Renal ultrasonography, 51–53
  color flow Doppler, 53
  intrarenal resistance to blood flow assessment
    in, 53
  medullary rim sign in, 53
  in monitoring renal allografts, 53
  utility of, 52
    in ethylene glycol intoxication, 52–53, 100–101,
      100f
Renal-dose dopamine, 84
Renin-angiotensin-aldosterone syndrome, in
  chronic kidney disease, 166
Resistant bacterial urinary infections, treatment of,
  262–264
Resource checklist and client action plan, 315f–318f
Retrograde urinary catheter placement, in male
  cats, 362–366, 364f, 364b–365b
Retrograde urohydropropulsion, for dislodging
  urethral calculi, 289, 290f
Rhabdomyosarcoma, 439, 439f
Rottweiler
  familial renal disease of, 198t–199t, 209
  primary sphincter incompetence in, 417–427

Samoyed, familial renal disease of, 198t–199t,
  210–211, 230
Sensipar. *See* Cinacalcet.
Serum amyloid A protein, 228–229
Serum calcitriol concentration, in chronic kidney
  disease, 166
Serum calcium concentration, in chronic kidney
  disease, 161–162, 161b
Serum creatinine concentration
  in acute intrinsic renal failure, 76
  in chronic kidney disease, 159
  and glomerular filtration rate, 37–39, 38t
  increased, in loss of renal mass, 37b
  laboratory evaluation, 36–37, 37b
  in uroperitoneum, 396–398, 397b, 400–402, 400b
Serum phosphorus concentration
  in acute intrinsic renal failure, 76
  in chronic kidney disease, 161
  control of, in acute intrinsic renal failure, 81–82
  laboratory evaluation of, 41, 41b
Serum potassium concentration
  in acute intrinsic renal failure, 76
  in chronic kidney disease, 159–161
Serum sodium concentration, in chronic kidney
  disease, 159
Sevelamer HCl, as phosphorus binder, 177–178

Shar pei, familial renal disease of, 198t–199t, 211, 230
Shih tzu
    familial renal disease of, 198t–199t, 208
    urate urolithiasis in, 281–283
Siamese cat, familial renal disease of, 198t–199t, 230
Silicate urolithiasis, 284–285
    signalment in, 285
    treatment of, 301
Silicate uroliths, 275f
Simplicef. *See* Cefpodoxime.
Single nephron glomerular filtration rate (SNGFR), increased, 149–150, 149f
Sodium bicarbonate treatment, in chronic kidney disease, 180
Sodium chloride restriction, in chronic kidney disease, 179–180
Soft-coated Wheaten terrier, familial renal disease of, 198t–199t, 211–212, 229
Solutes, in urine, 272–274
Specific gravity reagent pad reaction, 15
Spironolactone, for chronic kidney disease, 189–190
Squamous cell carcinoma, of renal pelvis, 437
Squamous epithelial cells, in urinary sediment, 19
Standard poodle, familial renal disease of, 198t–199t, 212
Struvite calculi, cystic, 276f
Struvite crystalloid(s), 275
    in urine specimen, 27, 29f
Struvite urolithiasis
    dietary treatment of, 293–294
    medical treatment of, 292–294
    pathophysiology of, 275–277, 276f, 276b
    signalment in, 285
Subcapsular lymphosarcoma, in cat, 438f
Sucralfate
    dosage, as gastroprotectant, 182
    as phosphorus binder, 177
Sulfonamides, contraindications to use of, 256, 256b
Super nephron, 149f
Systemic complications, and progression of chronic kidney disease, 153
Systemic hypertension, in chronic kidney disease, 157–158

Terminology, used in clinical evaluation, 32, 33t
Texas NAV dog, familial renal disease of, 198t–199t
Thiazide diuretics, for hyposthenuric disorders, 483
Thiol disulfide exchange drugs (D-penicillamine, 2-MPG), 300–301, 300f
Thirst, 465
Torbugesic. *See* Butorphanol.
Transitional cell papilloma, 437
Transitional epithelial cells, in urinary sediment, 19–20, 20f
Tribrissen. *See* Trimethoprim-potentiated sulfonamides.

Tricyclic antidepressants, for feline idiopathic cystitis, 334
Trimethoprim-potentiated sulfonamides, for urinary tract infections, 256
Tube cystostomy, for urethral obstruction in male cats, 375
Tubular backleak, 69f
Tubular dysfunction, familial trait, 198t–199t
    in Basenji, 204
Tubular function, 44f
    laboratory evaluation of, 44–47
Tumors, urinary system, 434
    bladder neoplasia in, 438–441
    canine transitional cell carcinoma in, 441–459
    renal neoplasia in, 434–438
    suggested readings on, 463
    urethral neoplasia in, 459–460
Ultrasonography, 51–54
    of bladder, 53–54
    of prostate gland, 54
    renal, 51–53
    of ureters, 53
    of urethra, 54
Upper motor neuron incontinence, 427–428
Upper urinary tract disease. *See* Renal disease.
Urate calculi, 281, 281f
Urate crystalluria, 27, 30f
Urate urolithiasis, 281–283
    medical treatment of, 298–300
        allopurinol in, 298
        dietary therapy in, 299
        sodium bicarbonate in, 298–299
    signalment in, 285
Ureaplasma, in recurrent urinary infections, 262
Uremia, 32
    in chronic kidney disease, 148
Ureter(s)
    calculi in. *See also* Ureterolithiasis
        history in, 286
        physical findings in, 287
    rupture of, treatment of, 404
    ultrasonography of, 53
Ureterolithiasis, in cats, 380
    imaging findings in, 385, 382f–383f
    treatment of, 380
        decision making regarding, 384
Urethra
    biopsy of, 57–58
    infections of
        in dogs, 240. *See also* Urinary tract infection
        idiopathic, in cats, 342–343
    neoplasms of, 459–460, 459f–460f
    rupture of

Urethra *(Continued)*
  contrast radiography of, 401f
  treatment of, 404
  stricture of, 348, 348f
  ultrasonography of, 54
Urethral calculi
  in cats, 347–348, 347f. *See also* Feline idiopathic
    cystitis; Feline interstitial cystitis
  in dogs, 272–305. *See also* Urolithiasis
    history in, 286
    physical findings in, 287
Urethral obstruction
  in dogs, 240–271, 272–305, 376–377. *See also*
    Urinary tract infection; Urolithiasis
    treatment of, 377
  in male cats, 343–375. *See also* Urethral calculi;
    Urethral plugs
  alternatives to euthanasia for, 374–375, 374b
  bladder overdistension in, 369
  causes of, 343–348, 344t, 347b
  diagnosis of
    contrast radiography in, 354
    hyperkalemia and effects in, 350, 350b–351b
    hypocalcemia and effects in, 352, 352b
    physical examination in, 350–351
    radiographic imaging in, 353–354, 353b
    serum biochemistry in, 351–353, 351b
    signalment and history in, 348–350, 348b
    ultrasonography in, 354, 354b
    urethroscopy in, 354
    urinalysis in, 353
    urine culture in, 353, 353b
  perineal urethrostomy in, 373, 373b
  postobstructive diuresis in, 366–368
  postprocedural intravenous fluid management
    in, 366–367, 367t, 367b
  postprocedural medical management in, 368,
    368b
  postprocedural urine output in, 368–369, 369b
  prognosis for acute, 372
  prognosis for chronic, 372
  recurrent, prevention of, 371–372
  syndromes associated with, 349, 349f, 349b
  treatment of, 354–375, 355f–356f
    acidosis management in, 357
    amitriptyline in, 375
    anesthesia protocols in, 360f, 361–362, 361b
    antegrade urinary catheter placement in,
      366
    complications after, 369
    decompressive cystocentesis in, 358–361
    home care after, 371
    with hospitalization instead of
      catheterization, 373–374
    hydropulsion and urinary catheter
      placement for, 362–366, 364f, 364b–365b

Urethral obstruction *(Continued)*
    hyperkalemia management in, 356, 357b
    hypocalcemia management in, 357
    plug removal procedure for, 362
    sedation and analgesia in, 358, 359t
    stabilization of patient in, 356
    tube cystostomy in, 375
Urethral plugs, 343–347, 344f
  composition of, 345, 345f
  diagnosis of, 345, 346f
  differentiation of, from uroliths, 345
  frequency of obstruction by, 344t, 345b
  location of, 346f
  pathophysiology of, 346–347, 347b
Urethral pressure profile (UPP), 415–417, 416f–417f
Urethritis
  in dogs, 240. *See also* Urinary tract infection
  idiopathic, in cats, 342–343
Urethrography, positive contrast, 50
Uric acid, metabolic derivation of, 283, 283f
Urinalysis, 1
  common misconceptions about, 29–30
  in diagnosis of acute intrinsic renal failure, 75–76
  in diagnosis of chronic kidney disease, 166
  and differentiation of acute and chronic renal
    failure, 75–76, 75b
  frequently asked questions about, 30–31
  interpretation of, 9–29. *See also* Urine specimen
    chemical properties in, 11–15
    physical properties in, 9–11
    sediment in, 16–29
  specimen data and observation in, 7
  suggested readings on, 31
Urinary acidifiers, 260–261
  for struvite urolithiasis, 254
Urinary calculi. *See also* Urolithiasis.
  analysis of, 288
  nonsurgical retrieval of, for analysis or
    treatment, 289–291, 290f
Urinary catheters, for male cats, 363f
Urinary incontinence, 409, 409b
  common misconceptions about, 430–431
  diagnosis of, 429–430
    differential, 412, 413b
    history in, 414
    imaging in, 415
    laboratory findings in, 415
    physical examination in, 414–415, 414b
    signalment in, 413–414
    special studies in, 415–417, 415b
  frequently asked questions about, 431–433
  suggested readings on, 433
  treatment of, 429–430
    in anatomic abnormalities, 423–427
    future, 430
    in neurogenic etiology, 427–429

Urinary incontinence (*Continued*)
  in paradoxical (obstructive) incontinence, 427
  in primary sphincter incompetence, 417–427
  summary tips on, 431
  and vestibulovaginal stenosis, in female dogs,
    427, 427b
Urinary sediment, 16–29, 16b
  casts in, 20–25
  crystals in, 26–27, 27b, 28f–29f
  epithelial cells in, 18f, 19–20, 20f
  formed elements in, 18f
  microorganisms in, 25–26, 25f
  red blood cells in, 16–18, 17f
  white blood cells in, 18–19, 18f
Urinary tract, clinical evaluation of, 32, 58
  approach to, 33–34
  bladder and urethral biopsy in, 57–58
  common misconceptions about, 58–59
  cystoscopy in, 54–55
  diagnostic imaging in, 49–54
  frequently asked questions about, 59–61
  future developments in, 58
  history in, 33–34
  microbiology in, 47–48
  physical examination in, 35
  questions to be answered in, 32
  renal biopsy in, 55–57
  renal function findings in, 35–47. *See also*
    Laboratory evaluation
  suggested readings in, 61
Urinary tract infection, 240–241
  asymptomatic, 240, 240b
  common misconceptions about, 269
  complicated, 254
  diagnosis of
    hematology and serum biochemistry in, 249,
      249b
    imaging in, 251, 53–54
    summary tips in, 268–269
    urinalysis in, 249–251, 249b
    urine collection in, 48
    urine culture in, 47–48, 250–251, 251f, 268
  frequently asked questions about, 269–271
  gender differences in, 262
  history and clinical signs of, 248
  host defenses against, 243–244, 244b
  incidence of, 240–241, 240b
  pathogenesis of, 241–248
    bacteria associated with, 241–243,
      242b, 245f
    in cats, 242f
    in dogs, 241f
    common route of bacterial, 243b
    resistant or unique microorganisms in,
      262–263
  physical findings in, 248

Urinary tract infection (*Continued*)
  recurrent, 266–267
  reinfection and relapse in, differentiation of, 32,
    33t, 47, 55
  resistant and unique pathogens in, treatment
    of, 262–264
  risk for development of, 271, 245
    anatomic and functional, 246b
    catheterization in, 247, 247b
    metabolic, 246b
  treatment of, 254, 255b
    alternative and supplemental, 260–261
    antimicrobial agents and dosages in, 255–257,
      255t
    appropriate antimicrobial choice in, 255, 255b,
      257
    dietary, 257
    outcomes in, 264–265
    prophylactic, 261–262, 261b
    successful, 265, 265b
    supportive, 260
    unsuccessful, considerations in, 265–268,
      265b–266b
  uncomplicated, 254
  untreated, consequences of, 254
Urinary tract trauma, 391
  causes of, 393
  common misconceptions about, 406
  diagnosis of, 406
  diagnosis of uroperitoneum in, 396–403
    abdominocentesis in, 396–398
    differential, 402b
    imaging in, 398–400, 398f–400f
    methylene blue injection in, 398
    serum biochemistry in, 400–402
    urethral catheter passage in, 396, 396b
    urinalysis in, 402
  frequently asked questions about, 407
  history and clinical signs of, 394, 394b
  physical findings in, 394–396, 395f–396f
  syndromes resulting from, 393–394
  treatment of, 403–406
    future, 406
    stabilization before surgery in,
      404–405
    summary tips on, 407
    urine drainage from abdomen
      in, 405–406
Urination
  evaluation for clinical history, 34
  physiology of, 409–412
    parasympathetic, 410f
    somatic, 412f
    sympathetic, 411f
Urine alkalinization, for cysteine urolithiasis
  therapy, 301

Urine collection, 1–7
 catheterization in, 2–5
 cystocentesis in, 5–7
 manual expression in, 2
 midstream voided sample in, 1
 for quantitative microbiology, 48
Urine culture
 in determining urinary tract infection, 47–48,
  250–251
 in diagnosis of acute intrinsic renal failure, 76
 in differential diagnosis of urolithiasis, 288
 scheduling, in recurrent urinary tract infections,
  267t
 urine collection for, 48
Urine osmolality (Uosm), and tubular function,
  44–45, 44f
Urine protein, laboratory evaluation of, 41–42, 42b
Urine sediment, modified Wright stain of, 250
Urine specific gravity (USG), 10–11, 10b
 and tubular function, 44–45, 44f
 variation in dogs, with time of day, 45b
Urine specimen, 7
 appearance of, 10
 bilirubin in, 15
 collection technique for microbiology, 48
 color of, 9–10
 data form and expected results for normal cats
  and dogs, 8
 dip strip evaluation of, 11, 11b
 glucose concentration in, 13–14, 13b
 ketone concentration in, 14
 leukocyte esterase reaction in, 15
 miscellaneous elements and artifacts in, 27–29
 occult blood in, 14–15, 14b
 odor of, 10
 pH of, 12
 protein concentration in, 12–13, 12b
 sediment in, 16–29
 specific gravity of, 10–11, 10b
 specific gravity reagent pad reaction in, 15
Urine telomerase test, 449
Uroendoscopy, 54–55
Urohydropropulsion
 in male dog with urethral calculi, 342f, 377
 retrograde, for dislodging urethral calculi, 289, 290f
 and urinary catheter placement, in feline
  urethral obstruction, 362–366
 voiding, of bladder stones, 290–291, 291f
Urolith(s), 272
 crystalloid components of, 272, 273f
 lamellar pattern of, 273f
 location of, 272b
Urolithiasis, 272–275
 calculi analysis in, 288
 common misconceptions about, 302–303
 complications of, 302

Urolithiasis (Continued)
 cystine, 283–284
 development of, theories of, 274–275, 275f
 diagnosis of, 302
  hematology in, 288
  imaging in, 289
  microbiology in, 288
  serum biochemistry in, 288
  urinalysis in, 287, 287b
 frequently asked questions about, 303–304
 history in, 285–286
 induction of, 274
 inhibition of, 274
 medical treatment of, 292
  for cystine calculi, 300–301
  for oxalate calculi, 294–298
  for silicate calculi, 301
  for struvite calculi, 292–294
  for urate calculi, 298–300
 oxalate, 277–281
 physical findings in, 286–287
 prognosis in, 302
 selected readings on, 304
 signalment of, 285
 silicate, 284–285
 struvite, 275–277
 treatment of, 289–291
  medical, 292
  surgical, 291–292, 292b
 urate, 281–283
Uropathy, and nephropathy
 canine cystitis and urethritis in, 240. See also
  Urinary tract infection
 canine obstructive, 272, 342–343. See also
  Urolithiasis
 feline non-obstructive, 306. See also Feline
  idiopathic cystitis; Feline interstitial
  cystitis
 feline obstructive, 341. See also Urethral
  obstruction; Urethral plugs
 micturition and urinary incontinence in, 409.
  See also Micturition disorders; Urinary
  incontinence
 miscellaneous syndromes of, 487
 polydipsia and polyuria as clinical signs of,
  465–486. See also Polyuria, and polydipsia
 renal disease in, 32
  acute, 63. See also Acute intrinsic renal failure;
   Acute renal failure
  chronic, 145. See also Chronic kidney disease
  familial, 197. See also Familial renal disease(s)
  glomerular, 218. See also Glomerular disease
 after trauma, 391. See also Renal trauma; Urinary
  tract trauma; Uroperitoneum
 tumors in, 434. See also Bladder neoplasia;
  Renal neoplasia; Urethral neoplasia

Uroperitoneum, 393
  clinical cases of, in small animals, 402
  diagnosis of, 396–403, 406
    abdominocentesis in, 396–398
    differential, 402b
    imaging in, 398–400, 398f–400f
    methylene blue injection in, 398
    serum biochemistry in, 400–402
    urethral catheter passage in, 396, 396b
    urinalysis in, 402
  experimental, in dogs, data summary,
      402–403
  frequently asked questions about, 407
  treatment of, 403–406
    stabilization before surgery in, 404–405
    summary tips about, 407
    urine drainage from abdomen in, 405–406

Veloquinol. *See* Azodyl.
Vestibulovaginal stenosis in, in female dogs, 427,
  427b
Visceral epithelial cells, of glomerulus, 219
Voiding urohydropropulsion, of bladder stones,
  273f, 290–291, 291f

Vomiting and inappetence, in chronic kidney
    disease, 181–182
  treatment of
    anti-emetics in, 181
    gastric acid suppression in, 181
    gastroprotectants in, 182
    percutaneous esophagostomy in, 182, 182b

Water deprivation test, 45–46
  contraindications to performance of, 45b
Water intake
  increased, 466–468. *See also* Polyuria, and
      polydipsia
  normal, 34, 34b, 465, 465b
Waxy casts, in urinary sediment, 24–25, 24f
Welsh corgi, familial renal disease of, 198t–199t, 212
West Highland white terrier, familial renal disease
    of, 198t–199t, 205
White blood cell casts, in urinary sediment, 22, 23f
White blood cells, in urinary sediment, 18–19, 18f
Wilms tumor, 436–437
Yorkshire terrier, urate urolithiasis in, 281–283
Zeniquin. *See* Marbofloxacin.
Zinc carnosine, dosage, as gastroprotectant, 182